Neurogenesis in the Adult Brain

Neurogenesis in the Adult Brain

Editor: Alfred Carter

MURPHY & MOORE
www.murphy-moorepublishing.com

www.murphy-moorepublishing.com

MURPHY & MOORE

Cataloging-in-Publication Data

Neurogenesis in the adult brain / edited by Alfred Carter.
p. cm.
Includes bibliographical references and index.
ISBN 978-1-63987-384-5
1. Developmental neurobiology. 2. Neurons--Growth. 3. Neurobiology. 4. Nervous system--Evolution. I. Carter, Alfred.
QP363.5 .N48 2022
612.8--dc23

Murphy & Moore Publishing,
1 Rockefeller Plaza,
New York City, NY 10020, USA

ISBN 978-1-63987-384-5 (Hardback)

Contents

Preface

Neurogenesis refers to the process of production of neurons by neural stem cells. There are different types of neural stem cells such as radial glial cells, neuroepithelial cells, intermediate neuronal precursors, basal progenitors, subgranular zone radial astrocytes and subventricular zone astrocytes. Neural stem cells are self-renewing and multipotent cells. Neurogenesis is responsible for producing all the different types of neurons within an individual. It is most active during embryonic development but continues throughout adult life. Adult neurogenesis is different from prenatal neurogenesis. Formation of new neurons in adults takes place in two regions of the brain, namely, subgranular zone and subventricular zone. This book strives to provide a fair idea about neurogenesis in adult brain and helps to develop a better understanding of the latest advances within this field. It presents researches and studies performed by experts across the globe. This book will serve as a valuable source of reference for graduate and post graduate students.

This book is a comprehensive compilation of works of different researchers from varied parts of the world. It includes valuable experiences of the researchers with the sole objective of providing the readers (learners) with a proper knowledge of the concerned field. This book will be beneficial in evoking inspiration and enhancing the knowledge of the interested readers.

In the end, I would like to extend my heartiest thanks to the authors who worked with great determination on their chapters. I also appreciate the publisher's support in the course of the book. I would also like to deeply acknowledge my family who stood by me as a source of inspiration during the project.

Editor

1

The Contradictory Effects of Neuronal Hyperexcitation on Adult Hippocampal Neurogenesis

José R. Pineda[1] *and Juan M. Encinas*[1,2*]

[1] *Laboratory of Neural Stem Cells and Neurogenesis, Achucarro Basque Center for Neuroscience, Zamudio, Spain,*
[2] *IKERBASQUE, The Basque Foundation for Science, Bilbao, Spain*

Adult hippocampal neurogenesis is a highly plastic process that responds swiftly to neuronal activity. Adult hippocampal neurogenesis can be regulated at the level of neural stem cell recruitment and activation, progenitor proliferation, as well as newborn cell survival and differentiation. An "excitation-neurogenesis" rule was proposed after the demonstration of the capability of cultured neural stem and progenitor cells to intrinsically sense neuronal excitatory activity. *In vivo*, this property has remained elusive although recently the direct response of neural stem cells to GABA in the hippocampus via $GABA_A$ receptors has evidenced a mechanism for a direct talk between neurons and neural stem cells. As it is pro-neurogenic, the effect of excitatory neuronal activity has been generally considered beneficial. But what happens in situations of neuronal hyperactivity in which neurogenesis can be dramatically boosted? In animal models, electroconvulsive shock markedly increases neurogenesis. On the contrary, in epilepsy rodent models, seizures induce the generation of misplaced neurons with abnormal morphological and electrophysiological properties, namely aberrant neurogenesis. We will herein discuss what is known about the mechanisms of influence of neurons on neural stem cells, as well as the severe effects of neuronal hyperexcitation on hippocampal neurogenesis.

Keywords: neurogenesis, hippocampus, neural stem cells, hyperexcitation, epilepsy

Edited by:
Alino Martinez-Marcos,
Universidad de Castilla, Spain

Reviewed by:
Ashok K. Shetty,
Texas A&M Health Science Center College of Medicine, USA
Carlos Vicario-Abejón,
Consejo Superior de Investigaciones Científicas, Spain
Helena Mira,
Instituto de Salud Carlos III, Spain

***Correspondence:**
Juan M. Encinas
jm.encinas@ikerbasque.org

INTRODUCTION

Neurogenesis in the hippocampus starts with the activation of quiescent neural stem cells (NSCs), the first regulatory step that will determine the amount of new neurons generated in a given time point. Although neurogenesis is tightly linked to the level of hippocampal circuitry activity it has only been recently unveiled how gamma-aminobutyric acid (GABA) plays an essential role into translating neuronal activity into NSCs activation, as we will explain below. The question that we want to address in this review is what occurs when neuronal activity is increased to abnormal hyperexcitatory levels, especially in the clinically relevant context of epilepsy or electroconvulsive therapy (ECT) and its animal model, electroconvulsive shock (ECS). Two aspects make this question important. First, the possibility that enhanced activation of NSCs leads to a premature exhaustion of the NSC population and of neurogenesis; and second the existence of aberrant neurogenesis, i.e., the generation of neurons with ectopic location and different morphological and electrophysiological properties that can contribute to epilepsy.

NSCs, in rodents, have been shown to be able to divide symmetrically to generate more copies of themselves (Bonaguidi et al., 2011), and therefore the possibility exist that they can expand their pool. However, in normal conditions, this capability does not counteract the depletion of the NSC population that associates with age (Encinas and Enikolopov, 2008; Bonaguidi et al., 2011; Walter et al., 2011; Andersen et al., 2014). The depletion of the population is based on the activation-coupled astrocytic differentiation of NSCs. Most of the NSCs remain quiescent but once they get activated they undergo a round of several asymmetric divisions to generate neuronal precursors that either die by apoptosis and are removed by microglia, or become mature granule cells (Sierra et al., 2010). At least in mice, after finishing their round of asymmetric cell divisions NSCs differentiate into astrocytes losing their stem cell capabilities (Encinas et al., 2011). Thus, the level of activation of NSCs not only determines the level of neurogenesis but also the rate of depletion of NSCs. The prediction derived from this model is that increased activation of NSCs would lead to an initial boost of neurogenesis followed by diminished neurogenesis in the long term. This model would explain the seemingly contradictory results regarding hippocampal cell proliferation and neurogenesis in human epilepsy. Noteworthy, the dynamics of neurogenesis decline in normal conditions in humans might be different as pointed out by carbon-14-based methods (Spalding et al., 2013).

Several *in vivo* manipulations or brain alterations that influence electrical activity also affect adult neurogenesis. Seizures trigger an early increase of cell proliferation that involved NSCs (Huttmann et al., 2003; Indulekha et al., 2010). Also, ECS has been consistently reported (Segi-Nishida et al., 2008; Jun et al., 2015) to increase NSC recruitment and activation of NSCs. However, long-term studies addressing the fate of dividing NSCs as well as the chronic effect on the neurogenic niche are still missing. Both models of hyperexcitation are usually accompanied with the induction of neuronal death in granule cells (Zarubenko et al., 2005; Dingledine et al., 2014), which in turn might affect neurogenesis. We will focus on two aspects of neurogenesis that seem to be key regarding neuronal hyperexcitation in the hippocampus, activation and exhaustion of NSCs, and the induction of aberrant neurogenesis.

ACTIVATION AND EXHAUSTION OF NSCs

We have recently shown that in mice seizures trigger a dramatic response in the dentate gyrus (DG) leading to a swift and almost complete disruption of the neurogenic niche (Sierra et al., 2015). The main effect of seizures is to activate NSCs and induce them to differentiate into reactive astrocytes. Thus, the neurogenic potential is abandoned and the NSC pool rapidly depletes. Even though seizures trigger an initial boost of cell proliferation, mainly accounted for the activation of NSCs, in following weeks cell proliferation and neurogenesis diminish to a minimum (Sierra et al., 2015). These results could explain the chronic impairment observed in two rat models of temporal lobe epilepsy (TLE; Hattiangady et al., 2004; Hattiangady and Shetty, 2010). They also are in agreement with part of the data obtained from human samples and provide and explanation for them. Because mesial TLE (MTLE) is often resistant to drugs, surgical resection of the hippocampus as a last-resort therapeutic strategy to stop seizures is frequently performed. These samples represent a valuable source of tissue that can be analyzed without any of the drawbacks of postmortem tissue, such as degradation and overfixation.

Nestin-positive radial cells considered as putative NCSs were not found in samples from adult MTLE patients, leading the authors to suggest that the neural stem/progenitor pool might be depleted by chronic seizure activity in humans (Blümcke et al., 2001), a hypothesis that is supported in rodents by studies showing how seizure indeed recruit and activate NSCs in significantly manner (Huttmann et al., 2003) that later translates into an almost total depletion of the NSC pool (Sierra et al., 2015). Furthermore, *ex vivo* analysis of hippocampal neurogenesis showed that even though the epileptic human hippocampus could contain neural progenitors (Blümcke et al., 2001), these were absent in epilepsy patients with hippocampal sclerosis (Paradisi et al., 2010). The data obtained, however, are not consistent and sometimes are even contradictory when measuring other parameters. Using these samples from intractable-MTLE patients it has been shown that the immunoreactivity for PSA-NCAM (polysialic acid neural cell adhesion molecule) a specific marker of neuroblasts, or immature neurons, was lost in the neurogenic niche of the dentate gyrus (Mikkonen et al., 1998). A similar result was reported later, describing how the frequency and early onset of seizures correlated with decreased adult neurogenesis (Mathern et al., 2002). The mRNA expression of another marker of neuroblasts, doublecortin (DCX), was also decreased in MTLE patients compared to age-matched controls (Fahrner et al., 2007). The protein levels, however, did not change significantly. In contrast, an increase in the number of neural progenitors in MTLE has been suggested based on the expression of Musashi, a stem cell marker functionally related to self-renewal (Crespel et al., 2005). However, the precise cell type expressing Musashi, as well as the function of this protein in the adult hippocampus has not been explored. More conflicting evidence regarding proliferation in the MTLE hippocampus has been reported. For instance, no significant change in proliferation was found by labeling with Ki67 or minichromosome 2 (mcm2; Fahrner et al., 2007), a DNA replication licensing protein; although another study reported increased proliferation employing mcm2 (Thom et al., 2005). In general it might be inferred that an initial wave of proliferation could be followed by diminished cell division and neurogenesis, and that the age of onset, frequency and severity of the seizures will determine the neurogenic outcome in the long run. It must be considered also that human samples are obtained from individuals resistant to pharmacological treatment, which might represent only a particular subset of patients of MTLE.

Aberrant Neurogenesis

One of the most common findings in experimental models of MTLE, as well as in human samples is aberrant neurogenesis, i.e., the generation of neurons with ectopic location (located mostly into the hilus but also in the molecular layer), with abnormal ultrastructural (Dashtipour et al., 2001) and morphological features including network reorganization through mossy fiber sprouting (Parent et al., 1997), and with altered electrophysiological properties (Scharfman, 2000; Scharfman et al., 2003). One explanation for the ectopic location of neurons in MTLE could be the loss of reelin. Seizures cause death of the reelin-expressing interneurons that populate the hilus; PSA-NCAM neuroblasts express the downstream reelin signaling molecule Dab1; and *in vitro*, the migration of neuronal precursors is altered by manipulating the levels of reelin (Gong et al., 2007). The involvement of reelin could explain the existence of different levels of aberrant neurogenesis even when neurogenesis is greatly impaired (Murphy et al., 2012; Sierra et al., 2015).It has also been shown, that in mice lacking fibroblast growth factor (FGF) 22, ectopic location of newborn neurons is significantly reduced, suggestion that FGF22 might be playing a role in seizure-induced abnormal migration of neuroblasts (Lee and Umemori, 2013). Newly-born and developing granule cells are more sensitive to seizures than the mature and preexistent ones, and undergo noticeable changes such as the abnormal development of basal dendrites (Walter et al., 2007). The contribution of aberrant neurogenesis to MTLE is still not fully understood. A positive correlation between the number of ectopic newborn granule cells, mossy fiber sprouting, and loss of mossy cells; and the frequency of seizures was found in the intraperitoneal-pilocarpine model of mouse epilepsy (Hester and Danzer, 2013). No conclusions on causality can be extracted form that study. However, it has been recently shown that reducing neurogenesis by triggering apoptosis in dividing nestin-expressing cell reduced aberrant neurogenesis and lead to a reduction of the frequency of chronic seizures, but not of the severity or duration (Cho et al., 2015). This positive effect could not be attributed only to decreased aberrant neurogenesis, as "normal" neurogenesis was reduced as well. Importantly, the positive effect on the frequency of spontaneous seizures was abolished when the generation of reactive astrocytes following the induction of seizures was impaired.

POTENTIAL MECHANISMS

GABA Signaling

Confirming previous results obtained *in vitro*, showing that $GABA_A$ receptors are expressed in neural progenitors *in vitro* (Farrant and Nusser, 2005; Ge et al., 2007), it has been more recently reported how NSCs respond directly to GABA via $GABA_A$ and $GABA_B$ receptors (Song et al., 2012; Giachino et al., 2014). GABA released by paravalbumin-expressing interneurons acts tonically on NSCs maintaining them in quiescence. Administration of the $GABA_A$ receptor agonist muscimol reduces the number of NSCs that enter the cell cycle whereas knocking down of the γ2 subunit of the $GABA_A$ receptor induces the activation of a higher number of NSCs. Interestingly, blocking the action of GABA in NSCs not only increases activation but also promotes symmetrical cell division (Song et al., 2012). In the context of MTLE, and assuming that the results found in mice regarding the massive activation and loss of NSCs (Sierra et al., 2015) could be similar in humans, treatments based on activating $GABA_A$ receptors (such as benzodiazepines) could be directly beneficial as they would preserve neurogenesis by promoting quiescence, and therefore preserving the NSC population. In a similar fashion, both the knock-out of the $GABA_{B1}$ receptor and the infusion of its antagonist CGP54626A increased NSC activation, although in this case an expansion of the NSCs population, expected if symmetric division was augmented, was not found. Administration of the $GABA_{B1}$ receptor baclofen decreased the number of NSCs in division (Giachino et al., 2014). Interestingly neuroblasts are a major source of GABA suggesting a retro-control or feedback mechanism for NSC quiescence as GABA exerts a tonic inhibitory control of NSC proliferation (Liu et al., 2005). In the SVZ, it was shown *in vivo* that treatments with the $GABA_AR$ agonist muscimol decreased cell proliferation and the number of label-retaining stem cells (LRSCs), whereas the blockade of $GABA_AR$ signaling with the specific inhibitor bicuculline increased mitosis and the number of LRSCs (Fernando et al., 2011). The authors concluded that the inhibitor bicuculline primarily increased the rate of division of already cycling stem cells. However, more recent data in which cycling cells were eradicated by using exposure to γ-radiation, showed that muscimol or bicuculline delayed and increased (respectively) the entry of quiescent NSCs into the cell cycle (Daynac et al., 2013). In the hippocampus, during the progression of the MTLE alterations of the GABAergic neuronal circuitry also take place (Maru and Ura, 2014), which in turn could affect directly NSCs. Interestingly tonic GABAergic signaling from PV can prevent their proliferation and subsequent maturation or return them to quiescence if previously activated (Moss and Toni, 2013; Song et al., 2013). Moreover, PV interneurons are capable of suppress neurogenesis during periods of high network activity and, on the other hand, facilitate neurogenesis when network activity is low (Song et al., 2012). The efficacy of GABAergic synaptic inhibition is a principal factor in controlling neuronal activity. Recent studies demonstrated that $GABA_A$-based synaptic inhibition is decreased in the hippocampal CA1 area of patients with intractable MTLE (Maru and Ura, 2014). It remains to be elucidated what happens in local PV circuitry during seizures and if stimulation of PV in this context could be a therapeutic tool to control NSC massive activation.

Finally, another manner in which GABAergic interneurons regulate excitability is through direct action of a 36-amino acid peptide called neuropeptide Y (NPY; Colmers and El Bahh, 2003) and norepinephrine (NE; Jhaveri et al., 2015). Both are potent endogenous anticonvulsants (Erickson et al., 1996; Baraban et al., 1997; Woldbye et al., 1997; Szot et al., 1999; Weinshenker et al., 2001). Gene expression of NPY has been found to be upregulated in the hippocampus either after induction of seizures or ECS (Gruber et al., 1994; Kragh et al., 1994). It has been speculated that both transmitters, NPY and NE, likely dampen excessive excitation of neurons in brain regions implicated in epileptic seizures. However, recent findings have been demonstrated that both peptides are able to independently promote proliferation of hippocampal neural stem and progenitor cells (Decressac et al., 2011; Jhaveri et al., 2015). These findings propose that aberrant neural activity is a master key to provoke deregulation of the fine-tuning control of NSC activation and progenitor proliferation. Therefore, GABAergic input seems to be a key regulator of NSCs activation and neurogenesis, as it also has effects on other steps of the neurogenic cascade, namely survival and differentiation of neuronal progenitors (Ge et al., 2007; Song et al., 2012; Giachino et al., 2014). However, other regulatory pathways might exist and unveiling their interplay will provide the ultimate understanding of NSC activation in physiological conditions.

Other Mechanisms

Up to date it was believed that mitogenic factors participating on the induction of neurogenesis were released by dying neurons and reactive glia. In severe epilepsy such as MTLE the progression of the disease leads to a severe neuronal loss in the hippocampus (Dericioglu et al., 2013). The release of mitogenic factors can be, however, faster. After generation of seizures Shh protein from Hedgehog signaling pathway, growth factors such as FGF-2, neurotrophins such as BDNF were found to be acutely upregulated in hippocampal tissue before there was neuronal loss and then progressively diminished in chronic epilepsy (Riva et al., 1992; Lowenstein et al., 1993; Gall et al., 1994; Shetty et al., 2003, 2004; Hattiangady et al., 2004). The majority of these factors were upregulated during acute seizures, potentially reflecting an initial response to neural activity (as it happens also in ECS), independently of neuronal cell death.

BDNF Neurotrophin

Hippocampal network activity stimulates transcription of the Brain-derived neurotrophic factor (BDNF) gene and the translation of *Bdnf* mRNA (Mattson, 2008; Kazanis et al., 2010). BDNF is neuroprotective in a wide variety of brain pathologies (Zeev et al., 2009; Zuccato and Cattaneo, 2009). In the hippocampus BDNF is able to modulate synaptic transmission (Huang and Reichardt, 2001; Waterhouse and Xu, 2009), and in the cortex, it participates in the maturation of GABAergic inhibitory networks (Huang et al., 1999; Hong et al., 2008). Locally synthesized BDNF in dendrites of granule cells promotes differentiation and maturation of progenitor cells in the SGZ by enhancing GABA release from PV GABAergic interneurons (Waterhouse et al., 2012). Several studies have determined that seizure activity is able to increase both mRNA and protein levels (Bengzon et al., 1993). Other studies suggest that an upregulation of BDNF levels could contribute to epileptogenesis (Binder, 2004; Lähteinen et al., 2004), although at the same time it was proposed that its upregulation could be protective for neurons from excitotoxicity (Wu et al., 2004; Pérez-Navarro et al., 2005). Regarding neurogenesis, BDNF is a neurotrophin that promotes proliferation of human fetal neural stem and progenitor cells *in vitro* (Zhang et al., 2011) and it is a potent regulator of the survival and differentiation of adult NSCs (Park and Poo, 2013), suggesting another mechanism linking the effect of hyperexcitotoxycity on stem cell activation and neurogenesis. I has been shown that in glioma-cell populations containing cancer stem cells BDNF is able to increase directly cell division through Akt activation and PTEN inactivation (Tamura et al., 1999; Bertrand et al., 2009). Although Akt and PTEN also has been independently implicated in the proliferation of neural stem and progenitor cells (Amiri et al., 2012; Cai et al., 2014) it remains to be elucidated whether BDNF is the direct regulator.

Stimulation by FGF

Neuronal activity also can regulate growth factors such as basic FGF(bFGF) and FGF-2 (Riva et al., 1992). FGF-2 overexpression increases excitability and seizure susceptibility (Zucchini et al., 2008) and is acutely overexpressed after seizures (Indulekha et al., 2010). It is well stablished that the morphology of reactive astrocytes is controlled by FGF signaling. In a recent work Goldshmit et al. demonstrated this pleiotropic cytokine is able to decrease gliosis and increase radial glia and neural progenitor cells in spinal cord injury (Goldshmit et al., 2014). However, Kang et al. demonstrated that FGF signaling in brain is responsible for astrocyte hypertrophy in response to an inflammatory stimulus (Kang et al., 2014). Previous studies demonstrated that the expression of FGF-2 and its receptors is induced in astrocytes after epileptiform activity using KA injections in rats (Van Der Wal et al., 1994). FGF signaling is a strong mitogenic factor *in vitro* and *in vivo* when injected subcutaneously or in an intravitreal manner, stimulating cellular proliferation including astrocytes (Lewis et al., 1992; Wagner et al., 1999). In addition, in FGF-2 knock-out mice, intraperitoneal KA injection fails to trigger an increase in cell proliferation, as it does in wild-type mice (Yoshimura et al., 2001). These results support the idea that endogenously synthesized FGF-2 is necessary to stimulate adult hippocampal neurogenesis after brain insult. Interestingly, in the early phase of acute epilepsy FGF-2-expressing reactive astrocytes are observed (Erkanli et al., 2007). However, FGF-2 expression declines considerably in human chronic epilepsy (Hattiangady et al., 2004), with a decrease in parallel of the number FGF-2-positive reactive astrocytes (Erkanli et al., 2007). Reactive astrocytes persist in the chronically epileptic hippocampus, but it remains unclear whether reactive astrocytes that emerge in the early phase after SE persist for prolonged periods of time, or there is turnover and new reactive astrocytes are added progressively. The involvement of FGF signaling in the transformation of NSCs into hypertrophic reactive astrocytes (Sierra et al., 2015) has not yet been addressed.

Sonic Hedgehog Signaling

Sonic hedgehog (Shh) signal acts directly on the astrocytes and is sufficient to provoke stem cell response in both models *in vitro* and *in vivo* (Sirko et al., 2013). Shh is one of three ligands for hedegehog (Hh) signaling in mammals (Washington Smoak et al., 2005). When secreted glycoprotein Shh binds Ptc receptor on the cell surface it relieves the inhibition of Smo. Activated Smo goes to the nucleus and triggers the activation of transcription factors, which regulate proliferation, migration, and differentiation. Mice lacking Smo in NSC during development have a small DG with reduced proliferation and reduced generation of neurons (Breunig et al., 2008; Han et al., 2008).

Previous studies of ECS observed a strong and robust increase of Hh signaling through Ptc upregulation and a rapid and reduction of Smo in the hippocampal DG, proposing that both acute and chronic ECS enhanced Shh signaling in the adult hippocampus (Banerjee et al., 2005). In other experiments using the Smo antagonist cyclopamine Lai et al. observed a reduction of hippocampal neural progenitor proliferation *in vivo* (Lai et al.,

2003). In agreement with the effects of ECS, synaptic activity involving glutamatergic transmission is proposed to regulate Smo protein, suggesting additional roles for Hh signaling in the control of hippocampal functions (Palma et al., 2005). In the KA model of epilepsy, Shh expression and release by astrocytes induces its own activation in a positive feedback loop, boosting further autocrine Shh release which translates ultimately into increased astrocytes proliferation and conversion into reactive astrocytes (Pitter et al., 2014). One study documented increased expression of Shh by neurons in the epileptic temporal lobe of human and experimental rats, although the consequences of elevated Shh were not studied (Fang et al., 2011).

CONCLUSIONS

Even though the relationship between epilepsy affecting the hippocampus and adult hippocampal neurogenesis has been known for almost two decades, many basic questions remain unsolved. One of the characteristics of the studies published so far is the apparent differential or even contradictory results among them. More than perceiving these controversial results as fruit of inconsistencies due to different animal models and the impossibility to control certain variables (especially when analyzing human tissue), we believe that they are reflecting the overwhelming biological plasticity of neurogenesis. Alterations of neurogenesis in different directions (excessive, aberrant and impaired neurogenesis) in the pathophysiology of epilepsy might be relevant to explain at least some of the cognitive symptoms associated to this disorder and we therefore conclude that further research should be carried out with an open mind in lieu of the variety of possible outcomes.

AUTHOR CONTRIBUTIONS

All authors listed, have made substantial, direct and intellectual contribution to the work, and approved it for publication.

FUNDING

This work was supported by a grant from the Spanish Ministry of Economy and Competitiveness (MINECO) with FEDER funds to JE (SAF2012-40085), and with MINECO Ramón y Cajal contracts to JE (RyC-2012-11185) and JP (RyC-2013-13450).

REFERENCES

Amiri, A., Cho, W., Zhou, J., Birnbaum, S. G., Sinton, C. M., McKay, R. M., et al. (2012). Pten deletion in adult hippocampal neural stem/progenitor cells causes cellular abnormalities and alters neurogenesis. *J. Neurosci.* 32, 5880–5890. doi: 10.1523/JNEUROSCI.5462-11.2012

Andersen, J., Urbán, N., Achimastou, A., Ito, A., Simic, M., Ullom, K., et al. (2014). A transcriptional mechanism integrating inputs from extracellular signals to activate hippocampal stem cells. *Neuron* 83, 1085–1097. doi: 10.1016/j.neuron.2014.08.004

Banerjee, S. B., Rajendran, R., Dias, B. G., Ladiwala, U., Tole, S., and Vaidya, V. A. (2005). Recruitment of the Sonic hedgehog signalling cascade in electroconvulsive seizure-mediated regulation of adult rat hippocampal neurogenesis. *Eur. J. Neurosci.* 22, 1570–1580. doi: 10.1111/j.1460-9568.2005.04317.x

Baraban, S. C., Hollopeter, G., Erickson, J. C., Schwartzkroin, P. A., and Palmiter, R. D. (1997). Knock-out mice reveal a critical antiepileptic role for neuropeptide Y. *J. Neurosci.* 17, 8927–8936.

Bengzon, J., Kokaia, Z., Ernfors, P., Kokaia, M., Leanza, G., Nilsson, O. G., et al. (1993). Regulation of neurotrophin and trkA, trkB and trkC tyrosine kinase receptor messenger RNA expression in kindling. *Neuroscience* 53, 433–446. doi: 10.1016/0306-4522(93)90207-V

Bertrand, J., Begaud-Grimaud, G., Bessette, B., Verdier, M., Battu, S., and Jauberteau, M.-O. (2009). Cancer stem cells from human glioma cell line are resistant to Fas-induced apoptosis. *Int. J. Oncol.* 34, 717–727. doi: 10.3892/ijo_00000198

Binder, D. K. (2004). The role of BDNF in epilepsy and other diseases of the mature nervous system. *Adv. Exp. Med. Biol.* 548, 34–56. doi: 10.1007/978-1-4757-6376-8_3

Blümcke, I., Schewe, J. C., Normann, S., Brüstle, O., Schramm, J., Elger, C. E., et al. (2001). Increase of nestin-immunoreactive neural precursor cells in the dentate gyrus of pediatric patients with early-onset temporal lobe epilepsy. *Hippocampus* 11, 311–321. doi: 10.1002/hipo.1045

Bonaguidi, M. A., Wheeler, M. A., Shapiro, J. S., Stadel, R. P., Sun, G. J., Ming, G. L., et al. (2011). *In vivo* clonal analysis reveals self-renewing and multipotent adult neural stem cell characteristics. *Cell* 145, 1142–1155. doi: 10.1016/j.cell.2011.05.024

Breunig, J. J., Sarkisian, M. R., Arellano, J. I., Morozov, Y. M., Ayoub, A. E., Sojitra, S., et al. (2008). Primary cilia regulate hippocampal neurogenesis by mediating sonic hedgehog signaling. *Proc. Natl. Acad. Sci. U.S.A.* 105, 13127–13132. doi: 10.1073/pnas.0804558105

Cai, M., Zhou, Y., Zhou, B., and Lou, S. (2014). Hypoxic conditioned medium from rat cerebral cortical cells enhances the proliferation and differentiation of neural stem cells mainly through PI3-K/Akt pathways. *PLoS ONE* 9:e111938. doi: 10.1371/journal.pone.0111938

Cho, K.-O., Lybrand, Z. R., Ito, N., Brulet, R., Tafacory, F., Zhang, L., et al. (2015). Aberrant hippocampal neurogenesis contributes to epilepsy and associated cognitive decline. *Nat. Commun.* 6, 6606. doi: 10.1038/ncomms 7606

Colmers, W. F., and El Bahh, B. (2003). Neuropeptide Y and Epilepsy. *Epilepsy Curr.* 3, 53–58. doi: 10.1046/j.1535-7597.2003.03208.x

Crespel, A., Rigau, V., Coubes, P., Rousset, M. C., de Bock, F., Okano, H., et al. (2005). Increased number of neural progenitors in human temporal lobe epilepsy. *Neurobiol. Dis.* 19, 436–450. doi: 10.1016/j.nbd.2005.01.020

Dashtipour, K., Tran, P. H., Okazaki, M. M., Nadler, J. V., and Ribak, C. E. (2001). Ultrastructural features and synaptic connections of hilar ectopic granule cells in the rat dentate gyrus are different from those of granule cells in the granule cell layer. *Brain Res.* 890, 261–271. doi: 10.1016/S0006-8993(00)03119-X

Daynac, M., Chicheportiche, A., Pineda, J. R., Gauthier, L. R., Boussin, F. D., and Mouthon, M.-A. (2013). Quiescent neural stem cells exit dormancy upon alteration of GABAAR signaling following radiation damage. *Stem Cell Res.* 11, 516–528. doi: 10.1016/j.scr.2013.02.008

Decressac, M., Wright, B., David, B., Tyers, P., Jaber, M., Barker, R. A., et al. (2011). Exogenous neuropeptide Y promotes *in vivo* hippocampal neurogenesis. *Hippocampus* 21, 233–238. doi: 10.1002/hipo.20765

Dericioglu, N., Soylemezoglu, F., Gursoy-Ozdemir, Y., Akalan, N., Saygi, S., and Dalkara, T. (2013). Cell death and survival mechanisms are concomitantly active in the hippocampus of patients with mesial temporal sclerosis. *Neuroscience* 237, 56–65. doi: 10.1016/j.neuroscience.2013.01.050

Dingledine, R., Varvel, N. H., and Dudek, F. E. (2014). When and how do seizures kill neurons, and is cell death relevant to epileptogenesis? *Adv. Exp. Med. Biol.* 813, 109–122. doi: 10.1007/978-94-017-8914-1_9

Encinas, J. M., and Enikolopov, G. (2008). Identifying and quantitating neural stem and progenitor cells in the adult brain. *Methods Cell Biol.* 85, 243–272. doi: 10.1016/S0091-679X(08)85011-X

Encinas, J. M., Michurina, T. V., Peunova, N., Park, J. H., Tordo, J., Peterson, D. A., et al. (2011). Division-coupled astrocytic differentiation and age-related depletion of neural stem cells in the adult hippocampus. *Cell Stem Cell* 8, 566–579. doi: 10.1016/j.stem.2011.03.010

Erickson, J. C., Clegg, K. E., and Palmiter, R. D. (1996). Sensitivity to leptin and susceptibility to seizures of mice lacking neuropeptide Y. *Nature* 381, 415–421. doi: 10.1038/381415a0

Erkanli, G., Ercan, F., Sirvanci, S., Yananli, H. R., Onat, F., and San, T. (2007). Time-dependent changes in distribution of basic fibroblast growth factor immunoreactive cells in rat hippocampus after status epilepticus. *Neurol. Res.* 29, 816–823. doi: 10.1179/174313213X13789811969229

Fahrner, A., Kann, G., Flubacher, A., Heinrich, C., Freiman, T. M., Zentner, J., et al. (2007). Granule cell dispersion is not accompanied by enhanced neurogenesis in temporal lobe epilepsy patients. *Exp. Neurol.* 203, 320–332. doi: 10.1016/j.expneurol.2006.08.023

Fang, M., Lu, Y., Chen, G.-J., Shen, L., Pan, Y.-M., and Wang, X.-F. (2011). Increased expression of sonic hedgehog in temporal lobe epileptic foci in humans and experimental rats. *Neuroscience* 182, 62–70. doi: 10.1016/j.neuroscience.2011.02.060

Farrant, M., and Nusser, Z. (2005). Variations on an inhibitory theme: phasic and tonic activation of GABA(A) receptors. *Nat. Rev. Neurosci.* 6, 215–229. doi: 10.1038/nrn1625

Fernando, R. N., Eleuteri, B., Abdelhady, S., Nussenzweig, A., Andäng, M., and Ernfors, P. (2011). Cell cycle restriction by histone H2AX limits proliferation of adult neural stem cells. *Proc. Natl. Acad. Sci. U.S.A.* 108, 5837–5842. doi: 10.1073/pnas.1014993108

Gall, C. M., Berschauer, R., and Isackson, P. J. (1994). Seizures increase basic fibroblast growth factor mRNA in adult rat forebrain neurons and glia. *Brain Res. Mol. Brain Res.* 21, 190–205. doi: 10.1016/0169-328X(94)90250-X

Ge, S., Pradhan, D. A., Ming, G.-L. L., and Song, H. (2007). GABA sets the tempo for activity-dependent adult neurogenesis. *Trends Neurosci.* 30, 1–8. doi: 10.1016/j.tins.2006.11.001

Giachino, C., Barz, M., Tchorz, J. S., Tome, M., Gassmann, M., Bischofberger, J., et al. (2014). GABA suppresses neurogenesis in the adult hippocampus through GABAB receptors. *Development* 141, 83–90. doi: 10.1242/dev.102608

Goldshmit, Y., Frisca, F., Pinto, A. R., Pébay, A., Tang, J.-K. K. Y., Siegel, A. L., et al. (2014). Fgf2 improves functional recovery-decreasing gliosis and increasing radial glia and neural progenitor cells after spinal cord injury. *Brain Behav.* 4, 187–200. doi: 10.1002/brb3.172

Gong, C., Wang, T.-W., Huang, H. S., and Parent, J. M. (2007). Reelin regulates neuronal progenitor migration in intact and epileptic hippocampus. *J. Neurosci.* 27, 1803–1811. doi: 10.1523/JNEUROSCI.3111-06.2007

Gruber, B., Greber, S., Rupp, E., and Sperk, G. (1994). Differential NPY mRNA expression in granule cells and interneurons of the rat dentate gyrus after kainic acid injection. *Hippocampus* 4, 474–482. doi: 10.1002/hipo.450040409

Han, Y.-G., Spassky, N., Romaguera-Ros, M., Garcia-Verdugo, J.-M., Aguilar, A., Schneider-Maunoury, S., et al. (2008). Hedgehog signaling and primary cilia are required for the formation of adult neural stem cells. *Nat. Neurosci.* 11, 277–284. doi: 10.1038/nn2059

Hattiangady, B., Rao, M. S., and Shetty, A. K. (2004). Chronic temporal lobe epilepsy is associated with severely declined dentate neurogenesis in the adult hippocampus. *Neurobiol. Dis.* 17, 473–490. doi: 10.1016/j.nbd.2004.08.008

Hattiangady, B., and Shetty, A. K. (2010). Decreased neuronal differentiation of newly generated cells underlies reduced hippocampal neurogenesis in chronic temporal lobe epilepsy. *Hippocampus* 20, 97–112. doi: 10.1002/hipo.20594

Hester, M. S., and Danzer, S. C. (2013). Accumulation of abnormal adult-generated hippocampal granule cells predicts seizure frequency and severity. *J. Neurosci.* 33, 8926–8936. doi: 10.1523/JNEUROSCI.5161-12.2013

Hong, E. J., McCord, A. E., and Greenberg, M. E. (2008). A biological function for the neuronal activity-dependent component of Bdnf transcription in the development of cortical inhibition. *Neuron* 60, 610–624. doi: 10.1016/j.neuron.2008.09.024

Huang, E. J., and Reichardt, L. F. (2001). Neurotrophins: roles in neuronal development and function. *Annu. Rev. Neurosci.* 24, 677–736. doi: 10.1146/annurev.neuro.24.1.677

Huang, Z. J., Kirkwood, A., Pizzorusso, T., Porciatti, V., Morales, B., Bear, M. F., et al. (1999). BDNF regulates the maturation of inhibition and the critical period of plasticity in mouse visual cortex. *Cell* 98, 739–755. doi: 10.1016/S0092-8674(00)81509-3

Huttmann, K., Sadgrove, M., Wallraff, A., Hinterkeuser, S., Kirchhoff, F., Steinhauser, C., et al. (2003). Seizures preferentially stimulate proliferation of radial glia-like astrocytes in the adult dentate gyrus: functional and immunocytochemical analysis. *Eur. J. Neurosci.* 18, 2769–2778. doi: 10.1111/j.1460-9568.2003.03002.x

Indulekha, C. L., Sanalkumar, R., Thekkuveettil, A., and James, J. (2010). Seizure induces activation of multiple subtypes of neural progenitors and growth factors in hippocampus with neuronal maturation confined to dentate gyrus. *Biochem. Biophys. Res. Commun.* 393, 864–871. doi: 10.1016/j.bbrc.2010.02.101

Jhaveri, D. J., O'Keeffe, I., Robinson, G. J., Zhao, Q.-Y., Zhang, Z. H., Nink, V., et al. (2015). Purification of neural precursor cells reveals the presence of distinct, stimulus-specific subpopulations of quiescent precursors in the adult mouse hippocampus. *J. Neurosci.* 35, 8132–8144. doi: 10.1523/JNEUROSCI.0504-15.2015

Jun, H., Hussaini, S. M. Q., Cho, C. H., Welby, J., and Jang, M.-H. (2015). Gadd45b mediates electroconvulsive shock induced proliferation of hippocampal neural stem cells. *Brain Stimul.* 8, 1021–1024. doi: 10.1016/j.brs.2015.07.036

Kang, K., Lee, S.-W., Han, J. E., Choi, J. W., and Song, M.-R. (2014). The complex morphology of reactive astrocytes controlled by fibroblast growth factor signaling. *Glia* 62, 1328–1344. doi: 10.1002/glia.22684

Kazanis, I., Lathia, J. D., Vadakkan, T. J., Raborn, E., Wan, R., Mughal, M. R., et al. (2010). Quiescence and activation of stem and precursor cell populations in the subependymal zone of the mammalian brain are associated with distinct cellular and extracellular matrix signals. *J. Neurosci.* 30, 9771–9781. doi: 10.1523/JNEUROSCI.0700-10.2010

Kragh, J., Tønder, N., Finsen, B. R., Zimmer, J., and Bolwig, T. G. (1994). Repeated electroconvulsive shocks cause transient changes in rat hippocampal somatostatin and neuropeptide Y immunoreactivity and mRNA *in situ* hybridization signals. *Exp. Brain Res.* 98, 305–313. doi: 10.1007/BF00228418

Lähteinen, S., Pitkänen, A., Knuuttila, J., Törönen, P., and Castrén, E. (2004). Brain-derived neurotrophic factor signaling modifies hippocampal gene expression during epileptogenesis in transgenic mice. *Eur. J. Neurosci.* 19, 3245–3254. doi: 10.1111/j.0953-816X.2004.03440.x

Lai, K., Kaspar, B. K., Gage, F. H., and Schaffer, D. V. (2003). Sonic hedgehog regulates adult neural progenitor proliferation *in vitro* and *in vivo*. *Nat. Neurosci.* 6, 21–27. doi: 10.1038/nn983

Lee, C. H., and Umemori, H. (2013). Suppression of epileptogenesis-associated changes in response to seizures in FGF22-deficient mice. *Front. Cell. Neurosci.* 7:43. doi: 10.3389/fncel.2013.00043

Lewis, G. P., Erickson, P. A., Guérin, C. J., Anderson, D. H., and Fisher, S. K. (1992). Basic fibroblast growth factor: a potential regulator of proliferation and intermediate filament expression in the retina. *J. Neurosci.* 12, 3968–3978.

Liu, X., Wang, Q., Haydar, T. F., and Bordey, A. (2005). Nonsynaptic GABA signaling in postnatal subventricular zone controls proliferation of GFAP-expressing progenitors. *Nat. Neurosci.* 8, 1179–1187. doi: 10.1038/nn1522

Lowenstein, D. H., Seren, M. S., and Longo, F. M. (1993). Prolonged increases in neurotrophic activity associated with kainate-induced hippocampal synaptic reorganization. *Neuroscience* 56, 597–604. doi: 10.1016/0306-4522(93)90359-N

Maru, E., and Ura, H. (2014). [GABA(A) receptor trafficking and epilepsy]. *Nihon Rinsho.* 72, 790–795.

Mathern, G. W., Leiphart, J. L., De Vera, A., Adelson, P. D., Seki, T., Neder, L., et al. (2002). Seizures decrease postnatal neurogenesis and granule cell development in the human fascia dentata. *Epilepsia* 43(Suppl. 5), 68–73. doi: 10.1046/j.1528-1157.43.s.5.28.x

Mattson, M. P. (2008). Glutamate and neurotrophic factors in neuronal plasticity and disease. *Ann. N.Y. Acad. Sci.* 1144, 97–112. doi: 10.1196/annals.1418.005

Mikkonen, M., Soininen, H., Kälviänen, R., Tapiola, T., Ylinen, A., Vapalahti, M., et al. (1998). Remodeling of neuronal circuitries in human temporal lobe epilepsy: increased expression of highly polysialylated neural cell adhesion molecule in the hippocampus and the entorhinal cortex. *Ann. Neurol.* 44, 923–934. doi: 10.1002/ana.410440611

Moss, J., and Toni, N. (2013). A circuit-based gatekeeper for adult neural stem cell proliferation: Parvalbumin-expressing interneurons of the dentate gyrus control the activation and proliferation of quiescent adult neural stem cells. *Bioessays* 35, 28–33. doi: 10.1002/bies.201200136

Murphy, B. L., Hofacer, R. D., Faulkner, C. N., Loepke, A. W., and Danzer, S. C. (2012). Abnormalities of granule cell dendritic structure are a prominent feature of the intrahippocampal kainic acid model of epilepsy despite reduced postinjury neurogenesis. *Epilepsia* 53, 908–921. doi: 10.1111/j.1528-1167.2012.03463.x

Palma, V., Lim, D. A., Dahmane, N., Sánchez, P., Brionne, T. C., Herzberg, C. D., et al. (2005). Sonic hedgehog controls stem cell behavior in the postnatal and adult brain. *Development* 132, 335–344. doi: 10.1242/dev.01567

Paradisi, M., Fernández, M., Del Vecchio, G., Lizzo, G., Marucci, G., Giulioni, M., et al. (2010). *Ex vivo* study of dentate gyrus neurogenesis in human pharmacoresistant temporal lobe epilepsy. *Neuropathol. Appl. Neurobiol.* 36, 535–550. doi: 10.1111/j.1365-2990.2010.01102.x

Parent, J. M., Yu, T. W., Leibowitz, R. T., Geschwind, D. H., Sloviter, R. S., and Lowenstein, D. H. (1997). Dentate granule cell neurogenesis is increased by seizures and contributes to aberrant network reorganization in the adult rat hippocampus. *J. Neurosci.* 17, 3727–3738.

Park, H., and Poo, M. (2013). Neurotrophin regulation of neural circuit development and function. *Nat. Rev. Neurosci.* 14, 7–23. doi: 10.1038/nrn3379

Pérez-Navarro, E., Gavaldà, N., Gratacòs, E., and Alberch, J. (2005). Brain-derived neurotrophic factor prevents changes in Bcl-2 family members and caspase-3 activation induced by excitotoxicity in the striatum. *J. Neurochem.* 92, 678–691. doi: 10.1111/j.1471-4159.2004.02904.x

Pitter, K. L., Tamagno, I., Feng, X., Ghosal, K., Amankulor, N., Holland, E. C., et al. (2014). The SHH/Gli pathway is reactivated in reactive glia and drives proliferation in response to neurodegeneration-induced lesions. *Glia* 62, 1595–1607. doi: 10.1002/glia.22702

Riva, M. A., Gale, K., and Mocchetti, I. (1992). Basic fibroblast growth factor mRNA increases in specific brain regions following convulsive seizures. *Brain Res. Mol. Brain Res.* 15, 311–318. doi: 10.1016/0169-328X(92)90123-S

Scharfman, H. E. (2000). Epileptogenesis in the parahippocampal region. Parallels with the dentate gyrus. *Ann. N.Y. Acad. Sci.* 911, 305–327. doi: 10.1111/j.1749-6632.2000.tb06734.x

Scharfman, H. E., Sollas, A. L., Berger, R. E., and Goodman, J. H. (2003). Electrophysiological evidence of monosynaptic excitatory transmission between granule cells after seizure-induced mossy fiber sprouting. *J. Neurophysiol.* 90, 2536–2547. doi: 10.1152/jn.00251.2003

Segi-Nishida, E., Warner-Schmidt, J. L., and Duman, R. S. (2008). Electroconvulsive seizure and VEGF increase the proliferation of neural stem-like cells in rat hippocampus. *Proc. Natl. Acad. Sci. U.S.A.* 105, 11352–11357. doi: 10.1073/pnas.0710858105

Shetty, A. K., Rao, M. S., Hattiangady, B., Zaman, V., and Shetty, G. A. (2004). Hippocampal neurotrophin levels after injury: relationship to the age of the hippocampus at the time of injury. *J. Neurosci. Res.* 78, 520–532. doi: 10.1002/jnr.20302

Shetty, A. K., Zaman, V., and Shetty, G. A. (2003). Hippocampal neurotrophin levels in a kainate model of temporal lobe epilepsy: a lack of correlation between brain-derived neurotrophic factor content and progression of aberrant dentate mossy fiber sprouting. *J. Neurochem.* 87, 147–159. doi:10.1046/j.1471-4159.2003.01979.x

Sierra, A., Encinas, J. M., Deudero, J. J. P., Chancey, J. H., Enikolopov, G., Overstreet-Wadiche, L. S., et al. (2010). Microglia shape adult hippocampal neurogenesis through apoptosis-coupled phagocytosis. *Cell Stem Cell* 7, 483–495. doi: 10.1016/j.stem.2010.08.014

Sierra, A., Martín-suárez, S., Valcárcel-martín, R., Pascual, J., Anderson, A. E., Baekelandt, V., et al. (2015). Neuronal hyperactivity accelerates depletion of neural stem cells and impairs hippocampal neurogenesis. *Cell Stem Cell* 16, 488–503. doi: 10.1016/j.stem.2015.04.003

Sirko, S., Behrendt, G., Johansson, P. A., Tripathi, P., Costa, M., Bek, S., et al. (2013). Reactive glia in the injured brain acquire stem cell properties in response to sonic hedgehog glia. *Cell Stem Cell* 12, 426–439. doi: 10.1016/j.stem.2013.01.019

Song, J., Sun, J., Moss, J., Wen, Z., Sun, G. J., Hsu, D., et al. (2013). Parvalbumin interneurons mediate neuronal circuitry-neurogenesis coupling in the adult hippocampus. *Nat. Neurosci.* 16, 1728–1730. doi: 10.1038/nn.3572

Song, J., Zhong, C., Bonaguidi, M. A., Sun, G. J., Hsu, D., Gu, Y., et al. (2012). Neuronal circuitry mechanism regulating adult quiescent neural stem-cell fate decision. *Nature* 489, 150–154. doi: 10.1038/nature11306

Spalding, K. L., Bergmann, O., Alkass, K., Bernard, S., Salehpour, M., Huttner, H. B., et al. (2013). Dynamics of hippocampal neurogenesis in adult humans. *Cell* 153, 1219–1227. doi: 10.1016/j.cell.2013.05.002

Szot, P., Weinshenker, D., White, S. S., Robbins, C. A., Rust, N. C., Schwartzkroin, P. A., et al. (1999). Norepinephrine-deficient mice have increased susceptibility to seizure-inducing stimuli. *J. Neurosci.* 19, 10985–10992.

Tamura, M., Gu, J., Danen, E. H., Takino, T., Miyamoto, S., and Yamada, K. M. (1999). PTEN interactions with focal adhesion kinase and suppression of the extracellular matrix-dependent phosphatidylinositol 3-kinase/Akt cell survival pathway. *J. Biol. Chem.* 274, 20693–20703. doi: 10.1074/jbc.274.29.20693

Thom, M., Martinian, L., Williams, G., Stoeber, K., and Sisodiya, S. M. (2005). Cell proliferation and granule cell dispersion in human hippocampal sclerosis. *J. Neuropathol. Exp. Neurol.* 64, 194–201. doi: 10.1093/jnen/64.3.194

Van Der Wal, E. A., Gomez-Pinilla, F., and Cotman, C. W. (1994). Seizure-associated induction of basic fibroblast growth factor and its receptor in the rat brain. *Neuroscience* 60, 311–323. doi: 10.1016/0306-4522(94)90245-3

Wagner, J. P., Black, I. B., and DiCicco-Bloom, E. (1999). Stimulation of neonatal and adult brain neurogenesis by subcutaneous injection of basic fibroblast growth factor. *J. Neurosci.* 19, 6006–6016.

Walter, C., Murphy, B. L., Pun, R. Y. K., Spieles-Engemann, A. L., and Danzer, S. C. (2007). Pilocarpine-induced seizures cause selective time-dependent changes to adult-generated hippocampal dentate granule cells. *J. Neurosci.* 27, 7541–7552. doi: 10.1523/JNEUROSCI.0431-07.2007

Walter, J., Keiner, S., Witte, O. W., and Redecker, C. (2011). Age-related effects on hippocampal precursor cell subpopulations and neurogenesis. *Neurobiol. Aging* 32, 1906–1914. doi: 10.1016/j.neurobiolaging.2009.11.011

Washington Smoak, I., Byrd, N. A., Abu-Issa, R., Goddeeris, M. M., Anderson, R., Morris, J., et al. (2005). Sonic hedgehog is required for cardiac outflow tract and neural crest cell development. *Dev. Biol.* 283, 357–372. doi: 10.1016/j.ydbio.2005.04.029

Waterhouse, E. G., An, J. J., Orefice, L. L., Baydyuk, M., Liao, G.-Y., Zheng, K., et al. (2012). BDNF promotes differentiation and maturation of adult-born neurons through GABAergic transmission. *J. Neurosci.* 32, 14318–14330. doi: 10.1523/JNEUROSCI.0709-12.2012

Waterhouse, E. G., and Xu, B. (2009). New insights into the role of brain-derived neurotrophic factor in synaptic plasticity. *Mol. Cell. Neurosci.* 42, 81–89. doi: 10.1016/j.mcn.2009.06.009

Weinshenker, D., Szot, P., Miller, N. S., Rust, N. C., Hohmann, J. G., Pyati, U., et al. (2001). Genetic comparison of seizure control by norepinephrine and neuropeptide Y. *J. Neurosci.* 21, 7764–7769.

Woldbye, D. P., Larsen, P. J., Mikkelsen, J. D., Klemp, K., Madsen, T. M., and Bolwig, T. G. (1997). Powerful inhibition of kainic acid seizures by neuropeptide Y via Y5-like receptors. *Nat. Med.* 3, 761–764. doi: 10.1038/nm0797-761

Wu, X., Zhu, D., Jiang, X., Okagaki, P., Mearow, K., Zhu, G., et al. (2004). AMPA protects cultured neurons against glutamate excitotoxicity through a phosphatidylinositol 3-kinase-dependent activation in extracellular signal-regulated kinase to upregulate BDNF gene expression. *J. Neurochem.* 90, 807–818. doi: 10.1111/j.1471-4159.2004.02526.x

Yoshimura, S., Takagi, Y., Harada, J., Teramoto, T., Thomas, S. S., Waeber, C., et al. (2001). FGF-2 regulation of neurogenesis in adult hippocampus after brain injury. *Proc. Natl. Acad. Sci. U.S.A.* 98, 5874–5879. doi: 10.1073/pnas.101034998

Zarubenko, I. I., Yakovlev, A. A., Stepanichev, M. Y., and Gulyaeva, N. V. (2005). Electroconvulsive shock induces neuron death in the mouse hippocampus: correlation of neurodegeneration with convulsive activity. *Neurosci. Behav. Physiol.* 35, 715–721. doi: 10.1007/s11055-005-0115-0

Zeev, B. B., Bebbington, A., Ho, G., Leonard, H., de Klerk, N., and Christodoulou, J. (2009). The common BDNF polymorphism may be a modifier of disease severity in Rett syndrome. *Neurology* 72, 1242–1247. doi: 10.1212/01.wnl.0000345664.72220.6a

Zhang, Q., Liu, G., Wu, Y., Sha, H., Zhang, P., and Jia, J. (2011). BDNF promotes EGF-induced proliferation and migration of human fetal neural stem/progenitor cells via the PI3K/Akt pathway. *Molecules* 16, 10146–10156. doi: 10.3390/molecules161210146

Zuccato, C., and Cattaneo, E. (2009). Brain-derived neurotrophic factor in neurodegenerative diseases. *Nat. Rev. Neurol.* 5, 311–322. doi: 10.1038/nrneurol.2009.54

Zucchini, S., Buzzi, A., Barbieri, M., Rodi, D., Paradiso, B., Binaschi, A., et al. (2008). Fgf-2 overexpression increases excitability and seizure susceptibility but decreases seizure-induced cell loss. *J. Neurosci.* 28, 13112–13124. doi: 10.1523/JNEUROSCI.1472-08.2008

2

Can Exercise make you Smarter, Happier, and have more Neurons? A Hormetic Perspective

Simona Gradari, Anna Pallé, Kerry R. McGreevy, Ángela Fontán-Lozano and José L. Trejo *

Laboratory of Adult Neurogenesis, Department of Molecular, Cellular and Developmental Neurobiology, Cajal Institute, Consejo Superior de Investigaciones Científicas, Madrid, Spain

Exercise can make you smarter, happier and have more neurons depending on the dose (intensity) of the training program. It is well recognized that exercise protocols induce both positive and negative effects depending on the intensity of the exercise, among other key factors, a process described as a hormetic-like biphasic dose-response. However, no evidences have been reported till very recently about the biphasic response of some of the potential mediators of the exercise-induced actions. This hypothesis and theory will focus on the adult hippocampal neurogenesis (AHN) as a putative physical substrate for hormesis responses to exercise in the context of exercise-induced actions on cognition and mood, and on the molecular pathways which might potentially be mediating these actions.

Edited by:
João O. Malva, University of Coimbra, Portugal

Reviewed by:
Stefano Farioli Vecchioli, Consiglio Nazionale delle Ricerche, Italy
Gerd Kempermann, German Center for Neurodegenerative Disease (DZNE) Dresden, Germany

***Correspondence:**
José L. Trejo
jltrejo@cajal.csic.es

Keywords: exercise, adult hippocampal neurogenesis, biphasic dose-response, hormesis, molecular mechanisms, cognition, mood

INTRODUCTION

Physical activity induces pleiotropic effects for the whole organism including brain (Dishman et al., 2006). The effects of physical exercise can be described by means of a hormetic (biphasic) dose-response curve both on cognition and mood (Mattson, 2012a), and many of these effects have been closely related to the adult hippocampal neurogenesis (AHN) in the last decade (Kempermann, 2011). AHN is a phenomenon consisting of the formation of new neurons during adult life, and certainly these new neurons are highly responsive to exercise. AHN has also been related, independently of their response to exercise, to some hippocampus-dependent behaviors and mood (Kempermann, 2011).

Taking this knowledge into consideration, we have reviewed first the literature related to the hormetic profile effects of both the exercise and its molecular mediators on the brain. Following these evidences, we have posed and discussed the hypothesis whether AHN responses display a biphasic/hormetic dose-response to exercise and whether some putative mechanisms underlying this response profile may be detected in the literature.

The answer to this question is relevant for our knowledge about the neurobiology of exercise, but nevertheless, also to raise a property of AHN (hormesis), that can easily influence and improve our attempts to manipulate adult neurogenesis beyond exercise (drugs or other interventions).

EXERCISE AND BRAIN

Physical activity is an essential component of everyday life. Searching for food or sexual partners, chasing preys or running away from predators, seasonal migrations, and almost any regular activity related to maintaining life is usually mediated by some kind of physical activity. These life-sustaining activities involving a physical component are intimately associated to cognitive activities. The processing of information about the surrounding environment where the organism is living and moving, learning, and storing such information, and its application for decision making are cognitive processes naturally occuring at the same time the organisms are moving.

Furthermore, the relationship between physical activity and brain information processing is more relevant than a mere correlational event. The way the brain processes information changes along with the level of physical activity of the organism (Foster, 2015), but even more important, physical activity effectively changes the brain, both at a morphological and functional levels. This adaptive brain plasticity responds to the different levels of information processing demand in the way of adjusting neural resources available to process that information level (Chen and Tonegawa, 1997). These neural resources and the available changes range from neural cell metabolism and gene expression, cell and processes size, neuronal dendrite and synapse number, and blood-brain barrier properties, to synaptic plasticity. While all these changes involve existing cells, neural resources also include a form of metaplasticity (named adult neurogenesis): the capability to recruit, in some specific areas of the adult brain, more neurons which show cellular and synaptic plasticity abilities (Garcia-Segura, 2009).

In this scenario, it is not surprising that physical exercise training has been largely reported as increasing synaptic plasticity, neural cells metabolism and blood supply in an active brain area-specific way, and increasing neural processing abilities, even in humans (in adults, children, and adolescents). Besides, in human beings a specific capability for endurance running, compared to the other primates has been postulated (Mattson, 2012b). Comparisons between animal and human studies are, therefore, difficult. However, common mechanisms underlie the aspects discussed in the present work, as for example, the inflection point for the effects of different intensity levels of exercise around the anaerobic threshold (lactate threshold) used in both laboratory rodent and human studies (see below). An increasing body of literature has long demonstrated benefits of exercise for cognition in humans (reviewed by Hillman et al., 2008). In experiments with laboratory rodents, it has been long demonstrated that exercise increases cognitive performance in almost any brain area, especially at hippocampus-dependent tasks, by means of synaptic plasticity and neurogenesis increments. It increases complexity of neuronal dendrites and synapse numbers. Regular exercise induces neuroprotection in all brain areas analyzed; it improves different parameters related to neurodegenerative diseases (age of onset, progression, and severity of symptoms) both in animal models and in humans. Finally, exercise has also been reported as a useful tool to recover the symptomatology of some neurodegenerative diseases and from different brain damages and insults (Dishman et al., 2006; Mattson, 2015). From a mechanistic point of view, exercise is able to increase blood flow (Lucas et al., 2015) and oxygen consumption (Rooks et al., 2010), modulate the growth factor signaling cascade (especially IGF1 Llorens-Martin et al., 2009, BDNF Gomez-Pinilla and Hillman, 2013, and VEGF During and Cao, 2006), and increase neurotransmitter availability and function (especially dopamine, glutamate, norepinephrine, and serotonin Meeusen, 2012).

Nevertheless, exercise displays inseparable negative effects. These stressors range from thermal, metabolic, hypoxic, and oxidative, to mechanical stress (reviewed by Peake et al., 2015). These effects have been reported both in animal and human studies. The higher capacity for endurance running showed by human beings (Mattson, 2012b) would just be one stage of the hormetic response by which a low dose of a stressful stimulus activates an adaptive response that increases the resistance to a moderate-to-severe level of stress (Calabrese et al., 2007). However, a number of different approaches have demonstrated inverted-U performance curves on cognition after exercise in humans (Tomporowski, 2003). The relationship is not simple because it clearly depends on the duration of the bouts (typically intense but brief, leading to a rapid recovery of the individual's capacity) and on the individual's fitness level previous to the study, a factor under the lack of clear effects of brief bouts of intense exercise (Tomporowski, 2003), and on the motivation to participate in both acute bouts of exercise or long endurance training regimes, a factor that surely distorts any conclusion about relationships between exercise and cognitive performance in humans. On the other side, steady-state aerobic exercise causes impaired information processing and cognition depending on the level of dehydration, in turn depending on the duration of the exercise (Cian et al., 2001). As the most outstanding factor, exercise increases oxidative stress, as expected as it consists of a physical increased activity of oxygen-consuming organisms and this effect is intimately associated to variations in energy metabolism (Coyle, 2000). This aspect of exercise programs can well be underlying the negative effects of strenuous physical activity (Nieman et al., 1990; Lee et al., 1995; Andersen et al., 2013). As it is well-known that exercise displays this kind of hormetic-like non-monotonic response curve for most outcomes analyzed (Radak et al., 2005), it is relevant to take into account that this biphasic response strongly depends on oxidative stress, oxygen consumption and mitochondrial metabolism. All these evidences are related to the effects on the whole body, mainly muscle and cardiovascular systems. As for the brain, it is important to take into account that exercise induces increased generation of ROS but also antioxidant enzymes and redox signaling in the body (Powers and Jackson, 2008; Radak et al., 2013), and oxidative stress can be induced into the brain by circulating factors (Calabrese et al., 2010). As general positive effects of exercise on brain's oxidative stress has long been recognized due to an increased activity of antioxidant enzymes (reviewed by Radak et al., 2014), it has been suggested that a complex regulation and balance between exercise-induced generation of sistemic ROS-related factors and brain antioxidant enzymes are mediating the effects of exercise on the brain in a hormetic, bell-shaped curve, where high levels of ROS cause oxidative damage, while moderate amounts would induce an adaptive response to oxidative challenge (Radak et al., 2014).

Moreover intense, above lactate threshold level exercise induces brain mitochondrial dysfunction and decreased BDNF levels in mice (Aguiar et al., 2008), increased activity of hypothalamic paraventricular nucleus and concomitant increase in CRH expression (Timofeeva et al., 2003), suggesting a direct activation of stress responses, while others have found only positive effects of intense exercise in aged mice (Lezi et al., 2014).

A word of caution is worth to be taking into account at this time. For the present work, we have considered that the broad range of parameters related to exercise are the same for humans, rats and mice, although subtle differences exist, not only between species, but also between mouse strains, gender and even inter-individual variability. Therefore, aerobic capacity, lactate and anaerobic thresholds and critical speed show similar features and the same curve profiles for human, rats and mice (Billat et al., 2005), as well as similar characteristics of maximal lactate steady state (MLSS; Ferreira et al., 2007), although noticeable differences do exist, such as a different sensitivity of MLSS for mice to endurance training compared to humans and rats (Beneke et al., 2000; Gobatto et al., 2001; Ferreira et al., 2007). All these works point to a very similar physiology of exercise and relevant parameters in laboratory rodents and humans, making the conclusions of this work relevant not only to know the specific features of rodent physiology but also to use animal models to study preclinical interventions. The most relevant distinction might be the subtle differences in the profile of aerobic–anaerobic transition between mice and both rats and humans. These differences are not critical for the topics discussed in the present work.

In this work, hormesis is considered the dual response of an individual's behavior, an organ or a cell's physiology or any other analyzed parameter in response to the graded intensity of a specific treatment/intervention (Mattson, 2008). In its most usual form, hormesis represents a dose-response curve with a biphasic profile: beneficial effects at a low dose/intensity and detrimental (inverted-J curve) or no effects (inverted-U curve) at a higher dose/intensity. Therefore, hormesis refers not only to negative effects at high doses, but also to a lack of moderate dose-induced positive effects at higher doses. As for exercise, hormesis adopts the features of pre-conditioning/adaptation to a mild, intermittent stress when coping with further higher stressors. This way, the hormesis curve is an adequate description of the effects of exercise (Radak et al., 2008). Therefore, it is relevant to consider the hormetic responses to physical exercise, focused on brain effects.

BIPHASIC RESPONSES TO EXERCISE ON COGNITION AND MOOD

It is not the aim of the present work to determine which are the specific characteristics that are optimal to obtain beneficial or detrimental effects with an exercise training protocol, both because the comparison between different works have been demonstrated very difficult in a number of meta-analysis, due to the inability to equate exercise intensity levels between studies, and because it is known only scarcely the many different parameters of the exercise regime influencing the exercise outcomes. What is most relevant for this work is whether authors have found biphasic responses independently of the applied protocol. Anyway, examples of reports with some of the most representative forced exercise protocols in animal studies and its both positive and negative effects on stress biomarkers, neuroplasticity and behavior are included in **Table 1**. Protocols vary especially when forced exercise is considered, because voluntary running protocols use to depend largely on the animals' motivation to run.

Physical exercise in human beings presents a biphasic dose-response curve for a huge number of cognition/mood parameters, depending on the intensity level of exercise program. Specifically, inverted U-shaped curves are found with an inflection point around the lactate or ventilatory thresholds. In a recent meta-analysis (Oliveira et al., 2015) on Feeling Scale (Hardy and Rejeski, 1989), it has been demonstrated that the intensity of the exercise is the main determinant to establish affective responses (no matter whether the exercise is self-selected or imposed). Beneficial effects of exercise in humans have been largely reported in a dose-response way (see Gomez-Pinilla and Hillman, 2013 for a recent review and Cotman and Berchtold, 2002; Dishman et al., 2006; Ang and Gomez-Pinilla, 2007; Mattson, 2012a,b). In a similar way, the subjective perception of the performance is decreased after an intense exercise (Grebot et al., 2003), and the stress associated to high intensity exercise has been reported to impair working and declarative memory (Taverniers et al., 2010).

In laboratory rodents, it is very well-known the high number of beneficial effects that a moderate exercise program can induce (Cotman and Berchtold, 2002; Kramer et al., 2006; Cotman et al., 2007). These beneficial effects include a variety of different tasks ranging from water maze (Ding et al., 2006), passive avoidance (Samorajski et al., 1985; Radak et al., 2006), contextual fear conditioning (Baruch et al., 2004; Burghardt et al., 2006) to radial arm maze (Schweitzer et al., 2006). On the contrary, it has been reported that high intensity exercise induces a variety of detrimental effects, including brain region-specific (amygdala - dorsal striatum becoming affected while hippocampus seem to be unaffected) and task-specific (differences found in some associative learning tasks-tone/shock conditioning-but not others-fear conditioning-and not in spatial reference and working memory tasks-water maze—) impairments in memory processing (Aguiar et al., 2010). Similar results have been found for passive avoidance tasks and contextual fear conditioning closely associated to brain oxidative stress (Rosa et al., 2007). Other authors have reported impairment of spatial-water maze-learning after high intensity exercise by using a different ergometer (treadmill running), although only at early acquisition phase (Blustein et al., 2006). High intensity levels of exercise can promote no improvements at all on cognition even after voluntary running and selective breeding for high levels of voluntary exercise (Rhodes et al., 2003). The deleterious effects of high intensity exercise can

TABLE 1 | Examples of positive, lack of positive, and negative effects of different forced training intensities on stress, behavior, and neurogenesis.

Animal model	Treadmill protocol	Stress biomarkers	Effects on cognition	Histological and molecular procedures	References
Brain ischemia rat model: Adult Sprague-Dawley (SD) rats	- Sedentary (SED) group: 0 m/min - Low-intensity exercise (LI) group: 8 m/min - High-intensity exercise (HI) group: 20 m/min Duration in each group: 30 min/day for 14 days.	Serum corticosterone (CORT) Only HI group presented higher serum CORT concentration (levels around 200 μg/ml) than SED group.	Morris Water Maze (MWM) task LI but not HI group demonstrated a better spatial memory performance than SED group by spending more time in the target (platform) quadrant.	BDNF, Synapsin-I, PSD-95 Only the LI but not HI group presented increased levels of BDNF, Synapsin-I and PSD-95 in the contralesional hippocampus compared to the SED group.	Shih et al., 2013
Adult male Sprague-Dawley (SD) with severe cortical impact	- Sedentary (Control) group: 0 m/min - Low-intensity (LI) group: Progressive speed until reaching a maximum of 8 m/min from day 8 to day 14 (end of the protocol). - High-intensity (HI) group: Progressive speed until reaching 12 m/min from day 4 to the end of the running protocol. Duration: 30 min/day for 14 days.	No stress biomarkers were assessed	MWM task LI group had a shorter latency to locate the platform and a better performance in spatial memory compared to the control group. The HI exercise group showed a longer latency and a mild improvement in spatial memory compared to the control group.	BDNF LI group had increased levels of BDNF in the contralateral hippocampus respect de control group. p-CREB LI group had increased levels of p-CREB in the contralateral hippocampus respect de control group.	Shen et al., 2013
Adult rats	Treadmill with speed paradigm based on the lactate threshold (LT being around 20 m/min) - Sedentary control (CONT) group: Duration: 6 weeks - Stress free mild exercise (ME, <LT) group: Duration: 6 weeks. - Intense exercise (IE, >LT) group: Duration: 6 weeks.	Only IE causes general adaptive syndrome (GAS): hypercorticosteronemia, adrenal hypertrophy, thymic atrophy.	MWM task ME led to enhanced memory, but not learning, compared with CONT. IE produced no changes in either learning capacities, probably due to GAS.	Adult Hippocampal Neurogenesis (AHN) 2 weeks of training with stress-free mild exercise (ME), but not intense exercise (IE), comprising exercise stress, promotes adult hippocampal neurogenesis.	Inoue et al., 2015a
Adult male Wistar rats	Treadmill with speed paradigm based on the lactate threshold - Sedentary control (CONT) group: 0 m/min - Supra-lactate threshold (Middle speed) group: 25 m/min. - Sub-lactate-threshold (Low speed) group: 15 m/min. Duration: 30 min/day for 2 weeks.	Serum ACTH levels Significant increases in plasma ACTH were observed during supra-LT running.	No behavioral tasks were performed	cFos induction Only supra-LT running significantly increased c-Fos induction in various hypothalamic regions.	Soya et al., 2007
Male albino Sprague-Dawley rats (4–6 weeks old)	For 4 weeks: intensity of 70% of maximal oxygen consumption, for 1 h/day, 5 day/week.	No stress biomarkers were assessed	One-trial step-through passive avoidance test: ↑ learning and memory.	No histological or molecular procedures were performed	Chen et al., 2008
Adult Wistar Rats	Treadmill with speed paradigm based on the lactate threshold - Sedentary control (CONT) group: 0 m/min	Plasma CORT Only IE had the higher CORT concentration than CONT group.	No behavioral tasks were performed	AHN ME was better suited to improve AHN, especially in regards to the survival and maturation of newborn neurons.	Inoue et al., 2015a

(Continued)

TABLE 1 | Continued

Animal model	Treadmill protocol	Stress biomarkers	Effects on cognition	Histological and molecular procedures	References
- Mild-exercise (ME, <LT) group: 15 m/min, 60 min/day. - Intense-exercise (IE, >LT) group: 40 m/min, 60 min/day. Duration: 6 weeks in total including the habituation period. Running took place during the dark phase (19:00 and 22:00).			DNA microarray - ME-influenced genes were principally related to lipid metabolism, protein synthesis and inflammatory response, which are recognized as associated with AHN - IE-influenced genes linked to an excessive inflammatory immune response, known to be negative regulator of hippocampal neuroadaptation, were identified.		
Sprague-Dawley rats (5-weeks-old)	Treadmill: initial speed of 9 m/min for 20–60 min per day, 5 days per week for the first week, followed by 60 min/day at the same speed, 5 days/week. Increasing speed about 3 m/min per week reaching 16 m/min at the end of the training period. Running Wheel: singly placed in cages.	No stress biomarkers were assessed	Fear conditioning: No changes in the acquisition of fear-evoked conditional responses and ↑ context-conditioned freezing responses in treadmill and running wheel. Only treadmill improved the cue-conditioned performance.	No histological or molecular procedures were performed	Lin et al., 2012
Male juvenile Sprague-Dawley rats (5 weeks old)	For 1 week: 30 min/day. Three groups: - low intensity (LI) group: ran at 5 m/min for the first 5 min, 8 m/min for the next 5 min and 11 m/min for the remaining 20 min; - moderate intensity (MI) group ran at 8 m/min for the first 5 min, 11 m/min for the next 5 min and 14 m/min for the remaining 20 min; - high intensity (HI) group ran at 8 m/min for the first 5 min, 11 m/min for the next 5 min and 22 m/min for the remaining 20 min.	No stress biomarkers were assessed	No behavioral tasks perfomed	AHN ↑↑↑↑ $BrdU^+$ and $BrdU^+/NeuN^+$ cells in the LI group; ↑↑↑ $BrdU^+$ and $BrdU^+/NeuN^+$ cells in the MI group; ↑↑ $BrdU^+$ cells in HI group; ↑ $BrdU^+$ and $BrdU^+/NeuN^+$ cells in the control group.	Lou et al., 2008
Male Sprague-Dawley rats (2 weeks of age): induction of autism-like with valproic acid injections.	30 min/day, five times a week for 4 weeks, starting postnatal day 28. Speed of 2 m/min for the first 5 min, at a speed of 5 m/min for the next 5 min, and then at a speed of 8 m/min for the last 20 min, with the 0° inclination.	No stress biomarkers were assessed	Open field and social interaction test: ↑ spatial learning memory in the autistic rats; Radial 8-arm maze test: ↑ working memory in the VPA-injected rats with exercise.	AHN ↑ number of $BrdU^+$ cells	Seo et al., 2013
Male Wistar rats subjected to surgery	For 1 week: 1h/day, 5-10 m/min.	No stress biomarkers were assessed	Object displacement task: ↑ spatial learning; Object substitution task: ↑ object recognition learning.	No histological or molecular procedures were performed	Griffin et al., 2009

(Continued)

TABLE 1 | Continued

Animal model	Treadmill protocol	Stress biomarkers	Effects on cognition	Histological and molecular procedures	References
C57BL/J6 mice	- Controls (CON): 0 m/min - Regular Runners (RR): 10 m/min, at the same time of the day until 28 days - Irregular Duration Runners (IDR): 10 m/min. Same time of the day but variable duration. - Irregular time-of-day runners (ITR): 10 m/min. Same duration but at different time of day.	Serum CORT levels Day 4: No differences were found among runners. Day 29: RR group had significantly lower levels of serum CORT (110-150ng/ml at 10:00 am).	MWM task The RR group had a lower escape latency in the acquisition compared to the CON or IDR group. Regarding memory consolidation, RR spent more time in the target quadrant compared to the other three groups.	RR group presented higher levels of BrdU$^+$ cells compared to the other groups.	Li et al., 2013
C57BL/J6 mice	Forced Walking Wheel System - Sedentary: 0m/min - Low impact runners (LIR): 10 m/min. 45 min/day. Duration: 10 weeks. - High impact runners (HIR): 21m/min, 45 min/day. Duration: 5 weeks.	No stress biomarkers were assessed	MWM task* In the acquisition phase, HIR had longer escape latencies compared to LIR group and sedentary controls. Regarding memory consolidation performance, LIR crossed the platform quadrant more than HIR. Rotorod test 5 weeks of HIR led to significant improvement in rotorod test performance.	No histological or molecular procedures were performed	Kennard and Woodruff-Pak, 2012
Adult male C57BL/6 mice	For 2 weeks: 7 days/week, 40 min/day, speed 12 m/min.	No stress biomarkers were assessed	No behavioral tasks perfomed	AHN ↑ number of BrdU$^+$ cell; ↑ density of spine of granule cells in the DG	Glasper et al., 2010
Adult male C57BL/6 mice	For 2 weeks: 5 days/week, 40 min/day, speed 12 m/min.	No stress biomarkers were assessed	No behavioral tasks perfomed	AHN No changes in the number of mature granule neurons; ↑ number of DCX$^+$/CLR$^-$ cells; ↑ number of (DCX$^+$/CLR$^+$)/Granule neurons; ↑ total DCX$^+$/Granule neurons; ↑ total CLR$^+$/Granule neurons	Llorens-Martín et al., 2006
Adult male C57BL/6J mice (5-weeks-old)	10 m/min, 20 min for the first day, with an increment of 10 min/day until reaching 60 min/day to fulfill the 70% of maximal oxygen consumption. The running duration was 60 min/day, and the running speed was increased gradually from 10 to 12 m/min. The speed was accelerated 1 m/min every 2 weeks.	No stress biomarkers were assessed	No behavioral tasks perfomed	AHN ↑ number of Nestin$^+$ cells in the SGZ; ↑ number of Ki67$^+$ cells; ↑ more DCX$^+$ cells, with prominently developed dendrites; ↑ pCREB expression; ↑ BDNF expression	Nam et al., 2014
Male BALB/c mice (3-months old)	For 4 weeks: 10 m/min, for 20-60 min/day, 5 days/week.	No stress biomarkers were assessed	One-trial passive avoidance: ↑ retention latency. Multiple-trial passive avoidance:	No histological or molecular procedures were performed	Liu et al., 2008

(Continued)

TABLE 1 | Continued

Animal model	Treadmill protocol	Stress biomarkers	Effects on cognition	Histological and molecular procedures	References
			↑ just the retention phase of memory (not the acquisition).		
C57BL/6 male mice (19 months)	For 8 weeks, 5 days/week, 2 sessions/day, 5° incline. For the first week, each session consisted of a 10-min warm-up at 15 m/min followed by 30 min at 18 m/min. During the following 7 weeks, treadmill speed was progressively increased every week. Specifically, for weeks 2, 3, 4, 5, 6, 7, and 8 the treadmill speed was set to 21 m/min, 22 m/min, 23 m/min, 24 m/min, 25 m/min, 25 m/min, and 26 m/min, respectively.	No stress biomarkers were assessed	No behavioral tasks perfomed	No changes in DCX mRNA levels; ↑ VEGF mRNA; No changes in BDNF mRNA levels	Lezi et al., 2014

In general, the highest intensities lead to a higher concentration of stress biomarkers, and either to a lower improvement, no improvement or negative effects (compared to sedentary controls) in behavioral performance and neurogenesis. Most authors designate the different intensities according to the velocity of running, based on the assumption that a correlation exists between running speed and lactate threshold (LT) although most of them do not measure lactate in their studies, so we have used the different running velocity as a classification criterion. LT, lactate threshold. References included in the Table and not in the text are: (Van Praag et al., 1999; Griesbach et al., 2004; Adlard et al., 2005; Bjørnebekk et al., 2005; Eadie et al., 2005; Redila and Christie, 2006; Kohl et al., 2007; Soya et al., 2007; Stranahan et al., 2007; Naylor et al., 2008; Leasure and Decker, 2009; Berchtold et al., 2010; Creer et al., 2010; Falls et al., 2010; Lafenêtre et al., 2010; Kennard and Woodruff-Pak, 2012; Li et al., 2013; Shen et al., 2013; Shih et al., 2013; Fischer et al., 2014; Inoue et al., 2015a,b; Radahmadi et al., 2015).

also rely on individual variability, depending on the basal performance level previous to training (Braszko et al., 2001).

To our knowledge, very few studies have reported beneficial effects of high intensity exercise on cognition. It is noteworthy to mention one work reporting an improved memory performance in both strenuous and over-training exercise programs in a passive avoidance test (Ogonovszky et al., 2005). Surprisingly, this work found an increase in the BDNF levels only in the group performing most intense exercise.

As for the biphasic dose-response to exercise in animal studies, a recent work has reported evidences of biphasic dose-response curves for exercise effects on cognition in laboratory mice. Memory retention in an object recognition task was significantly improved at low-moderate intensity exercise while high and very-high intensity exercise induced no and negative effects, respectively, on discrimination (García-Capdevila et al., 2009).

The features of inverted-U shaped dose-response curves (the maximum-hormetic-response, the width of hormetic zone, the No Observed (Adverse) Effect Level (NOAEL), the distance to NOAEL and the zero equivalent point (Calabrese, 2008) to exercise are quite relevant considering that they strongly depend on the animal's previous health, brain specific outcomes analyzed, and parameters of exercise programs including whether the exercise is voluntary or forced (Radák et al., 2001, and see below).

A very relevant aspect of the hormetic response to exercise is the biological meaning. As already stated, sedentary life has well-known detrimental effects on brain functioning, while exercise is one of the most outstanding conducts in order to maintain health as well as a healthy aging, both in animal and humans. It is plausible to postulate that exercise effects are increasingly positive within the range from sedentary life to moderate and high intensity exercise. This response to exercise would show a sigmoidal profile, due to a ceiling effect: beyond a given level of exercise intensity, training time, or frequency of training, no further positive effects would accumulate due to a maximum plastic capacity of our body and brain to change in response to activity and/or to a maximum ability to modify the body and brain's performance. The evidences reviewed above suggest that this is not the case. The response to exercise seems to fit better with a hormetic profile where increasing intensity, training time, or frequency of training cause the disappearance of the positive effects of low-to-moderate exercise. Why might this be so? As exposed above, exercise is a stress. The adaptive effects of exercise on both muscles, bones, immune system, cardiovascular system, and brain make the whole body healthier and resistant to further stress. But nevertheless, there is a threshold of intensity from where the exercise-induced stress leads to non-positive, even in some cases detrimental effects (an inverted-U or even an inverted-J hormetic curve) due to the canonical long-term actions of stress hormones in the whole body. Therefore, the inherent stress associated to physical exercise might be postulated under the hormetic profile of responses to exercise. Anyway, it will be below presented a second putative explanation for the biological evolutionary meaning of hormetic responses to exercise focused on AHN.

MOLECULAR MEDIATORS OF EXERCISE ACTIONS

A long list has been accounted with the factors responsible for the different effects of exercise on brain, both positive and negative. Among those most relevant, an activity-driven growth factors cascade including IGF1, BDNF, and VEGF (Cotman et al., 2007; Llorens-Martin et al., 2008; Pérez-Domper et al., 2013; Szuhany et al., 2015) has been postulated as responsible for most of the beneficial effects together with the anti-inflammatory actions (Silverman and Deuster, 2014), while the oxidative stress signaling has been pointed out as the most outstanding detrimental factor after exercise. Other factors with a clear, direct influence on the outcomes of exercise training protocols are diet and lifestyle (Gomez-Pinilla, 2008). It is far beyond the scope of this review to mention an extensive list of molecular mediators of exercise actions. A well-known consensus (Mattson et al., 2004) establishes physical-cognitive activity and dietary restriction as inducing a mild, metabolic stress on neural cells (through increased levels of intracellular calcium and reactive oxygen species). This pathway activates several transcription factors like CREB and NF-kB, controlling BDNF and anti-apoptotic gene (such as Bcl-2) expression. These factors drive cell survival, synaptic plasticity and neurogenesis processes.

In the present work, we aim to emphasize the increasing body of evidences showing that both positive and negative effects of exercise have usually been found mediated by the same factors in a hormetic-like biphasic dose-response. To cite just a few examples, many of the positive effects of exercise depend on the concomitant increases of BDNF (Marosi and Mattson, 2014) and IGF1 levels (Llorens-Martin et al., 2009), as well as calorie restriction interacts with the individual's activity level (Mattson, 2000; Dietrich and Horvath, 2012), while high levels of BDNF and IGF1 may induce negative effects on the brain (Gwag et al., 1995; Ramsden et al., 2003) and the energy intake is associated to the risk of developing neurodegenerative diseases in a biphasic dose-response. Furthermore, it is not casual that all these factors and lifestyles are directly related to energy balance.

While all the above-mentioned factors are directly involved in the effects of physical training on cognition and mood, in the last decade a growing literature has accumulated pointing to the adult neurogenesis to be closely related to these changes and under the direct action of those growth factors.

EXERCISE ACTIONS AND ADULT HIPPOCAMPAL NEUROGENESIS

Adult neurogenesis is the production of new functional neurons in the adult brain (Kempermann, 2011). It is well recognized that physical activity influences the level of adult neurogenesis in hippocampus as well as learning recruits newborn neurons in both hippocampus and olfactory system, and environmental enrichment increase immature neurons survival (see classical reviews by Kempermann et al., 1999; Mattson, 2000; Olson et al., 2006, and an extensive, recent review in Kempermann, 2011). Some evidence also suggests a potential effect of exercise on the olfactory system (Chae et al., 2014) although conflicting evidence has also been reported (Brown et al., 2003). This kind of experience-driven plasticity has even been proposed as a necessary process to the fine tuning of brain functioning (Opendak and Gould, 2015). A number of different mechanisms has been demonstrated in close relationship to this exercise actions on adult neurogenesis, the most outstanding being IGF1 (Trejo et al., 2001, 2008; Llorens-Martin et al., 2009; LLorens-Martín et al., 2010; Glasper et al., 2010), BDNF (Bekinschtein et al., 2011; Rothman and Mattson, 2013; Vivar et al., 2013), VEGF (Fabel et al., 2003; During and Cao, 2006), and Wnt pathway (Chen and Do, 2012; Bayod et al., 2014), to cite just a few. Examples of reports with some of the most representative exercise protocols and its effects on cognition and AHN are included for both forced (in **Table 1**) and voluntary exercise (in **Table 2**).

BIPHASIC RESPONSES OF ADULT HIPPOCAMPAL NEUROGENESIS

AHN has been reported displaying hormetic-like non-monotonic response curves after several treatments/interventions. One example of this biphasic response is driven by adrenal steroids, in turn one of the best known cases of biphasic responses in the brain (Joëls, 2006). A dual population of receptors mediates the mechanism with different affinities for the substrate and very different actions. At low concentrations, glucocorticoids induce supportive and survival actions on dentate granule neurons of the hippocampus by mean of the mineralocorticoid receptor, while at higher concentrations, a deleterious effect is achieved through the glucocorticoid receptor (Sapolsky et al., 1986; McEwen, 2012). A similar scenario takes place when considering the role of glucocorticoids and adult neurogenesis (Schoenfeld and Gould, 2013). While low levels of glucocorticoid receptor (GR) activation is maintained (as for example while living in an impoverished environment, or with a sedentary lifestyle), low levels of adult neurogenesis are observed (both cell proliferation and maturation), while an enriched environment, regular moderate exercise, or learning, generates a normal GR activation and consequently, basal levels of adult neurogenesis. On the other end, high GR activity driven by uncontrollable stress decreases dramatically the neurogenesis by affecting both precursor proliferation and immature neuron differentiation. This scenario adopts a well-known inverted U-shaped biphasic response (Saaltink and Vreugdenhil, 2014). The mechanisms of adrenal steroids-induced inhibition of cell proliferation in the dentate gyrus (Gould and Tanapat, 1999) are mediated by N-Methyl-D-aspartate receptor (Cameron et al., 1997).

Apart from this well-known example of hormetic response, a body of evidences has accumulated in recent years with further examples. Thus, neural stem cells treated with low levels of chemical, physical or pharmacological stimuli (otherwise high concentrations being toxic) have been shown to protect

TABLE 2 | Examples of voluntary exercise protocols (running wheel).

Animal model	Running wheel protocol	Behavior	AHN and neuroplasticity	References
Adult male Sprague-Dawley rats	For 2 weeks	No behavioral tasks perfomed	↑ cellular proliferation in the SGZ; ↑↑ number of Ki67$^+$ cells in the SGZ; ↑ total length of granule cells dendrites; ↑ spine density	Eadie et al., 2005
Adult male Sprague-Dawley rats	For 2 weeks	No behavioral tasks perfomed	↑ cell proliferation; ↑ granule cells with single primary processes	Redila and Christie, 2006
Adult male Sprague-Dawley rats	For 2 months	No behavioral tasks perfomed	↑ spines; ↑ dendrite length; ↑ arborization complexity in the DG	Stranahan et al., 2007
Female Long-Evans rats	In social isolation condition for 10 days	No behavioral tasks perfomed	No changes in the number of BrdU$^+$ cells	Leasure and Decker, 2009
Flinders sensitive line (FSL) rats (a genetic model of depression)	For 1 month	Forced Swim Test: ↓ time of immobility than sedentary control	4 days after Forced Swim Test: ↑ cell proliferation in SGZ	Bjørnebekk et al., 2005
Male Sprague-Dawley adult rats subjected to a lateral fluid percussion injury	From day 0 to day 6 post-injury	No behavioral tasks perfomed	↑ plasticity markers in the sham operates, but ↓ in the injured rats	Griesbach et al., 2004
Adult female C57BL/6 mice (3 months old)	For 2 to 4 months	Morris Water Maze (between day 30 and 49): with 2 trials/day, runners decrease path length and latency to the platform	↑ BrdU$^+$ and BrdU$^+$/NeuN$^+$ cells	Van Praag et al., 1999
Adult female C57BL/6JRj mice (10 weeks old)	For 5 days	No behavioral tasks perfomed	↑ proliferation; No changes in the S-phase and total cell cycle length; ↓ G1 phase	Fischer et al., 2014
Adult male C57bl/6 mice (2 months of age)	For 3 weeks	Radial Arm Water Maze: ↑ cognitive performance	No histological or molecular procedures were performed	Berchtold et al., 2010
Adult male C57bl/6 mice (2 months of age)	For 2 weeks	Fear conditioning: ↓startle amplitude in the absence of the tone both before and after conditioning; No changes in shock sensitization of startle; ↑ cued conditioned fear.	No histological or molecular procedures were performed	Falls et al., 2010
Adult male C57BL/6 mice (3 months old)	For 23 km	Pattern separation: ↑ enhanced spatial touch-screen performance when stimuli were presented in close proximity in adult mice	↑ number and density of BrdU$^+$ cells; No changes in number of BrdU$^+$/NeuN$^+$ cells	Creer et al., 2010
C57BL/6 mice subjected to 6-Gy irradiation at P9	Introduced to a running wheel at 9 weeks of age for 4 weeks	Open-field test: running alleviates irradiation-induced behavioral alterations.	Exercise after irradiation: ↑ number of BrdU$^+$/NeuN$^+$ cells; ↑number of GFAP$^+$/Sox2$^+$ cells; No changes in the number of DCX$^+$ cells	Naylor et al., 2008
Female TgCRND8 mouse line (encondes a double mutant form of APP 695)	For 1 month	Morris Water Maze: ↑ performance on day 1 and day 2; No changes in the probe trial	No histological or molecular procedures were performed	Adlard et al., 2005

(Continued)

TABLE 2 | Continued

Animal model	Running wheel protocol	Behavior	AHN and neuroplasticity	References
Female R6/2 mice (a transgenic model of Huntington's disease)	5 mice per cage with access to two running wheels for 4 weeks	No behavioral tasks perfomed	No changes in cell proliferation; No changes in the number of neural progenitor cells; No changes in the survival of newborn hippocampal neurons	Kohl et al., 2007
Female synRas (a mouse model with reduced neurogenesis) (2–3 months old)	For 12 days	Novel object recognition task: ↑ performance	↑ proliferation rate; ↑ density of DCX$^+$ cells; ↑dendritic arborization of the immature neurons	Lafenêtre et al., 2010

Voluntary running increases hippocampal neurogenesis and improves learning. References included in the Table and not in the text are: (Llorens-Martín et al., 2006; Chen et al., 2008; Liu et al., 2008; Glasper et al., 2010; Lin et al., 2012; Lezi et al., 2014; Nam et al., 2014).

these cell precursors when the brain becomes affected by a neurodegenerative disease (reviewed in Wang, 2013). One recent work has demonstrated that the proneurogenic effect of calorie restriction is mediated by the receptor for the orexigenic hormone acyl-ghrelin and the neurogenic transcription factor Egr1 (Hornsby et al., 2016). This receptor is involved in the hormetic-like response of the adult neurogenesis to energy balance. In a similar way, the neurogenic effect of some ginsenosides has been shown with a biphasic dose- and time-dependent regulation (Liu et al., 2007), a property shared by a growing number of phytochemicals (reviewed by Mattson et al., 2007). Certainly, the list of biphasic responses of AHN to different compounds is enormous, including oxytocin (Leuner et al., 2012), bisphenol (Kim et al., 2011), allopregnanolone (Wang, 2014), lead toxic exposition (White et al., 2007), statins (Chen et al., 2003), and even fluoxetin (Guilloux et al., 2013). Nevertheless, both VEGF and TGF-β display a biphasic action on neurogenesis. High doses of VEGF downregulates endogenous VEGF receptors (increasing neuronal differentiation and decreasing progenitor proliferation). Low dose upregulates VEGF receptors (with no clear effect in proliferation or differentiation, Meng et al., 2006). Low doses of TGF-β promote neurogenesis while high doses induce apoptosis in autonomic gangliogenesis (Hagedorn et al., 2000).

Therefore, as a body of evidences has been accumulated about biphasic responses to exercise of a variety of brain parameters including cognition and mood, and about biphasic responses of AHN to a variety of factors, and AHN has been postulated as a necessary mediator of many of the effects of exercise, the next question is whether biphasic responses of AHN exist to exercise.

HYPOTHESIS AND FIRST EVIDENCES SUPPORTING A BIPHASIC RESPONSE OF ADULT HIPPOCAMPAL NEUROGENESIS TO EXERCISE

Taking into account the above indirect evidences and two direct evidences recently reported (see below), we propose the hypothesis that adult neurogenesis might be a physical substrate for hormetic responses to exercise on cognition and mood. This hypothesis must be tested by analyzing the response of a battery of parameters associated to the AHN to increasing levels of exercise intensities, with higher intensities being above lactate (anaerobic) threshold (Billat et al., 2005). We suggest that this hypothesis would fit to the cited literature, to the direct evidences mentioned below, and to future data testing this possibility, best than the sigmoidal dose-response reported up to date. However, the dose-response of AHN to exercise is very well-known (Holmes et al., 2004). This response was initially found to be monotonic, as raising the exercise intensity (exercise volume) from the basal level of sedentary control animals rapidly leads to increases in neurogenesis rate. Not so many evidences have been accumulated for biphasic responses when exercise intensity reaches strenuous or very high levels. In fact, to our knowledge only a few works have reported evidences in this direction. A work reports enhanced neurogenesis (BrdU/NeuN-double immunoreactivity, no stereological methods) and increases in BDNF, NMDAR1, and Flk-1 mRNA only after low intensity exercise, while high intensity exercise brought all parameters back to control, sedentary levels (Lou et al., 2008). A second group, which had previously demonstrated a ceiling effect in the exercise actions above lactate threshold (intense exercise) in spatial memory and in AHN in rats (Inoue et al., 2015a,b), have also reported recently a significant inverted U-shaped dose-response of the BrdU/DCX-positive cells in the adult dentate gyrus to increasing levels of exercise (sedentary animals, subLactate threshold, and supraLactate threshold exercise), being the number of newborn, immature neurons increased only in the subLactate threshold, mild exercise group, together with no increase in ACTH or CORT levels (Okamoto et al., 2015). Interestingly, this neurogenesis-promoting effect of sub-stress threshold (mild) exercise depends on glucocorticoid receptor activation, suggesting a facilitative, permissive role of GC receptors, and moderate glucocorticoid levels during mild exercise. These evidences, together with the above mentioned hormetic-like responses to GC actions of hippocampus, make glucocorticoid receptors to be suggested a very plausible mechanism mediating the hormetic, biphasic dose-response of adult neurogenesis to the different intensity levels of exercise. But GRs might not be alone in these responses.

Finally, other work reported that other forms of hormetic U-shape responses of AHN to exercise exists, as a lack of significant pro-proliferative effects induced by exercise has been reported over time (Kronenberg et al., 2006). Therefore, hormetic responses to exercise of adult neurogenesis can be observed not only as a consequence of increasing doses but also after long-term trainings.

It is worth to consider what can the biological meaning of this profile response to exercise be. As discussed above in Section Biphasic Responses to Exercise on Cognition and Mood, the inherent stress associated to exercise can induce a detrimental increment in stress hormone levels, counteracting the positive actions of exercise beyond a given intensity level in the whole body including brain. The sensitivity to these hormones can even be more relevant in adult hippocampus as the higher brain region involved in the control of stress hormone levels in the body, as well as when considering the specific sensitivity of AHN to stress hormones concentration. Besides, we suggest a second further explanation for this profile specifically for adult-born neurons. It is tempting to speculate that an increasingly high number of newborn neurons in the adult hippocampus is not necessarily endlessly positive but much on the contrary, a very high number of newborn neurons can be detrimental for the functioning of the tri-synaptic hippocampal circuit. A too high number of newborn, immature neurons with specific and unique electrophysiological, morphological and connectivity properties into a fully mature circuit with mature granule neurons showing different physiological properties might cause an altered functioning of the system, after a very high intensity exercise. The evidences presented in this work may well be interpreted under the light of the proposed hypothesis, and as the adaptation of the system in response to very high intensity exercise to avoid the newborn neurons to accumulate beyond a given number, thereby the inverted-U response curve.

MECHANISMS OF BIPHASIC RESPONSES OF ADULT HIPPOCAMPAL NEUROGENESIS TO EXERCISE

As a second part of our hypothesis and taking into account the mentioned literature, we also propose that the growth factors (IGF1 and BDNF among the main key factors) mediating actions of exercise on AHN, may be potential candidates to mediate this response curve. Apart from GRs, some other molecular mediators of exercise actions on AHN have also been described displaying a hormetic-like dose-response for distinct parameters on brain, other than neurogenesis, thereby being putative candidates for the mediation of biphasic responses of neurogenesis. IGF1 has been reported as one of these factors, as a few exercise bouts induce no changes or even decrease serum levels (Kraemer et al., 1995), while long-term training increases IGF1 levels above pretraining values (Eliakim et al., 2006). IGF1 is able to induce neuronal rescue at low doses while no or opposite effects can be elicited at higher doses both *in vivo* (Johnston et al., 1996) and *in vitro* (Florini et al., 1986). No clear evidences exist about the mechanisms underlying this biphasic effect of IGF1 on brain, but a plausible suggestion is the well-known biphasic effect of insulin-like growth factor binding proteins, which are modulating the availability of IGFs for the canonical IGF receptors. In the choroid plexus, IGFBP2 enhances IGF1 biological actions at low levels while decrease the actions at higher concentrations (Delhanty and Han, 1993). These biphasic actions of IGF1 are also found in other organs like kidney (Wang et al., 2012), or muscle (Florini et al., 1986).

In the same way, secretion of VEGF in retinal epithelial cells to regulate cell proliferation displays a hormetic-like curve to hydroxynonenal in response to oxidative stress (Vatsyayan et al., 2012).

Finally but nevertheless, reactive oxygen species (ROS) can probably be mediators for hormesis in the responses to exercise (Radak et al., 2005; Goto and Radák, 2010). As explained before, ROS are compounds necessarily generated as a consequence of physical activity, in a dose-dependent manner. Oxidative stress is a basic, crucial response to the "alteration of redox homeostasis" generated by exercise (Nikolaidis et al., 2012). Depending on their concentration, their actions can be beneficial (as regulatory mediators in signaling processes or maintaining redox homeostasis) or detrimental for all major cellular components (Dröge, 2002). The stimulatory effects of low doses of ROS after moderate, intermittent stress, and the negative effects of high ROS dose after higher intensity exercise display a typical U-shaped dose-response curve. This hormetic profile is a major feature of adaptive stress responses, the underlying concept being that intermittent, moderate challenges increase the resistance of many different organ systems to chronic or higher levels of stress, and exercise-generated ROS, although inducing lipids, proteins and DNA oxidative damage, also induce the activation of redox sensitive transcription factors and signaling pathways necessary for the adaptive response (reviewed in Radak et al., 2008; Mattson, 2014).

OTHER FACTORS INFLUENCING THE EFFECT OF EXERCISE

Of course, other factors are involved in the body's response to exercise: the ergometer used, voluntary versus forced exercise, and the test used to analyze the behavior after the exercise protocol, among others. Very contradictory results have been reported when voluntary versus forced exercise are compared. Some works have reported an increase in locomotion after a voluntary running wheel while forced treadmill induced a decrease, together with the same opposite effect of these protocols on the number of GABAA receptors in striatum (Dishman et al., 1996). In the same line, other work reported an anxiogenic effect after forced treadmill exercise while voluntary exercise induced no effect (Leasure and Jones, 2008). Both works suggest an anxiogenic effect of forced but not voluntary exercise. Interestingly, in the latter work the authors observed the anxiogenic effect independently of the distance the animals ran, that was the same in both the voluntary wheel and the treadmill, and being the critical factor the speed of the exercise, consistenty higher in voluntary runners; this way the exercise took shorter time for voluntary runners in a daily basis. In parallel, AHN was significantly increased in both groups, voluntary and forced, being this increase higher in forced runners. This discrepancy between behavior and neurogenesis outcomes is in contradiction to most of the literature. It is relevant to take into account that both works used the open field alone to report locomotion or anxiety-like behaviors, and no other test to support the conclusions (elevated plus maze, or novelty suppressed feeding to mention just a few). On the contrary, other work has reported an anxiogenic effect of only voluntary wheel running compared to forced treadmill, by measuring contextual fear conditioning together with an increase in c-fos neuronal activation in amygdala (Burghardt et al., 2006).

All these studies and many others also point out to the duration of the daily exercise protocol and the duration of the whole exercise program (weeks or months) as another very relevant parameter for the different outcomes observed. Interestingly, the larger effects have been reported for the shorter durations of exercise protocols, concomitantly with the social isolation status of the animals (Hatchard et al., 2014). Motivation to run of the laboratory rodents used in the different studies, and the type of behavioral task used to test the animal conduct after the distinct exercise regimes are clearly determinant, key factors. Different tasks may require very different levels of motivation, and more relevantly, can recruit the activation of very distinct neural circuits and brain areas (see a review in García-Capdevila et al., 2009); brain region specific adaptations to exercise has also been recently reviewed (Morgan et al., 2015). Finally, to adequately compare works of voluntary versus forced exercise, different intensity levels, or human versus animal studies, measurement of VO_2 and VO_{2max} would greatly improve our ability to analyze different results and to distinguish confounding variables.

FINAL REMARKS

As for many other factors/drugs/interventions with hormetic-like biphasic dose-response curves, hormetic responses to exercise can be highly relevant to take into account. For example, it is well-known that forced treadmill exercise can induce detrimental effects when performed after a deep brain surgery (Jun et al., 2012). In our hands, physical exercise on a treadmill after a surgical intervention of adult male mice modifies the response both in hippocampus-dependent behaviors and in adult neurogenesis, by which the exercise intensity level usually promoting positive changes in neuron morphology, anxiolytic, and procognitive effects, induces after surgery no changes or changes in the opposite direction (forthcoming results). These findings can be easily interpreted in the way that surgery is diminishing the maximum positive response to exercise, and shortening the hormetic zone of exercise biphasic effects (Calabrese, 2008, all of them typical hormetic parameters). In the same line, some authors have recently reported that intensity level of exercise must be shifted down after a previous stress has been experienced, to obtain the usual positive effects typically measured by a variety of physiological parameters (Kim et al., 2015).

CONCLUSIONS

Some works have provided evidences that AHN might display hormetic-like biphasic dose-responses to exercise. A number of reports have also provided evidences that molecular mediators of exercise actions on neurogenesis, also respond with biphasic curves independently of their participation in the exercise-induced effects on AHN. Taking into account both groups of evidences, we propose the hypothesis that adult neurogenesis might be a physical substrate for hormetic responses to exercise on cognition and mood, and that the growth factors (IGF1 and BDNF among the main key factors) mediating actions of exercise on AHN, may be potential candidates to mediate this response curve, together with ROS.

AUTHOR CONTRIBUTIONS

SG, AP, KM, ÁF contributed to analyze the literature, made the Tables, and revise and made corrections to the draft of the manuscript. JT conceived the scientific main question, analyze the literature, wrote the draft and the final version of the manuscript, and is the correspondence author.

ACKNOWLEDGMENTS

The authors acknowledge the support of CSIC (Spanish Council for Scientific Investigation) and the Ministerio de Economía y Competitividad, Spain (research grant reference BFU2013-48907-R).

REFERENCES

Adlard, P. A., Perreau, V. M., Pop, V., and Cotman, C. W. (2005). Voluntary exercise decreases amyloid load in a transgenic model of Alzheimer's disease. *J. Neurosci.* 25, 4217–4221. doi: 10.1523/JNEUROSCI.0496-05.2005

Aguiar, A., Boemer, G., Rial, D., Cordova, F., Mancini, G., Walz, R., et al. (2010). High-intensity physical exercise disrupts implicit memory in mice: involvement of the striatal glutathione antioxidant system and intracellular signaling. *Neuroscience* 171, 1216–1227. doi: 10.1016/j.neuroscience.2010.09.053

Aguiar, A. S. Jr., Tuon, T., Pinho, C. A., Silva, L. A., Andreazza, A. C., Kapczinski, F., et al. (2008). Intense exercise induces mitochondrial dysfunction in mice brain. *Neurochem. Res.* 33, 51–58. doi: 10.1007/s11064-007-9406-x

Andersen, K., Farahmand, B., Ahlbom, A., Held, C., Ljunghall, S., Michaëlsson, K., et al. (2013). Risk of arrhythmias in 52 755 long-distance cross-country skiers: a cohort study. *Eur. Heart J.* 34, 3624–3631. doi: 10.1093/eurheartj/eht188

Ang, E., and Gomez-Pinilla, F. (2007). Potential therapeutic effects of exercise to the brain. *Curr. Med. Chem.* 14, 2564–2571. doi: 10.2174/0929867077820 23280

Baruch, D. E., Swain, R. A., and Helmstetter, F. J. (2004). Effects of exercise on Pavlovian fear conditioning. *Behav. Neurosci.* 118:1123. doi: 10.1037/0735-7044.118.5.1123

Bayod, S., Menella, I., Sanchez-Roige, S., Lalanza, J., Escorihuela, R., Camins, A., et al. (2014). Wnt pathway regulation by long-term moderate exercise in rat hippocampus. *Brain Res.* 1543, 38–48. doi: 10.1016/j.brainres.2013.10.048

Bekinschtein, P., Oomen, C. A., Saksida, L. M., and Bussey, T. J. (2011). Effects of environmental enrichment and voluntary exercise on neurogenesis, learning and memory, and pattern separation: BDNF as a critical variable? *Semin. Cell Dev. Biol.* 22, 536–542. doi: 10.1016/j.semcdb.2011.07.002

Beneke, R., Hütler, M., and Leithauser, R. M. (2000). Maximal lactate-steady-state independent of performance. *Med. Sci. Sports Exerc.* 32, 1135–1139. doi: 10.1097/00005768-200006000-00016

Berchtold, N. C., Castello, N., and Cotman, C. W. (2010). Exercise and time-dependent benefits to learning and memory. *Neuroscience* 167, 588–597. doi: 10.1016/j.neuroscience.2010.02.050

Billat, V. L., Mouisel, E., Roblot, N., and Melki, J. (2005). Inter- and intrastrain variation in mouse critical running speed. *J. Appl. Physiol. (1985)* 98, 1258–1263. doi: 10.1152/japplphysiol.00991.2004

Bjørnebekk, A., Mathé, A. A., and Brené, S. (2005). The antidepressant effect of running is associated with increased hippocampal cell proliferation. *Int. J. Neuro Psychopharmacol.* 8, 357–368. doi: 10.1017/s1461145705005122

Blustein, J. E., McLaughlin, M., and Hoffman, J. R. (2006). Exercise effects stress-induced analgesia and spatial learning in rats. *Physiol. Behav.* 89, 582–586. doi: 10.1016/j.physbeh.2006.07.017

Braszko, J. J., Kamiñski, K. A., Hryszko, T., Jedynak, W., and Brzósko, S. (2001). Diverse effects of prolonged physical training on learning of the delayed non-matching to sample by rats. *Neurosci. Res.* 39, 79–84. doi: 10.1016/S0168-0102(00)00207-8

Brown, J., Cooper-Kuhn, C. M., Kempermann, G., Van Praag, H., Winkler, J., Gage, F. H., et al. (2003). Enriched environment and physical activity stimulate hippocampal but not olfactory bulb neurogenesis. *Eur. J. Neurosci.* 17, 2042–2046. doi: 10.1046/j.1460-9568.2003.02647.x

Burghardt, P. R., Pasumarthi, R. K., Wilson, M. A., and Fadel, J. (2006). Alterations in fear conditioning and amygdalar activation following chronic wheel running in rats. *Pharmacol. Biochem. Behav.* 84, 306–312. doi: 10.1016/j.pbb.2006.05.015

Calabrese, E. J. (2008). Hormesis and medicine. *Br. J. Clin. Pharmacol.* 66, 594–617. doi: 10.1111/j.1365-2125.2008.03243.x

Calabrese, E. J., Bachmann, K. A., Bailer, A. J., Bolger, P. M., Borak, J., Cai, L., et al. (2007). Biological stress response terminology: integrating the concepts of adaptive response and preconditioning stress within a hormetic dose-response framework. *Toxicol. Appl. Pharmacol.* 222, 122–128. doi: 10.1016/j.taap.2007.02.015

Calabrese, V., Cornelius, C., Mancuso, C., Lentile, R., Stella, A. M., and Butterfield, D. A. (2010). Redox homeostasis and cellular stress response in aging and neurodegeneration. *Methods Mol. Biol.* 610, 285–308. doi: 10.1007/978-1-60327-029-8_17

Cameron, H., Tanapat, P., and Gould, E. (1997). Adrenal steroids and N-methyl-D-aspartate receptor activation regulate neurogenesis in the dentate gyrus of adult rats through a common pathway. *Neuroscience* 82, 349–354. doi: 10.1016/S0306-4522(97)00303-5

Chae, C. H., Jung, S. L., An, S. H., Park, B. Y., Kim, T. W., Wang, S. W., et al. (2014). Swimming exercise stimulates neuro-genesis in the subventricular zone via increase in synapsin I and nerve growth factor levels. *Biol. Sport* 31, 309–314. doi: 10.5604/20831862.1132130

Chen, C., and Tonegawa, S. (1997). Molecular genetic analysis of synaptic plasticity, activity-dependent neural development, learning, and memory in the mammalian brain. *Annu. Rev. Neurosci.* 20, 157–184. doi: 10.1146/annurev.neuro.20.1.157

Chen, H.-I., Lin, L.-C., Yu, L., Liu, Y.-F., Kuo, Y.-M., Huang, A.-M., et al. (2008). Treadmill exercise enhances passive avoidance learning in rats: the role of down-regulated serotonin system in the limbic system. *Neurobiol. Learn. Mem.* 89, 489–496. doi: 10.1016/j.nlm.2007.08.004

Chen, J., Zhang, Z. G., Li, Y., Wang, Y., Wang, L., Jiang, H., et al. (2003). Statins induce angiogenesis, neurogenesis, and synaptogenesis after stroke. *Ann. Neurol.* 53, 743–751. doi: 10.1002/ana.10555

Chen, M., and Do, H. (2012). Wnt signaling in neurogenesis during aging and physical activity. *Brain Sci.* 2, 745–768. doi: 10.3390/brainsci2040745

Cian, C., Barraud, P. A., Melin, B., and Raphel, C. (2001). Effects of fluid ingestion on cognitive function after heat stress or exercise-induced dehydration. *Int. J. Psychophysiol.* 42, 243–251. doi: 10.1016/S0167-8760(01)00142-8

Cotman, C. W., and Berchtold, N. C. (2002). Exercise: a behavioral intervention to enhance brain health and plasticity. *Trends Neurosci.* 25, 295–301. doi: 10.1016/S0166-2236(02)02143-4

Cotman, C. W., Berchtold, N. C., and Christie, L.-A. (2007). Exercise builds brain health: key roles of growth factor cascades and inflammation. *Trends Neurosci.* 30, 464–472. doi: 10.1016/j.tins.2007.06.011

Coyle, E. F. (2000). Physical activity as a metabolic stressor. *Am. J. Clin. Nutr. 72,* 512s–520s.

Creer, D. J., Romberg, C., Saksida, L. M., van Praag, H., and Bussey, T. J. (2010). Running enhances spatial pattern separation in mice. *Proc. Natl. Acad. Sci. U.S.A.* 107, 2367–2372. doi: 10.1073/pnas.0911725107

Delhanty, P., and Han, V. (1993). The expression of insulin-like growth factor (IGF)-binding protein-2 and IGF-II genes in the tissues of the developing ovine fetus. *Endocrinology* 132, 41–52.

Dietrich, M. O., and Horvath, T. L. (2012). Limitations in anti-obesity drug development: the critical role of hunger-promoting neurons. *Nat. Rev. Drug Discov.* 11, 675–691. doi: 10.1038/nrd3739

Ding, Q., Vaynman, S., Akhavan, M., Ying, Z., and Gomez-Pinilla, F. (2006). Insulin-like growth factor I interfaces with brain-derived neurotrophic factor-mediated synaptic plasticity to modulate aspects of exercise-induced cognitive function. *Neuroscience* 140, 823–833. doi: 10.1016/j.neuroscience.2006.02.084

Dishman, R. K., Berthoud, H. R., Booth, F. W., Cotman, C. W., Edgerton, V. R., Fleshner, M. R., et al. (2006). Neurobiology of exercise. *Obesity (Silver Spring)* 14, 345–356. doi: 10.1038/oby.2006.46

Dishman, R. K., Dunn, A. L., Youngstedt, S. D., Davis, J. M., Burgess, M. L., Wilson, S. P., et al. (1996). Increased open field locomotion and decreased striatal GABA A binding after activity wheel running. *Physiol. Behav.* 60, 699–705. doi: 10.1016/0031-9384(96)00102-3

Dröge, W. (2002). Free radicals in the physiological control of cell function. *Physiol. Rev.* 82, 47–95. doi: 10.1152/physrev.00018.2001

During, M. J., and Cao, L. (2006). VEGF, a mediator of the effect of experience on hippocampal neurogenesis. *Curr. Alzheimer Res.* 3, 29–33. doi: 10.2174/156720506775697133

Eadie, B. D., Redila, V. A., and Christie, B. R. (2005). Voluntary exercise alters the cytoarchitecture of the adult dentate gyrus by increasing cellular proliferation, dendritic complexity, and spine density. *J. Comp. Neurol.* 486, 39–47. doi: 10.1002/cne.20493

Eliakim, A., Nemet, D., Zaldivar, F., McMurray, R. G., Culler, F. L., Galassetti, P., et al. (2006). Reduced exercise-associated response of the GH-IGF-I axis and catecholamines in obese children and adolescents. *J. Appl. Physiol.* 100, 1630–1637. doi: 10.1152/japplphysiol.01072.2005

Fabel, K., Fabel, K., Tam, B., Kaufer, D., Baiker, A., Simmons, N., et al. (2003). VEGF is necessary for exercise-induced adult hippocampal neurogenesis. *Eur. J. Neurosci.* 18, 2803–2812. doi: 10.1111/j.1460-9568.2003.03041.x

Falls, W. A., Fox, J. H., and MacAulay, C. M. (2010). Voluntary exercise improves both learning and consolidation of cued conditioned fear in C57 mice. *Behav. Brain Res.* 207, 321–331. doi: 10.1016/j.bbr.2009.10.016

Ferreira, J. C., Rolim, N. P., Bartholomeu, J. B., Gobatto, C. A., Kokubun, E., and Brum, P. C. (2007). Maximal lactate steady state in running mice: effect of exercise training. *Clin. Exp. Pharmacol. Physiol.* 34, 760–765. doi: 10.1111/j.1440-1681.2007.04635.x

Fischer, T. J., Walker, T. L., Overall, R. W., Brandt, M. D., and Kempermann, G. (2014). Acute effects of wheel running on adult hippocampal precursor cells in mice are not caused by changes in cell cycle length or S phase length. *Front. Neurosci.* 8:314. doi: 10.3389/fnins.2014.00314

Florini, J. R., Ewton, D. Z., Falen, S. L., and Van Wyk, J. J. (1986). Biphasic concentration dependency of stimulation of myoblast differentiation by somatomedins. *Am. J. Physiol. Cell Physiol.* 250, C771–C778.

Foster, P. P. (2015). Role of physical and mental training in brain network configuration. *Front. Aging Neurosci.* 7:117. doi: 10.3389/fnagi.2015.00117

García-Capdevila, S., Portell-Cortés, I., Torras-Garcia, M., Coll-Andreu, M., and Costa-Miserachs, D. (2009). Effects of long-term voluntary exercise on learning and memory processes: dependency of the task and level of exercise. *Behav. Brain Res.* 202, 162–170. doi: 10.1016/j.bbr.2009.03.020

Garcia-Segura, L. M. (2009). *Hormones and Brain Plasticity.* New York, NY: Oxford University Press.

Glasper, E. R., Llorens–Martin, M. V., Leuner, B., Gould, E., and Trejo, J. L. (2010). Blockade of insulin–like growth factor–I has complex effects on structural plasticity in the hippocampus. *Hippocampus* 20, 706–712. doi: 10.1002/hipo.20672

Gobatto, C. A., de Mello, M. A., Sibuya, C. Y., de Azevedo, J. R., dos, Santos, L. A., and Kokubun, E. (2001). Maximal lactate steady state in rats submitted to swimming exercise. *Comp. Biochem. Physiol. A Mol. Integr. Physiol.* 130, 21–27. doi: 10.1016/S1095-6433(01)00362-2

Gomez-Pinilla, F. (2008). The influences of diet and exercise on mental health through hormesis. *Ageing Res. Rev.* 7, 49–62. doi: 10.1016/j.arr.2007.04.003

Gomez-Pinilla, F., and Hillman, C. (2013). The influence of exercise on cognitive abilities. *Compr. Physiol.* 3, 403–428. doi: 10.1002/cphy.c110063

Goto, S., and Radák, Z. (2010). Hormetic effects of reactive oxygen species by exercise: a view from animal studies for successful aging in human. *Dose Resp.* 8, 68–72. doi: 10.2203/dose-response.09-044.Goto

Gould, E., and Tanapat, P. (1999). Stress and hippocampal neurogenesis. *Biol. Psychiatry* 46, 1472–1479. doi: 10.1016/S0006-3223(99)00247-4

Grebot, C., Groslambert, A., Pernin, J.-N., Burtheret, A., and Rouillon, J.-D. (2003). Effects of exercise on perceptual estimation and short-term recall of shooting performance in a biathlon. *Percept. Mot. Skills* 97, 1107–1114. doi: 10.2466/PMS.97.8.1107-1114

Griesbach, G. S., Gomez-Pinilla, F., and Hovda, D. A. (2004). The upregulation of plasticity-related proteins following TBI is disrupted with acute voluntary exercise. *Brain Res.* 1016, 154–162. doi: 10.1016/j.brainres.2004.04.079

Griffin, E. W., Bechara, R. G., Birch, A. M., and Kelly, A. M. (2009). Exercise enhances hippocampal-dependent learning in the rat: evidence for a BDNF-related mechanism. *Hippocampus* 19, 973–980. doi: 10.1002/hipo.20631

Guilloux, J.-P., Mendez-David, I., Pehrson, A., Guiard, B. P., Repérant, C., Orvoën, S., et al. (2013). Antidepressant and anxiolytic potential of the multimodal antidepressant vortioxetine (Lu AA21004) assessed by behavioural and neurogenesis outcomes in mice. *Neuropharmacology* 73, 147–159. doi: 10.1016/j.neuropharm.2013.05.014

Gwag, B. J., Koh, J. Y., Chen, M. M., Dugan, L. L., Behrens, M. M., Lobner, D., et al. (1995). BDNF or IGF-I potentiates free radical-mediated injury in cortical cell cultures. *Neuroreport* 7, 93–96. doi: 10.1097/00001756-199512000-00022

Hagedorn, L., Floris, J., Suter, U., and Sommer, L. (2000). Autonomic neurogenesis and apoptosis are alternative fates of progenitor cell communities induced by TGFβ. *Dev. Biol.* 228, 57–72. doi: 10.1006/dbio.2000.9936

Hardy, C. J., and Rejeski, W. J. (1989). Not what, but how one feels: the measurement of affect during exercise. *J. Sport Exerc. Psychol.* 11, 304–317.

Hatchard, T., Ting, J. J., and Messier, C. (2014). Translating the impact of exercise on cognition: methodological issues in animal research. *Behav. Brain Res.* 273, 177–188. doi: 10.1016/j.bbr.2014.06.043

Hillman, C. H., Erickson, K. I., and Kramer, A. F. (2008). Be smart, exercise your heart: exercise effects on brain and cognition. *Nat. Rev. Neurosci.* 9, 58–65. doi: 10.1038/nrn2298

Holmes, M. M., Galea, L. A., Mistlberger, R. E., and Kempermann, G. (2004). Adult hippocampal neurogenesis and voluntary running activity: circadian and dose–dependent effects. *J. Neurosci. Res.* 76, 216–222. doi: 10.1002/jnr.20039

Hornsby, A. K., Redhead, Y. T., Rees, D. J., Ratcliff, M. S., Reichenbach, A., Wells, T., et al. (2016). Short-term calorie restriction enhances adult hippocampal neurogenesis and remote fear memory in a Ghsr-dependent manner. *Psychoneuroendocrinology* 63, 198–207. doi: 10.1016/j.psyneuen.2015.09.023

Inoue, K., Hanaoka, Y., Nishijima, T., Okamoto, M., Chang, H., Saito, T., et al. (2015a). Long-term mild exercise training enhances hippocampus-dependent memory in rats. *Int. J. Sports Med.* 36, 280–285. doi: 10.1055/s-0034-1390465

Inoue, K., Okamoto, M., Shibato, J., Lee, M. C., Matsui, T., Rakwal, R., et al. (2015b). Long-term mild, rather than intense, exercise enhances adult hippocampal neurogenesis and greatly changes the transcriptomic profile of the hippocampus. *PLoS ONE* 10:e0128720. doi: 10.1371/journal.pone.0128720

Joëls, M. (2006). Corticosteroid effects in the brain: U-shape it. *Trends Pharmacol. Sci.* 27, 244–250. doi: 10.1016/j.tips.2006.03.007

Johnston, B. M., Mallard, E. C., Williams, C. E., and Gluckman, P. D. (1996). Insulin-like growth factor-1 is a potent neuronal rescue agent after hypoxic-ischemic injury in fetal lambs. *J. Clin. Invest.* 97, 300. doi: 10.1172/JCI118416

Jun, H., Mohammed Qasim Hussaini, S., Rigby, M. J., and Jang, M. H. (2012). Functional role of adult hippocampal neurogenesis as a therapeutic strategy for mental disorders. *Neural Plast.* 2012, 854285. doi: 10.1155/2012/854285

Kempermann, G. (2011). *Adult Neurogenesis 2*. New York, NY: Oxford University Press.

Kempermann, G., van Praag, H., and Gage, F. H. (1999). Activity-dependent regulation of neuronal plasticity and self repair. *Prog. Brain Res.* 127, 35–48. doi: 10.1016/S0079-6123(00)27004-0

Kennard, J. A., and Woodruff-Pak, D. S. (2012). A comparison of low- and high-impact forced exercise: effects of training paradigm on learning and memory. *Physiol. Behav.* 106, 423–427. doi: 10.1016/j.physbeh.2012.02.023

Kim, M. E., Park, H. R., Gong, E. J., Choi, S. Y., Kim, H. S., and Lee, J. (2011). Exposure to bisphenol A appears to impair hippocampal neurogenesis and spatial learning and memory. *Food Chem. Toxicol.* 49, 3383–3389. doi: 10.1016/j.fct.2011.09.017

Kim, T.-K., Park, J.-Y., and Han, P.-L. (2015). Physiological parameters in the blood of a murine stress-induced depression model before and after repeated passive exercise. *Endocrinol. Metab. (Seoul).* 30, 371–380. doi: 10.3803/enm.2015.30.3.371

Kohl, Z., Kandasamy, M., Winner, B., Aigner, R., Gross, C., Couillard-Despres, S., et al. (2007). Physical activity fails to rescue hippocampal neurogenesis deficits in the R6/2 mouse model of Huntington's disease. *Brain Res.* 1155, 24–33. doi: 10.1016/j.brainres.2007.04.039

Kraemer, W. J., Aguilera, B. A., Terada, M., Newton, R. U., Lynch, J. M., Rosendaal, G., et al. (1995). Responses of IGF-I to endogenous increases in growth hormone after heavy-resistance exercise. *J. Appl. Physiol.* 79, 1310–1315.

Kramer, A. F., Erickson, K. I., and Colcombe, S. J. (2006). Exercise, cognition, and the aging brain. *J. Appl. Physiol.* 101, 1237–1242. doi: 10.1152/japplphysiol.00500.2006

Kronenberg, G., Bick-Sander, A., Bunk, E., Wolf, C., Ehninger, D., and Kempermann, G. (2006). Physical exercise prevents age-related decline in precursor cell activity in the mouse dentate gyrus. *Neurobiol. Aging* 27, 1505–1513. doi: 10.1016/j.neurobiolaging.2005.09.016

Lafenêtre, P., Leske, O., Ma-Högemeie, Z., Haghikia, A., Bichler, Z., Wahle, P., et al. (2010). Exercise can rescue recognition memory impairment in a model with reduced adult hippocampal neurogenesis. *Front. Behav. Neurosci.* 3:34. doi: 10.3389/neuro.08.034.2009

Leasure, J., and Jones, M. (2008). Forced and voluntary exercise differentially affect brain and behavior. *Neuroscience* 156, 456–465. doi: 10.1016/j.neuroscience.2008.07.041

Leasure, J. L., and Decker, L. (2009). Social isolation prevents exercise–induced proliferation of hippocampal progenitor cells in female rats. *Hippocampus* 19, 907–912. doi: 10.1002/hipo.20563

Lee, I. M., Hsieh, C. C., and Paffenbarger, R. S. Jr. (1995). Exercise intensity and longevity in men. The Harvard Alumni Health Study. *JAMA* 273, 1179–1184. doi: 10.1001/jama.1995.03520390039030

Leuner, B., Caponiti, J. M., and Gould, E. (2012). Oxytocin stimulates adult neurogenesis even under conditions of stress and elevated glucocorticoids. *Hippocampus* 22, 861–868. doi: 10.1002/hipo.20947

Lezi, E., Burns, J. M., and Swerdlow, R. H. (2014). Effect of high-intensity exercise on aged mouse brain mitochondria, neurogenesis, and inflammation. *Neurobiol. Aging* 35, 2574–2583. doi: 10.1016/j.neurobiolaging.2014.05.033

Li, H., Liang, A., Guan, F., Fan, R., Chi, L., and Yang, B. (2013). Regular treadmill running improves spatial learning and memory performance in young mice through increased hippocampal neurogenesis and decreased stress. *Brain Res.* 1531, 1–8. doi: 10.1016/j.brainres.2013.07.041

Lin, T.-W., Chen, S.-J., Huang, T.-Y., Chang, C.-Y., Chuang, J.-I., Wu, F.-S., et al. (2012). Different types of exercise induce differential effects on neuronal adaptations and memory performance. *Neurobiol. Learn. Mem.* 97, 140–147. doi: 10.1016/j.nlm.2011.10.006

Liu, J. W., Tian, S. J., de Barry, J., and Luu, B. (2007). Panaxadiol glycosides that induce neuronal differentiation in neurosphere stem cells. *J. Nat. Prod.* 70, 1329–1334. doi: 10.1021/np070135j

Liu, Y.-F., Chen, H.-I., Yu, L., Kuo, Y.-M., Wu, F.-S., Chuang, J.-I., et al. (2008). Upregulation of hippocampal TrkB and synaptotagmin is involved in treadmill exercise-enhanced aversive memory in mice. *Neurobiol. Learn. Mem.* 90, 81–89. doi: 10.1016/j.nlm.2008.02.005

Llorens-Martín, M., Torres-Alemán, I., and Trejo, J. L. (2006). Pronounced individual variation in the response to the stimulatory action of exercise on immature hippocampal neurons. *Hippocampus* 16, 480–490. doi: 10.1002/hipo.20175

Llorens-Martin, M., Torres-Alemán, I., and Trejo, J. L. (2008). Growth factors as mediators of exercise actions on the brain. *Neuromol. Med.* 10, 99–107. doi: 10.1007/s12017-008-8026-1

Lou, S.-J., Liu, J.-Y., Chang, H., and Chen, P.-J. (2008). Hippocampal neurogenesis and gene expression depend on exercise intensity in juvenile rats. *Brain Res.* 1210, 48–55. doi: 10.1016/j.brainres.2008.02.080

Lucas, S. J., Cotter, J. D., Brassard, P., and Bailey, D. M. (2015). High-intensity interval exercise and cerebrovascular health: curiosity, cause, and consequence. *J. Cereb. Blood Flow Metab.* 35, 902–911. doi: 10.1038/jcbfm.2015.49

Marosi, K., and Mattson, M. P. (2014). BDNF mediates adaptive brain and body responses to energetic challenges. *Trends Endocrinol. Metab.* 25, 89–98. doi: 10.1016/j.tem.2013.10.006

Llorens-Martin, M., Torres-Aleman, I., and Trejo, J. L. (2009). Reviews: mechanisms mediating brain plasticity: IGF1 and adult hippocampal neurogenesis. *Neuroscientist* 15, 134–148. doi: 10.1177/1073858408331371

LLorens-Martín, M., Torres-Alemán, I., and Trejo, J. L. (2010). Exercise modulates insulin-like growth factor 1-dependent and-independent effects on adult hippocampal neurogenesis and behaviour. *Mol. Cell. Neurosci.* 44, 109–117. doi: 10.1016/j.mcn.2010.02.006

Mattson, M. P. (2000). Neuroprotective signaling and the aging brain: take away my food and let me run. *Brain Res.* 886, 47–53. doi: 10.1016/S0006-8993(00)02790-6

Mattson, M. P. (2008). Hormesis defined. *Ageing Res. Rev.* 7, 1–7. doi: 10.1016/j.arr.2007.08.007

Mattson, M. P. (2012a). Energy intake and exercise as determinants of brain health and vulnerability to injury and disease. *Cell Metab.* 16, 706–722. doi: 10.1016/j.cmet.2012.08.012

Mattson, M. P. (2012b). Evolutionary aspects of human exercise—born to run purposefully. *Ageing Res. Rev.* 11, 347–352. doi: 10.1016/j.arr.2012.01.007

Mattson, M. P. (2014). Challenging oneself intermittently to improve health. *Dose Res.* 12, 600–618. doi: 10.2203/dose-response.14-028.Mattson

Mattson, M. P. (2015). Lifelong brain health is a lifelong challenge: from evolutionary principles to empirical evidence. *Ageing Res. Rev.* 20, 37–45. doi: 10.1016/j.arr.2014.12.011

Mattson, M. P., Duan, W., Wan, R., and Guo, Z. (2004). Prophylactic activation of neuroprotective stress response pathways by dietary and behavioral manipulations. *NeuroRx* 1, 111–116. doi: 10.1602/neurorx.1.1.111

Mattson, M. P., Son, T. G., and Camandola, S. (2007). Viewpoint: mechanisms of action and therapeutic potential of neurohormetic phytochemicals. *Dose Res.* 5, 174–186. doi: 10.2203/dose-response.07-004.Mattson

McEwen, B. S. (2012). The ever-changing brain: cellular and molecular mechanisms for the effects of stressful experiences. *Dev. Neurobiol.* 72, 878–890. doi: 10.1002/dneu.20968

Meeusen, R. F. V. (2012). "The monoaminergic system in animal models of exercise," in *Functional Neuroimaging in Exercise and Sport Sciences*, eds H. H. Boecker, C. H. Hillman, L. Scheef, and H. K. Strüder (New York, NY: Springer), 59–76.

Meng, H., Zhang, Z., Zhang, R., Liu, X., Wang, L., Robin, A. M., et al. (2006). Biphasic effects of exogenous VEGF on VEGF expression of adult neural progenitors. *Neurosci. Lett.* 393, 97–101. doi: 10.1016/j.neulet.2005.09.044

Morgan, J. A., Corrigan, F., and Baune, B. T. (2015). Effects of physical exercise on central nervous system functions: a review of brain region specific adaptations. *J. Mol. Psychiatry* 3, 3. doi: 10.1186/s40303-015-0010-8

Nam, S. M., Kim, J. W., Yoo, D. Y., Yim, H. S., Kim, D. W., Choi, J. H., et al. (2014). Physical exercise ameliorates the reduction of neural stem cell, cell proliferation and neuroblast differentiation in senescent mice induced by D-galactose. *BMC Neurosci.* 15:116. doi: 10.1186/s12868-014-0116-4

Naylor, A. S., Bull, C., Nilsson, M. K., Zhu, C., Björk-Eriksson, T., Eriksson, P. S., et al. (2008). Voluntary running rescues adult hippocampal neurogenesis after irradiation of the young mouse brain. *Proc. Natl. Acad. Sci. U.S.A.* 105, 14632–14637. doi: 10.1073/pnas.0711128105

Nieman, D. C., Johanssen, L. M., Lee, J., and Arabatzis, K. (1990). Infectious episodes in runners before and after the Los Angeles Marathon. *J. Sports Med. Phys. Fitness* 30, 316–328.

Nikolaidis, M. G., Kyparos, A., Spanou, C., Paschalis, V., Theodorou, A. A., and Vrabas, I. S. (2012). Redox biology of exercise: an integrative and comparative consideration of some overlooked issues. *J. Exp. Biol.* 215, 1615–1625. doi: 10.1242/jeb.067470

Ogonovszky, H., Berkes, I., Kumagai, S., Kaneko, T., Tahara, S., Goto, S., et al. (2005). The effects of moderate-, strenuous-and over-training on oxidative stress markers, DNA repair, and memory, in rat brain. *Neurochem. Int.* 46, 635–640. doi: 10.1016/j.neuint.2005.02.009

Okamoto, M., Yamamura, Y., Liu, Y.-F., Min-Chul, L., Matsui, T., Shima, T., et al. (2015). Hormetic effects by exercise on hippocampal neurogenesis with glucocorticoid signaling. *Brain Plast.* 1, 149–158. doi: 10.3233/BPL-150012

Oliveira, B. R., Deslandes, A. C., and Santos, T. M. (2015). Differences in exercise intensity seems to influence the affective responses in self-selected and imposed exercise: a meta-analysis. *Front. Psychol.* 6:1105. doi: 10.3389/fpsyg.2015.01105

Olson, A. K., Eadie, B. D., Ernst, C., and Christie, B. R. (2006). Environmental enrichment and voluntary exercise massively increase neurogenesis in the adult hippocampus via dissociable pathways. *Hippocampus* 16, 250–260. doi: 10.1002/hipo.20157

Opendak, M., and Gould, E. (2015). Adult neurogenesis: a substrate for experience-dependent change. *Trends Cogn. Sci.* 19, 151–161. doi: 10.1016/j.tics.2015.01.001

Peake, J. M., Markworth, J. F., Nosaka, K., Raastad, T., Wadley, G. D., and Coffey, V. G. (2015). Modulating exercise-induced hormesis: does less equal more? *J. Appl. Physiol.* 119, 172–189. doi: 10.1152/japplphysiol.01055.2014

Pérez-Domper, P., Gradari, S., and Trejo, J. L. (2013). The growth factors cascade and the dendrito-/synapto-genesis versus cell survival in adult hippocampal neurogenesis: the chicken or the egg. *Ageing Res. Rev.* 12, 777–785. doi: 10.1016/j.arr.2013.06.001

Powers, S. K., and Jackson, M. J. (2008). Exercise-induced oxidative stress: cellular mechanisms and impact on muscle force production. *Physiol. Rev.* 88, 1243–1276. doi: 10.1152/physrev.00031.2007

Radahmadi, M., Alaei, H., Sharifi, M. R., and Hosseini, N. (2015). Effect of forced exercise and exercise withdrawal on memory, serum and hippocampal corticosterone levels in rats. *Exp. Brain Res.* 233, 2789–2799. doi: 10.1007/s00221-015-4349-y

Radak, Z., Chung, H. Y., and Goto, S. (2005). Exercise and hormesis: oxidative stress-related adaptation for successful aging. *Biogerontology* 6, 71–75. doi: 10.1007/s10522-004-7386-7

Radak, Z., Chung, H. Y., Koltai, E., Taylor, A. W., and Goto, S. (2008). Exercise, oxidative stress and hormesis. *Ageing Res. Rev.* 7, 34–42. doi: 10.1016/j.arr.2007.04.004

Radak, Z., Ihasz, F., Koltai, E., Goto, S., Taylor, A. W., and Boldogh, I. (2014). The redox-associated adaptive response of brain to physical exercise. *Free Radic. Res.* 48, 84–92. doi: 10.3109/10715762.2013.826352

Radák, Z., Kaneko, T., Tahara, S., Nakamoto, H., Pucsok, J., Sasvári, M., et al. (2001). Regular exercise improves cognitive function and decreases oxidative damage in rat brain. *Neurochem. Int.* 38, 17–23. doi: 10.1016/S0197-0186(00)00063-2

Radak, Z., Toldy, A., Szabo, Z., Siamilis, S., Nyakas, C., Silye, G., et al. (2006). The effects of training and detraining on memory, neurotrophins and oxidative stress markers in rat brain. *Neurochem. Int.* 49, 387–392. doi: 10.1016/j.neuint.2006.02.004

Radak, Z., Zhao, Z., Koltai, E., Ohno, H., and Atalay, M. (2013). Oxygen consumption and usage during physical exercise: the balance between oxidative stress and ROS-dependent adaptive signaling. *Antioxid. Redox Signal.* 18, 1208–1246. doi: 10.1089/ars.2011.4498

Ramsden, M., Berchtold, N. C., Kesslak, J. P., Cotman, C. W., and Pike, C. J. (2003). Exercise increases the vulnerability of rat hippocampal neurons to kainate lesion. *Brain Res.* 971, 239–244. doi: 10.1016/S0006-8993(03)02365-5

Redila, V., and Christie, B. (2006). Exercise-induced changes in dendritic structure and complexity in the adult hippocampal dentate gyrus. *Neuroscience* 137, 1299–1307. doi: 10.1016/j.neuroscience.2005.10.050

Rhodes, J. S., Van Praag, H., Jeffrey, S., Girard, I., Mitchell, G. S., Garland T. Jr., et al. (2003). Exercise increases hippocampal neurogenesis to high levels but does not improve spatial learning in mice bred for increased voluntary wheel running. *Behav. Neurosci.* 117:1006. doi: 10.1037/0735-7044.117.5.1006

Rooks, C. R., Thom, N. J., McCully, K. K., and Dishman, R. K. (2010). Effects of incremental exercise on cerebral oxygenation measured by near-infrared spectroscopy: a systematic review. *Prog. Neurobiol.* 92, 134–150. doi: 10.1016/j.pneurobio.2010.06.002

Rosa, E. F., Takahashi, S., Aboulafia, J., Nouailhetas, V. L., and Oliveira, M. G. (2007). Oxidative stress induced by intense and exhaustive exercise impairs murine cognitive function. *J. Neurophysiol.* 98, 1820–1826. doi: 10.1152/jn.01158.2006

Rothman, S., and Mattson, M. (2013). Activity-dependent, stress-responsive BDNF signaling and the quest for optimal brain health and resilience throughout the lifespan. *Neuroscience* 239, 228–240. doi: 10.1016/j.neuroscience.2012.10.014

Saaltink, D.-J., and Vreugdenhil, E. (2014). Stress, glucocorticoid receptors, and adult neurogenesis: a balance between excitation and inhibition? *Cell. Mol. Life Sci.* 71, 2499–2515. doi: 10.1007/s00018-014-1568-5

Samorajski, T., Delaney, C., Durham, L., Ordy, J., Johnson, J., and Dunlap, W. (1985). Effect of exercise on longevity, body weight, locomotor performance, and passive-avoidance memory of C57BL/6J mice. *Neurobiol. Aging* 6, 17–24. doi: 10.1016/0197-4580(85)90066-1

Sapolsky, R. M., Krey, L. C., and McEwen, B. S. (1986). The neuroendocrinology of stress and aging: the glucocorticoid cascade hypothesis*. *Endocr. Rev.* 7, 284–301. doi: 10.1210/edrv-7-3-284

Schoenfeld, T. J., and Gould, E. (2013). Differential effects of stress and glucocorticoids on adult neurogenesis. *Curr. Top Behav. Neurosci.* 15, 139–164. doi: 10.1007/7854_2012_233

Schweitzer, N. B., Alessio, H. M., Berry, S. D., Roeske, K., and Hagerman, A. E. (2006). Exercise-induced changes in cardiac gene expression and its relation to spatial maze performance. *Neurochem. Int.* 48, 9–16. doi: 10.1016/j.neuint.2005.08.006

Seo, T. B., Cho, H. S., Shin, M. S., Kim, C. J., Ji, E. S., and Baek, S. S. (2013). Treadmill exercise improves behavioral outcomes and spatial learning memory through up-regulation of reelin signaling pathway in autistic rats. *J. Exerc. Rehabil.* 9, 220–229. doi: 10.12965/jer.130003

Shen, X., Li, A., Zhang, Y., Dong, X., Shan, T., Wu, Y., et al. (2013). The effect of different intensities of treadmill exercise on cognitive function deficit following a severe controlled cortical impact in rats. *Int. J. Mol. Sci.* 14, 21598–21612. doi: 10.3390/ijms141121598

Shih, P.-C., Yang, Y.-R., and Wang, R.-Y. (2013). Effects of exercise intensity on spatial memory performance and hippocampal synaptic plasticity in transient brain ischemic rats. *PLoS ONE* 8:e78163. doi: 10.1371/journal.pone.0078163

Silverman, M. N., and Deuster, P. A. (2014). Biological mechanisms underlying the role of physical fitness in health and resilience. *Interface Focus* 4, 20140040. doi: 10.1098/rsfs.2014.0040

Soya, H., Mukai, A., Deocaris, C. C., Ohiwa, N., Chang, H., Nishijima, T., et al. (2007). Threshold-like pattern of neuronal activation in the hypothalamus during treadmill running: establishment of a minimum running stress (MRS) rat model. *Neurosci. Res.* 58, 341–348. doi: 10.1016/j.neures.2007.04.004

Stranahan, A. M., Khalil, D., and Gould, E. (2007). Running induces widespread structural alterations in the hippocampus and entorhinal cortex. *Hippocampus* 17, 1017. doi: 10.1002/hipo.20348

Szuhany, K. L., Bugatti, M., and Otto, M. W. (2015). A meta-analytic review of the effects of exercise on brain-derived neurotrophic factor. *J. Psychiatr. Res.* 60, 56–64. doi: 10.1016/j.jpsychires.2014.10.003

Taverniers, J., Van Ruysseveldt, J., Smeets, T., and von Grumbkow, J. (2010). High-intensity stress elicits robust cortisol increases, and impairs working memory and visuo-spatial declarative memory in special forces candidates: a field experiment. *Stress* 13, 323–333. doi: 10.3109/10253891003642394

Timofeeva, E., Huang, Q., and Richard, D. (2003). Effects of treadmill running on brain activation and the corticotropin-releasing hormone system. *Neuroendocrinology* 77, 388–405. doi: 10.1159/000071311

Tomporowski, P. D. (2003). Effects of acute bouts of exercise on cognition. *Acta Psychol. (Amst)* 112, 297–324. doi: 10.1016/S0001-6918(02)00134-8

Trejo, J. L., Carro, E., and Torres-Aleman, I. (2001). Circulating insulin-like growth factor I mediates exercise-induced increases in the number of new neurons in the adult hippocampus. *J. Neurosci.* 21, 1628–1634.

Trejo, J. L., Llorens-Martin, M., and Torres-Alemán, I. (2008). The effects of exercise on spatial learning and anxiety-like behavior are mediated by an IGF-I-dependent mechanism related to hippocampal neurogenesis. *Mol. Cell. Neurosci.* 37, 402–411. doi: 10.1016/j.mcn.2007.10.016

Van Praag, H., Christie, B. R., Sejnowski, T. J., and Gage, F. H. (1999). Running enhances neurogenesis, learning, and long-term potentiation in mice. *Proc. Natl. Acad. Sci. U.S.A.* 96, 13427–13431. doi: 10.1073/pnas.96.23.13427

Vatsyayan, R., Lelsani, P. C. R., Chaudhary, P., Kumar, S., Awasthi, S., and Awasthi, Y. C. (2012). The expression and function of vascular endothelial growth factor in retinal pigment epithelial (RPE) cells is regulated by 4-hydroxynonenal (HNE) and glutathione S-transferaseA4-4. *Biochem. Biophys. Res. Commun.* 417, 346–351. doi: 10.1016/j.bbrc.2011.11.113

Vivar, C., Potter, M. C., and van Praag, H. (2013). All about running: synaptic plasticity, growth factors and adult hippocampal neurogenesis. *Curr. Top Behav. Neurosci.* 15, 189–210. doi: 10.1007/7854_2012_220

Wang, G. (2013). Hormesis, cell death, and regenerative medicine for neurodegenerative diseases. *Dose Response* 11, 238–254. doi: 10.2203/dose-response.12-019.Wang

Wang, J. M. (2014). Allopregnanolone and neurogenesis in the nigrostriatal tract. *Front. Cell. Neurosci.* 8:224. doi: 10.3389/fncel.2014.00224

Wang, L., Li, W., Kong, S., Wu, P., Zhang, C., Gu, L., et al. (2012). Insulin-like growth factor-1 (IGF-1) inhibits the basolateral Cl channels in the thick ascending limb of the rat kidney. *Biochim. Biophys. Acta* 1823, 1163–1169. doi: 10.1016/j.bbamcr.2012.04.015

White, L., Cory-Slechta, D., Gilbert, M., Tiffany-Castiglioni, E., Zawia, N., Virgolini, M., et al. (2007). New and evolving concepts in the neurotoxicology of lead. *Toxicol. Appl. Pharmacol.* 225, 1–27. doi: 10.1016/j.taap.2007.08.001

3

IGF-I: A Key Growth Factor that Regulates Neurogenesis and Synaptogenesis from Embryonic to Adult Stages of the Brain

Vanesa Nieto-Estévez [1,2], *Çağla Defterali* [1,2] *and Carlos Vicario-Abejón* [1,2*]

[1] *Consejo Superior de Investigaciones Científicas (CSIC), Instituto Cajal, Madrid, Spain,* [2] *Centro de Investigación Biomédica en Red sobre Enfermedades Neurodegenerativas (CIBERNED), Madrid, Spain*

Edited by:
Alino Martinez-Marcos, Universidad de Castilla, Spain

Reviewed by:
Jacques Epelbaum, Centre de Psychiatrie & Neurosciences, Université Paris Descartes, France
Jessica H. Brann, Loyola University Chicago, USA

***Correspondence:**
Carlos Vicario-Abejón
cvicario@cajal.csic.es

The generation of neurons in the adult mammalian brain requires the activation of quiescent neural stem cells (NSCs). This activation and the sequential steps of neuron formation from NSCs are regulated by a number of stimuli, which include growth factors. Insulin-like growth factor-I (IGF-I) exert pleiotropic effects, regulating multiple cellular processes depending on their concentration, cell type, and the developmental stage of the animal. Although IGF-I expression is relatively high in the embryonic brain its levels drop sharply in the adult brain except in neurogenic regions, i.e., the hippocampus (HP) and the subventricular zone-olfactory bulb (SVZ-OB). By contrast, the expression of IGF-IR remains relatively high in the brain irrespective of the age of the animal. Evidence indicates that IGF-I influences NSC proliferation and differentiation into neurons and glia as well as neuronal maturation including synapse formation. Furthermore, recent studies have shown that IGF-I not only promote adult neurogenesis by regulating NSC number and differentiation but also by influencing neuronal positioning and migration as described during SVZ-OB neurogenesis. In this article we will revise and discuss the actions reported for IGF-I signaling in a variety of *in vitro* and *in vivo* models, focusing on the maintenance and proliferation of NSCs/progenitors, neurogenesis, and neuron integration in synaptic circuits.

Keywords: IGF-I, neurogenesis, proliferation, survival, differentiation, maturation, migration, IGF-IR

INSULIN-LIKE GROWTH FACTOR I (IGF-I)

IGF-I belongs to the insulin family which is divided in two groups of peptides: one includes insulin and the IGFs and the other relaxin and insulin-like hormones. In the insulin group, each peptide binds to a specific receptor with high affinity, although it can also bind to the other receptor with low affinity (**Table 1**). Furthermore, the insulin receptor and the IGF-I receptor (IGF-IR) can form heterodimers with similar affinity for both growth factors (Hernández-Sánchez et al., 2008). The IGF-IR has the higher affinity for IGF-I but its affinity is 10 times lower for IGF-II and 250 times lower for insulin (Versteyhe et al., 2013). In addition, there are at least seven IGF-binding proteins (IGFBPs) that increase the half-life of the peptide by preventing its proteolysis and modulating the interaction with the receptor (**Table 1**; Ocrant et al., 1990; Hwa et al., 1999; Bondy and Cheng, 2004; Agis-Balboa et al., 2011; Fernandez and Torres-Alemán, 2012; Agis-Balboa and Fischer, 2014).

TABLE 1 | The insulin group of growth factors.

Ligand	Receptor	Binding proteins
Insulin	Insulin receptor (IR: high affinity) and IGF-IR (low affinity)	Not known
IGF-I	IGF-IR (high affinity), IR (low affinity), and IGF-IIR (very low affinity)	IGFBP1–5 (high affinity) and IGFBP6-7 (low affinity)
IGF-II	IGF-IIR (high affinity), IGF-IR (low affinity), and IR (very low affinity)	IGFBP6-7 (high affinity) and IGFB1–5 (low affinity)

The mature IGF-I is a single polypeptide chain of 70 amino acids (7.5 kDa) with 57 amino acids being identical in mammals, birds, and amphibians (Liu et al., 1993; Russo et al., 2005; Annunziata et al., 2011). The IGF-IR is a tyrosine kinase receptor characterized by tetramers, which are composed of two α subunits and two β subunits (Russo et al., 2005; Annunziata et al., 2011; Vogel, 2013).

EXPRESSION OF IGF-I AND IGF-I RECEPTOR

IGF-I is abundantly produced during embryonic development in many tissues, but its expression is markedly reduced during postnatal life. In the adult individual, IGF-I is mainly synthesized in the liver via a process regulated by the growth hormone (GH). Furthermore, there is a small local production in tissues including brain regions such as the SVZ, the OB, the HP, and the cerebellum (CB; Rotwein et al., 1988; Ye et al., 1997). In the brain, IGF-I can be synthesized by neurons independently of GH action (Bartlett et al., 1991, 1992; Bondy and Cheng, 2004; Russo et al., 2005; Fernandez and Torres-Alemán, 2012). Systemic IGF-I can pass from the blood to the cerebrospinal fluid through the lipoprotein receptor-related protein 2 (LRP2). In addition, IGF-I can cross the blood-brain-barrier by binding to the IGF-IR present on endothelial cells and later it is picked up either by astrocytes to be transferred to neurons or directly by neurons (Nishijima et al., 2010; Fernandez and Torres-Alemán, 2012). Therefore, IGF-I can act in the brain in an endocrine, paracrine or autocrine manner.

IGF-IR expression begins early during embryonic development in regions that include the cortex, OB, HP, CB, hypothalamus (HT), and spinal cord (Bondy et al., 1990). Postnatally, IGF-IR levels are slightly reduced and in the adult, its expression is clearly detected in the SVZ, OB, HP, CB, and the choroid plexus (Bondy and Cheng, 2004; Russo et al., 2005; Fernandez and Torres-Alemán, 2012).

IGF-I/IGF-IR SIGNALING PATHWAYS

The specific IGF-I binding to IGF-IR triggers the auto phosphorylation of the receptor and the activation of the insulin receptor substrates (IRS). These activated IRSs are auto-phosphorylated and in turn activate the intracellular signaling pathways including PI3K and MAP kinase pathways (Liu et al., 1993; Bondy and Cheng, 2004; Bateman and McNeill, 2006; Fernandez and Torres-Alemán, 2012; Puche and Castilla-Cortázar, 2012).

The phosphatidylinositol 3-kinase (PI3K) phophorylates the serine/threonine protein kinase (Akt) through the phosphoinositide-dependent protein kinase (PDK). Phospho-Akt promotes the translocation of the glucose transporters to the plasma membrane affecting cell metabolism (Bondy and Cheng, 2004; Fernandez and Torres-Alemán, 2012). Another Akt substrate is the mammalian target of rapamycin (mTOR). mTOR1 activates p70S6K, regulating protein synthesis while mTOR2 activates a series of kinases (including Akt), affecting proliferation, cell migration, and positioning (Hurtado-Chong et al., 2009; Iwanami et al., 2009; Onuma et al., 2011; Fernandez and Torres-Alemán, 2012; Paliouras et al., 2012; Pun et al., 2012). Akt also promotes the activation of fork head transcription factor (FOXO), which regulates cell proliferation, oxidative stress and apoptosis (Bateman and McNeill, 2006; Fernandez and Torres-Alemán, 2012; O'Kusky and Ye, 2012). Moreover, Akt can activate the cAMP responsive element binding protein (CREB) regulating the transcription of genes involved in cell cycle progression, survival, and differentiation. The binding of IGF-I to the IGF-IR can also promote the activation of Son of sevenless (SOS) triggering the phosphorylation of RAS, which in turn promotes the activation of MAPK. Later, MAPK produces the phosphorylation of ERK inducing proliferation of multiple cell types (Baltensperger et al., 1993; Skolnik et al., 1993; Bateman and McNeill, 2006; Cundiff et al., 2009; Fernandez and Torres-Alemán, 2012).

IGF-I FUNCTIONS

Body and Organ Growth

IGF-I is a pleiotropic factor involved in multiple processes, so its actions are different depending on its concentration, the cell type, and the developmental stage of the animal.

IGF-I is necessary very early during pregnancy because it promotes embryo implantation in the uterus (O'Kusky and Ye, 2012). Later, IGF-I is important for the proper prenatal growth and postnatal survival of the animal. This fact is reflected in the smaller size of the global *Igf-I* Knockout (KO) mice and *Igf-Ir* KO mice compared to their control littermates after birth. The liver-specific *Igf-I*-deficient (LID) mice have a similar body size compared to the control animals, suggesting that IGF-I affects tissue growth in an autocrine or paracrine manner (Yakar et al., 2002). Interestingly, exogenously administrated IGF-I can compensate for most autocrine/paracrine actions of this growth factor (Wu et al., 2009). The large majority of global *Igf-I* KO mice die soon after birth due to insufficient lung maturation, although the death rate depends on the mouse strains (Liu et al., 1993; Moreno-Barriuso et al., 2006; Kappeler et al., 2008; Hurtado-Chong et al., 2009; Pais et al., 2013). The muscles, brain, bones and skin are affected by the lack of IGF-I, as reflected by the muscle hypoplasia and the reduced brain size, ossification, and skin thickness found in the KO mice (Baker et al., 1993; Liu et al., 1993; Powell-Braxton et al., 1993; Beck et al., 1995; Pichel et al., 2003). This phenotype is also observed in the few surviving postnatal KO mice which show a reduction in body and brain size, lower development of ossification centers, infertility, and deafness (Baker et al., 1993; Wang et al., 1999; Yakar et al., 2002; Fernández-Moreno et al., 2004; Cediel et al., 2006; Stratikopoulos et al., 2008; Hurtado-Chong et al., 2009; Wu et al., 2009; O'Kusky and Ye, 2012; Rodríguez-de la Rosa et al., 2015).

In humans, mutations in the *IGF-I* and *IGF-IR* genes cause growth retardation including microcephaly (Roback et al., 1991; Woods et al., 1996; Walenkamp et al., 2005, 2013; van Duyvenvoorde et al., 2010; Burkhardt et al., 2015). Furthermore, the congenital deficiency of *IGF-I* or *IGF-IR* are features of the Laron syndrome, which also includes growth hormone receptor (GHR) deficiency and/or the alteration of molecules of the GH and IGF-I signaling pathways. Patients with this syndrome experience less growth after birth and this becomes more severe with age, leading to smaller brain size, smaller heart, less muscle development, among other deficits (Puche and Castilla-Cortázar, 2012). Although short stature is a common feature of the individuals bearing *IGF-I* and/or *IGF-IR* mutations, a recent study has described intragenic deletions of the *IGF-IR* associated to a developmental delay and intellectual disability of five people that do not have a significant short stature (Witsch et al., 2013).

During central nervous system (CNS) development and adult neurogenesis, the IGF-I/IGF-IR system regulates the proliferation and survival of neural progenitors, as well as the generation, differentiation, and maturation of neurons in multiple ways (Beck et al., 1995; Cheng et al., 2001; Pichel et al., 2003; Russo et al., 2005; Hurtado-Chong et al., 2009; Fernandez and Torres-Alemán, 2012; O'Kusky and Ye, 2012; Chaker et al., 2015). These aspects are discussed in depth below (**Figure 1**).

CELL PROLIFERATION

IGF-I promotes proliferation of neural cells by interacting with the IGF-IR which may activate the PI3K/Akt or the MAP kinase pathways (Otaegi et al., 2006; Mairet-Coello et al., 2009; Vogel, 2013; Yuan et al., 2015). During embryonic development, IGF-I promotes the proliferation of neuroepithelial progenitor cells both *in vitro* (Hernández-Sánchez et al., 1995; Arsenijevic et al., 2001; Vicario-Abejón et al., 2003; Cui and Almazan, 2007; Magariños et al., 2010; Ziegler et al., 2012) and *in vivo* (Popken et al., 2004; Ye and D'Ercole, 2006; Hu et al., 2012). This positive effect of IGF-I on cell proliferation was also observed postnatally and in the adult brain (Aberg et al., 2000, 2003; Trejo et al., 2001; Gago et al., 2003; Popken et al., 2004; Kalluri et al., 2007; Kouroupi et al., 2010; Pérez-Martín et al., 2010; Yuan et al., 2015), although enhanced proliferation was not found in the adult HP of an astrocyte-conditional IGF-I overexpressing mouse (Carlson et al., 2014). In contrast, mice that overexpress IGF-I under the regulation of the Nestin promoter, active in neural progenitors, show an increase in brain size both at E18 and postnatally (Popken et al., 2004) due to a shorter cell cycle produce by the decrease in the G1 phase length (Hodge et al., 2004).

During OB development, IGF-I can stimulate the proliferation of stem and progenitor cells as observed in embryonic olfactory bulb stem cells (eOBSCs) cultures where the addition of IGF-I

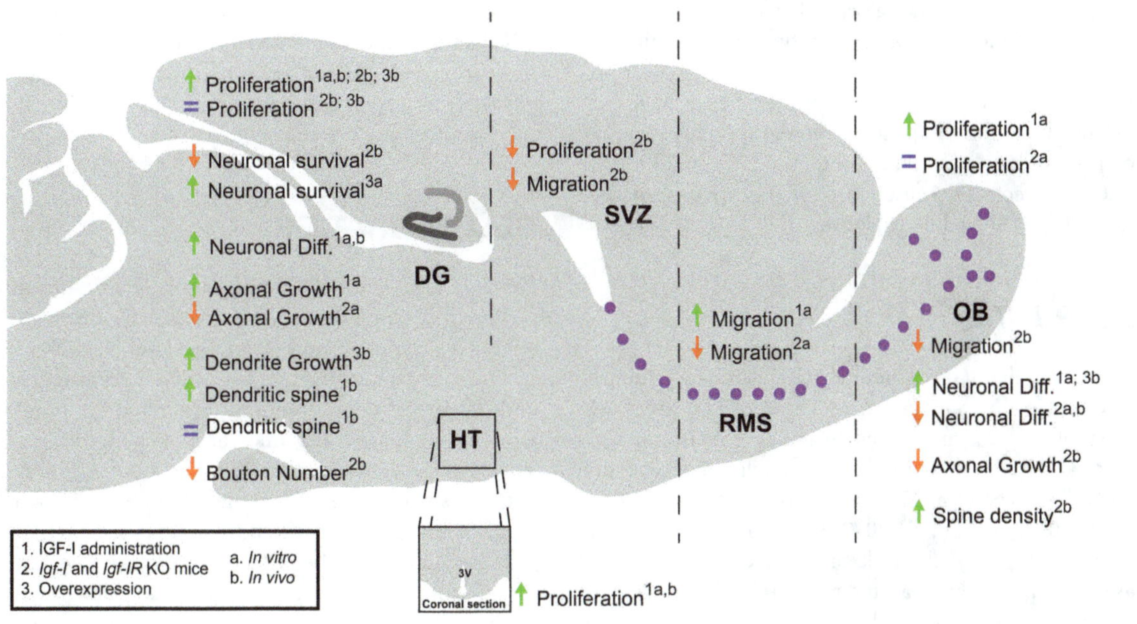

FIGURE 1 | A schematic summary of the role of IGF-I during postnatal-adult neurogenesis. The IGF-I is a pleiotropic factor that affect a variety of cellular processes. The administration of IGF-I enhances cell proliferation and neurogenesis in the OB, DG, and HT *in vitro* and *in vivo*. However, the use of transgenic mice that overexpress IGF-I or lack the *Igf-I* and *Igf-IR* genes has revealed contradictory effects of IGF-I signaling on these processes. IGF-I promotes cell migration in the SVZ-OB and the survival and axonal growth of neurons in both the SVZ-OB and DG. In contrast, the effects on dendritic spines and synapse formation may depend on the neuron type and developmental stage of the cell and animal. DG, dentate gyrus; Diff., differentiation; OB, olfactory bulb; RMS, rostral migratory stream; SVZ, subventricular zone; HT, hypothalamus; 3V, third ventricle.

increases the number of proliferative cells and of neurospheres compared to untreated cultures. However, when eOBSCs were isolated from *Igf-I* KO embryos, there was no difference in the percentage of BrdU$^+$ cells compared to wildtype (WT) cells (Vicario-Abejón et al., 2003). In contrast, a decrease in the number of cells in the M phase of cell cycle was observed in the SVZ of *Igf-I* adult KO mice (Hurtado-Chong et al., 2009; **Figure 1**).

IGF-I also affects cell proliferation in the dentate gyrus (DG) of the HP (**Figure 1**). In fact, in cultures of adult rat DG progenitor cells an increase in the number of dividing cells was found after IGF-I treatment (Aberg et al., 2003). In addition, when mice were administered with IGF-I peripherally, more BrdU$^+$ cells in the DG were detected (Aberg et al., 2000). A similar effect was observed after physical exercise, a condition that enhances IGF-I entry into the brain (Trejo et al., 2001, 2008; Glasper et al., 2010; Fernandez and Torres-Alemán, 2012). However, in the *Igf-I* KO mice the lack of IGF-I produced an increase in the number of proliferative cells in DG (Cheng et al., 2001) whereas both GH/IGF-I deficiency and deleting the IGF-IR in neural progenitors did not specifically affect proliferation in the postnatal-adult DG (Lichtenwalner et al., 2006; Liu et al., 2009).

In sum, the majority of these findings have shown that an increase in the IGF-I levels promotes cell proliferation both *in vitro* and *in vivo*. However, deleting this growth factor and/or its receptor in KO mouse has produced contrasting effects that are not completely elucidated yet (**Figure 1**). The expression of insulin, IGF-II and of truncated IGF-I-related peptides in the KO mice might partially explain the discrepancy obtained in different studies. Although the majority of truncated peptides are thought to be non-functional, we cannot completely exclude that in certain KO mice lines they could affect the results described. The development of new technologies such as the CRISPR-Cas9 system, which allows the complete deletion of specific genes, and the generation of double or triple KO mouse lines could help to understand the effect of the deletion of IGF-I or its receptor in cell proliferation during adult neurogenesis.

CELL SURVIVAL

Evidence indicates that IGF-I promotes cell survival by inhibiting apoptosis both *in vivo* and *in vitro*. These effects have been observed in neural progenitors and in multiple neuronal types such as cortical cells, motoneurons, Purkinje cells, or optic neural progenitor cells (Gago et al., 2003; Vicario-Abejón et al., 2004; Hodge et al., 2007; Croci et al., 2010; Aburto et al., 2012; Lunn et al., 2015). In the DG, the lack of IGF-I or IGF-IR causes a decrease in neuronal survival under basal conditions (Cheng et al., 2001; Lichtenwalner et al., 2006; Liu et al., 2009) or after ischemia (Liu et al., 2011) whereas IGF-I overexpression rescued neuronal survival in the lesioned HP (Carlson et al., 2014; **Figure 1**).

Moreover, IGF-I could prevent neuronal death in neurodegenerative diseases such as Alzheimer, regulating the accumulation of amyloid-β, and Tau proteins (Carro et al., 2002; Puche and Castilla-Cortázar, 2012). In fact, IGF-I enhances the transport of amyloid-β carrier proteins such as albumin and transthyretin, promoting its degradation (Carro et al., 2002). Moreover, this factor activates Akt which inhibits GSK3β, preventing Tau hyperphosporilation (Bondy and Cheng, 2004). In addition to the accumulation of amyloid-β and phosphorylated Tau proteins, the cognitive decline found in Alzheimer's patients might be attributable to decreased dentate gyrus neurogenesis. In contrast, an increase in IGF-I levels enhances neurogenesis (see below) and ameliorates the age-related cognitive malfunction in the brain. Therefore, restoring hippocampal neurogenesis by IGF-I may be a strategy for reversing age-related cerebral dysfunction. However, other studies have reported that IGF-I can promote the production of amyloid-β (Araki et al., 2009) and that knocking-out IGF-IR in neurons of a mouse model of Alzheimer's disease (AD) favors amyloid-β clearance probably by preserving autophagy and improves spatial memory (Gontier et al., 2015). This potential neuroprotective effect of reducing IGF-I/IGF-IR signaling has also been proposed for spinal muscular atrophy (SMA; Biondi et al., 2015). Therefore, the role of IGF-I in AD and motor neuron disease requires further investigation.

IGF-I can also prevent the gradual loss of other physiological functions associated with aging produced by oxidative stress and DNA damage, among others (Puche and Castilla-Cortázar, 2012). However, some *Igf-I* deficient mice, which have low levels of circulating IGF-I, exhibit an increased lifespan possibly due to alterations in energy metabolism and a transient enhancement in neurogenesis (Sun et al., 2005; Sun, 2006; Junnila et al., 2013; Chaker et al., 2015). These mice show an upregulation of local IGF-I levels in the hippocampus which could explain the increase in neurogenesis (Sun et al., 2005). All these data reveal that the effect of circulating and local IGF-I may be different but the full mechanisms have not been elucidated.

CELL MIGRATION

IGF-I is also involved in the regulation of the migration of certain cell types. In neuroblastoma cell line cultures, IGF-I stimulates cell migration (Puglianiello et al., 2000; Russo et al., 2005). The first demonstration that IGF-I regulates cell migration and positioning *in vivo* was described by Hurtado-Chong et al. through *Igf-I* KO mice and explant cultures (**Figure 1**). These studies showed that IGF-I is necessary for the exit of neuroblasts from the SVZ to the OB and for the radial neuronal migration in the OB (Hurtado-Chong et al., 2009). These effects were mediated by the activation of the PI3K pathway and by phosphorylation of the reelin signal transducer, homolog 1 (Dab1; Hurtado-Chong et al., 2009). These findings indicate that IGF-I promotes adult neurogenesis not only by regulating NSC number and differentiation but also by directing neuronal positioning and migration (**Figure 1**). Successively, IGF-I has been related to the migration of doublecortin$^+$ immature neurons in the SVZ-RMS, dorsal root ganglion neurons and cerebellar neurons in rodents, and neural crest cells in the zebrafish (Onuma et al., 2011; Xiang et al., 2011; Li et al., 2012; Maucksch et al., 2013).

NEURONAL GENERATION, DIFFERENTIATION, AND MATURATION

The IGF-I/IGF-IR system regulates the differentiation and maturation of neurons generated from NSCs and progenitors both during embryonic development and in the adult brain largely via the PI3K/Akt pathway (Aberg et al., 2000; Brooker et al., 2000; O'Kusky et al., 2000; Trejo et al., 2001; Vicario-Abejón et al., 2003; Otaegi et al., 2006; Carlson et al., 2014; Zhang et al., 2014; Yuan et al., 2015). Furthermore, IGF-I also influences the development of astrocytes and oligodendrocytes (Ye and D'Ercole, 2006; O'Kusky and Ye, 2012). Indeed, IGF-I promotes the differentiation of neural progenitors into mature oligodendrocytes that produce myelin (Carson et al., 1993; Ye et al., 1995; Gago et al., 2003; Hsieh et al., 2004) and stimulates the proliferation and differentiation of astrocytes under physiological conditions and after injury (Cao et al., 2003; Ye et al., 2004).

In *Igf-I* and *Igf-IR* KO mice, a reduction in the number of neurons during embryonic development and postnatal-adult neurogenesis in SVZ-OB and HP has been described (Baker et al., 1993; Liu et al., 1993, 2009; Powell-Braxton et al., 1993; Beck et al., 1995; Hurtado-Chong et al., 2009). When IGF-I was added to eOBSCs in culture, it produced an increase in the number of neurons, astrocytes and oligodendrocytes, whereas there was a decrease in the differentiation of eOBSCs isolated from the *Igf-I* KO mice (Vicario-Abejón et al., 2003; Otaegi et al., 2006). In the postnatal-adult OB of *Igf-I* KO animals, reductions in the number of interneuron populations were observed, possibly due to the altered neuroblast exit and migration from the SVZ, as mentioned above (Hurtado-Chong et al., 2009). By contrast, animals that overexpress *Igf-I* exhibit an increase in the number of neurons in the HP (O'Kusky et al., 2000; Popken et al., 2004; Carlson et al., 2014; **Figure 1**).

In addition to its role in the main neurogenic adult brain regions IGF-I also increases neurogenesis in the hypothalamus. After intra-cerebroventricular treatment with IGF-I, the number of neurons and astrocytes labeled with BrdU was significantly increased in the whole hypothalamus (Pérez-Martín et al., 2010). A similar effect of this growth factor was also found in hypothalamic cell cultures and explants (Torres-Aleman et al., 1990; Pérez-Martín et al., 2010).

IGF-I may regulate neuronal maturation, affecting axonal and dendritic growth, and establishing synapses in different brain areas independently of cell survival (O'Kusky et al., 2000; Cao et al., 2011; **Figure 1**). Thus, *Igf-I* KO animals have a lower development in the peripheral nerves (Gao et al., 1999), an altered innervation of the sensory cells of the organ of Corti (Camarero et al., 2001) and a lower density of spines in neurons of layers II-III of the cortex (Cheng et al., 2003). In the OB of *Igf-I* KO mice, the pattern of the axonal projections of sensory olfactory neurons is altered, because IGF-I acts as a chemoattractant for axonal growth cones (Scolnick et al., 2008). In the HP, IGF-I is involved in the establishment of neuronal polarity and the initial growth of the axonal cone, through the Akt pathway (Laurino et al., 2005; Sosa et al., 2006). Although the structure of the CB is preserved in E18.5 *Igf-I* KO mice (Vicario-Abejón et al., 2004), it has been shown that IGF-I promotes the establishment of cerebellar synapses whereas lack of IGF-I facilitates its removal during postnatal development (Kakizawa et al., 2003). Likewise, IGF-I overexpression in transgenic mouse promotes dendrite growth and synaptogenesis in the DG (O'Kusky et al., 2000; Carlson et al., 2014).

Exercise produces an increase in the IGF-I levels in adults which then stimulates an increase in the density of spines in the basal dendrites of CA1 pyramidal neurons but does not affect either the granule neurons in the GD or the CA3 pyramidal neurons (Glasper et al., 2010). Similarly, when IGF-I is administered by ventricular infusion no effect was observed in the number of synapses in CA3 (Poe et al., 2001). However, a decrease in the serum IGF-I levels causes a reduction of glutamatergic boutons in the HP (Trejo et al., 2007). This finding suggests that IGF-I entry to the HP can promote synapse formation and/or maintenance and as such can be beneficial for spatial learning and to reduce anxiety-like behavior (Llorens-Martín et al., 2010; Baldini et al., 2013). In contrast, it has been recently reported that the suppression of IGF-IR signaling in KO mice enhances olfactory function in aged males but not in females, adding new levels of complexity to the understanding of the role of IGF-I/IGF-IR in the regulation of neurogenesis, synaptogenesis and function in the adult brain (Chaker et al., 2015; **Figure 1**).

CONCLUSIONS AND FUTURE PERSPECTIVES

The IGF-I affects the proliferation of progenitor cells, the survival of both progenitors and neurons, differentiation, and maturation of neurons in the neurogenic areas of the adult brain (**Figure 1**). In addition it regulates neuronal positioning and migration in the SVZ-OB. However, the studies performed have reported that the action of IGF-I signaling could be different or even opposite depending on the experimental approach used, the point in development and/or cell type affected. The production of cell-specific transgenic mouse lines, double KO for IGF-I and IGF-IR in combination with new technologies such as CRISPR-Cas9, optogenetics, and pharmacogenetics might contribute to the deeper understanding of the role and mechanisms of action of IGF-I/IGF-IR signaling during postnatal-adult neurogenesis. They also could help to elucidate the role of local and systemic IGF-I in this process and to identify new molecules regulated by this growth factor.

AUTHOR CONTRIBUTIONS

VN Manuscript writing. ÇD Revision of the manuscript. CV Manuscript writing Financial support Final approval of the manuscript.

ACKNOWLEDGMENTS

The work in Carlos Vicario laboratory was funded by grants from the Spanish Ministerio de Ciencia e Innovación and Ministerio de Economía y Competitividad (MICINN and MINECO; BFU2007-61230, BFU2010-1963 and SAF2013-4759R, the Instituto de Salud Carlos III (ISCIII; CIBERNED CB06/05/0065), and the Comunidad de Madrid (S2011/BMD-2336) to CV. VN and ÇD were supported by a FPI Fellowship from the MICINN and MINECO and grants from CIBERNED and the European Union in the 7th framework program.

REFERENCES

Aberg, M. A., Aberg, N. D., Hedbäcker, H., Oscarsson, J., and Eriksson, P. S. (2000). Peripheral infusion of IGF-I selectively induces neurogenesis in the adult rat hippocampus. *J. Neurosci.* 20, 2896–2903.

Aberg, M. A., Aberg, N. D., Palmer, T. D., Alborn, A. M., Carlsson-Skwirut, C., Bang, P., et al. (2003). IGF-I has a direct proliferative effect in adult hippocampal progenitor cells. *Mol. Cell. Neurosci.* 24, 23–40. doi: 10.1016/S1044-7431(03)00082-4

Aburto, M. R., Magariños, M., Leon, Y., Varela-Nieto, I., and Sanchez-Calderon, H. (2012). AKT signaling mediates IGF-I survival actions on otic neural progenitors. *PLoS ONE* 7:e30790. doi: 10.1371/journal.pone.0030790

Agis-Balboa, R. C., Arcos-Diaz, D., Wittnam, J., Govindarajan, N., Blom, K., Burkhardt, S., et al. (2011). A hippocampal insulin-growth factor 2 pathway regulates the extinction of fear memories. *EMBO J.* 30, 4071–4083. doi: 10.1038/emboj.2011.293

Agis-Balboa, R. C., and Fischer, A. (2014). Generating new neurons to circumvent your fears: the role of IGF signaling. *Cell. Mol. Life Sci.* 71, 21–42. doi: 10.1007/s00018-013-1316-2

Annunziata, M., Granata, R., and Ghigo, E. (2011). The IGF system. *Acta Diabetol.* 48, 1–9. doi: 10.1007/s00592-010-0227-z

Araki, W., Kume, H., Oda, A., Tamaoka, A., and Kametani, F. (2009). IGF-1 promotes beta-amyloid production by a secretase-independent mechanism. *Biochem. Biophys. Res. Commun.* 380, 111–114. doi: 10.1016/j.bbrc.2009.01.044

Arsenijevic, Y., Weiss, S., Schneider, B., and Aebischer, P. (2001). Insulin-like growth factor-I is necessary for neural stem cell proliferation and demonstrates distinct actions of epidermal growth factor and fibroblast growth factor-2. *J. Neurosci.* 21, 7194–7202.

Baker, J., Liu, J. P., Robertson, E. J., and Efstratiadis, A. (1993). Role of insulin-like growth factors in embryonic and postnatal growth. *Cell* 75, b73–b82. doi: 10.1016/S0092-8674(05)80085-6

Baldini, S., Restani, L., Baroncelli, L., Coltelli, M., Franco, R., Cenni, M. C., et al. (2013). Enriched early life experiences reduce adult anxiety-like behavior in rats: a role for insulin-like growth factor 1. *J. Neurosci.* 33, 11715–11723. doi: 10.1523/JNEUROSCI.3541-12.2013

Baltensperger, K., Kozma, L. M., Cherniack, A. D., Klarlund, J. K., Chawla, A., Banerjee, U., et al. (1993). Binding of the Ras activator son of sevenless to insulin receptor substrate-1 signaling complexes. *Science* 260, 1950–1952. doi: 10.1126/science.8391166

Bartlett, W. P., Li, X. S., and Williams, M. (1992). Expression of IGF-1 mRNA in the murine subventricular zone during postnatal development. *Brain Res. Mol. Brain Res.* 12, 285–291. doi: 10.1016/0169-328X(92)90131-T

Bartlett, W. P., Li, X. S., Williams, M., and Benkovic, S. (1991). Localization of insulin-like growth factor-1 mRNA in murine central nervous system during postnatal development. *Dev. Biol.* 147, 239–250. doi: 10.1016/S0012-1606(05)80021-1

Bateman, J. M., and McNeill, H. (2006). Insulin/IGF signalling in neurogenesis. *Cell. Mol. Life Sci.* 63, 1701–1705. doi: 10.1007/s00018-006-6036-4

Beck, K. D., Powell-Braxton, L., Widmer, H. R., Valverde, J., and Hefti, F. (1995). Igf1 gene disruption results in reduced brain size, CNS hypomyelination, and loss of hippocampal granule and striatal parvalbumin-containing neurons. *Neuron* 14, 717–730. doi: 10.1016/0896-6273(95)90216-3

Biondi, O., Branchu, J., Ben Salah, A., Houdebine, L., Bertin, L., Chali, F., et al. (2015). IGF-1R reduction triggers neuroprotective signaling pathways in spinal muscular atrophy mice. *J. Neurosci.* 35, 12063–12079. doi: 10.1523/JNEUROSCI.0608-15.2015

Bondy, C. A., and Cheng, C. M. (2004). Signaling by insulin-like growth factor 1 in brain. *Eur. J. Pharmacol.* 490, 25–31. doi: 10.1016/j.ejphar.2004.02.042

Bondy, C. A., Werner, H., Roberts, C. T. Jr., and LeRoith, D. (1990). Cellular pattern of insulin-like growth factor-I (IGF-I) and type I IGF receptor gene expression in early organogenesis: comparison with IGF-II gene expression. *Mol. Endocrinol.* 4, 1386–1398. doi: 10.1210/mend-4-9-1386

Brooker, G. J., Kalloniatis, M., Russo, V. C., Murphy, M., Werther, G. A., and Bartlett, P. F. (2000). Endogenous IGF-1 regulates the neuronal differentiation of adult stem cells. *J. Neurosci. Res.* 59, 332–341. doi: 10.1002/(SICI)1097-4547(20000201)59:3<332::AID-JNR6>3.0.CO;2-2

Burkhardt, S., Gesing, J., Kapellen, T. M., Kovacs, P., Kratzsch, J., Schlicke, M., et al. (2015). Novel heterozygous IGF1R mutation in two brothers with developing impaired glucose tolerance. *J. Pediatr. Endocrinol. Metab.* 28, 217–225. doi: 10.1515/jpem-2014-0132

Camarero, G., Avendano, C., Fernandez-Moreno, C., Villar, A., Contreras, J., de Pablo, F., et al. (2001). Delayed inner ear maturation and neuronal loss in postnatal Igf-1-deficient mice. *J. Neurosci.* 21, 7630–7641.

Cao, P., Maximov, A., and Südhof, T. C. (2011). Activity-dependent IGF-1 exocytosis is controlled by the Ca(2+)-sensor synaptotagmin-10. *Cell* 145, 300–311. doi: 10.1016/j.cell.2011.03.034

Cao, Y., Gunn, A. J., Bennet, L., Wu, D., George, S., Gluckman, P. D., et al. (2003). Insulin-like growth factor (IGF)-1 suppresses oligodendrocyte caspase-3 activation and increases glial proliferation after ischemia in near-term fetal sheep. *J. Cereb. Blood Flow Metab.* 23, 739–747. doi: 10.1097/01.WCB.0000067720.12805.6F

Carlson, S. W., Madathil, S. K., Sama, D. M., Gao, X., Chen, J., and Saatman, K. E. (2014). Conditional overexpression of insulin-like growth factor-1 enhances hippocampal neurogenesis and restores immature neuron dendritic processes after traumatic brain injury. *J. Neuropathol. Exp. Neurol.* 73, 734–746. doi: 10.1097/NEN.0000000000000092

Carro, E., Trejo, J. L., Gomez-Isla, T., LeRoith, D., and Torres-Aleman, I. (2002). Serum insulin-like growth factor I regulates brain amyloid-beta levels. *Nat. Med.* 8, 1390–1397. doi: 10.1038/nm1202-793

Carson, M. J., Behringer, R. R., Brinster, R. L., and McMorris, F. A. (1993). Insulin-like growth factor I increases brain growth and central nervous system myelination in transgenic mice. *Neuron* 10, 729–740. doi: 10.1016/0896-6273(93)90173-O

Cediel, R., Riquelme, R., Contreras, J., Díaz, A., and Varela-Nieto, I. (2006). Sensorineural hearing loss in insulin-like growth factor I-null mice: a new model of human deafness. *Eur. J. Neurosci.* 23, 587–590. doi: 10.1111/j.1460-9568.2005.04584.x

Croci, L., Barili, V., Chia, D., Massimino, L., van Vugt, R., Masserdotti, G., et al. (2010). Local insulin-like growth factor I expression is essential for Purkinje neuron survival at birth. *Cell Death Differ.* 18, 48–59. doi: 10.1038/cdd.2010.78

Cui, Q. L., and Almazan, G. (2007). IGF-I-induced oligodendrocyte progenitor proliferation requires PI3K/Akt, MEK/ERK, and Src-like tyrosine kinases. *J. Neurochem.* 100, 1480–1493. doi: 10.1111/j.1471-4159.2006.04329.x

Cundiff, P., Liu, L., Wang, Y., Zou, J., Pan, Y. W., Abel, G., et al. (2009). ERK5 MAP kinase regulates neurogenin1 during cortical neurogenesis. *PLoS ONE* 4:e5204. doi: 10.1371/journal.pone.0005204

Chaker, Z., Aïd, S., Berry, H., and Holzenberger, M. (2015). Suppression of IGF-I signals in neural stem cells enhances neurogenesis and olfactory function during aging. *Aging Cell* 14, 847–856. doi: 10.1111/acel.12365

Cheng, C. M., Cohen, M., Tseng, V., and Bondy, C. A. (2001). Endogenous IGF1 enhances cell survival in the postnatal dentate gyrus. *J. Neurosci. Res.* 64, 341–347. doi: 10.1002/jnr.1084

Cheng, C. M., Mervis, R. F., Niu, S. L., Salem, N. Jr., Witters, L. A., Tseng, V., et al. (2003). Insulin-like growth factor 1 is essential for normal dendritic growth. *J. Neurosci. Res.* 73, 1–9. doi: 10.1002/jnr.10634

Fernández-Moreno, C., Pichel, J. G., Chesnokova, V., and De Pablo, F. (2004). Increased leptin and white adipose tissue hypoplasia are sexually dimorphic in Lif null/Igf-I haploinsufficient mice. *FEBS Lett.* 557, 64–68. doi: 10.1016/S0014-5793(03)01445-5

Fernandez, A. M., and Torres-Alemán, I. (2012). The many faces of insulin-like peptide signalling in the brain. *Nat. Rev. Neurosci.* 13, 225–239. doi: 10.1038/nrn3209

Gago, N., Avellana-Adalid, V., Baron-Van Evercooren A., and Schumacher, M. (2003). Control of cell survival and proliferation of postnatal PSA-NCAM(+) progenitors. *Mol. Cell. Neurosci.* 22, 162–178. doi: 10.1016/S1044-7431(02)00030-1

Gao, W. Q., Shinsky, N., Ingle, G., Beck, K., Elias, K. A., and Powell-Braxton, L. (1999). IGF-I deficient mice show reduced peripheral nerve conduction velocities and decreased axonal diameters and respond to exogenous IGF-I treatment. *J. Neurobiol.* 39, 142–152.

Glasper, E. R., Llorens-Martin, M. V., Leuner, B., Gould, E., and Trejo, J. L. (2010). Blockade of insulin-like growth factor-I has complex effects on structural plasticity in the hippocampus. *Hippocampus* 20, 706–712. doi: 10.1002/hipo.20672

Gontier, G., George, C., Chaker, Z., Holzenberger, M., and Aïd, S. (2015). Blocking IGF signaling in adult neurons alleviates alzheimer's disease pathology through amyloid-beta clearance. *J. Neurosci.* 35, 11500–11513. doi: 10.1523/JNEUROSCI.0343-15.2015

Hernández-Sánchez, C., López-Carranza, A., Alarcón, C., de La Rosa, E. J., and de Pablo, F. (1995). Autocrine/paracrine role of insulin-related growth factors in neurogenesis: local expression and effects on cell proliferation and differentiation in retina. *Proc. Natl. Acad. Sci. U.S.A.* 92, 9834–9838. doi: 10.1073/pnas.92.21.9834

Hernández-Sánchez, C., Mansilla, A., de Pablo, F., and Zardoya, R. (2008). Evolution of the insulin receptor family and receptor isoform expression in vertebrates. *Mol. Biol. Evol.* 25, 1043–1053. doi: 10.1093/molbev/msn036

Hodge, R. D., D'Ercole, A. J., and O'Kusky, J. R. (2004). Insulin-like growth factor-I accelerates the cell cycle by decreasing G1 phase length and increases cell cycle reentry in the embryonic cerebral cortex. *J. Neurosci.* 24, 10201–10210. doi: 10.1523/JNEUROSCI.3246-04.2004

Hodge, R. D., D'Ercole, A. J., and O'Kusky, J. R. (2007). Insulin-like growth factor-I (IGF-I) inhibits neuronal apoptosis in the developing cerebral cortex *in vivo*. *Int. J. Dev. Neurosci.* 25, 233–241. doi: 10.1016/j.ijdevneu.2007.03.004

Hsieh, J., Aimone, J. B., Kaspar, B. K., Kuwabara, T., Nakashima, K., and Gage, F. H. (2004). IGF-I instructs multipotent adult neural progenitor cells to become oligodendrocytes. *J. Cell Biol.* 164, 111–122. doi: 10.1083/jcb.200308101

Hu, Q., Lee, S. Y., O'Kusky, J. R., and Ye, P. (2012). Signaling through the type 1 insulin-like Growth Factor Receptor (IGF1R) interacts with canonical Wnt signaling to promote neural proliferation in developing brain. *ASN Neuro* 4:e00092. doi: 10.1042/AN20120009

Hurtado-Chong, A., Yusta-Boyo, M. J., Vergaño-Vera, E., Bulfone, A., de Pablo, F., and Vicario-Abejón, C. (2009). IGF-I promotes neuronal migration and positioning in the olfactory bulb and the exit of neuroblasts from the subventricular zone. *Eur. J. Neurosci.* 30, 742–755. doi: /10.1111/j.1460-9568.2009.06870.x

Hwa, V., Oh, Y., and Rosenfeld, R. G. (1999). The insulin-like growth factor-binding protein (IGFBP) superfamily. *Endocr. Rev.* 20, 761–787. doi: 10.1210/er.20.6.761

Iwanami, A., Cloughesy, T. F., and Mischel, P. S. (2009). Striking the balance between PTEN and PDK1: it all depends on the cell context. *Genes Dev.* 23, 1699–1704. doi: 10.1101/gad.1832909

Junnila, R. K., List, E. O., Berryman, D. E., Murrey, J. W., and Kopchick, J. J. (2013). The GH/IGF-1 axis in ageing and longevity. *Nat. Rev. Endocrinol.* 9, 366–376. doi: 10.1038/nrendo.2013.67

Kakizawa, S., Yamada, K., Iino, M., Watanabe, M., and Kano, M. (2003). Effects of insulin-like growth factor I on climbing fibre synapse elimination during cerebellar development. *Eur. J. Neurosci.* 17, 545–554. doi: 10.1046/j.1460-9568.2003.02486.x

Kalluri, H. S., Vemuganti, R., and Dempsey, R. J. (2007). Mechanism of insulin-like growth factor I-mediated proliferation of adult neural progenitor cells: role of Akt. *Eur. J. Neurosci.* 25, 1041–1048. doi: 10.1111/j.1460-9568.2007.05336.x

Kappeler, L., De Magalhaes Filho, C., Dupont, J., Leneuve, P., Cervera, P., Périn, L., et al. (2008). Brain IGF-1 receptors control mammalian growth and lifespan through a neuroendocrine mechanism. *PLoS Biol.* 6:e254. doi: 10.1371/journal.pbio.0060254

Kouroupi, G., Lavdas, A. A., Gaitanou, M., Thomaidou, D., Stylianopoulou, F., and Matsas, R. (2010). Lentivirus-mediated expression of insulin-like growth factor-I promotes neural stem/precursor cell proliferation and enhances their potential to generate neurons. *J. Neurochem.* 115, 460–474. doi: 10.1111/j.1471-4159.2010.06939.x

Laurino, L., Wang, X. X., de la Houssaye, B. A., Sosa, L., Dupraz, S., Cáceres, A., et al. (2005). PI3K activation by IGF-1 is essential for the regulation of membrane expansion at the nerve growth cone. *J. Cell Sci.* 118, 3653–3662. doi: 10.1242/jcs.02490

Li, Y., Komuro, Y., Fahrion, J. K., Hu, T., Ohno, N., Fenner, K. B., et al. (2012). Light stimuli control neuronal migration by altering of insulin-like growth factor 1 (IGF-1) signaling. *Proc. Natl. Acad. Sci. U.S.A.* 109, 2630–2635. doi: 10.1073/pnas.1111326109

Lichtenwalner, R. J., Forbes, M. E., Sonntag, W. E., and Riddle, D. R. (2006). Adult-onset deficiency in growth hormone and insulin-like growth factor-I decreases survival of dentate granule neurons: insights into the regulation of adult hippocampal neurogenesis. *J. Neurosci. Res.* 83, 199–210. doi: 10.1002/jnr.20719

Liu, J. P., Baker, J., Perkins, A. S., Robertson, E. J., and Efstratiadis, A. (1993). Mice carrying null mutations of the genes encoding insulin-like growth factor I (Igf-1) and type 1 IGF receptor (Igf1r). *Cell* 75, 59–72. doi: 10.1016/s0092-8674(05)80084-4

Liu, W., D'Ercole, J. A., and Ye, P. (2011). Blunting type 1 insulin-like growth factor receptor expression exacerbates neuronal apoptosis following hypoxic/ischemic injury. *BMC Neurosci.* 12:64. doi: 10.1186/1471-2202-12-64

Liu, W., Ye, P., O'Kusky, J. R., and D'Ercole, A. J. (2009). Type 1 insulin-like growth factor receptor signaling is essential for the development of the hippocampal formation and dentate gyrus. *J. Neurosci. Res.* 87, 2821–2832. doi: 10.1002/jnr.22129

Lunn, J. S., Sakowski, S. A., McGinley, L. M., Pacut, C., Hazel, T. G., Johe, K., et al. (2015). Autocrine production of IGF-I increases stem cell-mediated neuroprotection. *Stem Cells* 33, 1480–1489. doi: 10.1002/stem.1933

Llorens-Martín, M., Torres-Aleman, I., and Trejo, J. L. (2010). Exercise modulates insulin-like growth factor 1-dependent and -independent effects on adult hippocampal neurogenesis and behaviour. *Mol. Cell. Neurosci.* 44, 109–117. doi: 10.1016/j.mcn.2010.02.006

Magariños, M., Aburto, M. R., Sánchez-Calderón, H., Muñoz-Agudo, C., Rapp, U. R., and Varela-Nieto, I. (2010). RAF kinase activity regulates neuroepithelial cell proliferation and neuronal progenitor cell differentiation during early inner ear development. *PLoS ONE* 5:e14435. doi: 10.1371/journal.pone.0014435

Mairet-Coello, G., Tury, A., and DiCicco-Bloom, E. (2009). Insulin-like growth factor-1 promotes G(1)/S cell cycle progression through bidirectional regulation of cyclins and cyclin-dependent kinase inhibitors via the phosphatidylinositol 3-kinase/Akt pathway in developing rat cerebral cortex. *J. Neurosci.* 29, 775–788. doi: 10.1523/JNEUROSCI.1700-08.2009

Maucksch, C., McGregor, A. L., Yang, M., Gordon, R. J., Yang, M., and Connor, B. (2013). IGF-I redirects doublecortin-positive cell migration in the normal adult rat brain. *Neuroscience* 241, 106–115. doi: 10.1016/j.neuroscience.2013.03.021

Moreno-Barriuso, N., López-Malpartida, A. V., de Pablo, F., and Pichel, J. G. (2006). Alterations in alveolar epithelium differentiation and vasculogenesis in lungs of LIF/IGF-I double deficient embryos. *Dev. Dyn.* 235, 2040–2050. doi: 10.1002/dvdy.20842

Nishijima, T., Piriz, J., Duflot, S., Fernandez, A. M., Gaitan, G., Gomez-Pinedo, U., et al. (2010). Neuronal activity drives localized blood-brain-barrier transport of serum insulin-like growth factor-I into the CNS. *Neuron* 67, 834–846. doi: 10.1016/j.neuron.2010.08.007

O'Kusky, J., and Ye, P. (2012). Neurodevelopmental effects of insulin-like growth factor signaling. *Front. Neuroendocrinol.* 33:2. doi: 10.1016/j.yfrne.2012.06.002

O'Kusky, J. R., Ye, P., and D'Ercole, A. J. (2000). Insulin-like growth factor-I promotes neurogenesis and synaptogenesis in the hippocampal dentate gyrus during postnatal development. *J. Neurosci.* 20, 8435–8442.

Ocrant, I., Fay, C. T., and Parmelee, J. T. (1990). Characterization of insulin-like growth factor binding proteins produced in the rat central nervous system. *Endocrinology* 127, 1260–1267. doi: 10.1210/endo-127-3-1260

Onuma, T. A., Ding, Y., Abraham, E., Zohar, Y., Ando, H., and Duan, C. (2011). Regulation of temporal and spatial organization of newborn GnRH neurons by IGF signaling in zebrafish. *J. Neurosci.* 31, 11814–11824. doi: 10.1523/JNEUROSCI.6804-10.2011

Otaegi, G., Yusta-Boyo, M. J., Vergaño-Vera, E., Méndez-Gómez, H. R., Carrera, A. C., Abad, J. L., et al. (2006). Modulation of the PI 3-kinase-Akt signalling pathway by IGF-I and PTEN regulates the differentiation of neural stem/precursor cells. *J. Cell Sci.* 119, 2739–2748. doi: 10.1242/jcs.03012

Pais, R. S., Moreno-Barriuso, N., Hernández-Porras, I., López, I. P., De Las Rivas, J., and Pichel, J. G. (2013). Transcriptome analysis in prenatal IGF1-deficient mice identifies molecular pathways and target genes involved in distal lung differentiation. *PLoS ONE* 8:e83028. doi: 10.1371/journal.pone.0083028

Paliouras, G. N., Hamilton, L. K., Aumont, A., Joppé, S. E., Barnabé-Heider, F., and Fernandes, K. J. (2012). Mammalian target of rapamycin signaling is a key regulator of the transit-amplifying progenitor pool in the adult and aging forebrain. *J. Neurosci.* 32, 15012–15026. doi: 10.1523/JNEUROSCI.2248-12.2012

Pérez-Martín, M., Cifuentes, M., Grondona, J. M., López-Avalos, M. D., Gómez-Pinedo, U., García-Verdugo, J. M., et al. (2010). IGF-I stimulates neurogenesis in the hypothalamus of adult rats. *Eur. J. Neurosci.* 31, 1533–1548. doi: 10.1111/j.1460-9568.2010.07220.x

Pichel, J. G., Fernández-Moreno, C., Vicario-Abejón, C., Testillano, P. S., Patterson, P. H., and de Pablo, F. (2003). Developmental cooperation of leukemia inhibitory factor and insulin-like growth factor I in mice is tissue-specific and essential for lung maturation involving the transcription factors Sp3 and TTF-1. *Mech. Dev.* 120, 349–361. doi: 10.1016/S0925-4773(02)00449-5

Poe, B. H., Linville, C., Riddle, D. R., Sonntag, W. E., and Brunso-Bechtold, J. K. (2001). Effects of age and insulin-like growth factor-1 on neuron and synapse numbers in area CA3 of hippocampus. *Neuroscience* 107, 231–238. doi: 10.1016/S0306-4522(01)00341-4

Popken, G. J., Hodge, R. D., Ye, P., Zhang, J., Ng, W., O'Kusky, J. R., et al. (2004). *In vivo* effects of insulin-like growth factor-I (IGF-I) on prenatal and early postnatal development of the central nervous system. *Eur. J. Neurosci.* 19, 2056–2068. doi: 10.1111/j.0953-816X.2004.03320.x

Powell-Braxton, L., Hollingshead, P., Warburton, C., Dowd, M., Pitts-Meek, S., Dalton, D., et al. (1993). IGF-I is required for normal embryonic growth in mice. *Genes Dev.* 7, 2609–2617. doi: 10.1101/gad.7.12b.2609

Puche, J. E., and Castilla-Cortázar, I. (2012). Human conditions of insulin-like growth factor-I (IGF-I) deficiency. *J. Transl. Med.* 10, 224. doi: 10.1186/1479-5876-10-224

Puglianiello, A., Germani, D., Rossi, P., and Cianfarani, S. (2000). IGF-I stimulates chemotaxis of human neuroblasts. Involvement of type 1 IGF receptor, IGF binding proteins, phosphatidylinositol-3 kinase pathway and plasmin system. *J. Endocrinol.* 165, 123–131. doi: 10.1677/joe.0.1650123

Pun, R. Y., Rolle, I. J., Lasarge, C. L., Hosford, B. E., Rosen, J. M., Uhl, J. D., et al. (2012). Excessive activation of mTOR in postnatally generated granule cells is sufficient to cause epilepsy. *Neuron* 75, 1022–1034. doi: 10.1016/j.neuron.2012.08.002

Roback, E. W., Barakat, A. J., Dev, V. G., Mbikay, M., Chrétien, M., and Butler, M. G. (1991). An infant with deletion of the distal long arm of chromosome 15 (q26.1—-qter) and loss of insulin-like growth factor 1 receptor gene. *Am. J. Med. Genet.* 38, 74–79. doi: 10.1002/ajmg.1320380117

Rodríguez-de la Rosa, L., Sánchez-Calderón, H., Contreras, J., Murillo-Cuesta, S., Falagan, S., Avendaño, C., et al. (2015). Comparative gene expression study of the vestibular organ of the *Igf1* deficient mouse using whole-transcript arrays. *Hear. Res.* 330(Pt A), 62–77. doi: 10.1016/j.heares.2015.08.016

Rotwein, P., Burgess, S. K., Milbrandt, J. D., and Krause, J. E. (1988). Differential expression of insulin-like growth factor genes in rat central nervous system. *Proc. Natl. Acad. Sci. U.S.A.* 85, 265–269. doi: 10.1073/pnas.85.1.265

Russo, V. C., Gluckman, P. D., Feldman, E. L., and Werther, G. A. (2005). The insulin-like growth factor system and its pleiotropic functions in brain. *Endocr. Rev.* 26, 916–943. doi: 10.1210/er.2004-0024

Scolnick, J. A., Cui, K., Duggan, C. D., Xuan, S., Yuan, X.-B., Efstratiadis, A., et al. (2008). Role of IGF signaling in olfactory sensory map formation and axon guidance. *Neuron* 57, 847–857. doi: 10.1016/j.neuron.2008.01.027

Skolnik, E. Y., Lee, C. H., Batzer, A., Vicentini, L. M., Zhou, M., Daly, R., et al. (1993). The SH2/SH3 domain-containing protein GRB2 interacts with tyrosine-phosphorylated IRS1 and Shc: implications for insulin control of ras signalling. *EMBO J.* 12, 1929–1936.

Sosa, L., Dupraz, S., Laurino, L., Bollati, F., Bisbal, M., Cáceres, A., et al. (2006). IGF-1 receptor is essential for the establishment of hippocampal neuronal polarity. *Nat. Neurosci.* 9, 993–995. doi: 10.1038/nn1742

Stratikopoulos, E., Szabolcs, M., Dragatsis, I., Klinakis, A., and Efstratiadis, A. (2008). The hormonal action of IGF1 in postnatal mouse growth. *Proc. Natl. Acad. Sci. U.S.A.* 105, 19378–19383. doi: 10.1073/pnas.0809223105

Sun, L. Y. (2006). Hippocampal IGF-1 expression, neurogenesis and slowed aging: clues to longevity from mutant mice. *Age (Dordr).* 28, 181–189. doi: 10.1007/s11357-006-9009-5

Sun, L. Y., Evans, M. S., Hsieh, J., Panici, J., and Bartke, A. (2005). Increased neurogenesis in dentate gyrus of long-lived Ames dwarf mice. *Endocrinology* 146, 1138–1144. doi: 10.1210/en.2004-1115

Torres-Aleman, I., Naftolin, F., and Robbins, R. J. (1990). Trophic effects of basic fibroblast growth factor on fetal rat hypothalamic cells: interactions with insulin-like growth factor I. *Brain Res. Dev. Brain Res.* 52, 253–257. doi: 10.1016/0165-3806(90)90242-Q

Trejo, J. L., Carro, E., and Torres-Aleman, I. (2001). Circulating insulin-like growth factor I mediates exercise-induced increases in the number of new neurons in the adult hippocampus. *J. Neurosci.* 21, 1628–1634.

Trejo, J. L., Llorens-Martín, M. V., and Torres-Alemán, I. (2008). The effects of exercise on spatial learning and anxiety-like behavior are mediated by an IGF-I-dependent mechanism related to hippocampal neurogenesis. *Mol. Cell. Neurosci.* 37, 402–411. doi: 10.1016/j.mcn.2007.10.016

Trejo, J. L., Piriz, J., Llorens-Martin, M. V., Fernandez, A. M., Bolós, M., LeRoith, D., et al. (2007). Central actions of liver-derived insulin-like growth factor I underlying its pro-cognitive effects. *Mol. Psychiatry* 12, 1118–1128. doi: 10.1038/sj.mp.4002076

van Duyvenvoorde, H. A., van Setten, P. A., Walenkamp, M. J., van Doorn, J., Koenig, J., Gauguin, L., et al. (2010). Short stature associated with a novel heterozygous mutation in the insulin-like growth factor 1 gene. *J. Clin. Endocrinol. Metab.* 95, E363–E367. doi: 10.1210/jc.2010-0511

Versteyhe, S., Klaproth, B., Borup, R., Palsgaard, J., Jensen, M., Gray, S. G., et al. (2013). IGF-I, IGF-II, and insulin stimulate different gene expression responses through binding to the IGF-I Receptor. *Front. Endocrinol. (Lausanne).* 4:98. doi: 10.3389/fendo.2013.00098

Vicario-Abejón, C., Fernandez-Moreno, C., Pichel, J. G., and de Pablo, F. (2004). Mice lacking IGF-I and LIF have motoneuron deficits in brain stem nuclei. *Neuroreport* 15, 2769–2772.

Vicario-Abejón, C., Yusta-Boyo, M. J., Fernández-Moreno, C., and de Pablo, F. (2003). Locally born olfactory bulb stem cells proliferate in response to insulin-related factors and require endogenous insulin-like growth factor-I for differentiation into neurons and glia. *J. Neurosci.* 23, 895–906.

Vogel, T. (2013). "Insulin/IGF-signalling in embryonic and adult neural proliferation and differentiation in the mammalian central nervous system," in *Trends in Cell Signaling Pathways in Neuronal Fate Decision,* ed S. Wislet-Gendebien (Rijeka: InTech), 37–73.

Walenkamp, M. J., Karperien, M., Pereira, A. M., Hilhorst-Hofstee, Y., van Doorn, J., Chen, J. W., et al. (2005). Homozygous and heterozygous expression of a novel insulin-like growth factor-I mutation. *J. Clin. Endocrinol. Metab.* 90, 2855–2864. doi: 10.1210/jc.2004-1254

Walenkamp, M. J., Losekoot, M., and Wit, J. M. (2013). Molecular IGF-1 and IGF-1 receptor defects: from genetics to clinical management. *Endocr. Dev.* 24, 128–137. doi: 10.1159/000342841

Wang, J., Zhou, J., Powell-Braxton, L., and Bondy, C. (1999). Effects of Igf1 gene deletion on postnatal growth patterns. *Endocrinology* 140, 3391–3394. doi: 10.1210/endo.140.7.7045

Witsch, J., Szafranski, P., Chen, C. A., Immken, L., Simpson Patel, G., Hixson, P., et al. (2013). Intragenic deletions of the IGF1 receptor gene in five individuals with psychiatric phenotypes and developmental delay. *Eur. J. Hum. Genet.* 21, 1304–1307. doi: 10.1038/ejhg.2013.42

Woods, K. A., Camacho-Hübner, C., Savage, M. O., and Clark, A. J. (1996). Intrauterine growth retardation and postnatal growth failure associated with deletion of the insulin-like growth factor I gene. *N. Engl. J. Med.* 335, 1363–1367. doi: 10.1056/NEJM199610313351805

Wu, Y., Sun, H., Yakar, S., and LeRoith, D. (2009). Elevated levels of insulin-like growth factor (IGF)-I in serum rescue the severe growth retardation of IGF-I null mice. *Endocrinology* 150, 4395–4403. doi: 10.1210/en.2009-0272

Xiang, Y., Ding, N., Xing, Z., Zhang, W., Liu, H., and Li, Z. (2011). Insulin-like growth factor-1 regulates neurite outgrowth and neuronal migration from organotypic cultured dorsal root ganglion. *Int. J. Neurosci.* 121, 101–106. doi: 10.3109/00207454.2010.535935

Yakar, S., Rosen, C. J., Beamer, W. G., Ackert-Bicknell, C. L., Wu, Y., Liu, J.-L., et al. (2002). Circulating levels of IGF-1 directly regulate bone growth and density. *J. Clin. Invest.* 110, 771–781. doi: 10.1172/JCI0215463

Ye, P., Carson, J., and D'Ercole, A. J. (1995). *In vivo* actions of insulin-like growth factor-I (IGF-I) on brain myelination: studies of IGF-I and IGF binding protein-1 (IGFBP-1) transgenic mice. *J. Neurosci.* 15, 7344–7356.

Ye, P., and D'Ercole, A. J. (2006). Insulin-like growth factor actions during development of neural stem cells and progenitors in the central nervous system. *J. Neurosci. Res.* 83, 1–6. doi: 10.1002/jnr.20688

Ye, P., Popken, G. J., Kemper, A., McCarthy, K., Popko, B., and D'Ercole, A. J. (2004). Astrocyte-specific overexpression of insulin-like growth factor-I promotes brain overgrowth and glial fibrillary acidic protein expression. *J. Neurosci. Res.* 78, 472–484. doi: 10.1002/jnr.20288

Ye, P., Umayahara, Y., Ritter, D., Bunting, T., Auman, H., Rotwein, P., et al. (1997). Regulation of insulin-like growth factor I (IGF-I) gene expression in brain of transgenic mice expressing an IGF-I-luciferase fusion gene. *Endocrinology* 138, 5466–5475. doi: 10.1210/en.138.12.5466

Yuan, H., Chen, R., Wu, L., Chen, Q., Hu, A., Zhang, T., et al. (2015). The regulatory mechanism of neurogenesis by IGF-1 in adult mice. *Mol. Neurobiol.* 51, 512–522. doi: 10.1007/s12035-014-8717-6

Zhang, X., Zhang, L., Cheng, X., Guo, Y., Sun, X., Chen, G., et al. (2014). IGF-1 promotes Brn-4 expression and neuronal differentiation of neural stem cells via the PI3K/Akt pathway. *PLoS ONE* 9:e113801. doi: 10.1371/journal.pone.0113801

Ziegler, A. N., Schneider, J. S., Qin, M., Tyler, W. A., Pintar, J. E., Fraidenraich, D., et al. (2012). IGF-II promotes stemness of neural restricted precursors. *Stem Cells* 30, 1265–1276. doi: 10.1002/stem.1095

4

Alzheimer's Disease and Hippocampal Adult Neurogenesis: Exploring Shared Mechanisms

*Carolyn Hollands†, Nancy Bartolotti† and Orly Lazarov**

Department of Anatomy and Cell Biology, College of Medicine, The University of Illinois at Chicago, Chicago, IL, USA

Edited by:
Laura López-Mascaraque, Spanish National Research Council, Spain

Reviewed by:
Stefano Farioli Vecchioli, National Research Council, Italy
María Llorens-Martín, Spanish National Research Council, Spain

***Correspondence:**
Orly Lazarov
olazarov@uic.edu

† These authors have contributed equally to this work.

New neurons incorporate into the granular cell layer of the dentate gyrus throughout life. Neurogenesis is modulated by behavior and plays a major role in hippocampal plasticity. Along with older mature neurons, new neurons structure the dentate gyrus, and determine its function. Recent data suggest that the level of hippocampal neurogenesis is substantial in the human brain, suggesting that neurogenesis may have important implications for human cognition. In support of that, impaired neurogenesis compromises hippocampal function and plays a role in cognitive deficits in Alzheimer's disease mouse models. We review current work suggesting that neuronal differentiation is defective in Alzheimer's disease, leading to dysfunction of the dentate gyrus. Additionally, alterations in critical signals regulating neurogenesis, such as presenilin-1, Notch 1, soluble amyloid precursor protein, CREB, and β-catenin underlie dysfunctional neurogenesis in Alzheimer's disease. Lastly, we discuss the detectability of neurogenesis in the live mouse and human brain, as well as the therapeutic implications of enhancing neurogenesis for the treatment of cognitive deficits and Alzheimer's disease.

Keywords: hippocampus, neurogenesis, Alzheimer's disease, cognition, learning and memory

INTRODUCTION

In early development neurons are rapidly produced to form the intricate complexity of the brain and peripheral nervous system. Postnatally, the role of neurogenesis is shifted from brain development into brain plasticity. From then on, neurogenesis takes place only in specific niches in the adult brain, in the subgranular zone (SGZ) of the dentate gyrus (DG) of the hippocampus and the subventricular zone (Kempermann et al., 2015). Recent evidence suggests substantial levels of hippocampal neurogenesis in the human brain, estimating about 700 new neurons a day in the DG (Spalding et al., 2013). Humans replace ~35% of the DG, while rodents are estimated to replace only 10% (Ninkovic and Gotz, 2007; Imayoshi et al., 2008). Recent information also suggests that in humans, the striatum may be a source of adult neurogenesis as well (Ernst et al., 2014). The existence of adult neurogenesis in the human brain supports the notion that neurogenesis has important functional significance and implications for cognitive disorders and their therapy (Eriksson et al., 1998; Ninkovic and Gotz, 2007; Imayoshi et al., 2008; Lazarov and Marr, 2013; Spalding et al., 2013).

The circuitry of the DG, of which new neurons are part, promotes several important functions, namely, pattern separation, conjunctive encoding of multiple sensory output to the dorsal CA3, facilitation of encoding of spatial information based on its output to the dorsal CA3, and encoding of time in new memories (for review, Lazarov and Hollands, 2016).

In support of the role of hippocampal neurogenesis in plasticity, learning and memory, increasing evidence suggests that cognitive deficits, difficulty learning new information and memory loss, as occurs in Alzheimer's disease (AD), may be, at least in part, due to impairments in adult neurogenesis (Demars et al., 2010, 2013; Lazarov and Marr, 2010; Lazarov et al., 2010). Some of the foundation for the association between impairments in adult hippocampal neurogenesis and cognitive deficits leading to AD might be due to the fact that several key signals implicated in AD play a role in regulation of hippocampal neurogenesis (**Figure 1**).

NEUROGENESIS IN AGING, DISEASE STATE, AND COGNITIVE DYSFUNCTION

In the rodent brain, neurogenesis is dramatically decreased during adulthood and further declines during aging (Demars et al., 2013). Recent evidence suggests that in wild type mice reduced proliferation of neural progenitor cells (NPCs) might be one of the processes underlying this phenomenon (Demars et al., 2013). However, other mechanisms, such as altered signaling, increased quiescence of neural stem cells (NSCs) and differentiation toward non-neuronal subtypes have been proposed [see for example Hattiangady and Shetty, 2008]. In humans, the dynamics are less clear. A recent study suggests that there is a moderate decline in neurogenesis with aging (Spalding et al., 2013). However, as of yet, it is unclear how this decline impacts cognitive function in humans or whether similar memory paradigms are regulated by adult neurogenesis as they are in rodents. Observations in humans using high resolution fMRI (Brickman et al., 2014) and cognitive studies (Toner et al., 2009; Stark et al., 2010; Yassa et al., 2011; Brickman et al., 2012) suggest that age-related memory loss begins in the DG. These changes are believed to stem from a decline in the support of the neurogenic niche as well as intrinsic characteristics of NSC (for review Silva-Vargas et al., 2013). Many processes decline in the aging brain along with a decrease in adult neurogenesis. For example, in both rodents and humans the density of synaptic contacts onto granular cells in the DG decreases with age (Flood et al., 1996; Geinisman et al., 2001, 2004). It will be important to determine whether age-dependent decline in neurogenesis compromises the function of the DG and induces susceptibility to memory impairments.

Deficits in adult neurogenesis with age may compromise the structure and function of the entorhinal-hippocampal circuit. This area is particularly vulnerable and heavily affected in AD, the most common form of dementia. AD is characterized by progressive memory loss and cognitive dysfunction (Baulac et al., 2003). Rare, Familail AD (FAD) is caused by mutations in the *amyloid precursor protein* (*APP*) and *presenilin 1* and *2* (*PS1,2*) (Selkoe and Wolfe, 2007). However, the majority of AD cases are sporadic and aging is the greatest risk factor for AD. Research done in mouse models of FAD suggests that declining neurogenesis is an early stage event that can be observed as early as 2–3 months of age (Rodriguez et al., 2008; Demars et al., 2010; Hamilton et al., 2010)(for review Lazarov and Marr, 2010, 2013). Nevertheless, it is important to note that some FAD mouse lines, mostly lines that overexpress APP, exhibit enhanced, rather than reduced, neurogenesis (Jin et al., 2004; Chuang, 2010). As discussed below, this might be attributed to the overexpression of soluble APP (sAPP), a proliferation factor of NPCs (Demars et al., 2011, 2013; Lazarov and Demars, 2012). The manifestations of neurogenic impairments in FAD mice are diverse. They include defective maturation/reduced rate of survival of new neurons in the granular cell layer (GCL), compromised dendritic tree branching (Sun et al., 2009; Bonds et al., 2015), imbalance of GABAergic and glutamatergic input onto new granular neurons (Sun et al., 2009), expression of the less potent proliferation factor sAPPβ at the expense of sAPPα in the neurogenic niche (Demars et al., 2011, 2013) and loss of γ-secretase function in NPCs and new neurons (Gadadhar et al., 2011; Bonds et al., 2015).

Below, we highlight several key signaling factors that are implicated in AD and were recently described to regulate neurogenesis. These factors play a role in aging-dependent behavior, circadian rhythm, inflammation, oxidative stress, neurotrophic signaling, hormonal signaling, neurotransmission, vascular signaling, and others. Thus, the multi- factorial effect on neurogenesis exposes the complex relationship between neurogenesis and the progression of AD pathology (for review Lazarov and Marr, 2010, 2013; Lazarov et al., 2010).

ALTERATIONS IN MOLECULAR SIGNALS DURING AGING AND COGNITIVE DYSFUNCTION ACCOMPANYING NEURODEGENERATIVE DISEASE

Presenillin-1 (PS1) is the catalytic core of γ-secretase, an aspartyl protease, which cleaves numerous substrates, including APP and Notch (De Strooper et al., 1998, 1999). Mutations in PS1 cause FAD, presumably due to loss of γ-secretase function (Xia et al., 2015). A recent paper suggests that PS1 undergoes a conformational change during aging and sporadic AD, and this change may have downstream effects on the processing of its substrates APP and Notch (Wahlster et al., 2013). PS1 regulates NPC differentiation in the adult brain (Gadadhar et al., 2011) via β-catenin, Notch1 and CREB (Bonds et al., 2015). Down regulation of PS1 in hippocampal NPCs compromises the maturation of new neurons, manifested by deficits in their dendritic tree branching, leading to learning and memory deficits (Bonds et al., 2015), suggesting that PS1-induced dysfunction of neurogenesis can impair cognitive function in AD. Transgenic expression of FAD-linked mutant variants of PS1 also impairs neurogenesis and the neurogenic response to experience in an enriched environment (EE) (Wang et al., 2004; Wen et al., 2004; Chevallier et al., 2005; Choi et al., 2008).

Amyloid precursor protein (APP)- APP is a substrate of γ-secretase. Misregulated cleavage of APP in the amyloidogenic pathway is implicated in FAD. While the physiological role of APP is yet to be fully understood, numerous studies suggest a role in synaptic plasticity and neurogenesis (Lazarov and Demars, 2012). The soluble form of APP (sAPPα) regulates NPC proliferation and survival (Demars et al., 2011, 2013). In fact, neurogenesis can be upregulated in the aging mouse

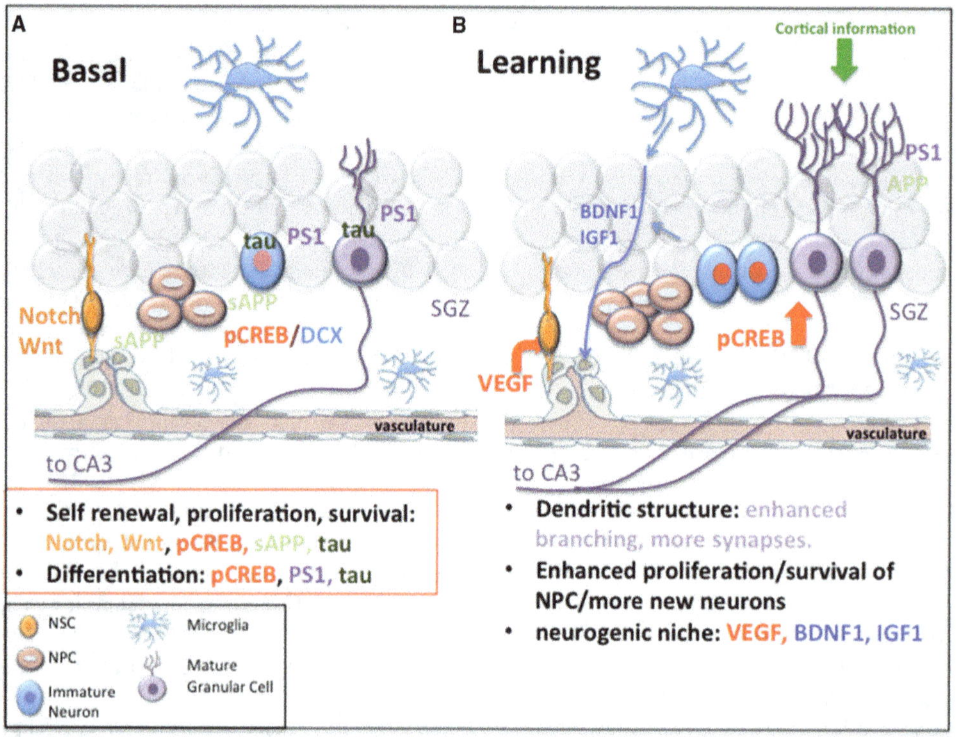

FIGURE 1 | Common mechanisms of neurogenesis and Alzheimer's disease and the implications for learning. (A) Signals that play a role in neurogenesis, such as Notch-1, Wnt/β-catenin, CREB, sAPP, tau, and presenilin-1 are implicated in Alzheimer's disease. **(B)** Following learning, changes in the neurogenic niche include alterations in Notch and sAPP, increased expression of neurotrophins such as VEGF, BDNF, and IGF which enhance angiogenesis and provide support for the neurogenic niche and lead to increased neurogenesis. Upregulation of CREB signaling by neural progenitor cells and neurons may promote survival and maturation of NPCs. Increased dendritic branching of mature neurons and synaptic plasticity may be mediated by presenilin-1 and APP. The factors mediating these processes are dysfunctional or compromised in Alzheimer's disease, suggesting that defective neurogenesis may affect hippocampal function in Alzheimer's disease.

brain following injection of sAPPα into the SVZ (Demars et al., 2013). While APP is extensively researched in regards to AD, the regulation of APP with aging is less well studied. However, there is some evidence that APP processing may be altered during aging, perhaps through dysregulation of the circadian system (Dobrowolska et al., 2014). In FAD, there is upregulation of the less potent sAPPβ counterpart at the expense of sAPPα, which may compromise proliferation of NPCs (Demars et al., 2011, 2013). Interestingly, sAPPα plays an important role in migration of NPC during brain development (Young-Pearse et al., 2007, 2008). Other metabolites of APP, such as AICD and Aβ have been suggested to regulate neurogenesis (for review see Lazarov et al., 2010), but more studies are warranted in order to establish their role.

Tau- is a neuronal microtubule-associated protein, the hyperphosphorylation and aggregation of which plays a key role in AD pathology. Significantly, adult born neurons transiently express the tau-3R isoform during development, overlapping with DCX and NeuN co-expression in the DG (Bullmann et al., 2007; Llorens-Martin et al., 2012). Tau phosphorylation in the DG is also temporally and spatially linked to DCX and neuroD expression with activated GSK-β believed to be the main tau kinase in newborn neurons (Fuster-Matanzo et al., 2009; Hong et al., 2010). The genomic based hTau mouse model exhibited reduction in adult neurogenesis, as a result of decreased proliferation, as early as 2 months of age before the appearance of significant tau pathology (Komuro et al., 2015), which may suggest that either impaired hippocampal neurogenesis is an early hallmark of tau pathology in AD or that there is an association between tau pathology and defective neurogenesis in AD. For a comprehensive review about tau and adult neurogenesis see (Fuster-Matanzo et al., 2012).

Notch 1- is a critical neurogenic signal and a substrate of γ-secretase. The intracellular domain cleavage product, NICD, translocates to the nucleus and drives transcription of factors important for maintaining the NSC pool such as *Hes* and *ErbB2* (for review Pierfelice et al., 2011). Notch signaling occurs when the Notch receptor is activated by one of its ligands in the Jagged or Delta-like family of proteins (for review Kopan and Ilagan, 2009). Following physical activity, NPC proliferation is increased in a Notch-dependent manner in the SGZ of the DG, even in aged mice (Lugert et al., 2010). In contrast, Notch signaling is decreased with age, including in the hippocampus (Lugert et al., 2010; Tseng et al., 2014). Down regulation of PS1 in hippocampal

NPC results in reduced levels of NICD (Bonds et al., 2015). In mature neurons Notch levels are low, and its function is not fully elucidated (for review see Marathe and Alberi, 2015; Marathe et al., 2015).

Wnt/β-catenin- are critical signaling factors in the regulation of hippocampal neurogenesis (Chenn and Walsh, 2003; Sato et al., 2004; Lie et al., 2005; Shimizu et al., 2008). Wnt3 is expressed in the SGZ of the DG, and overexpression of Wnt3 is sufficient to increase neurogenesis (Lie et al., 2005). Wnts are produced by astrocytes in the adult hippocampal niche and support the proliferation and differentiation of neuronally-restricted NPCs (Lie et al., 2005). Wnts regulate NSC self-renewal by inactivating Glycogen synthase kinase 3 (GSK3) and stabilizing β-catenin (Shimizu et al., 2008). Further, β-catenin promotes NPC proliferation through the activation of LEF/TCF transcription factors (Shimizu et al., 2008). Interestingly, nuclear accumulated β-catenin also induces anti-neurogenic hes1 gene expression through the enhancement of Notch1- and RBP-J-mediated transcription. β-catenin can associate with the NICD, and it is present in a nuclear protein-DNA complex containing the hes1 gene promoter. The β-catenin–NICD complex is efficiently formed when transcriptional coactivators p300 and P/CAF are present. Also, significantly, following its cleavage, the PS1CTF/NTF forms a complex with GSK3 and β-catenin (Tesco et al., 1998; Tesco and Tanzi, 2000). PS1 has been implicated as a negative regulator of the Wnt/β-catenin signaling pathway (Xia et al., 2001). Wnt-independent interaction of β-catenin and PS1 has also been described (Kang et al., 2002). Downregulation of PS1 in adult NPCs compromises the phosphorylation of β-catenin, which may affect β-catenin translocation to the nucleus, leading to alterations in the normal development of NPC (Bonds et al., 2015).

CREB- Cyclic-AMP Response Element Binding protein (CREB) is a critical signaling factor for adult brain plasticity and learning (for review Kandel, 2012). Activation of CREB by phosphorylation on Ser133 (pCREB) is observed in the hippocampus and cortical areas following learning and memory tasks (for review Mayr and Montminy, 2001). Importantly, NPCs, neuroblasts and immature neurons constitutively express pCREB, suggesting that pCREB is a critical component of neurogenesis. Indeed, CREB plays a role in neuronal maturation and survival in hippocampal neurogenesis (for review Ge et al., 2006; Jagasia et al., 2009; Herold et al., 2011; Merz et al., 2011). In rodents, CREB signaling components in the hippocampus decrease with age (Chung et al., 2002; Kudo et al., 2005; Porte et al., 2008). However, these observations were made primarily in mature neurons. Thus, the impact of aging on NPC-specific CREB signaling remains unclear. Also unclear is how aging causes a decrease in CREB signaling, although hypotheses suggest that this could occur either by aging-dependent increased levels of reactive oxygen species, or via decreased NMDA receptor and BDNF expression, which are both important for CREB activation (Chung et al., 2002; Kudo et al., 2005; Porte et al., 2008; Ozgen et al., 2010). Interestingly, exposure to young blood increased CREB activation and neurogenesis in the aged hippocampus, suggesting that systemic factors that are altered with aging may play an important role in CREB signaling and neurogenesis in the brain (Villeda et al., 2011; Villeda and Wyss-Coray, 2013). Impaired CREB signaling in AD has been the subject of much study. CREB signaling is dysregulated in both human AD and in mouse models of FAD (Vitolo et al., 2002; Ma et al., 2007; Caccamo et al., 2010; Bartolotti et al., 2015). In addition, down regulation of PS1 expression in NPCs compromises pCREB expression, leading to defective maturation of new neurons and induction of cognitive deficits (Bonds et al., 2015). While the role of CREB signaling in memory via mature neurons is well documented, the contribution of CREB signaling in NPCs to memory is not fully elucidated, and separating out the contribution of CREB to learning and memory via mature neurons or via NPC function is technically challenging and remains to be investigated (for review see Scott Bitner, 2012; Ortega-Martinez, 2015). Likewise, most of the work on CREB signaling in AD has focused on the transient activation in mature neurons during the formation of long-term memories, and so the contribution of CREB signaling in NPC in the context of AD also remains an open question.

NEUROGENESIS AS A BIOMARKER OF COGNITIVE FUNCTION AND AS A THERAPEUTIC APPROACH

While it is clear that hippocampal neurogenesis takes place in the human brain and that the number of new neurons generated is significant (Spalding et al., 2013), information concerning the fate of neurogenesis in aging and cognitively impaired individuals is scarce. Current techniques allow the examination of neurogenesis postmortem. However, because of the dynamic modulation neurogenesis can undergo following numerous stimuli, such as progressive pathology, the development of methodologies for the detection of neurogenesis in live individuals will be crucial. Up to the present time, tools for the detection of neurogenesis in live humans have been limited. The level of ^{14}C in genomic DNA has been used for the estimation of date of birth of hippocampal neurons and their quantification in postmortem tissue (Spalding et al., 2013). A previous study suggests that adult neurogenesis can be specifically detected by proton nuclear magnetic resonance spectroscopy (^{1}H-MRS, Manganas et al., 2007). However, this method was challenged by Loewenbruck et al. (2011), thus, more studies are warranted for the determination of the specificity, sensitivity and feasibility of ^{1}H-MRS for the detection and quantification of neurogenesis.

The association between decline in neurogenesis and cognitive deterioration during aging, coupled with disruption in neurogenesis and cognitive dysfunction in FAD mouse models suggests that enhancing neurogenesis may be a feasible therapeutic approach (**Figure 2**). Successful attempts to enhance neurogenesis in rodents have been described. For example Sahay et al. used genetic manipulation of neurogenic pathways, excising the pro-apoptotic gene *Bax*, to enhance survival of nestin expressing cells (Sahay et al., 2011). They observed enhanced performance in the DG-dependent pattern separation task, where animals must distinguish between two similar contexts. Wang et al. also enhanced cell survival, neuronal differentiation,

Enhancing Neurogenesis	Prospective Readouts of Neurogenesis
Environmental Enrichment; Cognitively complex experiences, Aerobic exercise, social interaction	**Postmortem;** Radioactive isotopes, analysis of neurogenic cellular markers
Anti-depressants; SSRI's	**Imaging;** specific imaging techniques to be developed
Pro-neurogenic small molecules	**Functional MRI;** Behavioral tests (e.g. pattern separation)
Manipulation of neurogenic pathway	**Plasma biomarkers** (learning and memory signals, inflammatory, cytokines, neurogenic signals)
Hormones, neurotransmitters	**Other?**

FIGURE 2 | Therapeutic and translational potential of neurogenesis. Examples of current and prospective methods for the modulation and detection of neurogenesis. Means of enhancing neurogenesis include noninvasive, environmental modulations like cognitively complex activities and exercise, as well as molecular interventions like anti-depressants, pro-neurogenic small molecules, hormones or neurotransmitters, or other manipulations of the neurogenic pathways. While readouts of human neurogenesis are typically done in postmortem tissue using radioactive isotopes or analysis of neurogeneic cell markers, imaging techniques such as fMRI, or blood biomarkers will offer non-invasive avenues to determine neurogenesis during life.

and dendritic complexity in neurogenic regions through activation of ERK5 map kinase (Wang et al., 2014). Following this manipulation, animals had increased performance in spatial learning and memory in the Morris Water Maze (MWM) task. In MWM and the novel object recognition task they also probed long-term memory and saw improvements as well, suggesting that adult neurogenesis may be a key therapeutic target.

Given the evidence from genetic manipulation of neurogenesis in rodents, it is important to consider how neurogenesis could be modulated in humans. One approach is the modulation of lifestyle factors, termed environmental enrichment (EE). Evidence from rodents suggests that EE and running are effective ways to enhance hippocampal plasticity and neurogenesis in particular (Kempermann et al., 1997; van Praag et al., 1999a,b). These behavioral interventions have been found to enhance neurogenesis and ameliorate pathology in AD mouse models (Lazarov et al., 2005; Lazarov and Larson, 2007; Hu et al., 2010, 2013). Significantly, studies have shown that exercise can improve cognitive performance in the elderly (Ahlskog et al., 2011). Brief increases in physical activity (6–12 months) upregulates hippocampal volume and improves both episodic and spatial memory (Klusmann et al., 2010; Erickson et al., 2011; Ruscheweyh et al., 2011). In rodents it has also been shown that EE can increase many of the molecular factors involved in neurogenesis, such as pCREB expression and CRE-gene transcription in the hippocampus of wild-type mice (Hu et al., 2013; Bartolotti et al., 2015). While this observation was not specific to new neurons, it raises the possibility that enhanced CREB signaling may be one mechanism by which EE may increase the survival of new neurons. Nevertheless, EE and running do not target neurogenesis specifically, but have numerous effects on the hippocampus. Several studies describe the manipulation of neurogenesis using small molecules (Longo et al., 2006; Schneider et al., 2008; McNeish et al., 2010; Pieper et al., 2010; Lange et al., 2011; MacMillan et al., 2011; Neely et al., 2012; Petrik et al., 2012; Shi et al., 2013) or pharmacological agents, such as SSRI's or modulators of neurogenic pathways [For example, see Warner-Schmidt and Duman, 2007]. Some of these have been shown to enhance neurogenesis and reverse memory deficits. However, to this point the use of these compounds in AD mouse models has not been explored. In future experiments it will be important to consider the mechanism by which these molecules modulate adult neurogenesis in light of the signaling cascades we have described here. Particularly considering how these cascades are altered in aging and AD, both in rodent models and in humans.

AUTHOR CONTRIBUTIONS

This manuscript is based on data produced by Dr. CH and Mrs. NB. Dr. CH and Ms. NB and Prof. OL wrote this mini-review.

ACKNOWLEDGMENTS

This work was supported by NIA R01AG033570, Department of Defense 10917352, NIA 1RC1AG036208-01 ARR, CCTS-0512-06 (OL), PECTS Award CCTS Pre-doctoral Education (NB).

REFERENCES

Ahlskog, J. E., Geda, Y. E., Graff-Radford, N. R., and Petersen, R. C. (2011). Physical exercise as a preventive or disease-modifying treatment of dementia and brain aging. *Mayo Clin. Proc.* 86, 876–884. doi: 10.4065/mcp.2011.0252

Bartolotti, N., Segura, L., and Lazarov, O. (2015). Diminished CRE-induced plasticity is linked to memory deficits in familial Alzheimer's Disease mice. *J. Alzheimers Dis.* 50, 477–489. doi: 10.3233/JAD-150650

Baulac, S., LaVoie, M. J., Kimberly, W. T., Strahle, J., Wolfe, M. S., Selkoe, D. J., et al. (2003). Functional gamma-secretase complex assembly in Golgi/trans-Golgi network: interactions among presenilin, nicastrin, Aph1, Pen-2, and gamma-secretase substrates. *Neurobiol. Dis.* 14, 194–204. doi: 10.1016/S0969-9961(03)00123-2

Bonds, J. A., Kuttner-Hirshler, Y., Bartolotti, N., Tobin, M. K., Pizzi, M., Marr, R., et al. (2015). Presenilin-1 dependent neurogenesis regulates hippocampal learning and memory. *PLoS ONE* 10:e0131266. doi: 10.1371/journal.pone.0131266

Brickman, A. M., Khan, U. A., Provenzano, F. A., Yeung, L. K., Suzuki, W., Schroeter, H., et al. (2014). Enhancing dentate gyrus function with dietary flavanols improves cognition in older adults. *Nat. Neurosci.* 17, 1798–1803. doi: 10.1038/nn.3850

Brickman, A. M., Meier, I. B., Korgaonkar, M. S., Provenzano, F. A., Grieve, S. M., Siedlecki, K. L., et al. (2012). Testing the white matter retrogenesis hypothesis of cognitive aging. *Neurobiol. Aging* 33, 1699–1715. doi: 10.1016/j.neurobiolaging.2011.06.001

Bullmann, T., de Silva, R., Holzer, M., Mori, H., and Arendt, T. (2007). Expression of embryonic tau protein isoforms persist during adult neurogenesis in the hippocampus. *Hippocampus* 17, 98–102. doi: 10.1002/hipo.20255

Caccamo, A., Maldonado, M. A., Bokov, A. F., Majumder, S., and Oddo, S. (2010). CBP gene transfer increases BDNF levels and ameliorates learning and memory deficits in a mouse model of Alzheimer's disease. *Proc. Natl. Acad. Sci. U.S.A.* 107, 22687–22692. doi: 10.1073/pnas.1012851108

Chenn, A., and Walsh, C. A. (2003). Increased neuronal production, enlarged forebrains and cytoarchitectural distortions in beta-catenin overexpressing transgenic mice. *Cereb. Cortex* 13, 599–606. doi: 10.1093/cercor/13.6.599

Chevallier, N. L., Soriano, S., Kang, D. E., Masliah, E., Hu, G., and Koo, E. H. (2005). Perturbed neurogenesis in the adult hippocampus associated with presenilin-1 A246E mutation. *Am. J. Pathol.* 167, 151–159. doi: 10.1016/S0002-9440(10)62962-8

Choi, S. H., Veeraraghavalu, K., Lazarov, O., Marler, S., Ransohoff, R. M., Ramirez, J. M., et al. (2008). Non-cell-autonomous effects of presenilin 1 variants on enrichment-mediated hippocampal progenitor cell proliferation and differentiation. *Neuron* 59, 568–580. doi: 10.1016/j.neuron.2008.07.033

Chuang, T. T. (2010). Neurogenesis in mouse models of Alzheimer's disease. *Biochim. Biophys. Acta* 1802, 872–880. doi: 10.1016/j.bbadis.2009.12.008

Chung, Y. H., Kim, E. J., Shin, C. M., Joo, K. M., Kim, M. J., Woo, H. W., et al. (2002). Age-related changes in CREB binding protein immunoreactivity in the cerebral cortex and hippocampus of rats. *Brain Res.* 956, 312–318. doi: 10.1016/S0006-8993(02)03562-X

Demars, M., Hu, Y. S., Gadadhar, A., and Lazarov, O. (2010). Impaired neurogenesis is an early event in the etiology of familial Alzheimer's disease in transgenic mice. *J. Neurosci. Res.* 88, 2103–2117. doi: 10.1002/jnr.22387

Demars, M. P., Bartholomew, A., Strakova, Z., and Lazarov, O. (2011). Soluble amyloid precursor protein: a novel proliferation factor of adult progenitor cells of ectodermal and mesodermal origin. *Stem Cell Res. Ther.* 2, 36. doi: 10.1186/scrt77

Demars, M. P., Hollands, C., Zhao, K. D., and Lazarov, O. (2013). Soluble amyloid precursor protein-alpha rescues age-linked decline in neural progenitor cell proliferation. *Neurobiol. Aging.* 34, 2431–2440. doi: 10.1016/j.neurobiolaging.2013.04.016

De Strooper, B., Annaert, W., Cupers, P., Saftig, P., Craessaerts, K., Mumm, J. S., et al. (1999). A presenilin-1-dependent gamma-secretase-like protease mediates release of Notch intracellular domain. *Nature* 398, 518–522. doi: 10.1038/19083

De Strooper, B., Saftig, P., Craessaerts, K., Vanderstichele, H., Guhde, G., Annaert, W., et al. (1998). Deficiency of presenilin-1 inhibits the normal cleavage of amyloid precursor protein. *Nature* 391, 387–390. doi: 10.1038/34910

Dobrowolska, J. A., Michener, M. S., Wu, G., Patterson, B. W., Chott, R., Ovod, V., et al. (2014). CNS amyloid-beta, soluble APP-alpha and -beta kinetics during BACE inhibition. *J. Neurosci.* 34, 8336–8346. doi: 10.1523/JNEUROSCI.0540-14.2014

Erickson, K. I., Voss, M. W., Prakash, R. S., Basak, C., Szabo, A., Chaddock, L., et al. (2011). Exercise training increases size of hippocampus and improves memory. *Proc. Natl. Acad. Sci. U.S.A.* 108, 3017–3022. doi: 10.1073/pnas.1015950108

Eriksson, P. S., Perfilieva, E., Björk-Eriksson, T., Alborn, A. M., Nordborg, C., Peterson, D. A., et al. (1998). Neurogenesis in the adult human hippocampus. *Nat. Med.* 4, 1313–1317. doi: 10.1038/3305

Ernst, A., Alkass, K., Bernard, S., Salehpour, M., Perl, S., Tisdale, J., et al. (2014). Neurogenesis in the striatum of the adult human brain. *Cell* 156, 1072–1083. doi: 10.1016/j.cell.2014.01.044

Flood, J. F., Harris, F. J., and Morley, J. E. (1996). Age-related changes in hippocampal drug facilitation of memory processing in SAMP8 mice. *Neurobiol. Aging* 17, 15–24. doi: 10.1016/0197-4580(95)02007-1

Fuster-Matanzo, A., de Barreda, E. G., Dawson, H. N., Vitek, M. P., Avila, J., and Hernández, F. (2009). Function of tau protein in adult newborn neurons. *FEBS Lett.* 583, 3063–3068. doi: 10.1016/j.febslet.2009.08.017

Fuster-Matanzo, A., Llorens-Martín, M., Jurado-Arjona, J., Avila, J., and Hernández, F. (2012). Tau protein and adult hippocampal neurogenesis. *Front. Neurosci.* 6:104. doi: 10.3389/fnins.2012.00104

Gadadhar, A., Marr, R., and Lazarov, O. (2011). Presenilin-1 regulates neural progenitor cell differentiation in the adult brain. *J. Neurosci.* 31, 2615–2623. doi: 10.1523/JNEUROSCI.4767-10.2011

Ge, S., Goh, E. L., Sailor, K. A., Kitabatake, Y., Ming, G. L., and Song, H. (2006). GABA regulates synaptic integration of newly generated neurons in the adult brain. *Nature* 439, 589–593. doi: 10.1038/nature04404

Geinisman, Y., Berry, R. W., Disterhoft, J. F., Power, J. M., and Van der Zee, E. A. (2001). Associative learning elicits the formation of multiple-synapse boutons. *J. Neurosci.* 21, 5568–5573.

Geinisman, Y., Ganeshina, O., Yoshida, R., Berry, R. W., Disterhoft, J. F., and Gallagher, M. (2004). Aging, spatial learning, and total synapse number in the rat CA1 stratum radiatum. *Neurobiol. Aging* 25, 407–416. doi: 10.1016/j.neurobiolaging.2003.12.001

Hamilton, L. K., Aumont, A., Julien, C., Vadnais, A., Calon, F., and Fernandes, K. J. (2010). Widespread deficits in adult neurogenesis precede plaque and tangle formation in the 3xTg mouse model of Alzheimer's disease. *Eur. J. Neurosci.* 32, 905–920. doi: 10.1111/j.1460-9568.2010.07379.x

Hattiangady, B., and Shetty, A. K. (2008). Aging does not alter the number or phenotype of putative stem/progenitor cells in the neurogenic region of the hippocampus. *Neurobiol. Aging* 29, 129–147. doi: 10.1016/j.neurobiolaging.2006.09.015

Herold, S., Jagasia, R., Merz, K., Wassmer, K., and Lie, D. C. (2011). CREB signalling regulates early survival, neuronal gene expression and morphological development in adult subventricular zone neurogenesis. *Mol. Cell Neurosci.* 46, 79–88. doi: 10.1016/j.mcn.2010.08.008

Hong, X. P., Peng, C. X., Wei, W., Tian, Q., Liu, Y. H., Yao, X. Q., et al. (2010). Essential role of tau phosphorylation in adult hippocampal neurogenesis. *Hippocampus* 20, 1339–1349. doi: 10.1002/hipo.20712

Hu, Y. S., Long, N., Pigino, G., Brady, S. T., and Lazarov, O. (2013). Molecular mechanisms of environmental enrichment: impairments in Akt/GSK3beta, neurotrophin-3 and CREB signaling. *PLoS ONE* 8:e64460. doi: 10.1371/journal.pone.0064460

Hu, Y. S., Xu, P., Pigino, G., Brady, S. T., Larson, J., and Lazarov, O. (2010). Complex environment experience rescues impaired neurogenesis, enhances synaptic plasticity, and attenuates neuropathology in familial Alzheimer's disease-linked APPswe/PS1{Delta}E9 mice. *FASEB J.* 24, 1667–1681. doi: 10.1096/fj.09-136945

Imayoshi, I., Sakamoto, M., Ohtsuka, T., Takao, K., Miyakawa, T., Yamaguchi, M., et al. (2008). Roles of continuous neurogenesis in the structural and functional integrity of the adult forebrain. *Nat. Neurosci.* 11, 1153–1161. doi: 10.1038/nn.2185

Jagasia, R., Steib, K., Englberger, E., Herold, S., Faus-Kessler, T., Saxe, M., et al. (2009). GABA-cAMP response element-binding protein signaling regulates maturation and survival of newly generated neurons in the adult hippocampus. *J. Neurosci.* 29, 7966–7977. doi: 10.1523/JNEUROSCI.1054-09.2009

Jin, K., Peel, A. L., Mao, X. O., Xie, L., Cottrell, B. A., Henshall, D. C., et al. (2004). Increased hippocampal neurogenesis in Alzheimer's disease. *Proc. Natl. Acad. Sci. U.S.A.* 101, 343–347. doi: 10.1073/pnas.2634794100

Kandel, E. R. (2012). The molecular biology of memory: cAMP, PKA, CRE, CREB-1, CREB-2, and CPEB. *Mol. Brain* 5:14. doi: 10.1186/1756-6606-5-14

Kang, D. E., Soriano, S., Xia, X., Eberhart, C. G., De Strooper, B., Zheng, H., et al. (2002). Presenilin couples the paired phosphorylation of beta-catenin independent of axin: implications for beta-catenin activation in tumorigenesis. *Cell* 110, 751–762. doi: 10.1016/S0092-8674(02)00970-4

Kempermann, G., Kuhn, H. G., and Gage, F. H. (1997). More hippocampal neurons in adult mice living in an enriched environment. *Nature* 386, 493–495. doi: 10.1038/386493a0

Kempermann, G., Song, H., and Gage, F. H. (2015). Neurogenesis in the Adult Hippocampus. *Cold Spring Harb. Perspect. Med.* 5:a018812. doi: 10.1101/cshperspect.a018812

Klusmann, V., Evers, A., Schwarzer, R., Schlattmann, P., Reischies, F. M., Heuser, I., et al. (2010). Complex mental and physical activity in older women and cognitive performance: a 6-month randomized controlled trial. *J. Gerontol. A Biol. Sci. Med. Sci.* 65, 680–688. doi: 10.1093/gerona/glq053

Komuro, Y., Xu, G., Bhaskar, K., and Lamb, B. T. (2015). Human tau expression reduces adult neurogenesis in a mouse model of tauopathy. *Neurobiol. Aging* 36, 2034–2042. doi: 10.1016/j.neurobiolaging.2015.03.002

Kopan, R., and Ilagan, M. X. G. (2009). The canonical Notch signaling pathway: unfolding the activation mechanism. *Cell* 137, 216–233. doi: 10.1016/j.cell.2009.03.045

Kudo, K., Wati, H., Qiao, C., Arita, J., and Kanba, S. (2005). Age-related disturbance of memory and CREB phosphorylation in CA1 area of hippocampus of rats. *Brain Res.* 1054, 30–37. doi: 10.1016/j.brainres.2005.06.045

Lange, C., Mix, E., Frahm, J., Glass, A., Müller, J., Schmitt, O., et al. (2011). Small molecule GSK-3 inhibitors increase neurogenesis of human neural progenitor cells. *Neurosci. Lett.* 488, 36–40. doi: 10.1016/j.neulet.2010.10.076

Lazarov, O., and Demars, M. P. (2012). All in the family: how the APPs regulate neurogenesis. *Front. Neurosci.* 6:81. doi: 10.3389/fnins.2012.00081

Lazarov, O., and Hollands, C. (2016). Hippocampal neurogenesis: learning to remember. *Prog Neurobiol.* 138-140:1-18. doi: 10.1016/j.pneurobio.2015.12.006

Lazarov, O., and Larson, J. (2007). "Research progress in Alzheimer's disease and dementia," in *Environmental Enrichment: from Mouse AD Model to AD Therapy, Vol. 3.* (New York, NY: Nova Science Publishers, Inc.), 303–328.

Lazarov, O., and Marr, R. A. (2010). Neurogenesis and Alzheimer's disease: at the crossroads *Exp. Neurol.* 223, 267–281. doi: 10.1016/j.expneurol.2009.08.009

Lazarov, O., and Marr, R. A. (2013). Of mice and men: neurogenesis, cognition and Alzheimer's disease. *Front. Aging Neurosci.* 5:43. doi: 10.3389/fnagi.2013.00043

Lazarov, O., Mattson, M. P., Peterson, D. A., Pimplikar, S. W., and van Praag, H. (2010). When neurogenesis encounters aging and disease. *Trends Neurosci.* 33, 569–579. doi: 10.1016/j.tins.2010.09.003

Lazarov, O., Robinson, J., Tang, Y. P., Hairston, I. S., Korade-Mirnics, Z., Lee, V. M., et al. (2005). Environmental enrichment reduces Abeta levels and amyloid deposition in transgenic mice. *Cell* 120, 701–713. doi: 10.1016/j.cell.2005.01.015

Lie, D. C., Colamarino, S. A., Song, H. J., Désiré, L., Mira, H., Consiglio, A., et al. (2005). Wnt signalling regulates adult hippocampal neurogenesis. *Nature* 437, 1370–1375. doi: 10.1038/nature04108

Llorens-Martin, M., Teixeira, C. M., Fuster-Matanzo, A., Jurado-Arjona, J., Borrell, V., Soriano, E., et al. (2012). Tau isoform with three microtubule binding domains is a marker of new axons generated from the subgranular zone in the hippocampal dentate gyrus: implications for Alzheimer's disease. *J. Alzheimers. Dis.* 29, 921–930. doi: 10.3233/JAD-2012-112057.

Loewenbruck, K. F., Fuchs, B., Hermann, A., Brandt, M., Werner, A., Kirsch, M., et al. (2011). Proton MR spectroscopy of neural stem cells: does the proton-NMR peak at 1.28 ppm function as a biomarker for cell type or state? *Rejuvenation Res.* 14, 371–381. doi: 10.1089/rej.2010.1102

Longo, F. M., Yang, T., Xie, Y., and Massa, S. M. (2006). Small molecule approaches for promoting neurogenesis. *Curr. Alzheimer Res.* 3, 5–10. doi: 10.2174/156720506775697089

Lugert, S., Basak, O., Knuckles, P., Haussler, U., Fabel, K., Götz, M., et al. (2010). Quiescent and active hippocampal neural stem cells with distinct morphologies respond selectively to physiological and pathological stimuli and aging. *Cell Stem Cell* 6, 445–456. doi: 10.1016/j.stem.2010.03.017

Ma, Q. L., Harris-White, M. E., Ubeda, O. J., Simmons, M., Beech, W., Lim, G. P., et al. (2007). Evidence of Abeta- and transgene-dependent defects in ERK-CREB signaling in Alzheimer's models. *J. Neurochem.* 103, 1594–1607. doi: 10.1111/j.1471-4159.2007.04869.x

MacMillan, K. S., Naidoo, J., Liang, J., Melito, L., Williams, N. S., Morlock, L., et al. (2011). Development of proneurogenic, neuroprotective small molecules. *J. Am. Chem. Soc.* 133, 1428–1437. doi: 10.1021/ja108211m

Manganas, L. N., Zhang, X., Li, Y., Hazel, R. D., Smith, S. D., Wagshul, M. E., et al. (2007). Magnetic resonance spectroscopy identifies neural progenitor cells in the live human brain. *Science* 318, 980–985. doi: 10.1126/science.1147851

Marathe, S., and Alberi, L. (2015). Notch in memories: points to remember. *Hippocampus* 25, 1481–1488. doi: 10.1002/hipo.22426

Marathe, S., Liu, S., Brai, E., Kaczarowski, M., and Alberi, L. (2015). Notch signaling in response to excitotoxicity induces neurodegeneration via erroneous cell cycle reentry. *Cell Death Differ.* 22, 1775–1784. doi: 10.1038/cdd.2015.23

Mayr, B., and Montminy, M. (2001). Transcriptional regulation by the phosphorylation-dependent factor CREB. *Nat. Rev. Mol. Cell Biol.* 2, 599–609. doi: 10.1038/35085068

McNeish, J., Roach, M., Hambor, J., Mather, R. J., Weibley, L., Lazzaro, J., et al. (2010). High-throughput screening in embryonic stem cell-derived neurons identifies potentiators of alpha-amino-3-hydroxyl-5-methyl-4-isoxazolepropionate-type glutamate receptors. *J. Biol. Chem.* 285, 17209–17217. doi: 10.1074/jbc.M109.098814

Merz, K., Herold, S., and Lie, D. C. (2011). CREB in adult neurogenesis–master and partner in the development of adult-born neurons? *Eur. J. Neurosci.* 33, 1078–1086. doi: 10.1111/j.1460-9568.2011.07606.x

Neely, M. D., Litt, M. J., Tidball, A. M., Li, G. G., Aboud, A. A., Hopkins, C. R., et al. (2012). DMH1, a highly selective small molecule BMP inhibitor promotes neurogenesis of hiPSCs: comparison of PAX6 and SOX1 expression during neural induction. *ACS Chem. Neurosci.* 3, 482–491. doi: 10.1021/cn300029t

Ninkovic, J., and Götz, M. (2007). Signaling in adult neurogenesis: from stem cell niche to neuronal networks. *Curr. Opin. Neurobiol.* 17, 338–344. doi: 10.1016/j.conb.2007.04.006

Ortega-Martínez, S. (2015). A new perspective on the role of the CREB family of transcription factors in memory consolidation via adult hippocampal neurogenesis. *Front. Mol. Neurosci.* 8:46. doi: 10.3389/fnmol.2015.00046

Ozgen, N., Lau, D. H., Shlapakova, I. N., Sherman, W., Feinmark, S. J., Danilo, P. Jr., et al. (2010). Determinants of CREB degradation and KChIP2 gene transcription in cardiac memory. *Heart Rhythm* 7, 964–970. doi: 10.1016/j.hrthm.2010.03.024

Petrik, D., Jiang, Y., Birnbaum, S. G., Powell, C. M., Kim, M. S., Hsieh, J., et al. (2012). Functional and mechanistic exploration of an adult neurogenesis-promoting small molecule. *FASEB J.* 26, 3148–3162. doi: 10.1096/fj.11-201426

Pieper, A. A., Xie, S., Capota, E., Estill, S. J., Zhong, J., Long, J. M., et al. (2010). Discovery of a proneurogenic, neuroprotective chemical. *Cell* 142, 39–51. doi: 10.1016/j.cell.2010.06.018

Pierfelice, T., Alberi, L., and Gaiano, N. (2011). Notch in the vertebrate nervous system: an old dog with new tricks. *Neuron* 69, 840–855. doi: 10.1016/j.neuron.2011.02.031

Porte, Y., Buhot, M. C., and Mons, N. (2008). Alteration of CREB phosphorylation and spatial memory deficits in aged 129T2/Sv mice. *Neurobiol. Aging* 29, 1533–1546. doi: 10.1016/j.neurobiolaging.2007.03.023

Rodríguez, J. J., Jones, V. C., Tabuchi, M., Allan, S. M., Knight, E. M., LaFerla, F. M., et al. (2008). Impaired adult neurogenesis in the dentate gyrus of a triple transgenic mouse model of Alzheimer's disease. *PLoS ONE* 3:e2935. doi: 10.1371/journal.pone.0002935

Ruscheweyh, R., Willemer, C., Krüger, K., Duning, T., Warnecke, T., Sommer, J., et al. (2011). Physical activity and memory functions: an interventional study. *Neurobiol. Aging* 32, 1304–1319. doi: 10.1016/j.neurobiolaging.2009.08.001

Sahay, A., Scobie, K. N., Hill, A. S., O'Carroll, C. M., Kheirbek, M. A., Burghardt, N. S., et al. (2011). Increasing adult hippocampal neurogenesis is sufficient to improve pattern separation. *Nature* 472, 466–470. doi: 10.1038/nature09817

Sato, N., Meijer, L., Skaltsounis, L., Greengard, P., and Brivanlou, A. H. (2004). Maintenance of pluripotency in human and mouse embryonic stem cells through activation of Wnt signaling by a pharmacological GSK-3-specific inhibitor. *Nat. Med.* 10, 55–63. doi: 10.1038/nm979

Schneider, J. W., Gao, Z., Li, S., Farooqi, M., Tang, T. S., Bezprozvanny, I., et al. (2008). Small-molecule activation of neuronal cell fate. *Nat. Chem. Biol.* 4, 408–410. doi: 10.1038/nchembio.95

Scott Bitner, R. (2012). Cyclic AMP response element-binding protein (CREB) phosphorylation: a mechanistic marker in the development of memory enhancing Alzheimer's disease therapeutics. *Biochem. Pharmacol.* 83, 705–714. doi: 10.1016/j.bcp.2011.11.009

Selkoe, D. J., and Wolfe, M. S. (2007). Presenilin: running with scissors in the membrane. *Cell* 131, 215–221. doi: 10.1016/j.cell.2007.10.012

Shi, J., Longo, F. M., and Massa, S. M. (2013). A small molecule p75(NTR) ligand protects neurogenesis after traumatic brain injury. *Stem Cells* 31, 2561–2574. doi: 10.1002/stem.1516

Shimizu, T., Kagawa, T., Inoue, T., Nonaka, A., Takada, S., Aburatani, H., et al. (2008). Stabilized beta-catenin functions through TCF/LEF proteins and the Notch/RBP-Jkappa complex to promote proliferation and suppress differentiation of neural precursor cells. *Mol. Cell Biol.* 28, 7427–7441. doi: 10.1128/MCB.01962-07

Silva-Vargas, V., Crouch, E. E., and Doetsch, F. (2013). Adult neural stem cells and their niche: a dynamic duo during homeostasis, regeneration, and aging. *Curr. Opin. Neurobiol.* 23, 935–942. doi: 10.1016/j.conb.2013.09.004

Spalding, K., Bergmann, O., Alkass, K., Bernard, S., Salehpour, M., Huttner, H., et al. (2013). Dynamics of hippocampal neurogenesis in adult humans *Cell.* 153, 1219–1227 doi: 10.1016/j.cell.2013.05.002

Stark, S. M., Yassa, M. A., and Stark, C. E. (2010). Individual differences in spatial pattern separation performance associated with healthy aging in humans. *Learn. Mem.* 17, 284–288. doi: 10.1101/lm.1768110

Sun, B., Halabisky, B., Zhou, Y., Palop, J. J., Yu, G., Mucke, L., et al. (2009). Imbalance between GABAergic and glutamatergic transmission impairs adult neurogenesis in an animal model of Alzheimer's Disease. *Cell Stem Cell* 5, 624–633. doi: 10.1016/j.stem.2009.10.003

Tesco, G., Kim, T. W., Diehlmann, A., Beyreuther, K., and Tanzi, R. E. (1998). Abrogation of the presenilin 1/beta-catenin interaction and preservation of the heterodimeric presenilin 1 complex following caspase activation. *J. Biol. Chem.* 273, 33909–33914. doi: 10.1074/jbc.273.51.33909

Tesco, G., and Tanzi, R. E. (2000). GSK3 beta forms a tetrameric complex with endogenous PS1-CTF/NTF and beta-catenin. Effects of the D257/D385A and FAD-linked mutations. *Ann. N.Y. Acad. Sci.* 920, 227–232. doi: 10.1111/j.1749-6632.2000.tb06927.x

Toner, C. K., Pirogovsky, E., Kirwan, C. B., and Gilbert, P. E. (2009). Visual object pattern separation deficits in nondemented older adults. *Learn. Mem.* 16, 338–342. doi: 10.1101/lm.1315109

Tseng, C. Y., Kao, S. H., Wan, C. L., Cho, Y., Tung, S. Y., and Hsu, H. J. (2014). Notch signaling mediates the age-associated decrease in adhesion of germline stem cells to the niche. *PLoS Genet.* 10:e1004888. doi: 10.1371/journal.pgen.1004888

van Praag, H., Christie, B. R., Sejnowski, T. J., and Gage, F. H. (1999a). Running enhances neurogenesis, learning, and long-term potentiation in mice. *Proc. Natl. Acad. Sci. U.S.A.* 96, 13427–13431. doi: 10.1073/pnas.96.23.13427

van Praag, H., Kempermann, G., and Gage, F. H. (1999b). Running increases cell proliferation and neurogenesis in the adult mouse dentate gyrus [see comments]. *Nat. Neurosci.* 2, 266–270. doi: 10.1038/6368

Villeda, S. A., Luo, J., Mosher, K. I., Zou, B., Britschgi, M., Bieri, G., et al. (2011). The ageing systemic milieu negatively regulates neurogenesis and cognitive function. *Nature* 477, 90–94. doi: 10.1038/nature10357

Villeda, S. A., and Wyss-Coray, T. (2013). The circulatory systemic environment as a modulator of neurogenesis and brain aging. *Autoimmun. Rev.* 12, 674–677. doi: 10.1016/j.autrev.2012.10.014

Vitolo, O. V., Sant'Angelo, A., Costanzo, V., Battaglia, F., Arancio, O., and Shelanski, M. (2002). Amyloid beta -peptide inhibition of the PKA/CREB pathway and long-term potentiation: reversibility by drugs that enhance cAMP signaling. *Proc. Natl. Acad. Sci. U.S.A.* 99, 13217–13221. doi: 10.1073/pnas.172504199

Wahlster, L., Arimon, M., Nasser-Ghodsi, N., Post, K. L., Serrano-Pozo, A., Uemura, K., et al. (2013). Presenilin-1 adopts pathogenic conformation in normal aging and in sporadic Alzheimer's disease. *Acta Neuropathol.* 125, 187–199. doi: 10.1007/s00401-012-1065-6

Wang, R., Dineley, K. T., Sweatt, J. D., and Zheng, H. (2004). Presenilin 1 familial Alzheimer's disease mutation leads to defective associative learning and impaired adult neurogenesis. *Neuroscience* 126, 305–312. doi: 10.1016/j.neuroscience.2004.03.048

Wang, W., Pan, Y. W., Zou, J., Li, T., Abel, G. M., Palmiter, R. D., et al. (2014). Genetic activation of ERK5 MAP kinase enhances adult neurogenesis and extends hippocampus-dependent long-term memory. *J. Neurosci.* 34, 2130–2147. doi: 10.1523/JNEUROSCI.3324-13.2014

Warner-Schmidt, J. L., and Duman, R. S. (2007). VEGF is an essential mediator of the neurogenic and behavioral actions of antidepressants. *Proc. Natl. Acad. Sci. U.S.A.* 104, 4647–4652. doi: 10.1073/pnas.0610282104

Wen, P. H., Hof, P. R., Chen, X., Gluck, K., Austin, G., Younkin, S. G., et al. (2004). The presenilin-1 familial Alzheimer disease mutant P117L impairs neurogenesis in the hippocampus of adult mice. *Exp. Neurol.* 188, 224–237. doi: 10.1016/j.expneurol.2004.04.002

Xia, D., Watanabe, H., Wu, B., Lee, S. H., Li, Y., Tsvetkov, E., et al. (2015). Presenilin-1 knockin mice reveal loss-of-function mechanism for familial Alzheimer's disease. *Neuron* 85, 967–981. doi: 10.1016/j.neuron.2015.02.010

Xia, X., Qian, S., Soriano, S., Wu, Y., Fletcher, A. M., Wang, X. J., et al. (2001). Loss of presenilin 1 is associated with enhanced beta-catenin signaling and skin tumorigenesis. *Proc. Natl. Acad. Sci. U.S.A.* 98, 10863–10868. doi: 10.1073/pnas.191284198

Yassa, M. A., Mattfeld, A. T., Stark, S. M., and Stark, C. E. (2011). Age-related memory deficits linked to circuit-specific disruptions in the hippocampus. *Proc. Natl. Acad. Sci. U.S.A.* 108, 8873–8878. doi: 10.1073/pnas.1101567108

Young-Pearse, T. L., Bai, J., Chang, R., Zheng, J. B., LoTurco, J. J., and Selkoe, D. J. (2007). A critical function for beta-amyloid precursor protein in neuronal migration revealed by in utero RNA interference. *J. Neurosci.* 27, 14459–14469. doi: 10.1523/JNEUROSCI.4701-07.2007

Young-Pearse, T. L., Chen, A. C., Chang, R., Marquez, C., and Selkoe, D. J. (2008). Secreted APP regulates the function of full-length APP in neurite outgrowth through interaction with integrin beta1. *Neural Dev.* 3:15. doi: 10.1186/1749-8104-3-15

5

Live Imaging of Adult Neural Stem Cells in Rodents

Felipe Ortega[1*] *and Marcos R. Costa*[2]

[1] *Biochemistry and Molecular Biology Department, Faculty of Veterinary Medicine, Complutense University, Madrid, Spain,*
[2] *Brain Institute, Federal University of Rio Grande do Norte, Natal, Brazil*

The generation of cells of the neural lineage within the brain is not restricted to early development. New neurons, oligodendrocytes, and astrocytes are produced in the adult brain throughout the entire murine life. However, despite the extensive research performed in the field of adult neurogenesis during the past years, fundamental questions regarding the cell biology of adult neural stem cells (aNSCs) remain to be uncovered. For instance, it is crucial to elucidate whether a single aNSC is capable of differentiating into all three different macroglial cell types *in vivo* or these distinct progenies constitute entirely separate lineages. Similarly, the cell cycle length, the time and mode of division (symmetric vs. asymmetric) that these cells undergo within their lineage progression are interesting questions under current investigation. In this sense, live imaging constitutes a valuable ally in the search of reliable answers to the previous questions. In spite of the current limitations of technology new approaches are being developed and outstanding amount of knowledge is being piled up providing interesting insights in the behavior of aNSCs. Here, we will review the state of the art of live imaging as well as the alternative models that currently offer new answers to critical questions.

Keywords: live imaging, aNSCs, neurogenic niches, timelapse videomicroscopy, lineage tracing

Edited by:
Laura López-Mascaraque, Instituto Cajal- Consejo Superior de Investigaciones Científicas, Spain

Reviewed by:
Olivier Raineteau, Institut National de la Santé et de la Recherche Médicale - Université de Lyon, France
Carlos Vicario-Abejón, Instituto Cajal, Consejo Superior de Investigaciones Científicas, Spain

***Correspondence:**
Felipe Ortega
fortegao@ucm.es

INTRODUCTION

Current Knowledge of the Cytoarchitecture of the Adult Neurogenic Niches; Subependymal Zone and Dentate Gyrus

Stem Cells are defined by their ability to self-renew, giving rise to new stem cells, and their capacity to generate diverse specialized cell types. In the adult nervous system, the term neural stem cells (NSCs) refers to cells that maintain the capacity to self-renew and generate neurons and macroglial cells both *in vitro* (Reynolds and Weiss, 1996; Costa et al., 2011) and *in vivo* (Lois and Alvarez-Buylla, 1993; Gould and Cameron, 1996; Kempermann et al., 1997; Menn et al., 2006; Sohn et al., 2015). Adult neural stem cells (aNSCs) continuously generate neurons oligodendrocytes and astrocytes in discrete niches in the brain, although it is unclear whether multipotent or unipotent aNSCs contribute all these different lineages. Historically, the adult neurogenesis has been associated, under physiological conditions, to two specific neurogenic niches: the subependymal zone (SEZ) in the lateral wall of the lateral ventricle, and the subgranular zone (SGZ) of the dentate gyrus in the hippocampus reviewed by Gage (2000) and Kriegstein and Alvarez-Buylla (2009). However, the presence of aNSCs in alternative domains of the adult brain should not be discarded. Indeed, multipotent progenitors have been isolated from the postnatal mouse cerebral cortex (Marmur et al., 1998; Belachew et al., 2003; Seaberg et al., 2005; Costa et al., 2007) or adult mouse cerebral cortex after traumatic and ischemic lesion

(Buffo et al., 2008; Sirko et al., 2013). Another interesting adult domain described to contain NSCs is the inner core of the olfactory bulb (OB) of both rodents and humans. Populations of NSCs expressing GFAP, Nestin, Sox2, and RC2 are located within the adult OB giving rise to neurons *in vivo*. Likewise they can be expanded *in vitro* as neurospheres, giving rise to astrocytes, oligodendrocytes and neurons. (Pagano et al., 2000; Gritti et al., 2002; Liu and Martin, 2003; Giachino and Taylor, 2009; Vergano-Vera et al., 2009; Moreno-Estelles et al., 2012). The same is applied for human temporal and frontal cortex, amygdala and hippocampus after resection due to a drug-resistant epilepsy, dysplasia, trauma, or brain edema (Arsenijevic et al., 2001). More recent evidence indicate that lesions may activate those "dormant" aNSCs through release of signaling molecules such as vascular endothelial growth factor (VEGF), basic fibroblast growth factor (bGFG), and sonic hedgehog (SHH; Sirko et al., 2013; Luo et al., 2015). Contribution of these quiescent aNSCs to a possible periodical and so far unnoticed turnover of their associated neuronal populations remains to be demonstrated **Figure 1**.

Focusing on the two main neurogenic niches of the adult brain, the SEZ harbors a population of aNSCs, known as type B cells, located beneath the ependymal cell layer of the lateral ventricles (Doetsch et al., 1999a,b). Type B has been proposed to share a common lineage with embryonic radial glia (RG) (Merkle et al., 2004). However, whether type B cells constitute the endpoint or RG lineage progression or whether the divergence arrives earlier is a matter of debate. Recent research went into detail about the relationship between RG and aNSCs (Fuentealba et al., 2015; Furutachi et al., 2015). Interestingly, evidences suggest that RG give rise to a subset of progenitors named pre-B1 cells at early stages of embryonic neural development (E 13.5-E 15.5). Pre-B1 cells remain quiescent until adulthood when they become reactivated. Furutachi and colleagues, points to the slowing down of the cell cycle of a subset of RG as the responsible for the origin to the adult pool of NSCs. Moreover, the cyclin-dependent kinase inhibitor p57 is proposed as the key regulator of the RG cell cycle. Selective deletion of p57 blocked the deceleration of the cell cycle, impairing the emergence of adult NSCs. These evidences are also supported by long-term *in vivo* experiments that described, using the STARTRACK tracing system, the presence of adult progenitors with embryonic origins (E-14), remaining as small, round and quiescent cells on the SEZ (Garcia-Marques and Lopez-Mascaraque, 2013). Type B cells are characterized by the expression of astroglial proteins such as the glial-fibrillary acidic protein (GFAP) and glutamate-aspartate transporter (GLAST; Doetsch et al., 1997; Platel et al., 2009). These cells contact the lateral ventricle through a single primary cilia located in the apical zone where they form junctional complexes among themselves (Mirzadeh et al., 2008). They also exhibit long basal processes that are closely associated with blood vessels, suggesting that vascular derived signals could play a role of the in the regulation of aNSC behavior (Mirzadeh et al., 2008; Shen et al., 2008; Tavazoie et al., 2008; Calvo et al., 2011). Regarding the cell cycle, type B cells are relatively quiescent (Doetsch et al., 1999a) but become activated giving rise to activated astroglia and type C cells or transit amplifying progenitors (TAPs; Pastrana et al., 2009; Costa et al., 2011). TAPs are more active in proliferation, undergoing several rounds of amplifying divisions (Costa et al., 2011; Ponti et al., 2013) before giving rise to neuroblasts or Type A cells. Subsequently, neuroblasts form a chain migrating along the rostral migratory stream toward the olfactory bulb (Lois et al., 1996). After reaching the olfactory bulb neuroblasts differentiate into different subtypes of neurons (Lledo et al., 2006; Fiorelli et al., 2015). The majority becomes GABAergic granule neurons and a minority becomes GABAergic periglomerular neurons. In addition, a small percentage of neuroblasts, generated in the dorsal wall of the SEZ, turn into short-axon glutamatergic, or GABAergic juxtaglomerular neurons (Kosaka and Kosaka, 2008; Brill et al., 2009; Kiyokage et al., 2010) Moreover, at least four subtypes of OB interneurons are generated at the anterior ventral SEZ, arising from microdomains that correlate with the expression domains of the Nkx6.2 and Zic family of transcription factors (Merkle et al., 2014).

Specific molecular markers to identify type B cells population have not been available for a long time. However recent publications employed interesting combinations of markers to differentiate between quiescent and activated type B cells, allowing for their isolation. Vascular cell adhesion molecule 1 (V-CAM1) has been recently described as a marker for quiescent type B cells (Kokovay et al., 2012). Likewise, combination of GFAP, prominin1 and the absence or presence of Epidermal growth factor (EGF) receptors has been suggested as a valid approach for isolation of quiescent and activated type B cells, respectively (Beckervordersandforth et al., 2010; Codega et al., 2014). The use of EGF fluorescent ligands, combined with the CD24 (Calaora et al., 1996) and GFAP expression has also been employed to successfully isolate aNSCs and their progeny from the SEZ (Pastrana et al., 2009). Along the same line, Daynac et al. (2015) employed a triple staining based on the stem cell marker Lewis X (LeX/ssea 1) (Capela and Temple, 2002), EGFR and the neuroblast marker CD24 to isolate the different populations comprised within the lineage progression.

Adult SEZ does not only provide the olfactory bulb with new neurons. In this region, astrocytes and oligodendrocytes are also generated and migrate toward the corpus callosum, rostral migratory stream, white matter tracts of the striatum and the fimbria fornix, under both physiological conditions (Hack et al., 2005; Menn et al., 2006; Gonzalez-Perez and Alvarez-Buylla, 2011; Sohn et al., 2015; Tong et al., 2015), and demyelinating pathologies (Picard-Riera et al., 2002).

The other main area of neurogenesis in the adult brain is the SGZ, which produce dentate gyrus granular neurons involved in learning and memory (Shors et al., 2002; Zhao et al., 2008). This area, located at the interface of the granule cell layer and the hilus, harbors two types of neuronal progenitors. Type 1 progenitors display a radial glia-like morphology with a long process that crosses the entire granule cell layer and small processes horizontally oriented along the SGZ. These progenitors are characterized by the expression of GFAP, Nestin, and Sox2 (Seri et al., 2001; Fukuda et al., 2003; Garcia et al., 2004). Type 2 is the second population of progenitors that may arise from type 1 cells, have only short processes and lack GFAP expression. Type

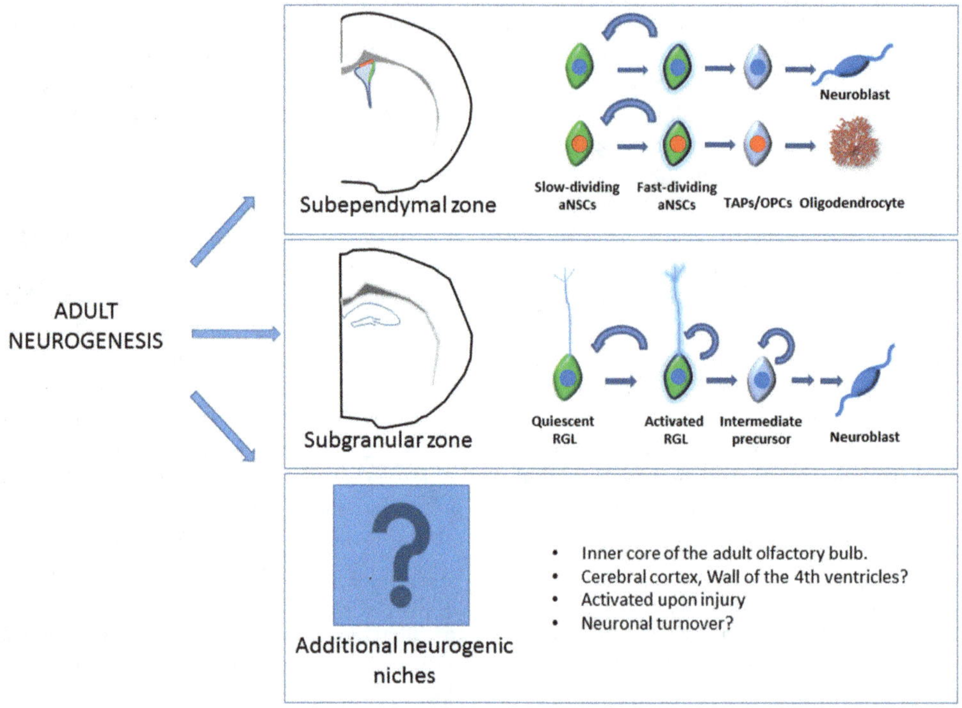

FIGURE 1 | Schematic representation of the adult neurogenesis. Here there are depicted the two main adult neurogenic niches, the subependymal zone in the lateral wall of the lateral ventricle and the subgranular zone in the hippocampus. Live imaging experiments have shown than within the SEZ, neurogenic, and oligodendrogliogenic lineage follows a similar pattern of lineage progression but constitutes independent lineages. Slow dividing astroglia (quiescent type B cells) give rise to fast dividing astroglia (activated type B cells) that subsequently generates Transit amplifying progenitors (TAPs) and finally neuroblast or oligodendrocytes. In the SGZ, quiescent radial glia like (RGL) progenitors become activated giving rise to intermediate progenitors and neuroblast that undergoes a complex process of maturation. Additional neurogenic niches like the olfactory bulb or the cerebral cortex have also been reported. The existence of undiscovered neurogenic niches should not be discarded. Several regions of the adult brain reactivate "dormant" aNSCs through signaling pathways released upon injury. Likewise, contribution of these quiescent aNSCs to the periodical turnover of neural populations still remains to be demonstrated.

1 and Type 2 progenitors give rise to intermediate progenitors, which in turn generate neuroblasts (Filippov et al., 2003; Fukuda et al., 2003). Subsequently, immature neurons migrate to the inner granule cell layer and differentiate into dentate granule cells in the hippocampus projecting axons through the hilus toward the CA3 region. These newborn neurons undergo a long process of maturation acquiring finally the electrophysiological and functional properties of their mature partners (reviewed by Ming and Song, 2011; Mongiat and Schinder, 2011; Kempermann et al., 2015).

The regulation of the cell fate specification of aNSCs is a critical point of discussion in which the balance between the role of intrinsic and extrinsic/environmental signaling is still not fully clarified. Recent studies have shown that within the SEZ internal programs would have a dominant role. According to these studies, SEZ seems to be highly regionalized, with neuronal progeny of distinct identity being generated at different areas along the dorsoventral and rostrocaudal axes (Hack et al., 2005; Merkle et al., 2007; Brill et al., 2009). Thus, aNSCs from the SEZ could be intrinsically specified on the basis of their location and they may display a limited potential of differentiation. Progenitors located along the SGZ on the other hand, seem to be more instructed by their microenvironment signals, regardless of the regional origin of the NSCs. For a detailed review of the existing knowledge of adult neurogenesis and the molecular mechanisms controlling it see (Zhao et al., 2008; Kriegstein and Alvarez-Buylla, 2009; Suh et al., 2009; Ming and Song, 2011).

In contrast to this more deterministic view, growing evidence suggest that SEZ progenitors exhibit a higher degree of plasticity, retaining the potential to generate larger diversity of neuronal subtypes (Sequerra et al., 2013; Fiorelli et al., 2015). Indeed, SHH signaling in the ventral SEZ is necessary for the generation of ventral-associated OB neurons (Ihrie et al., 2011; Merkle et al., 2014). Disruption of the SHH signaling redirects the ventral progenitors to a more dorsal cell fate, whereas overexpression of Smoothened leads to a "ventralization" of the dorsal SEZ (Ihrie et al., 2011). Likewise, exposure of postnatal and adult SEZ explants to an embryonic cortical environment, triggered an enhanced generation of glutamatergic neurons in addition to the predominant GABAergic subtypes (Sequerra et al., 2010). In addition, infusion of gamma amino butyric acid (GABA) into the OB induces the differentiation of newly generated cells into dopaminergic neurons (Akiba et al., 2009), suggesting a role for electrical activity in fate specification of those neurons. Thus, a parsimonious explanation for those data is that adult NSCs inherit genetic patterning of the embryonic RG (Merkle et al., 2007; Fuentealba et al., 2015), but this pattern is actively maintained by morphogenic signals and electrical activity in the adult SVZ. Changes in the external conditions could drive aNSCs into different neuronal lineages despite their embryonic origin and location in the SEZ.

Live Imaging of Adult Neural Stem Cells: Applications and Limitations

Understanding the mechanisms controlling the lineage progression of the adult neural stem cells (aNSCs) is critical for the future design of therapies against neurodegenerative diseases. However, the majority of the current knowledge regarding adult neurogenesis comes from population studies *in vivo*, leaving critical questions regarding the cell biology of the aNSCs unsolved. For example, how stem cells enact the decisions of self-renewal and differentiation on a single cell level is far from being understood. In fact, there is an ongoing discussion in the stem cell field whether such fate decisions are stochastic or deterministic in nature. Likewise, it is a matter of intense debate the concept of multipotency regarding aNSCs, i.e., whether a single aNSC is capable of differentiating into all the different cell types within their lineage or these distinct progenies constitute entirely separate lineages instead. Several studied reported that aNSCs exhibit multipotency when isolated *in vitro* from both rodents (Reynolds and Weiss, 1996; Gritti et al., 2002; Reynolds and Rietze, 2005; Vergano-Vera et al., 2009) and human brain (Sanai et al., 2004). However, this conclusion is mostly supported by experiments using the neurosphere assay, which has important caveats for assessing clonality (Singec et al., 2006; Pastrana et al., 2011). Moreover, as we will discuss in more details below, those studies also share the common feature of continuous exposure to mitogen factors, which can exert confounding effects on cell fate decisions (Doetsch et al., 2002; Costa et al., 2011). In contrast, recent evidences points to a more restricted outcome of the lineage progression, suggesting the bi-potency or even unipotency as the main hallmark of aNSCs in both the SEZ and the DG (Bonaguidi et al., 2011; Encinas et al., 2011; Ortega et al., 2013; Calzolari et al., 2015). That opens an interesting debate of which factors (as suggested by Ravin et al., 2008; Vergano-Vera et al., 2009) may re-direct the NSCs toward multipotency. Similarly, it is crucial to understand the mechanisms instructing aNSCs toward a specific cell fate *in vivo* and whether distinct populations of aNSCs contributing neurons or macroglial cells show different behaviors in lineage progression, such as cell cycle length, mode of cell division, and number of cell divisions (symmetric vs. asymmetric; Costa et al., 2011; Ortega et al., 2011, 2013; Ponti et al., 2013). Improved knowledge regarding all these questions will be determinant to understand how the generation of neurons, astrocytes, and oligodendrocytes is regulated in the adult germinative niches, allowing for the design of future therapeutic strategies focused on the replenishment of the cell loss due to pathological scenarios.

Lineage tracing, the identification, and monitoring of all the progeny of a single progenitor hold the key to elucidate these crucial interrogations. Ideal lineage tracing implies label retaining and specific marking of the founder of the clone (aNSC) and all its progeny without spreading the labeling to unrelated cells and without modifying the aNSC/progeny behavior. Several approaches have been used in order to perform lineage tracing: Dyes and radioactive tracers, viral transduction, transplantation, genetic recombination, and multicolor reporter constructs were used both *in vivo* and *in vitro*, in order to follow the NSCs and their progeny (reviewed by Kretzschmar and Watt, 2012). All these techniques enclose positive aspects but imply one main and critical drawback: the results and conclusions are based on still pictures along the lineage progression without comprising the whole sequence. This means that cell death, diffusion, dilution, spreading or low efficiency of the markers, among other important shortcomings could lead to incorrect conclusions **Figure 2**.

Although, constituting one of the oldest strategies for lineage tracing (Conklin, 1905; Sulston et al., 1983), live imaging followed by single cell tracking remains as the ideal method for the study of aNSCs lineage progression. Indeed, continuous observation of cell lineages over time allows studying the precise relations between a founder aNSC and its final clone, depicting in detail, with the adequate temporal resolution(Ravin et al., 2008; Eilken et al., 2009; Rieger et al., 2009), every intermediate step during the lineage progression. Using live imaging techniques *in vitro* we could predict crucial characteristics of the aNSCs cell biology (Costa et al., 2011; Ortega et al., 2011) later confirmed by BrdU-chasing or multicolor based clonal analysis *in vivo* (Ortega et al., 2013; Ponti et al., 2013; Calzolari et al., 2015). However, technical issues currently limit a comprehensive analysis of aNSCs lineage progression *in vivo* (see discussion below). Here, we will review some of the current techniques that have been developed to study the biology of the aNSCs by using live imaging in combination with single cell tracking. We will highlight the main advantages and limitations of both *in vitro* and *in vivo* approaches and discuss possible future directions toward a full understanding of aNSCs behavior, a crucial requirement in order to design future therapy strategies.

LIVE IMAGING OF aNSCs *IN VITRO*

Before describing in detail the present *in vitro* analysis that applied live imaging to the study of aNSCs, it is important to mention that the majority of the *in vitro* studies using aNSCs has been carried out by using the classical *in vitro* test for stem cell self-renewal, the neurosphere assay (Reynolds and Rietze, 2005). This method has been widely used to identify NSCs based on their capacity to evaluate self-renewal and differentiation at the single-cell level *in vitro*. However, as already discussed, several evidence indicate that the neurosphere assay may not be appropriate (Singec et al., 2006; Pastrana et al., 2011). Among several problems, is especially important the fact that clonality is not always guaranteed. Moreover, quiescent stem cells may not be detected by the neurosphere assay, in fact it was demonstrated that EGFR positive cells, i.e., activated type B cells and TAPs, are responsible for the generation of neurospheres (Doetsch et al., 2002; Pastrana et al., 2009). This clearly demonstrate that neurosphere assay does not reflect

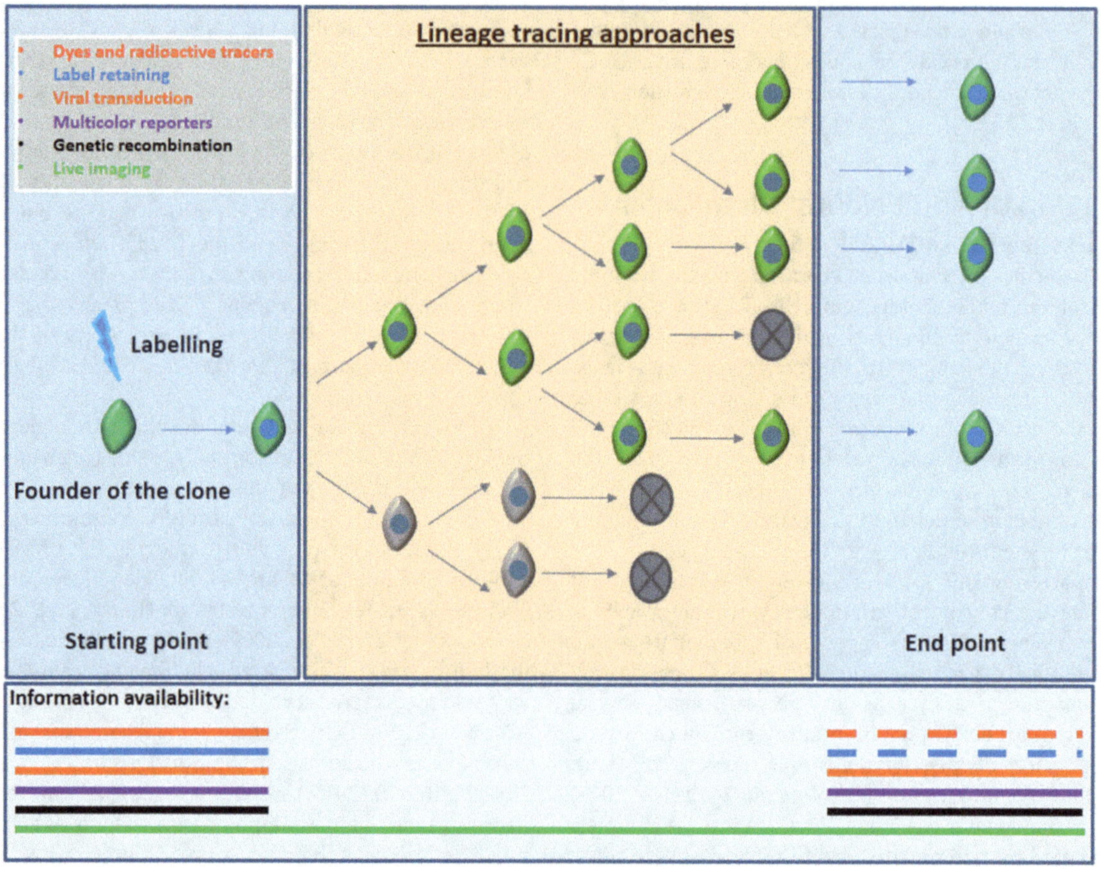

FIGURE 2 | Information available according to the lineage tracing approach employed. Most of the lineage tracers implies a readout based on static end-point experiments. That implies that information regarding cell death, proliferation, differentiation, cell fate decisions, and migration inside or outside of the field of view of cell populations might be missing. Discontinuous segments of lines depict the lack of information that may also occur when using dyes or label retaining due to the dilution of the signal after several rounds of proliferation. Conversely, direct observation by live imaging allows for the visualization of each event from the founder of the clone, till the clone is formed improving the strength of the conclusions obtained from the experiment.

an accurate readout of the number of stem cells *in vivo*. In addition, this approach does not allow addressing the question of the stem cell mode of cell division due to its high cell density. Finally, the assay depends on the exposure of NSCs to mitogenic growth factors with their well-known confounding effects on cell fate decisions (Doetsch et al., 2002; Costa et al., 2011).

Therefore, live imaging of aNSCs required the development of new methods to perform successful and reliable single cell tracking. As we previously mentioned, the ideal situation would be the long-term imaging of single cells in whole living organisms, in real time and using several molecular readouts. However, the present available technology makes impossible the long-range immobilization of the organism as well as the access to the adult neurogenic areas (SEZ and SGZ) without the employment of highly invasive, and thus non-viable, approaches. In contrast, live imaging can be performed up to weeks *in vitro*, which allows for the analysis and manipulation of several molecular properties of aNSCs. Moreover, *in vitro* analysis provides crucial information regarding cell morphology, cell growth, migration, cell divisions patterns, cell cycle length, and cell fate decisions undergone by aNSCs (Costa et al., 2011).

There are several requirements to perform a good quality long-term live imaging experiment (reviewed in Schroeder, 2011). Live imaging followed by single cell tracking requires a complex balance between the imaging optimizations and the viability of the culture. Long or frequent exposition to excitation light, periodical changes in cell culture medium, adequate regulation of the gas composition of the incubator, among others, are technical aspects that may influence cell stress and toxicity. Moreover, the researcher has to establish carefully the settings of several peripheral components. For example, long-term live imaging requires adequate microscope systems. Bright-field and phase contrast are the systems most frequently used, in combination with motorized components that make possible a level of automation, indispensable for long term experiments (i.e., stages, shutters, and filters). Likewise the researcher has to count on incubation and permeable plates system able to keep the correct conditions of CO_2 saturation and pH during the developing of the assay. Furthermore, the correct storage and subsequent processing of the results (i.e., images) requires expeditious hardware and software to deal properly with the huge amount of data that implies an experiment of live imaging. Finally, the accomplishment of the live imaging experiments depends often on the availability of specific fluorescent markers that allow the identification of the target population in real-time (Eilken et al., 2014).

Combining long term time-lapse video-microscopy with cultures seeded at clonal density Qian and colleagues provided important improvements in the knowledge of the behavior of embryonic NSCs. Culturing embryonic day (E)13 murine NSCs in medium supplemented with FGF2 they observed that the majority of the clones produced mainly neuroblast. These clones formed a heterogeneous population regarding their capacity of division, undergoing different rounds of amplifying divisions prior to the neuronal differentiation. Moreover, they were able to identify lineages containing both "neuroblast" and "glioblast" progenitors in these cultures (Qian et al., 1998). Lately, the use of time-lapse video-microscopy revealed that the production of neurons and glia followed a defined temporal pattern. Live imaging of different time points of embryonic NSCs isolated in culture indicated that neuroblast are generated first, whereas glia arise later. Furthermore, they confirmed that after the production of neuroblast and glioblast, NSCs in culture acquire features of postnatal progenitors, modifying their response to EGF (Qian et al., 2000). Recently, embryonic cultures (E12.5) in combination with time-lapse video-microscopy and computational processing and tracking have also been employed to elucidate behavioral differences between anterior (motor cortex-related) and posterior (visual cortex-related) neural progenitors (Winter et al., 2015). Single cell tracking of both populations indicate that posterior cortical progenitors exhibit higher speed in the cell cycle, increased cell size, and more motility than the anterior ones. As a consequence of the difference in the cell cycle length, the posterior progenitors generates larger clones that the anterior counterparts.

Clonal density cultures have been also used to image the lineage progression of rat or zebrafish embryonic retinal progenitor cells. Live imaging of single clones, controlling the composition of the extracellular environment and restricting completely the interaction between different clones demonstrated an unexpected degree of stochasticity in the progenitors regarding the decision between proliferation or differentiation into the different cell types located in the retina (Gomes et al., 2011; He et al., 2012). As we described previously for the aNSCs located in the SEZ, exits also an important line of research in retina suggesting that within the progenitor pool of the retina there is an important molecular heterogeneity. This heterogeneity would be determined by the presence of intrinsic genetic programs but also as a plastic response of progenitors to the influence of instructive extrinsic signals as Notch, Shh, GDF11 etc. (Cepko et al., 1996; Livesey and Cepko, 2001; Cayouette et al., 2006; Riesenberg et al., 2009).

Several modifications have been developed in order to improve the efficiency of the live imaging protocols. The use of extracellular matrix proteins in the coating defined a limited area where the cells are allowed to grow, creating then, a restricted environment that make the live imaging easier and more accurate. Combining this method with the manufacturing of a culture chamber that controls media and gas exchange over the microscope stage, Ravin and colleagues performed long term timelapse video-microscopy of E-14.5 NSCs. Manual reconstruction of the NSCs lineage trees revealed that under these culture conditions and in presence of FGF2, tripotent NSCs generate unipotent progenitors through an intermediate bipotent step, involving short phases of self-renewal within each independent stage. They also demonstrate that periodical passage of the progenitors in culture retrieve the tripotent capacity to the NSCs (Ravin et al., 2008).

Other significant improvements in the live imaging of NSCs involve techniques that allow the combination of time-lapse video-microscopy and single cell tracking in high density cultures instead of the previous clonal density. The application of these methods to the embryonic NSCs rendered the discovery of a new population of progenitors located in the marginal zone of the mouse cerebral cortex. This new embryonic niche harbors oligodendrogliogenic, astrogliogenic, and neurogenic progenitors as well as some bipotent NSCs (Costa et al., 2007). Another example was the descriptions of the role of Par-complex proteins in the lineage progression of embryonic NSCs (Costa et al., 2008). Par-complex proteins exhibit an apical gradual expression, being enriched in the ventricular radial glia and decreasing subsequently along the neurogenesis process. Time-lapse video-microscopy demonstrated that gain of function of Par3/Par6 proteins promoted self-renewal of ventricular progenitors whereas loss of function forced them to exit the cell cycle, regulating then, their mode of cell division (Costa et al., 2008). Finally, the use of high density cultures to further study the cell fate switch undergone by cortical NSCs during embryogenesis demonstrated that virtually all cortical progenitors generate neurons before giving rise to glia-committed progenitors (Costa et al., 2009).

Several researchers have tried to establish an automated method of tracking the lineage progression once the live imaging is accomplished. Different computational methods have been tested in murine embryonic NSCs cultures in order to monitor automatically the migration, proliferation, and cell growth of the clones along the timelapse video-microscopy, generating a lineage tree as a read out (Al-Kofahi et al., 2006; Winter et al., 2011). Likewise, Cohen and colleagues employed an automated algorithmic-information-theory-based method in order to obtain morphological and behavioral patterns. This data was used to predict with high levels of accuracy the mode of division (self-renewal vs. differentiation) and the cell fate decision (generated progeny) of rat retinal progenitors cells in culture (Cohen et al., 2010). However is important to mention here that, in contrast to retinal progenitors, most of the stem cells do not display an obvious characteristic morphology immediately after plating or along the culture. Although, some important improvements have been achieved in orders to reduce human validation in embryonic NSC cultures at clonal density (Winter et al., 2011, 2015), culture of NSCs requires often higher cell density, leading to a fast expansion and mixing of the clones generated depicting a much more complex scenario where current automated methods produce too many errors and requires of inevitable manual correction and interaction.

In contrast to their embryonic counterparts, aNSCs were mostly studied using neurosphere assay and other few culture systems conveying high concentrations of mitogenic factors (FGF2, EGF, or both) in culture medium. As we previously mentioned, these factors induce important alterations in the behavior of aNSCs (Doetsch et al., 2002; Costa et al., 2011) and may lead to inaccurate conclusions regarding the potency of these cells. Likewise, the use of live imaging on the study of the lineage progression of NSCs has long been restricted to the field of embryonic development, due to the technical limitations involved in singe-cell tracking in the neurosphere assay. To overcome these limitations, several laboratories developed adherent SEZ cultures that replicate some aspects of the SEZ *in vivo* (Lim and Alvarez-Buylla, 1999; Scheffler et al., 2005). Scheffler et al. reported an adherent culture, which involves expansion of stem/precursor cells in presence of EGF/FGF2 prior to differentiation (Scheffler et al., 2005). However, following this protocol, neural stem cells adopt tumorigenic properties (Walton et al., 2009), an effect that can be attributed to growth factor treatment (Kuhn et al., 1997; Doetsch et al., 2002). Lim and Alvarez-Buylla developed an interesting strategy of co-culturing adult SEZ cells with postnatal astroglia, which circumvent the necessity of growth factors for maintaining proliferation and neurogenesis. However, the requirement of such astroglial feeder introduces new uncontrollable variables: astroglia themselves secrete both growth factors and extracellular matrix molecules, likely affecting the intrinsic properties of adult neural stem cells; they introduce direct cell-contact mediated effects; they preclude analyse of direct effects of both intrinsic and extrinsic factor over SEZ cells, as astroglia feeder cells would also be affected; finally, due to the high cell density in such co-cultures single cell tracking becomes more cumbersome.

To circumvent these limitations, we recently developed a new method of culturing adult NSCs under adherent conditions and in absence of mitogenic factors (Costa et al., 2011; Ortega et al., 2011; see **Table 1**). Using this culture method, it was possible to monitor in real-time the lineage progression of aNSCs isolated from the lateral wall of the SEZ up to several days (Costa et al., 2011; Ponti et al., 2013). This technique allowed the direct observation of the intermediate steps between the progression from aNSCs to neurons: slow-dividing astroglia (type B cells) give rise to fast-dividing astroglia, which in turns generates TAPs. TAPs undergo subsequently several (up to 5) rounds of division giving rise to post-mitotic neuroblast in an orderly manner. These observations are in accordance with the sequence proposed by population-based studies *in vivo* (Doetsch et al., 1999a), but added two new pieces of information: (i) slow-dividing astroglia generate fast-dividing astroglial cells before TAPs and (ii) the number of cell divisions from aNSCs to the final neuronal progeny is limited. Moreover, this live-imaging system allowed the direct observation of asymmetric cell divisions within the lineage of aNSCs, providing a unique model for the study of NSC self-renewal. Interestingly, the asymmetry in the lineage is not observed in the first aNSC division, but rather at later points in the lineage. Finally, we could observe morphological changes characteristic of each cell type, such as the substantial cell growth prior to cell division of aNSCs, and the high motility of immature bipolar neuroblasts shortly after cell division.

This method was also applied to the study of other cell population generated in the adult SEZ, the oligodendrocytes (Menn et al., 2006; Gonzalez-Perez and Alvarez-Buylla, 2011). When the lateral and dorsal wall of the adult SEZ were cultured

TABLE 1 | Different methods employed for lineage tracing of aNSCs, highlighting some of their strongest advantages, and main weaknesses.

	Method	Strongest adventage	Main weakness
Cells not monitored by live imaging	Retroviral vector	Allows to label dividing cells *in vivo* and *in vitro*.	The entire clone is not labeled. Cell death, migration away of a labeled cell, or immigration of a non-related labeled cells to the field of view are not discriminated.
	Genetic recombination and multicolor reporter systems	Allows to discriminate clonally while labeling high numbers of progenitors.	Cell death, migration away of a labeled cell, or immigration of a non-related labeled cells to the field of view are not discriminated.
	Classical neurosphere assay	Classical assay to evaluate NSCs hallmarks. (Self-renewal and differentiation capacity).	Does not ensure clonality, does not guarantee to monitor the slow dividing NSCs. Mitogen factors exerts confounding effects on the NSCs.
Cells monitored by live imaging	*In vitro* live imaging in presence of feeder layers/mitogen factors	Allows for continuous monitoring. Presence of niche factors.	Mitogen factors exerts confounding effects on the NSCs.
	Mitogen-free *in vitro* live imaging system	Allows for continuous monitoring. Perfect tool to evaluate the effect of each niche factor at a time. *In vivo* studies confirm their conclusions.	Absence of niche environment.
	Live imaging by brain slices	Allows for continuous monitoring. Preserves neurogenic niche.	Usually comprises high doses of serum in the preparation protocol. Restricted time of preservation of the neurogenic niche properties.
	Live imaging *in vivo*	Intact neurogenic niche in an intact brain environment.	Not yet developed for a single cell resolution.

together, an increase in the number of oligodendroglial cells was observed, indicating, and enrichment of oligodendrogliogenic aNSCs in the dorsal aspect of the SEZ (Ortega et al., 2013). Timelapse video microscopy followed by single cell tracking revealed that aNSCs generating oligodendroglial progeny *in vitro* share several hallmarks (cell growth, slow cell cycle, etc.) with neurogenic aNSCs. Moreover, oligodendrogliogenic and the neurogenic aNSCs constitute strictly separate lineages, giving rise to either neurons and glia or oligodendrocytes and glia, respectively. Interestingly, we observed that the oligodendrogliogenic progeny is selectively activated by Wnt canonical signaling, known to be particularly prominent in the dorsal SEZ *in vivo* (Marinaro et al., 2012). Presence of Wnt recombinant proteins in the culture medium increased the rounds of amplifying divisions undergone by oligodendroglial progenitors by shortening their cell cycle. The expansion of the oligodendrogliogenic lineage induced by Wnt signaling within the SEZ has also been corroborated *in vivo* in both the adult (Ortega et al., 2013) and the postnatal (Azim et al., 2014) SEZ. It will be interesting to study the lineage progression of aNSCs when exposed to other extrinsic factors known to affect neurogenesis and oligodendrogenesis in the SEZ, such as BMP (ventral; Colak et al., 2008) and Shh (dorsal; Merkle et al., 2014; Tong et al., 2015).

One of the main criticisms regarding the study of cell behavior in culture is precisely that the progenitors are isolated from their "stem cell niche environment." Therefore, important signals that regulate the aNSCs lineage progression could be missing and then, their behavior could be altered. Nevertheless, live-imaging of adherent SEZ cells under serum-free culture conditions allow to reproduce important steps in the lineage-progression of aNSCs and to describe new phenomena previously unnoticed (Costa et al., 2011; Ortega et al., 2011). In fact, results *in vivo* (Ponti et al., 2013) confirmed our observations *in vitro* (Costa et al., 2011) regarding aNSCs lineage progression and the number of cell divisions enacted in the lineage, indicating that important features of aNSCs are maintained in our culture system, despite the absence of niche signals. It is likely that SEZ cells isolated and observed in our experiments had already received environmental influences and the main merit of the system is not to use factor affecting the development of cell lineages.

Organotypic-slice cultures also constitute an interesting *ex-vivo* approach to study cell-divison and migration over short periods of time in embryonic (Noctor et al., 2004), posnatal (Raineteau et al., 2004; Namba et al., 2007; Yokose et al., 2011), and adult brain (Kamada et al., 2004). Combination of organotypic cultures, time-lapse microscopy, and two-photon microscopy uncovered interesting features of the motility of the SEZ-derived neuroblast (Nam et al., 2007; James et al., 2011). Contrary to expectations, it was shown that neuroblast migratory chains remain stable and immotile for longer periods. Moreover, brain slice cultures were also employed to demonstrate that adult NSCs are capable to regulate the local blood flow within the neurogenic niche by releasing ATP and vasodilating factors (Lacar et al., 2012). Organotypic cultures were also used to described alternatives models of oligodendrocytic-dependent myelination (Sobottka et al., 2011). However, to the best of our knowledge, aNSC lineage progression has not been comprehensively studied in organotypic culture. One important challenge in this system is to maintain healthy slices over long periods of time. In fact, neural precursors have a limited capacity to differentiate into neurons and the structural integrity of the neurogenic niche seems to be compromised during the culture period (Namba et al., 2007). One possible explanation to these problems is the high concentration of serum required to keep slices alive. Lastly, it is important to consider that the different steps observed in the aNSC lineage start in the SEZ, progress over the RMS and end in the olfactory bulb. Therefore, the slice must keep all these structures intact and the live-imaging set up to follow all those steps must be able to image cells at long distances. Nevertheless, we believe that organotypic cultures could be improved, allowing longer survival periods and more physiologic neurogenic rates, and then used to monitor aNSC behavior within the SEZ.

LIVE IMAGING OF aNSCs *IN VIVO*

As discussed in the previous sections, one potential pitfall of studying aNSCs *in vitro* could be the absence of the niche. In fact, organotypic-slice cultures may keep some local relations, but do not maintain long-distance axonal influences involved in the control of aNSCs behavior (Tong et al., 2014). Thus, the perfect situation would be to be able to image aNSCs within their niche under physiological conditions *in vivo*. However, imaging techniques so far available to image the brain *in vivo* do not allow the study of aNSCs in a single-cell manner.

Up to date, there are three main imaging techniques used to image NSCs and neurogenesis in the adult live brain: Magnetic resonance imaging/spectroscopy (MRI/MRS); Positron emission tomography (PET); and optical imaging (fluorescence and bioluminiscence). However, as discussed below, each of these techniques has limitations that preclude their use to study the behavior of single cells in the live brain.

MRI offers a relatively high morphological resolution in deep regions of the brain (78 × 78 × 370 μm) (Weber et al., 2006). However, this resolution does not allow studying single cells. In fact, MRI has been mostly used to evaluate volumetric modifications in regions where neurogenesis occurs under physiological or pathological conditions and to correlate these changes with possible alterations in the rate of neurogenesis (Couillard-Despres and Aigner, 2011).

To identify specific cell population using MRI, some researches have used iron oxide particle labeling of neural stem and precursors cells *in vitro* and then transplanting labeled cells into aNSC niches *in vivo* (Hoehn et al., 2002). Using this technique, it has been possible to image transplanted cells over several weeks in the host brains and follow their migration. However, *in vitro* labeling of cells may lead to changes in several properties of the cells, hampering the enthusiasm regarding the use of such technique to study the physiological behavior of aNSCs.

In order to overcome this limitation, some groups have attempted to label endogenous neural stem/precursos cells *in vivo* through the injection of iron particles directly into the lateral ventricles or in the subventricular zone. These works have shown that particles can be uptaken by migrating neuroblasts, allowing the observation of their migration toward the olfactory bulb by MRI. Thus, particle-labeling of cells is a promising technique to study adult neurogenesis *in vivo* by non-invasive imaging (Panizzo et al., 2009; Granot et al., 2011; Iordanova and Ahrens, 2012).

Nevertheless, several issues must be taken into consideration in these studies: (i) uptake of particles by SVZ cells is unspecific, in other words, it is not possible to distinguish which type of cell (ependymal, type B, C, or A cell) is being observed; (ii) injection of iron particles *in vivo* may lead to cell toxicity (Crabbe et al., 2010; Vreys et al., 2010); and (iii) iron particles may be uptaken by other cells following death of the primary-carrier cells, which could cause a great confusion in the analysis of data. Together, these technical issues embody serious limitations to the use of MRI to study aNSC behavior *in vivo*.

An elegant way to identify specific cell populations has been proposed by Manganas et al. (2007). They used MRS to identify possible "metabolic biomarkers" for different cell types in the adult hippocampus. For example, they reported a MRS peak, detected at 1.28 ppm (parts per million), which seemed to correlate with the presence of neural stem cells (Manganas et al., 2007). The authors reported an increase in the 1.28-ppm biomarker in the dentate gyrus of rodents following electric convulsive shock, which could be interpreted as a sign for increased endogenous neurogenesis. Conversely, they described a reduction of the 1.28-ppm biomarker in the hippocampus of adult humans, as compared to preadolescents and adolescents. Based on these findings, they concluded that the 1.28-ppm biomarker could be applied to track and analyze endogenous NSCs *in vivo* (Manganas et al., 2007). However, Ramm et al. (2009) demonstrated that the 1.28-ppm peak was also evident in mesenchymal stem cells and in non-stem cell lines. Notably, this peak could only be observed in neural progenitor cells cultured under conditions favoring growth arrest or apoptosis, suggesting that such peak could be caused by the appearance of mobile lipid droplets during apoptosis (Ramm et al., 2009). Therefore, the validity of the 1.28-ppm biomarker as a measure for NSCs and neurogenesis requires additional evidence.

PET has also been used to study neurogenesis in the rodent adult brain (Rueger et al., 2010). Using the ^{18}F-labeled 3′-deoxy-3′-fluorothymidine (FLT), a thymidine analog incorporated to newly synthesized DNA molecules, they could observe an increase in the PET signal both in the hippocampus and subventricular regions in the ipsilateral hemisphere subjected to ischaemic lesion (Rueger et al., 2010). However, although such increase has been interpreted as readout for augmented neurogenesis, the signal intensity observed in the hippocampus and SVZ seemed very similar, even though neurogenesis in the SVZ is 10-100 times higher. One possible explanation for this discrepancy could be the low resolution of PET in comparison to MRI.

Needless to say, incorporation of ^{18}F-FLT is unspecific and, consequently, does not allow the identification of cell types imaged by PET. Thus, the use this technique to study endogenous NSCs and neurogenesis *in vivo* remains a forthcoming alternative.

Compared to MRI/MRS and PET, optical imaging based in fluorescence or bioluminescence is a cheaper and more versatile method to study cells *in vivo*. Using any microscope equipped for epifluorescence acquisition, for instance, it is possible to exploit all the advantages of transgenic animals expressing fluorescent proteins controlled by specific promoters or virally-transduced markers, prompting the identification of specific cell types, and achieve resolution sufficient for morphological studies at cellular and subcellular levels.

Although, light penetration in the live brain is an important drawback for fluorescence live imaging in the SVZ and hippocampus, the advent of multi-photon confocal microscopy has significantly improved the quality of fluorescence imaging in deep regions of the brain (Lendvai et al., 2000; Grutzendler et al., 2002; Trachtenberg et al., 2002). In a seminal work, Mizrahi et al. used two-photon microscopy to image the olfactory bulb of transgenic mice expressing GFP in juxtaglomerular neurons (JGNs), a population that undergoes adult neurogenesis, over periods of up to 3 months, *in vivo*. Based on GFP identification, they could perform time-lapse analysis and demonstrate that JGNs in the olfactory bulb have a turnover rate of about 3% per month (Mizrahi et al., 2006). Recently, this imaging technique has been combined to treatment with calcium indicators and used to study the functional integration of newly generated neurons in the adult rodent olfactory bulb (Kovalchuk et al., 2015).

However, neurogenic niches in the SVZ and hippocampal DG exist in much deeper brain regions as compared to the regions studied in the above cited work (Lendvai et al., 2000; Grutzendler et al., 2002; Trachtenberg et al., 2002; Mizrahi et al., 2006), hampering the use of two-photon microscopy to study endogenous aNSCs.

Recently, however, the group of David W. Tank has developed a preparation to image adult hippocampal cells in wake animals (Dombeck et al., 2010). In order to image neuron activity in CA1 during navigation, the authors removed the overlaying cortical tissue by aspiration and placed a stainless cannula that functioned as a window to CA1 of adult rats. Two-photon time-lapse microscopy of CA1 neurons labeled with the calcium indicator GCaMP3 during navigation in a virtual reality system allowed the identification of place cells and the correlation between the location of their place fields in the virtual environment and their anatomical location in the local circuit (Dombeck et al., 2010).

These data indicate that deeper regions of the brain can be imaged following removal of covering structures. However, to the best of our knowledge, this has not yet been tested to image aNSCs either in the DG or SVZ. Furthermore, it is important to keep in mind that surgical procedures to remove brain tissue may have critical influences in aNSC behavior and neurogenesis. In fact, several models have shown changes in the rate of proliferation within neurogenic niches following injury (Arvidsson et al., 2002; Collin et al., 2005; Aponso et al., 2008; Saha et al., 2013).

IMAGING OF LOCAL PROGENITORS IN THE CEREBRAL CORTEX

It has also been proposed that cells with stem/progenitor potential reside within the cortical parenchyma and could be activated under specific condition, such as injuries. Because these cells are located in superficial regions of the brain, it is possible to study their behavior by two-photon time-lapse microscopy.

The cerebral cortex layer 1, the most superficial layer of the cerebral cortex, for example, harbors a population of progenitors capable of generating neurons and glial cells during development (Costa et al., 2007; Breunig et al., 2012). Although, neurogenesis from layer 1 progenitors seems to be restricted to embryonic and postnatal stages under physiological conditions, these progenitors may resume proliferation after ischemic injury in adult animals and generate neurons (Ohira et al., 2010). Given the matchless superficial location of layer 1 progenitors, they are good candidates to imaging by two-photon microscopy.

Another interesting cell population for imaging in the adult brain is the parenchymal astroglia. Following traumatic and ischemic injury, astroglial cells proliferate, and acquire several hallmarks of neural stem cells (Buffo et al., 2008; Sirko et al., 2013), leading to the suggestion that parenchymal astroglia could be an interesting source for neuronal replacement under different neurological conditions (Robel et al., 2011; Chouchane and Costa, 2012).

In a recent work, Bardehle et al. (2013) used *in vivo* two-photon laser-scanning microscopy to follow the response of GFP-labeled astrocytes in the adult mouse cerebral cortex over several weeks after acute injury. The authors described a selective proliferation of juxtavascular astrocytes after the introduction of a lesion, indicating that astrocyte recruitment after injury relies solely on proliferation in a specific niche (Bardehle et al., 2013). If these proliferating astrocytes are the cells acquiring neural stem cell properties *in vitro*, two-photon time-lapse imaging of these cells might bring some insights about aNSC behavior *in vivo*.

CONCLUSION

Live-imaging of isolated SVZ cells *in vitro* has contribute to deepen our knowledge about the lineage-progression of adult NSCs. However, *in vivo* imaging systems still lack resolution to resolve single-cell lineages. Future studies should address the contribution of individual NSCs to different neuronal lineages and the possible influence of signaling molecules in this process, both *in vitro* and *in vivo*. Long-term imaging *in vivo*, however, awaits future developments in microscopy that will permit the observation of cells generated in the SVZ and the following up of these cells through the RMS and in the OB. Alternatively, short time live-imaging of aNSCs within the SEZ *in vivo* combined with multicolored fate-mapping could help to describe how the progeny of single NSCs, identified in the olfactory bulb by multicolor codes, is generated.

AUTHOR CONTRIBUTIONS

FO organized and coordinated the preparation of the present review. FO and MC contributed to the writing of the manuscript.

FUNDING

FO was supported by research grants MICINN (BFU2011-24743), Consolider-Ingenio 2010 "Spanish Ion Channel Initiative" (CSD2008-00005), MEC (BFU2014-53654-P), and BRADE-CM (S2013/ICE-2958) and the Ramon y Cajal Program of the Spanish Ministry of Economy and competitiveness (MEC) (RYC-2013-13290). MC is supported by CNPq, CAPES, and Fundação de Amparo à Pesquisa do Rio de Grande do Norte (FAPERN).

REFERENCES

Akiba, Y., Sasaki, H., Huerta, P. T., Estevez, A. G., Baker, H., and Cave, J. W. (2009). gamma-Aminobutyric acid-mediated regulation of the activity-dependent olfactory bulb dopaminergic phenotype. *J. Neurosci. Res.* 87, 2211–2221. doi: 10.1002/jnr.22055

Al-Kofahi, O., Radke, R. J., Goderie, S. K., Shen, Q., Temple, S., and Roysam, B. (2006). Automated cell lineage construction: a rapid method to analyze clonal development established with murine neural progenitor cells. *Cell Cycle* 5, 327–335. doi: 10.4161/cc.5.3.2426

Aponso, P. M., Faull, R. L., and Connor, B. (2008). Increased progenitor cell proliferation and astrogenesis in the partial progressive 6-hydroxydopamine model of Parkinson's disease. *Neuroscience* 151, 1142–1153. doi: 10.1016/j.neuroscience.2007.11.036

Arsenijevic, Y., Villemure, J. G., Brunet, J. F., Bloch, J. J., Deglon, N., Kostic, C., et al. (2001). Isolation of multipotent neural precursors residing in the cortex of the adult human brain. *Exp. Neurol.* 170, 48–62. doi: 10.1006/exnr.2001.7691

Arvidsson, A., Collin, T., Kirik, D., Kokaia, Z., and Lindvall, O. (2002). Neuronal replacement from endogenous precursors in the adult brain after stroke. *Nat. Med.* 8, 963–970. doi: 10.1038/nm747

Azim, K., Fischer, B., Hurtado-Chong, A., Draganova, K., Cantu, C., Zemke, M., et al. (2014). Persistent Wnt/beta-catenin signaling determines dorsalization of the postnatal subventricular zone and neural stem cell specification into oligodendrocytes and glutamatergic neurons. *Stem Cells* 32, 1301–1312. doi: 10.1002/stem.1639

Bardehle, S., Kruger, M., Buggenthin, F., Schwausch, J., Ninkovic, J., Clevers, H., et al. (2013). Live imaging of astrocyte responses to acute injury reveals selective juxtavascular proliferation. *Nat. Neurosci.* 16, 580–586. doi: 10.1038/nn.3371

Beckervordersandforth, R., Tripathi, P., Ninkovic, J., Bayam, E., Lepier, A., Stempfhuber, B., et al. (2010). *In vivo* fate mapping and expression analysis reveals molecular hallmarks of prospectively isolated adult neural stem cells. *Cell Stem Cell* 7, 744–758. doi: 10.1016/j.stem.2010.11.017

Belachew, S., Chittajallu, R., Aguirre, A. A., Yuan, X., Kirby, M., Anderson, S., et al. (2003). Postnatal NG2 proteoglycan-expressing progenitor cells are intrinsically multipotent and generate functional neurons. *J. Cell Biol.* 161, 169–186. doi: 10.1083/jcb.200210110

Bonaguidi, M. A., Wheeler, M. A., Shapiro, J. S., Stadel, R. P., Sun, G. J., Ming, G. L., et al. (2011). *In vivo* clonal analysis reveals self-renewing and multipotent adult neural stem cell characteristics. *Cell* 145, 1142–1155. doi: 10.1016/j.cell.2011.05.024

Breunig, J. J., Gate, D., Levy, R., Rodriguez, J. Jr., Kim, G. B., Danielpour, M., et al. (2012). Rapid genetic targeting of pial surface neural progenitors and immature neurons by neonatal electroporation. *Neural Dev* 7:26. doi: 10.1186/1749-8104-7-26

Brill, M. S., Ninkovic, J., Winpenny, E., Hodge, R. D., Ozen, I., Yang, R., et al. (2009). Adult generation of glutamatergic olfactory bulb interneurons. *Nat. Neurosci.* 12, 1524–1533. doi: 10.1038/nn.2416

Buffo, A., Rite, I., Tripathi, P., Lepier, A., Colak, D., Horn, A. P., et al. (2008). Origin and progeny of reactive gliosis: a source of multipotent cells in the injured brain. *Proc. Natl. Acad. Sci. U.S.A.* 105, 3581–3586. doi: 10.1073/pnas.0709002105

Calaora, V., Chazal, G., Nielsen, P. J., Rougon, G., and Moreau, H. (1996). mCD24 expression in the developing mouse brain and in zones of secondary neurogenesis in the adult. *Neuroscience* 73, 581–594. doi: 10.1016/0306-4522(96)00042-5

Calvo, C. F., Fontaine, R. H., Soueid, J., Tammela, T., Makinen, T., Alfaro-Cervello, C., et al. (2011). Vascular endothelial growth factor receptor 3 directly regulates murine neurogenesis. *Genes Dev.* 25, 831–844. doi: 10.1101/gad.615311

Calzolari, F., Michel, J., Baumgart, E. V., Theis, F., Gotz, M., and Ninkovic, J. (2015). Fast clonal expansion and limited neural stem cell self-renewal in the adult subependymal zone. *Nat. Neurosci.* 18, 490–492. doi: 10.1038/nn.3963

Capela, A., and Temple, S. (2002). LeX/ssea-1 is expressed by adult mouse CNS stem cells, identifying them as nonependymal. *Neuron* 35, 865–875. doi: 10.1016/S0896-6273(02)00835-8

Cayouette, M., Poggi, L., and Harris, W. A. (2006). Lineage in the vertebrate retina. *Trends Neurosci.* 29, 563–570. doi: 10.1016/j.tins.2006.08.003

Cepko, C. L., Austin, C. P., Yang, X., Alexiades, M., and Ezzeddine, D. (1996). Cell fate determination in the vertebrate retina. *Proc. Natl. Acad. Sci. U.S.A.* 93, 589–595. doi: 10.1073/pnas.93.2.589

Chouchane, M., and Costa, M. R. (2012). Cell therapy for stroke: use of local astrocytes. *Front. Cell. Neurosci.* 6:49. doi: 10.3389/fncel.2012.00049

Codega, P., Silva-Vargas, V., Paul, A., Maldonado-Soto, A. R., Deleo, A. M., Pastrana, E., et al. (2014). Prospective identification and purification of quiescent adult neural stem cells from their *in vivo* niche. *Neuron* 82, 545–559. doi: 10.1016/j.neuron.2014.02.039

Cohen, A. R., Gomes, F. L., Roysam, B., and Cayouette, M. (2010). Computational prediction of neural progenitor cell fates. *Nat. Methods* 7, 213–218. doi: 10.1038/nmeth.1424

Colak, D., Mori, T., Brill, M. S., Pfeifer, A., Falk, S., Deng, C., et al. (2008). Adult neurogenesis requires Smad4-mediated bone morphogenic protein signaling in stem cells. *J. Neurosci.* 28, 434–446. doi: 10.1523/JNEUROSCI.4374-07.2008

Collin, T., Arvidsson, A., Kokaia, Z., and Lindvall, O. (2005). Quantitative analysis of the generation of different striatal neuronal subtypes in the adult brain following excitotoxic injury. *Exp. Neurol.* 195, 71–80. doi: 10.1016/j.expneurol.2005.03.017

Conklin, E. G. (1905). The organization and cell lineage of the ascidian egg. *J. Acad. Nat. Schi. Phila.* 12, 1–19.

Costa, M. R., Bucholz, O., Schroeder, T., and Gotz, M. (2009). Late origin of glia-restricted progenitors in the developing mouse cerebral cortex. *Cereb. Cortex* 19(Suppl 1), i135–i143. doi: 10.1093/cercor/bhp046

Costa, M. R., Kessaris, N., Richardson, W. D., Gotz, M., and Hedin-Pereira, C. (2007). The marginal zone/layer I as a novel niche for neurogenesis and gliogenesis in developing cerebral cortex. *J. Neurosci.* 27, 11376–11388. doi: 10.1523/JNEUROSCI.2418-07.2007

Costa, M. R., Ortega, F., Brill, M. S., Beckervordersandforth, R., Petrone, C., Schroeder, T., et al. (2011). Continuous live imaging of adult neural stem cell division and lineage progression *in vitro*. *Development* 138, 1057–1068. doi: 10.1242/dev.061663

Costa, M. R., Wen, G., Lepier, A., Schroeder, T., and Gotz, M. (2008). Par-complex proteins promote proliferative progenitor divisions in the developing mouse cerebral cortex. *Development* 135, 11–22. doi: 10.1242/dev.009951

Couillard-Despres, S., and Aigner, L. (2011). *In vivo* imaging of adult neurogenesis. *Eur. J. Neurosci.* 33, 1037–1044. doi: 10.1111/j.1460-9568.2011.07601.x

Crabbe, A., Vandeputte, C., Dresselaers, T., Sacido, A. A., Verdugo, J. M., Eyckmans, J., et al. (2010). Effects of MRI contrast agents on the stem cell phenotype. *Cell Transplant.* 19, 919–936. doi: 10.3727/096368910X494623

Daynac, M., Morizur, L., Kortulewski, T., Gauthier, L. R., Ruat, M., Mouthon, M. A., et al. (2015). Cell sorting of neural stem and progenitor cells from the adult mouse subventricular zone and live-imaging of their cell cycle dynamics. *J. Vis. Exp.* 103:e53247. doi: 10.3791/53247

Doetsch, F., Caille, I., Lim, D. A., Garcia-Verdugo, J. M., and Alvarez-Buylla, A. (1999a). Subventricular zone astrocytes are neural stem cells in the adult mammalian brain. *Cell* 97, 703–716. doi: 10.1016/S0092-8674(00)80783-7

Doetsch, F., Garcia-Verdugo, J. M., and Alvarez-Buylla, A. (1997). Cellular composition and three-dimensional organization of the subventricular germinal zone in the adult mammalian brain. *J. Neurosci.* 17, 5046–5061.

Doetsch, F., Garcia-Verdugo, J. M., and Alvarez-Buylla, A. (1999b). Regeneration of a germinal layer in the adult mammalian brain. *Proc. Natl. Acad. Sci. U.S.A.* 96, 11619–11624. doi: 10.1073/pnas.96.20.11619

Doetsch, F., Petreanu, L., Caille, I., Garcia-Verdugo, J. M., and Alvarez-Buylla, A. (2002). EGF converts transit-amplifying neurogenic precursors in the adult brain into multipotent stem cells. *Neuron* 36, 1021–1034. doi: 10.1016/S0896-6273(02)01133-9

Dombeck, D. A., Harvey, C. D., Tian, L., Looger, L. L., and Tank, D. W. (2010). Functional imaging of hippocampal place cells at cellular resolution during virtual navigation. *Nat. Neurosci.* 13, 1433–1440. doi: 10.1038/nn.2648

Eilken, H., Rieger, M., Hoppe, P. S., Hermann, A., Smejkal, B., Drew, E., Thum, M., et al. (2014). Continuous long-term detection of live cell surface markers by 'in culture' antibody staining. *Protoc. Exch.* doi: 10.1038/protex.2011.205. [Epub ahead of print].

Eilken, H. M., Nishikawa, S., and Schroeder, T. (2009). Continuous single-cell imaging of blood generation from haemogenic endothelium. *Nature* 457, 896–900. doi: 10.1038/nature07760

Encinas, J. M., Michurina, T. V., Peunova, N., Park, J. H., Tordo, J., Peterson, D. A., et al. (2011). Division-coupled astrocytic differentiation and age-related depletion of neural stem cells in the adult hippocampus. *Cell Stem Cell* 8, 566–579. doi: 10.1016/j.stem.2011.03.010

Filippov, V., Kronenberg, G., Pivneva, T., Reuter, K., Steiner, B., Wang, L. P., et al. (2003). Subpopulation of nestin-expressing progenitor cells in the adult murine hippocampus shows electrophysiological and morphological characteristics of astrocytes. *Mol. Cell. Neurosci.* 23, 373–382. doi: 10.1016/S1044-7431(03)00060-5

Fiorelli, R., Azim, K., Fischer, B., and Raineteau, O. (2015). Adding a spatial dimension to postnatal ventricular-subventricular zone neurogenesis. *Development* 142, 2109–2120. doi: 10.1242/dev.119966

Fuentealba, L. C., Rompani, S. B., Parraguez, J. I., Obernier, K., Romero, R., Cepko, C. L., et al. (2015). Embryonic origin of postnatal neural stem cells. *Cell* 161, 1644–1655. doi: 10.1016/j.cell.2015.05.041

Fukuda, S., Kato, F., Tozuka, Y., Yamaguchi, M., Miyamoto, Y., and Hisatsune, T. (2003). Two distinct subpopulations of nestin-positive cells in adult mouse dentate gyrus. *J. Neurosci.* 23, 9357–9366.

Furutachi, S., Miya, H., Watanabe, T., Kawai, H., Yamasaki, N., Harada, Y., et al. (2015). Slowly dividing neural progenitors are an embryonic origin of adult neural stem cells. *Nat. Neurosci.* 18, 657–665. doi: 10.1038/nn.3989

Gage, F. H. (2000). Mammalian neural stem cells. *Science* 287, 1433–1438. doi: 10.1126/science.287.5457.1433

Garcia, A. D., Doan, N. B., Imura, T., Bush, T. G., and Sofroniew, M. V. (2004). GFAP-expressing progenitors are the principal source of constitutive neurogenesis in adult mouse forebrain. *Nat. Neurosci.* 7, 1233–1241. doi: 10.1038/nn1340

Garcia-Marques, J., and Lopez-Mascaraque, L. (2013). Clonal identity determines astrocyte cortical heterogeneity. *Cereb. Cortex* 23, 1463–1472. doi: 10.1093/cercor/bhs134

Giachino, C., and Taylor, V. (2009). Lineage analysis of quiescent regenerative stem cells in the adult brain by genetic labelling reveals spatially restricted neurogenic niches in the olfactory bulb. *Eur. J. Neurosci.* 30, 9–24. doi: 10.1111/j.1460-9568.2009.06798.x

Gomes, F. L., Zhang, G., Carbonell, F., Correa, J. A., Harris, W. A., Simons, B. D., et al. (2011). Reconstruction of rat retinal progenitor cell lineages *in vitro* reveals a surprising degree of stochasticity in cell fate decisions. *Development* 138, 227–235. doi: 10.1242/dev.059683

Gonzalez-Perez, O., and Alvarez-Buylla, A. (2011). Oligodendrogenesis in the subventricular zone and the role of epidermal growth factor. *Brain Res. Rev.* 67, 147–156. doi: 10.1016/j.brainresrev.2011.01.001

Gould, E., and Cameron, H. A. (1996). Regulation of neuronal birth, migration and death in the rat dentate gyrus. *Dev. Neurosci.* 18, 22–35. doi: 10.1159/000111392

Granot, D., Scheinost, D., Markakis, E. A., Papademetris, X., and Shapiro, E. M. (2011). Serial monitoring of endogenous neuroblast migration by cellular MRI. *Neuroimage* 57, 817–824. doi: 10.1016/j.neuroimage.2011.04.063

Gritti, A., Bonfanti, L., Doetsch, F., Caille, I., Alvarez-Buylla, A., Lim, D. A., et al. (2002). Multipotent neural stem cells reside into the rostral extension and olfactory bulb of adult rodents. *J. Neurosci.* 22, 437–445.

Grutzendler, J., Kasthuri, N., and Gan, W. B. (2002). Long-term dendritic spine stability in the adult cortex. *Nature* 420, 812–816. doi: 10.1038/nature01276

Hack, M. A., Saghatelyan, A., De Chevigny, A., Pfeifer, A., Ashery-Padan, R., Lledo, P. M., et al. (2005). Neuronal fate determinants of adult olfactory bulb neurogenesis. *Nat. Neurosci.* 8, 865–872. doi: 10.1038/nn1479

He, J., Zhang, G., Almeida, A. D., Cayouette, M., Simons, B. D., and Harris, W. A. (2012). How variable clones build an invariant retina. *Neuron* 75, 786–798. doi: 10.1016/j.neuron.2012.06.033

Hoehn, M., Kustermann, E., Blunk, J., Wiedermann, D., Trapp, T., Wecker, S., et al. (2002). Monitoring of implanted stem cell migration *in vivo*: a highly resolved *in vivo* magnetic resonance imaging investigation of experimental stroke in rat. *Proc. Natl. Acad. Sci. U.S.A.* 99, 16267–16272. doi: 10.1073/pnas.242435499

Ihrie, R. A., Shah, J. K., Harwell, C. C., Levine, J. H., Guinto, C. D., Lezameta, M., et al. (2011). Persistent sonic hedgehog signaling in adult brain determines neural stem cell positional identity. *Neuron* 71, 250–262. doi: 10.1016/j.neuron.2011.05.018

Iordanova, B., and Ahrens, E. T. (2012). *In vivo* magnetic resonance imaging of ferritin-based reporter visualizes native neuroblast migration. *Neuroimage* 59, 1004–1012. doi: 10.1016/j.neuroimage.2011.08.068

James, R., Kim, Y., Hockberger, P. E., and Szele, F. G. (2011). Subventricular zone cell migration: lessons from quantitative two-photon microscopy. *Front. Neurosci.* 5:30. doi: 10.3389/fnins.2011.00030

Kamada, M., Li, R. Y., Hashimoto, M., Kakuda, M., Okada, H., Koyanagi, Y., et al. (2004). Intrinsic and spontaneous neurogenesis in the postnatal slice culture of rat hippocampus. *Eur. J. Neurosci.* 20, 2499–2508. doi: 10.1111/j.1460-9568.2004.03721.x

Kempermann, G., Kuhn, H. G., and Gage, F. H. (1997). More hippocampal neurons in adult mice living in an enriched environment. *Nature* 386, 493–495. doi: 10.1038/386493a0

Kempermann, G., Song, H., and Gage, F. H. (2015). Neurogenesis in the adult hippocampus. *Cold Spring Harb. Perspect. Med.* 5:a018812. doi: 10.1101/cshperspect.a018812

Kiyokage, E., Pan, Y. Z., Shao, Z., Kobayashi, K., Szabo, G., Yanagawa, Y., et al. (2010). Molecular identity of periglomerular and short axon cells. *J. Neurosci.* 30, 1185–1196. doi: 10.1523/JNEUROSCI.3497-09.2010

Kokovay, E., Wang, Y., Kusek, G., Wurster, R., Lederman, P., Lowry, N., et al. (2012). VCAM1 is essential to maintain the structure of the SVZ niche and acts as an environmental sensor to regulate SVZ lineage progression. *Cell Stem Cell* 11, 220–230. doi: 10.1016/j.stem.2012.06.016

Kosaka, T., and Kosaka, K. (2008). Tyrosine hydroxylase-positive GABAergic juxtaglomerular neurons are the main source of the interglomerular connections in the mouse main olfactory bulb. *Neurosci. Res.* 60, 349–354. doi: 10.1016/j.neures.2007.11.012

Kovalchuk, Y., Homma, R., Liang, Y., Maslyukov, A., Hermes, M., Thestrup, T., et al. (2015). *In vivo* odourant response properties of migrating adult-born neurons in the mouse olfactory bulb. *Nat. Commun.* 6, 6349. doi: 10.1038/ncomms7349

Kretzschmar, K., and Watt, F. M. (2012). Lineage tracing. *Cell* 148, 33–45. doi: 10.1016/j.cell.2012.01.002

Kriegstein, A., and Alvarez-Buylla, A. (2009). The glial nature of embryonic and adult neural stem cells. *Annu. Rev. Neurosci.* 32, 149–184. doi: 10.1146/annurev.neuro.051508.135600

Kuhn, H. G., Winkler, J., Kempermann, G., Thal, L. J., and Gage, F. H. (1997). Epidermal growth factor and fibroblast growth factor-2 have different effects on neural progenitors in the adult rat brain. *J. Neurosci.* 17, 5820–5829.

Lacar, B., Herman, P., Platel, J. C., Kubera, C., Hyder, F., and Bordey, A. (2012). Neural progenitor cells regulate capillary blood flow in the postnatal subventricular zone. *J. Neurosci.* 32, 16435–16448. doi: 10.1523/JNEUROSCI.1457-12.2012

Lendvai, B., Stern, E. A., Chen, B., and Svoboda, K. (2000). Experience-dependent plasticity of dendritic spines in the developing rat barrel cortex *in vivo*. *Nature* 404, 876–881. doi: 10.1038/35009107

Lim, D. A., and Alvarez-Buylla, A. (1999). Interaction between astrocytes and adult subventricular zone precursors stimulates neurogenesis. *Proc. Natl. Acad. Sci. U.S.A.* 96, 7526–7531. doi: 10.1073/pnas.96.13.7526

Liu, Z., and Martin, L. J. (2003). Olfactory bulb core is a rich source of neural progenitor and stem cells in adult rodent and human. *J. Comp. Neurol.* 459, 368–391. doi: 10.1002/cne.10664

Livesey, F. J., and Cepko, C. L. (2001). Vertebrate neural cell-fate determination: lessons from the retina. *Nat. Rev. Neurosci.* 2, 109–118. doi: 10.1038/35053522

Lledo, P. M., Alonso, M., and Grubb, M. S. (2006). Adult neurogenesis and functional plasticity in neuronal circuits. *Nat. Rev. Neurosci.* 7, 179–193. doi: 10.1038/nrn1867

Lois, C., and Alvarez-Buylla, A. (1993). Proliferating subventricular zone cells in the adult mammalian forebrain can differentiate into neurons and glia. *Proc. Natl. Acad. Sci. U.S.A.* 90, 2074–2077. doi: 10.1073/pnas.90.5.2074

Lois, C., Garcia-Verdugo, J. M., and Alvarez-Buylla, A. (1996). Chain migration of neuronal precursors. *Science* 271, 978–981. doi: 10.1126/science.271.5251.978

Luo, Y., Coskun, V., Liang, A., Yu, J., Cheng, L., Ge, W., et al. (2015). Single-cell transcriptome analyses reveal signals to activate dormant neural stem cells. *Cell* 161, 1175–1186. doi: 10.1016/j.cell.2015.04.001

Manganas, L. N., Zhang, X., Li, Y., Hazel, R. D., Smith, S. D., Wagshul, M. E., et al. (2007). Magnetic resonance spectroscopy identifies neural progenitor cells in the live human brain. *Science* 318, 980–985. doi: 10.1126/science.1147851

Marinaro, C., Pannese, M., Weinandy, F., Sessa, A., Bergamaschi, A., Taketo, M. M., et al. (2012). Wnt signaling has opposing roles in the developing and the adult brain that are modulated by Hipk1. *Cereb. Cortex* 22, 2415–2427. doi: 10.1093/cercor/bhr320

Marmur, R., Mabie, P. C., Gokhan, S., Song, Q., Kessler, J. A., and Mehler, M. F. (1998). Isolation and developmental characterization of cerebral cortical multipotent progenitors. *Dev. Biol.* 204, 577–591. doi: 10.1006/dbio.1998.9099

Menn, B., Garcia-Verdugo, J. M., Yaschine, C., Gonzalez-Perez, O., Rowitch, D., and Alvarez-Buylla, A. (2006). Origin of oligodendrocytes in the subventricular zone of the adult brain. *J. Neurosci.* 26, 7907–7918. doi: 10.1523/JNEUROSCI.1299-06.2006

Merkle, F. T., Fuentealba, L. C., Sanders, T. A., Magno, L., Kessaris, N., and Alvarez-Buylla, A. (2014). Adult neural stem cells in distinct microdomains generate previously unknown interneuron types. *Nat. Neurosci.* 17, 207–214. doi: 10.1038/nn.3610

Merkle, F. T., Mirzadeh, Z., and Alvarez-Buylla, A. (2007). Mosaic organization of neural stem cells in the adult brain. *Science* 317, 381–384. doi: 10.1126/science.1144914

Merkle, F. T., Tramontin, A. D., Garcia-Verdugo, J. M., and Alvarez-Buylla, A. (2004). Radial glia give rise to adult neural stem cells in the subventricular zone. *Proc. Natl. Acad. Sci. U.S.A.* 101, 17528–17532. doi: 10.1073/pnas.0407893101

Ming, G. L., and Song, H. (2011). Adult neurogenesis in the mammalian brain: significant answers and significant questions. *Neuron* 70, 687–702. doi: 10.1016/j.neuron.2011.05.001

Mirzadeh, Z., Merkle, F. T., Soriano-Navarro, M., Garcia-Verdugo, J. M., and Alvarez-Buylla, A. (2008). Neural stem cells confer unique pinwheel architecture to the ventricular surface in neurogenic regions of the adult brain. *Cell Stem Cell* 3, 265–278. doi: 10.1016/j.stem.2008.07.004

Mizrahi, A., Lu, J., Irving, R., Feng, G., and Katz, L. C. (2006). *In vivo* imaging of juxtaglomerular neuron turnover in the mouse olfactory bulb. *Proc. Natl. Acad. Sci. U.S.A.* 103, 1912–1917. doi: 10.1073/pnas.0506297103

Mongiat, L. A., and Schinder, A. F. (2011). Adult neurogenesis and the plasticity of the dentate gyrus network. *Eur. J. Neurosci.* 33, 1055–1061. doi: 10.1111/j.1460-9568.2011.07603.x

Moreno-Estelles, M., Gonzalez-Gomez, P., Hortiguela, R., Diaz-Moreno, M., San Emeterio, J., Carvalho, A. L., et al. (2012). Symmetric expansion of neural stem cells from the adult olfactory bulb is driven by astrocytes via WNT7A. *Stem Cells* 30, 2796–2809. doi: 10.1002/stem.1243

Nam, S. C., Kim, Y., Dryanovski, D., Walker, A., Goings, G., Woolfrey, K., et al. (2007). Dynamic features of postnatal subventricular zone cell motility: a two-photon time-lapse study. *J. Comp. Neurol.* 505, 190–208. doi: 10.1002/cne.21473

Namba, T., Mochizuki, H., Onodera, M., Namiki, H., and Seki, T. (2007). Postnatal neurogenesis in hippocampal slice cultures: early *in vitro* labeling of neural precursor cells leads to efficient neuronal production. *J. Neurosci. Res.* 85, 1704–1712. doi: 10.1002/jnr.21295

Noctor, S. C., Martinez-Cerdeno, V., Ivic, L., and Kriegstein, A. R. (2004). Cortical neurons arise in symmetric and asymmetric division zones and migrate through specific phases. *Nat. Neurosci.* 7, 136–144. doi: 10.1038/nn1172

Ohira, K., Furuta, T., Hioki, H., Nakamura, K. C., Kuramoto, E., Tanaka, Y., et al. (2010). Ischemia-induced neurogenesis of neocortical layer 1 progenitor cells. *Nat. Neurosci.* 13, 173–179. doi: 10.1038/nn.2473

Ortega, F., Costa, M. R., Simon-Ebert, T., Schroeder, T., Gotz, M., and Berninger, B. (2011). Using an adherent cell culture of the mouse subependymal zone to study the behavior of adult neural stem cells on a single-cell level. *Nat. Protoc.* 6, 1847–1859. doi: 10.1038/nprot.2011.404

Ortega, F., Gascon, S., Masserdotti, G., Deshpande, A., Simon, C., Fischer, J., et al. (2013). Oligodendrogliogenic and neurogenic adult subependymal zone neural stem cells constitute distinct lineages and exhibit differential responsiveness to Wnt signalling. *Nat. Cell Biol.* 15, 602–613. doi: 10.1038/ncb2736

Pagano, S. F., Impagnatiello, F., Girelli, M., Cova, L., Grioni, E., Onofri, M., et al. (2000). Isolation and characterization of neural stem cells from the adult human olfactory bulb. *Stem Cells* 18, 295–300. doi: 10.1634/stemcells.18-4-295

Panizzo, R. A., Kyrtatos, P. G., Price, A. N., Gadian, D. G., Ferretti, P., and Lythgoe, M. F. (2009). *In vivo* magnetic resonance imaging of endogenous neuroblasts labelled with a ferumoxide-polycation complex. *Neuroimage* 44, 1239–1246. doi: 10.1016/j.neuroimage.2008.10.062

Pastrana, E., Cheng, L. C., and Doetsch, F. (2009). Simultaneous prospective purification of adult subventricular zone neural stem cells and their progeny. *Proc. Natl. Acad. Sci. U.S.A.* 106, 6387–6392. doi: 10.1073/pnas.0810407106

Pastrana, E., Silva-Vargas, V., and Doetsch, F. (2011). Eyes wide open: a critical review of sphere-formation as an assay for stem cells. *Cell Stem Cell* 8, 486–498. doi: 10.1016/j.stem.2011.04.007

Picard-Riera, N., Decker, L., Delarasse, C., Goude, K., Nait-Oumesmar, B., Liblau, R., et al. (2002). Experimental autoimmune encephalomyelitis mobilizes neural progenitors from the subventricular zone to undergo oligodendrogenesis in adult mice. *Proc. Natl. Acad. Sci. U.S.A.* 99, 13211–13216. doi: 10.1073/pnas.192314199

Platel, J. C., Gordon, V., Heintz, T., and Bordey, A. (2009). GFAP-GFP neural progenitors are antigenically homogeneous and anchored in their enclosed mosaic niche. *Glia* 57, 66–78. doi: 10.1002/glia.20735

Ponti, G., Obernier, K., Guinto, C., Jose, L., Bonfanti, L., and Alvarez-Buylla, A. (2013). Cell cycle and lineage progression of neural progenitors in the ventricular-subventricular zones of adult mice. *Proc. Natl. Acad. Sci. U.S.A.* 110, E1045–E1054. doi: 10.1073/pnas.1219563110

Qian, X., Goderie, S. K., Shen, Q., Stern, J. H., and Temple, S. (1998). Intrinsic programs of patterned cell lineages in isolated vertebrate CNS ventricular zone cells. *Development* 125, 3143–3152.

Qian, X., Shen, Q., Goderie, S. K., He, W., Capela, A., Davis, A. A., et al. (2000). Timing of CNS cell generation: a programmed sequence of neuron and glial cell production from isolated murine cortical stem cells. *Neuron* 28, 69–80. doi: 10.1016/S0896-6273(00)00086-6

Raineteau, O., Rietschin, L., Gradwohl, G., Guillemot, F., and Gahwiler, B. H. (2004). Neurogenesis in hippocampal slice cultures. *Mol. Cell. Neurosci.* 26, 241–250. doi: 10.1016/j.mcn.2004.01.003

Ramm, P., Couillard-Despres, S., Plotz, S., Rivera, F. J., Krampert, M., Lehner, B., et al. (2009). A nuclear magnetic resonance biomarker for neural progenitor cells: is it all neurogenesis? *Stem Cells* 27, 420–423. doi: 10.1634/stemcells.2008-0816

Ravin, R., Hoeppner, D. J., Munno, D. M., Carmel, L., Sullivan, J., Levitt, D. L., et al. (2008). Potency and fate specification in CNS stem cell populations *in vitro*. *Cell Stem Cell* 3, 670–680. doi: 10.1016/j.stem.2008.09.012

Reynolds, B. A., and Rietze, R. L. (2005). Neural stem cells and neurospheres–re-evaluating the relationship. *Nat. Methods* 2, 333–336. doi: 10.1038/nmeth758

Reynolds, B. A., and Weiss, S. (1996). Clonal and population analyses demonstrate that an EGF-responsive mammalian embryonic CNS precursor is a stem cell. *Dev. Biol.* 175, 1–13. doi: 10.1006/dbio.1996.0090

Rieger, M. A., Hoppe, P. S., Smejkal, B. M., Eitelhuber, A. C., and Schroeder, T. (2009). Hematopoietic cytokines can instruct lineage choice. *Science* 325, 217–218. doi: 10.1126/science.1171461

Riesenberg, A. N., Liu, Z., Kopan, R., and Brown, N. L. (2009). Rbpj cell autonomous regulation of retinal ganglion cell and cone photoreceptor fates in the mouse retina. *J. Neurosci.* 29, 12865–12877. doi: 10.1523/JNEUROSCI.3382-09.2009

Robel, S., Berninger, B., and Gotz, M. (2011). The stem cell potential of glia: lessons from reactive gliosis. *Nat. Rev. Neurosci.* 12, 88–104. doi: 10.1038/nrn2978

Rueger, M. A., Backes, H., Walberer, M., Neumaier, B., Ullrich, R., Simard, M. L., et al. (2010). Noninvasive imaging of endogenous neural stem cell mobilization *in vivo* using positron emission tomography. *J. Neurosci.* 30, 6454–6460. doi: 10.1523/JNEUROSCI.6092-09.2010

Saha, B., Peron, S., Murray, K., Jaber, M., and Gaillard, A. (2013). Cortical lesion stimulates adult subventricular zone neural progenitor cell proliferation and migration to the site of injury. *Stem Cell Res.* 11, 965–977. doi: 10.1016/j.scr.2013.06.006

Sanai, N., Tramontin, A. D., Quinones-Hinojosa, A., Barbaro, N. M., Gupta, N., Kunwar, S., et al. (2004). Unique astrocyte ribbon in adult human brain contains neural stem cells but lacks chain migration. *Nature* 427, 740–744. doi: 10.1038/nature02301

Scheffler, B., Walton, N. M., Lin, D. D., Goetz, A. K., Enikolopov, G., Roper, S. N., et al. (2005). Phenotypic and functional characterization of adult brain neuropoiesis. *Proc. Natl. Acad. Sci. U.S.A.* 102, 9353–9358. doi: 10.1073/pnas.0503965102

Schroeder, T. (2011). Long-term single-cell imaging of mammalian stem cells. *Nat. Methods* 8, S30–S35. doi: 10.1038/nmeth.1577

Seaberg, R. M., Smukler, S. R., and Van Der Kooy, D. (2005). Intrinsic differences distinguish transiently neurogenic progenitors from neural stem cells in the early postnatal brain. *Dev. Biol.* 278, 71–85. doi: 10.1016/j.ydbio.2004.10.017

Sequerra, E. B., Costa, M. R., Menezes, J. R., and Hedin-Pereira, C. (2013). Adult neural stem cells: plastic or restricted neuronal fates? *Development* 140, 3303–3309. doi: 10.1242/dev.093096

Sequerra, E. B., Miyakoshi, L. M., Froes, M. M., Menezes, J. R., and Hedin-Pereira, C. (2010). Generation of glutamatergic neurons from postnatal and adult subventricular zone with pyramidal-like morphology. *Cereb. Cortex* 20, 2583–2591. doi: 10.1093/cercor/bhq006

Seri, B., Garcia-Verdugo, J. M., Mcewen, B. S., and Alvarez-Buylla, A. (2001). Astrocytes give rise to new neurons in the adult mammalian hippocampus. *J. Neurosci.* 21, 7153–7160.

Shen, Q., Wang, Y., Kokovay, E., Lin, G., Chuang, S. M., Goderie, S. K., et al. (2008). Adult SVZ stem cells lie in a vascular niche: a quantitative analysis of niche cell-cell interactions. *Cell Stem Cell* 3, 289–300. doi: 10.1016/j.stem.2008.07.026

Shors, T. J., Townsend, D. A., Zhao, M., Kozorovitskiy, Y., and Gould, E. (2002). Neurogenesis may relate to some but not all types of hippocampal-dependent learning. *Hippocampus* 12, 578–584. doi: 10.1002/hipo.10103

Singec, I., Knoth, R., Meyer, R. P., Maciaczyk, J., Volk, B., Nikkhah, G., et al. (2006). Defining the actual sensitivity and specificity of the neurosphere assay in stem cell biology. *Nat. Methods* 3, 801–806. doi: 10.1038/nmeth926

Sirko, S., Behrendt, G., Johansson, P. A., Tripathi, P., Costa, M., Bek, S., et al. (2013). Reactive glia in the injured brain acquire stem cell properties in response to sonic hedgehog. [corrected]. *Cell Stem Cell* 12, 426–439. doi: 10.1016/j.stem.2013.01.019

Sobottka, B., Ziegler, U., Kaech, A., Becher, B., and Goebels, N. (2011). CNS live imaging reveals a new mechanism of myelination: the liquid croissant model. *Glia* 59, 1841–1849. doi: 10.1002/glia.21228

Sohn, J., Orosco, L., Guo, F., Chung, S. H., Bannerman, P., Mills Ko, E., et al. (2015). The subventricular zone continues to generate corpus callosum and rostral migratory stream astroglia in normal adult mice. *J. Neurosci.* 35, 3756–3763. doi: 10.1523/JNEUROSCI.3454-14.2015

Suh, H., Deng, W., and Gage, F. H. (2009). Signaling in adult neurogenesis. *Annu. Rev. Cell Dev. Biol.* 25, 253–275. doi: 10.1146/annurev.cellbio.042308.113256

Sulston, J. E., Schierenberg, E., White, J. G., and Thomson, J. N. (1983). The embryonic cell lineage of the nematode Caenorhabditis elegans. *Dev. Biol.* 100, 64–119. doi: 10.1016/0012-1606(83)90201-4

Tavazoie, M., Van Der Veken, L., Silva-Vargas, V., Louissaint, M., Colonna, L., Zaidi, B., et al. (2008). A specialized vascular niche for adult neural stem cells. *Cell Stem Cell* 3, 279–288. doi: 10.1016/j.stem.2008.07.025

Tong, C. K., Chen, J., Cebrian-Silla, A., Mirzadeh, Z., Obernier, K., Guinto, C. D., et al. (2014). Axonal control of the adult neural stem cell niche. *Cell Stem Cell* 14, 500–511. doi: 10.1016/j.stem.2014.01.014

Tong, C. K., Fuentealba, L. C., Shah, J. K., Lindquist, R. A., Ihrie, R. A., Guinto, C. D., et al. (2015). A dorsal SHH-dependent domain in the V-SVZ produces large numbers of oligodendroglial lineage cells in the postnatal brain. *Stem Cell Rep.* 5, 461–470. doi: 10.1016/j.stemcr.2015.08.013

Trachtenberg, J. T., Chen, B. E., Knott, G. W., Feng, G., Sanes, J. R., Welker, E., et al. (2002). Long-term *in vivo* imaging of experience-dependent synaptic plasticity in adult cortex. *Nature* 420, 788–794. doi: 10.1038/nature01273

Vergano-Vera, E., Mendez-Gomez, H. R., Hurtado-Chong, A., Cigudosa, J. C., and Vicario-Abejon, C. (2009). Fibroblast growth factor-2 increases the expression of neurogenic genes and promotes the migration and differentiation of neurons derived from transplanted neural stem/progenitor cells. *Neuroscience* 162, 39–54. doi: 10.1016/j.neuroscience.2009.03.033

Vreys, R., Vande Velde, G., Krylychkina, O., Vellema, M., Verhoye, M., Timmermans, J. P., et al. (2010). MRI visualization of endogenous neural progenitor cell migration along the RMS in the adult mouse brain: validation of various MPIO labeling strategies. *Neuroimage* 49, 2094–2103. doi: 10.1016/j.neuroimage.2009.10.034

Walton, N. M., Snyder, G. E., Park, D., Kobeissy, F., Scheffler, B., and Steindler, D. A. (2009). Gliotypic neural stem cells transiently adopt tumorigenic properties during normal differentiation. *Stem Cells* 27, 280–289. doi: 10.1634/stemcells.2008-0842

Weber, T., Vroemen, M., Behr, V., Neuberger, T., Jakob, P., Haase, A., et al. (2006). *In vivo* high-resolution MR imaging of neuropathologic changes in the injured rat spinal cord. *AJNR Am. J. Neuroradiol.* 27, 598–604.

Winter, M., Wait, E., Roysam, B., Goderie, S. K., Ali, R. A., Kokovay, E., et al. (2011). Vertebrate neural stem cell segmentation, tracking and lineaging with validation and editing. *Nat. Protoc.* 6, 1942–1952. doi: 10.1038/nprot.2011.422

Winter, M. R., Liu, M., Monteleone, D., Melunis, J., Hershberg, U., Goderie, S. K., et al. (2015). Computational image analysis reveals intrinsic multigenerational differences between anterior and posterior cerebral cortex neural progenitor cells. *Stem Cell Rep.* 5, 609–620. doi: 10.1016/j.stemcr.2015.08.002

Yokose, J., Ishizuka, T., Yoshida, T., Aoki, J., Koyanagi, Y., and Yawo, H. (2011). Lineage analysis of newly generated neurons in organotypic culture of rat hippocampus. *Neurosci. Res.* 69, 223–233. doi: 10.1016/j.neures.2010.11.010

Zhao, C., Deng, W., and Gage, F. H. (2008). Mechanisms and functional implications of adult neurogenesis. *Cell* 132, 645–660. doi: 10.1016/j.cell.2008.01.033

6

Discerning Neurogenic vs. Non-Neurogenic Postnatal Lateral Ventricular Astrocytes via Activity-Dependent Input

Elena W. Adlaf[1], *Aaron Mitchell-Dick*[1,2] *and Chay T. Kuo*[1,2,3,4,5,6*]

[1] *Department of Cell Biology, Duke University School of Medicine, Durham, NC, USA,* [2] *Cellular and Molecular Biology Graduate Training Program, Duke University School of Medicine, Durham, NC, USA,* [3] *Brumley Neonatal Perinatal Research Institute, Duke University School of Medicine, Durham, NC, USA,* [4] *Department of Neurobiology, Duke University School of Medicine, Durham, NC, USA,* [5] *Preston Robert Tisch Brain Tumor Center, Duke University School of Medicine, Durham, NC, USA,* [6] *Duke Institute for Brain Sciences, Duke University, Durham, NC, USA*

Edited by:
Laura López-Mascaraque, Instituto Cajal-CSIC, Spain

Reviewed by:
Francis G. Szele, Oxford University, UK
Juan Manuel Encinas, Ikerbasque and University of the Basque Country, Spain

***Correspondence:**
Chay T. Kuo
chay.kuo@duke.edu

Throughout development, neural stem cells (NSCs) give rise to differentiated neurons, astrocytes, and oligodendrocytes which together modulate perception, memory, and behavior in the adult nervous system. To understand how NSCs contribute to postnatal/adult brain remodeling and repair after injury, the lateral ventricular (LV) neurogenic niche in the rodent postnatal brain serves as an excellent model system. It is a specialized area containing self-renewing GFAP$^+$ astrocytes functioning as NSCs generating new neurons throughout life. In addition to this now well-studied regenerative process, the LV niche also generates differentiated astrocytes, playing an important role for glial scar formation after cortical injury. While LV NSCs can be clearly distinguished from their neuroblast and oligodendrocyte progeny via molecular markers, the astrocytic identity of NSCs has complicated their distinction from terminally-differentiated astrocytes in the niche. Our current models of postnatal/adult LV neurogenesis do not take into account local astrogenesis, or the possibility that cellular markers may be similar between non-dividing GFAP$^+$ NSCs and their differentiated astrocyte daughters. Postnatal LV neurogenesis is regulated by NSC-intrinsic mechanisms interacting with extracellular/niche-driven cues. It is generally believed that these local effects are responsible for sustaining neurogenesis, though behavioral paradigms and disease states have suggested possibilities for neural circuit-level modulation. With recent experimental findings that neuronal stimulation can directly evoke responses in LV NSCs, it is possible that this exciting property will add a new dimension to identifying postnatal/adult NSCs. Here, we put forth a notion that neural circuit-level input can be a distinct characteristic defining postnatal/adult NSCs from non-neurogenic astroglia.

Keywords: adult neurogenesis, neural stem cells (NSCs), cholinergic circuit, lateral ventricles, astrogenesis

INTRODUCTION

During embryonic neurogenesis, the brain is constructed in a systematic and reproducible way by the division of NSCs, and the migration/differentiation of their progeny (Ma et al., 2009; Urbán and Guillemot, 2014). The requirements for neurogenesis to persist in distinct regions of the adult mammalian brain, which include the subgranular zone (SGZ) of the hippocampus and the lateral wall of the LV, but not others, are still not fully understood. It is generally believed that proliferation of adult NSCs to generate new neurons serves the functional needs of established neural circuits in a region-specific and stimulus-dependent manner. Thus, it is possible that network activity, driven by environmental stimuli, instructs the proliferation, migration and differentiation of postnatal NSCs. In this fashion, postnatal/adult neurogenesis may actively contribute to neural plasticity via a stimuli-driven feedback loop, in contrast to embryonic neurogenesis, which operates on a well-tuned timer for reproducible anatomical construction. Classically, for a cell to be defined as an NSC, it should possess the ability to undergo asymmetrical cell division for both self-renewal and generation of new neurons. How to positively identify NSCs from a seemingly heterogeneous population of cell types in the postnatal/adult neurogenic niche presents a significant challenge for experimental design and data interpretation. Currently, the most utilized methods for identifying adult NSCs based on morphological and molecular methods are perhaps overly inclusive or exclusive depending on context. When we visualize a GFAP$^+$ glia in the neurogenic niche, how do we tell whether it is neurogenic or not? What if the niche produced local, terminally-differentiated astrocytes with similar morphological and molecular characteristics as those defining NSCs? Our current models do not distinguish these important differences (**Figure 1**). This perspective summarizes emerging studies of LV astrogenesis as well as alternative strategies for defining postnatal NSCs and their potential drawbacks. We argue that circuit-level drive to sustain progenitor proliferation is an important aspect of adult neurogenesis/astrogenesis, and this property could be utilized to further define LV NSCs vs. terminally differentiated local astrocytes.

GLIAL IDENTITY OF LV NSCs

In a seminal 1999 study, Alvarez-Buylla and colleagues showed convincingly that a subset of LV cells expressing glial fibrillary acidic protein (GFAP) had the characteristics of NSCs (Doetsch et al., 1999a). GFAP$^+$ cells in the LV niche (also termed type B cells) were labeled with proliferation markers over long survival periods, and an intraventricularly-injected retrovirus targeting GFAP$^+$ cells resulted in labeled neuroblasts and neurons in the olfactory bulb. After elimination of proliferating LV cell types with the antimitotic agent Ara-C, GFAP$^+$ cells remained in the niche, began to divide and could be traced as the precursors of Mash1$^+$ transient amplifying cells (type C cells) and migrating neuroblasts (type A cells; Doetsch et al., 1999a; Alvarez-Buylla and Lim, 2004).

In addition to the neurogenic subset of type B astrocytes, designated type B1, GFAP$^+$ cells within the LV niche include type B2 astrocytes (García-Verdugo et al., 1998; Mirzadeh et al., 2008) and stellate astrocytes (Ma et al., 2005). These cell types are not always morphologically distinct (Garcia et al., 2004; Shen et al., 2008), and can be a challenge to distinguish during tissue experiments probing NSC function. In recent years, for simplicity, the process of adult LV neurogenesis has mostly been described in schematics to illustrate subependymal zone (SEZ) astrocytes functioning as NSCs. **Figure 2** shows native GFP fluorescence (without antibody staining) from an LV wholemount harvested from adult *GFAP-GFP* animal, showing

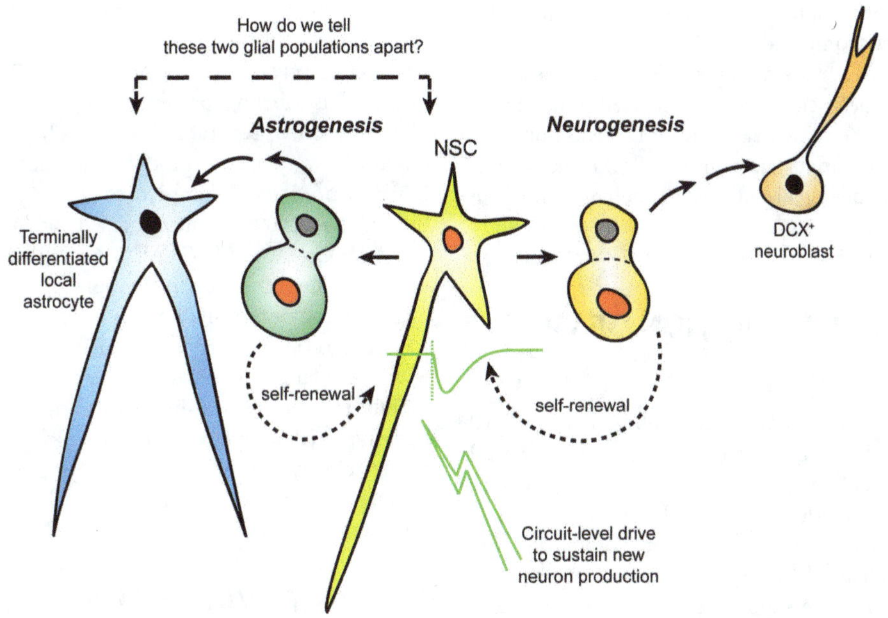

FIGURE 1 | Distinguishing neurogenic vs. non-neurogenic adult LV astrocytes. Schematic representation of an area of postnatal/adult LV neurogenesis needing reconsideration: the incorporation of astrogenesis in the context of ongoing neurogenesis. It is currently unclear how newly-generated (but terminally-differentiated) local astrocytes can be distinguished from NSCs that are not actively dividing. Response to neuronal activation may separate LV NSCs from other niche astrocytes.

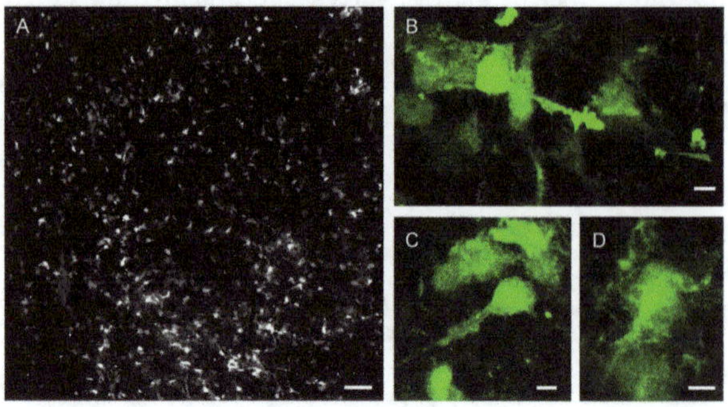

FIGURE 2 | Morphological diversity of postnatal LV niche GFAP-GFP$^+$ cells. LV lateral wall wholemount tissue preparation from P32 *GFAP-GFP* reporter mouse, imaged via endogenous GFP fluorescence. **(A)** Representative confocal enface view of lateral wall surface, at the level of anterior commissure, known to contain ependymal niche pinwheel-like structures. **(B–D)** Close-up views of example GFP$^+$ subependymal cells. Note the differences in cellular morphologies. Bars = 100 μm **(A)**, 5 μm **(B–D)**.

the difficulty in distinguishing different GFP$^+$ cell types based on morphology in real time. For simplicity during experimentation using live cells, GFAP and other astrocytic markers, such as GLAST1, have nonetheless been generalized in many instances as positive identifiers of NSCs within the SEZ of the LV niche.

Progress in moving away from such generalized astrocytic markers has been hindered by a lack of reliable, alternative expression markers that can clearly distinguish neurogenic vs. non-neurogenic LV astrocytes (Mamber et al., 2013). Further complicating this problem, adult NSCs can become quiescent *in vivo* over long timespans and change their proliferative profile/markers in the process (Doetsch et al., 1999b; Codega et al., 2014; Calzolari et al., 2015). Single-cell sequencing technology can be a powerful tool for expression profiling of LV NSCs in different states. Combined with fluorescent activated cell sorting (FACS) using cell surface markers, these approaches may provide the necessary specificity to more accurately characterize NSCs (Pastrana et al., 2009; Mich et al., 2014; Llorens-Bobadilla et al., 2015). However, an important consideration is that multi-genetic fluorescence labeling are difficult/time-consuming to generate for use in live tissue experiments, such as *in vitro* recording or live cell imaging.

MORPHOLOGICAL DEFINITION OF LV NSCs

Anatomical features of NSCs have been combined with GFAP expression to further refine the positional and morphological definition of a postnatal/adult LV NSC. B1 type astrocytes within the LV niche had originally been described to possess a primary cilium contacting the cerebrospinal fluid from the apical surface (Doetsch et al., 1997). Subsequent experiments revealed that they: (1) possess polarized and extended basal endfeet to contact blood vessels (Shen et al., 2008; Tavazoie et al., 2008); and (2) are arranged into a pinwheel-like architecture together with neighboring ependymal niche cells (Mirzadeh et al., 2008; Paez-Gonzalez et al., 2011). The combinatorial usage of astrocytic marker + anatomical features represents perhaps our current state-of-the-art in identifying LV niche NSCs in immunohistochemical experiments and their analyses. It has been well-described that the endfeet of stellate astrocytes also contact blood vessels and are an integral modulator of the blood-brain-barrier (Abbott et al., 2006). Also, the LV *medial* wall can be neurogenic (Merkle et al., 2007), although ependymal pinwheel-like niche structures have not been described in this brain region. Thus, it is difficult to conclude that contacting blood vessels and/or arranging into ependymal pinwheel structures are specific anatomical features for postnatal/adult LV NSCs.

GENETIC LINEAGE-TRACING OF POSTNATAL NSCS

While molecular markers and anatomical features are indispensable for NSC identification, they do not directly address the key cellular feature for these cells to generate neuronal progeny in the adult brain. Nestin is an intermediate filament protein expressed in nervous system cells during active division (Lendahl et al., 1990). To genetically define the cellular activity of postnatal/adult NSCs, we and others have generated tamoxifen-inducible Nestin-CreER transgenic drivers, together with Cre-driven reporters, to lineage-trace and understand the developmental process of neurogenesis (Kuo et al., 2006; Lagace et al., 2007; Aponso et al., 2008; Giachino and Taylor, 2009; Dhaliwal and Lagace, 2011; Benner et al., 2013; Faiz et al., 2015; Sohn et al., 2015). While this approach has been highly successful and widely adopted, Nestin-CreER also targets LV niche ependymal cells (Kuo et al., 2006), which are generally believed to be post-mitotic but express Nestin like their NSC counterpart. It is also important to note that, due to the nature of transgenic approaches, the different Nestin-CreER lines vary in NSC targeting efficiency as well as niche ependymal cells labeled (Kuo et al., 2006; Lagace et al., 2007; Giachino and Taylor, 2009). This labeling presents a significant challenge for NSC identification, as several publications have indicated neurogenic potential for ependymal niche cells under physiological and/or injury conditions (Johansson et al., 1999; Coskun et al., 2008; Carlén et al., 2009; Nomura et al., 2010; Luo et al., 2015).

GFAP-CreER and GLAST1-CreER lines have also been used to quantify the production of newborn neurons and oligodendrocytes from LV NSCs (Menn et al., 2006; Dhaliwal and Lagace, 2011; Calzolari et al., 2015). These drivers by definition will label mature astrocytes in the brain, and so they were used mainly to identify terminally-differentiated NSC progeny that had migrated away from the LV niche. However, these lines cannot clearly identify the cellular origins of newborn neurons or oligodendrocytes within the LV niche as both neurogenic and non-neurogenic astrocytes are targeted.

POSTNATAL/ADULT LV NICHE ASTROGENESIS

While it has long been observed that LV NSCs cultured in a dish can differentiate into GFAP$^+$ astrocytes, in contrast to neurogenesis, LV niche astrogenesis *in vivo* had been largely ignored. If there is significant baseline astrogenesis from LV NSCs and/or astrogenic progenitors, this will present significant challenges to NSC identification using glial markers since newly generated astrocytes may be indistinguishable. Nestin-CreER lineage-tracing experiments have recently revealed significant astrogenesis from the postnatal LV niche following cortical stroke (Benner et al., 2013; Faiz et al., 2015). While these migrating cells from the niche to cortical regions retain some cellular plasticity (Faiz et al., 2015), they mainly become reactive astrocytes important for normal glial scar formation at the injury site (Benner et al., 2013; Faiz et al., 2015). Additionally, the LV niche can also generate mature astrocytes under physiological conditions (Sohn et al., 2015). Further experimentation would benefit from a set of cellular markers for newborn LV niche astrocytes that are distinct from those used to identify NSCs.

NEUROTRANSMITTER AND ACTIVITY-DEPENDENT CONTROL IN THE LV NICHE

While the actual neural circuitry inputs to the LV niche are poorly understood and an important area for future study, there is mounting evidence that LV niche NSCs are controlled by neurotransmitters and neuronal activity. Several studies have shown that applications of synaptic and modulatory neurotransmitters to the LV niche alter the quantity of proliferative cells. (Banasr et al., 2004; Cooper-Kuhn et al., 2004; Van Kampen et al., 2004; Brazel et al., 2005; Liu et al., 2005; Mudò et al., 2007; O'Keeffe et al., 2009; Alfonso et al., 2012; Paez-Gonzalez et al., 2014; Tong et al., 2014). These results suggest that either the presence of neurotransmitters in the niche causes the release of factors that stimulate NSC proliferation, or that NSCs respond directly to network activity through membrane receptors. Slice electrophysiology experiments using GFAP-GFP reporter mice showed that GFAP$^+$ LV astrocytes respond directly to GABA (Liu et al., 2005). Another study performing *in vitro* whole-cell recording chose NSCs based on GFAP-GFP expression combined with the presence of a long cellular projection, and found that local application of serotonin (5HT) caused inward currents in B1 cells that were blocked by 5HT antagonists (Tong et al., 2014). These example studies and others verified the existence of neurotransmitter receptors on GFAP$^+$ cells in the LV niche. However, they do not rule out the possibility that non-neurogenic niche astrocytes express the same receptors. Furthermore, GFAP$^+$ LV cells have similar resting membrane potentials and input resistances to stellate astrocytes, thus NSCs may not be identified solely based on intrinsic membrane properties (Liu et al., 2005; Lacar et al., 2010; Tong et al., 2014).

We have recently identified a distinct population of cholinergic neurons residing within the postnatal/adult LV niche. Functional experiments utilizing optogenetics to examine circuit connectivity of cholinergic neurons to LV NSCs uncovered neuronal activity-dependent responses in NSCs. NSCs were chosen by a combination of Nestin-CreER lineage-tracing, cellular morphology, and Nestin expression. Acetylcholine (ACh) responses were seen in patch-clamped NSCs following light activation of channelrhodopsin-expressing ChAT$^+$ neurons (Paez-Gonzalez et al., 2014). Similar optogenetic activation of ChAT$^+$ neurons resulted in no noticeable responses in ependymal niche cells or transiently amplifying Mash1$^+$ cells, although there was a consistent response in DCX$^+$ neuroblasts. To our knowledge, this may perhaps be the first report of recorded response in a LV NSC as a result of direct neuronal activation. It remains unclear whether differentiated astrocytes in the LV niche have similar capacities to respond to ChAT$^+$ neuron activity.

CAN ACTIVITY RESPONSE BE UTILIZED TO DEFINE NSCs?

Whether the proliferation and differentiation of LV NSCs can be directly regulated by neural activity is a source of debate. In one view, NSCs are programmed to undergo mitosis and sustain cell division as a part of their identity, and the controlled environment of the niche is protected from outside signals by astrocytic boundaries (Ma et al., 2009). In the olfactory bulb (OB), the main target location for interneurons produced from the LV niche, enhanced sensory activation does not appear to stimulate LV NSC proliferation, suggesting that OB circuit activity is removed from NSC control (Rochefort et al., 2002). In fact, LV proliferation persists following complete bulbectomy (Kirschenbaum et al., 1999). On the other hand, increased LV NSC proliferation is observed after OB neuron cell death (Mandairon et al., 2003), as well as during odor-dependent behaviors such as paternal recognition (Mak and Weiss, 2010) and pheromone mating response (Mak et al., 2007). LV NSCs can also migrate to other brain regions and differentiate into varied cell types in response to cortical injury (Benner et al., 2013; Faiz et al., 2015), demyelination (El Waly et al., 2014), chemical lesions (Aponso et al., 2008), and electrical stimulation (Jahanshahi et al., 2013). Finally, if postnatal/adult NSCs are instructed to produce new neurons or glia for distinct neural circuits, theoretically it would be beneficial for NSCs to be in direct communication with those respective circuits. The finding that local cholinergic neurons can directly innervate LV NSCs is a step toward showing the existence of that neural circuit feedback. It remains possible that these responses may change depending on NSC states in quiescence vs. activation, and future exploration of these neuronal activity-dependent NSC responses may yet provide further refinements to our definitions for postnatal/adult NSC identity.

AUTHOR CONTRIBUTIONS

All authors listed, have made substantial, direct and intellectual contribution to the work, and approved it for publication.

ACKNOWLEDGMENTS

We thank Dominic Luciano and members of the Kuo laboratory for helpful discussions. This work was supported by N.I.H. grant MH105416, NS078192, The March of Dimes, and George and Jean Brumley Endowment (CK). AM is supported by a Fellowship from the Ruth K. Broad Biomedical Research Foundation.

REFERENCES

Abbott, N. J., Rönnbäck, L., and Hansson, E. (2006). Astrocyte-endothelial interactions at the blood-brain barrier. *Nat. Rev. Neurosci.* 7, 41–53. doi: 10.1038/nrn1824

Alfonso, J., Le Magueresse, C., Zuccotti, A., Khodosevich, K., and Monyer, H. (2012). Diazepam binding inhibitor promotes progenitor proliferation in the postnatal SVZ by reducing GABA signaling. *Cell Stem Cell* 10, 76–87. doi: 10.1016/j.stem.2011.11.011

Alvarez-Buylla, A., and Lim, D. A. (2004). For the long run: maintaining germinal niches in the adult brain. *Neuron* 41, 683–686. doi: 10.1016/S0896-6273(04)00111-4

Aponso, P. M., Faull, R. L., and Connor, B. (2008). Increased progenitor cell proliferation and astrogenesis in the partial progressive 6-hydroxydopamine model of Parkinson's disease. *Neuroscience* 151, 1142–1153. doi: 10.1016/j.neuroscience.2007.11.036

Banasr, M., Hery, M., Printemps, R., and Daszuta, A. (2004). Serotonin-induced increases in adult cell proliferation and neurogenesis are mediated through different and common 5-HT receptor subtypes in the dentate gyrus and the subventricular zone. *Neuropsychopharmacology* 29, 450–460. doi: 10.1038/sj.npp.1300320

Benner, E. J., Luciano, D., Jo, R., Abdi, K., Paez-Gonzalez, P., Sheng, H., et al. (2013). Protective astrogenesis from the SVZ niche after injury is controlled by Notch modulator Thbs4. *Nature* 497, 369–373. doi: 10.1038/nature12069

Brazel, C. Y., Nuñez, J. L., Yang, Z., and Levison, S. W. (2005). Glutamate enhances survival and proliferation of neural progenitors derived from the subventricular zone. *Neuroscience* 131, 55–65. doi: 10.1016/j.neuroscience.2004.10.038

Calzolari, F., Michel, J., Baumgart, E. V., Theis, F., Götz, M., and Ninkovic, J. (2015). Fast clonal expansion and limited neural stem cell self-renewal in the adult subependymal zone. *Nat. Neurosci.* 18, 490–492. doi: 10.1038/nn.3963

Carlén, M., Meletis, K., Göritz, C., Darsalia, V., Evergren, E., Tanigaki, K., et al. (2009). Forebrain ependymal cells are Notch-dependent and generate neuroblasts and astrocytes after stroke. *Nat. Neurosci.* 12, 259–267. doi: 10.1038/nn.2268

Codega, P., Silva-Vargas, V., Paul, A., Maldonado-Soto, A. R., Deleo, A. M., Pastrana, E., et al. (2014). Prospective identification and purification of quiescent adult neural stem cells from their *in vivo* niche. *Neuron* 82, 545–559. doi: 10.1016/j.neuron.2014.02.039

Cooper-Kuhn, C. M., Winkler, J., and Kuhn, H. G. (2004). Decreased neurogenesis after cholinergic forebrain lesion in the adult rat. *J. Neurosci. Res.* 77, 155–165. doi: 10.1002/jnr.20116

Coskun, V., Wu, H., Blanchi, B., Tsao, S., Kim, K., Zhao, J., et al. (2008). CD133+ neural stem cells in the ependyma of mammalian postnatal forebrain. *Proc. Natl. Acad. Sci. U.S.A.* 105, 1026–1031. doi: 10.1073/pnas.0710000105

Dhaliwal, J., and Lagace, D. C. (2011). Visualization and genetic manipulation of adult neurogenesis using transgenic mice. *Eur. J. Neurosci.* 33, 1025–1036. doi: 10.1111/j.1460-9568.2011.07600.x

Doetsch, F., Caillé, I., Lim, D. A., García-Verdugo, J. M., and Alvarez-Buylla, A. (1999a). Subventricular zone astrocytes are neural stem cells in the adult mammalian brain. *Cell* 97, 703–716. doi: 10.1016/S0092-8674(00)80783-7

Doetsch, F., García-Verdugo, J. M., and Alvarez-Buylla, A. (1999b). Regeneration of a germinal layer in the adult mammalian brain. *Proc. Natl. Acad. Sci. U.S.A.* 96, 11619–11624. doi: 10.1073/pnas.96.20.11619

Doetsch, F., García-Verdugo, J. M., and Alvarez-Buylla, A. (1997). Cellular composition and three-dimensional organization of the subventricular germinal zone in the adult mammalian brain. *J. Neurosci.* 17, 5046–5061.

El Waly, B., Macchi, M., Cayre, M., and Durbec, P. (2014). Oligodendrogenesis in the normal and pathological central nervous system. *Front. Neurosci.* 8:145. doi: 10.3389/fnins.2014.00145

Faiz, M., Sachewsky, N., Gascón, S., Bang, K. W., Morshead, C. M., and Nagy, A. (2015). Adult neural stem cells from the subventricular zone give rise to reactive astrocytes in the cortex after stroke. *Cell Stem Cell* 17, 624–634. doi: 10.1016/j.stem.2015.08.002

Garcia, A. D. R., Doan, N. B., Imura, T., Bush, T. G., and Sofroniew, M. V. (2004). GFAP-expressing progenitors are the principal source of constitutive neurogenesis in adult mouse forebrain. *Nat. Neurosci.* 7, 1233–1241. doi: 10.1038/nn1340

García-Verdugo, J. M., Doetsch, F., Wichterle, H., Lim, D. A., and Alvarez-Buylla, A. (1998). Architecture and cell types of the adult subventricular zone: in search of the stem cells. *J. Neurobiol.* 36, 234–248.

Giachino, C., and Taylor, V. (2009). Lineage analysis of quiescent regenerative stem cells in the adult brain by genetic labelling reveals spatially restricted neurogenic niches in the olfactory bulb. *Eur. J. Neurosci.* 30, 9–24. doi: 10.1111/j.1460-9568.2009.06798.x

Jahanshahi, A., Schonfeld, L., Janssen, M. L., Hescham, S., Kocabicak, E., Steinbusch, H. W., et al. (2013). Electrical stimulation of the motor cortex enhances progenitor cell migration in the adult rat brain. *Exp. Brain Res.* 231, 165–177. doi: 10.1007/s00221-013-3680-4

Johansson, C. B., Momma, S., Clarke, D. L., Risling, M., Lendahl, U., and Frisén, J. (1999). Identification of a neural stem cell in the adult mammalian central nervous system. *Cell* 96, 25–34. doi: 10.1016/S0092-8674(00)80956-3

Kirschenbaum, B., Doetsch, F., Lois, C., and Alvarez-Buylla, A. (1999). Adult subventricular zone neuronal precursors continue to proliferate and migrate in the absence of the olfactory bulb. *J. Neurosci.* 19, 2171–2180.

Kuo, C. T., Mirzadeh, Z., Soriano-Navarro, M., Rasin, M., Wang, D., Shen, J., et al. (2006). Postnatal deletion of Numb/Numblike reveals repair and remodeling capacity in the subventricular neurogenic niche. *Cell* 127, 1253–1264. doi: 10.1016/j.cell.2006.10.041

Lacar, B., Young, S. Z., Platel, J. C., and Bordey, A. (2010). Imaging and recording subventricular zone progenitor cells in live tissue of postnatal mice. *Front. Neurosci.* 4:43. doi: 10.3389/fnins.2010.00043

Lagace, D. C., Whitman, M. C., Noonan, M. A., Ables, J. L., DeCarolis, N. A., Arguello, A. A., et al. (2007). Dynamic contribution of nestin-expressing stem cells to adult neurogenesis. *J. Neurosci.* 27, 12623–12629. doi: 10.1523/JNEUROSCI.3812-07.2007

Lendahl, U., Zimmerman, L. B., and McKay, R. D. (1990). CNS stem cells express a new class of intermediate filament protein. *Cell* 60, 585–595. doi: 10.1016/0092-8674(90)90662-X

Liu, X., Wang, Q., Haydar, T. F., and Bordey, A. (2005). Nonsynaptic GABA signaling in postnatal subventricular zone controls proliferation of GFAP-expressing progenitors. *Nat. Neurosci.* 8, 1179–1187. doi: 10.1038/nn1522

Llorens-Bobadilla, E., Zhao, S., Baser, A., Saiz-Castro, G., Zwadlo, K., and Martin-Villalba, A. (2015). Single-cell transcriptomics reveals a population of dormant neural stem cells that become activated upon brain injury. *Cell Stem Cell* 17, 329–340. doi: 10.1016/j.stem.2015.07.002

Luo, Y., Coskun, V., Liang, A., Yu, J., Cheng, L., Ge, W., et al. (2015). Single-cell transcriptome analyses reveal signals to activate dormant neural stem cells. *Cell* 161, 1175–1186. doi: 10.1016/j.cell.2015.04.001

Ma, D. K., Kim, W. R., Ming, G. L., and Song, H. (2009). Activity-dependent extrinsic regulation of adult olfactory bulb and hippocampal neurogenesis. *Ann. N.Y. Acad. Sci.* 1170, 664–673. doi: 10.1111/j.1749-6632.2009.04373.x

Ma, D. K., Ming, G. L., and Song, H. (2005). Glial influences on neural stem cell development: cellular niches for adult neurogenesis. *Curr. Opin. Neurobiol.* 15, 514–520. doi: 10.1016/j.conb.2005.08.003

Mak, G. K., Enwere, E. K., Gregg, C., Pakarainen, T., Poutanen, M., Huhtaniemi, I., et al. (2007). Male pheromone-stimulated neurogenesis in the adult female brain: possible role in mating behavior. *Nat. Neurosci.* 10, 1003–1011. doi: 10.1038/nn1928

Mak, G. K., and Weiss, S. (2010). Paternal recognition of adult offspring mediated by newly generated CNS neurons. *Nat. Neurosci.* 13, 753–758. doi: 10.1038/nn.2550

Mamber, C., Kozareva, D. A., Kamphuis, W., and Hol, E. M. (2013). Shades of gray: the delineation of marker expression within the adult rodent subventricular zone. *Prog. Neurobiol.* 111, 1–16. doi: 10.1016/j.pneurobio.2013.07.003

Mandairon, N., Jourdan, F., and Didier, A. (2003). Deprivation of sensory inputs to the olfactory bulb up-regulates cell death and proliferation in the subventricular zone of adult mice. *Neuroscience* 119, 507–516. doi: 10.1016/S0306-4522(03)00172-6

Menn, B., Garcia-Verdugo, J. M., Yaschine, C., Gonzalez-Perez, O., Rowitch, D., and Alvarez-Buylla, A. (2006). Origin of oligodendrocytes in the subventricular zone of the adult brain. *J. Neurosci.* 26, 7907–7918. doi: 10.1523/JNEUROSCI.1299-06.2006

Merkle, F. T., Mirzadeh, Z., and Alvarez-Buylla, A. (2007). Mosaic organization of neural stem cells in the adult brain. *Science* 317, 381–384. doi: 10.1126/science.1144914

Mich, J. K., Signer, R. A., Nakada, D., Pineda, A., Burgess, R. J., Vue, T. Y., et al. (2014). Prospective identification of functionally distinct stem cells and neurosphere-initiating cells in adult mouse forebrain. *Elife* 3:e02669. doi: 10.7554/eLife.02669

Mirzadeh, Z., Merkle, F. T., Soriano-Navarro, M., Garcia-Verdugo, J. M., and Alvarez-Buylla, A. (2008). Neural stem cells confer unique pinwheel architecture to the ventricular surface in neurogenic regions of the adult brain. *Cell Stem Cell* 3, 265–278. doi: 10.1016/j.stem.2008.07.004

Mudò, G., Belluardo, N., Mauro, A., and Fuxe, K. (2007). Acute intermittent nicotine treatment induces fibroblast growth factor-2 in the subventricular zone of the adult rat brain and enhances neuronal precursor cell proliferation. *Neuroscience* 145, 470–483. doi: 10.1016/j.neuroscience.2006.12.012

Nomura, T., Göritz, C., Catchpole, T., Henkemeyer, M., and Frisén, J. (2010). EphB signaling controls lineage plasticity of adult neural stem cell niche cells. *Cell Stem Cell* 7, 730–743. doi: 10.1016/j.stem.2010.11.009

O'Keeffe, G. C., Tyers, P., Aarsland, D., Dalley, J. W., Barker, R. A., and Caldwell, M. A. (2009). Dopamine-induced proliferation of adult neural precursor cells in the mammalian subventricular zone is mediated through EGF. *Proc. Natl. Acad. Sci. U.S.A.* 106, 8754–8759. doi: 10.1073/pnas.0803955106

Paez-Gonzalez, P., Abdi, K., Luciano, D., Liu, Y., Soriano-Navarro, M., Rawlins, E., et al. (2011). Ank3-dependent SVZ niche assembly is required for the continued production of new neurons. *Neuron* 71, 61–75. doi: 10.1016/j.neuron.2011.05.029

Paez-Gonzalez, P., Asrican, B., Rodriguez, E., and Kuo, C. (2014). Identification of distinct $ChAT^+$ neurons and activity-dependent control of postnatal SVZ neurogenesis. *Nat. Neurosci.* 17, 934–942. doi: 10.1038/nn.3734

Pastrana, E., Cheng, L., and Doetsch, F. (2009). Simultaneous prospective purification of adult subventricular zone neural stem cells and their progeny. *Proc. Natl. Acad. Sci. U.S.A.* 106, 6387–6392. doi: 10.1073/pnas.081040

Rochefort, C., Gheusi, G., Vincent, J. D., and Lledo, P. M. (2002). Enriched odor exposure increases the number of newborn neurons in the adult olfactory bulb and improves odor memory. *J. Neurosci.* 22, 2679–2689.

Shen, Q., Wang, Y., Kokovay, E., Lin, G., Chuang, S. M., Goderie, S. K., et al. (2008). Adult SVZ stem cells lie in a vascular niche: a quantitative analysis of niche cell-cell interactions. *Cell Stem Cell* 3, 289–300. doi: 10.1016/j.stem.2008.07.026

Sohn, J., Orosco, L., Guo, F., Chung, S. H., Bannerman, P., Mills Ko, E., et al. (2015). The subventricular zone continues to generate corpus callosum and rostral migratory stream astroglia in normal adult mice. *J. Neurosci.* 35, 3756–3763. doi: 10.1523/JNEUROSCI.3454-14.2015

Tavazoie, M., Van der Veken, L., Silva-Vargas, V., Louissaint, M., Colonna, L., Zaidi, B., et al. (2008). A specialized vascular niche for adult neural stem cells. *Cell Stem Cell* 3, 279–288. doi: 10.1016/j.stem.2008.07.025

Tong, C. K., Chen, J., Cebrián-Silla, A., Mirzadeh, Z., Obernier, K., Guinto, C. D., et al. (2014). Axonal control of the adult neural stem cell niche. *Cell Stem Cell* 14, 500–511. doi: 10.1016/j.stem.2014.01.014

Urb´an, N., and Guillemot, F. (2014). Neurogenesis in the embryonic and adult brain: same regulators, different roles. *Front. Cell. Neurosci.* 8:396. doi: 10.3389/fncel.2014.00396

Van Kampen, J. M., Hagg, T., and Robertson, H. A. (2004). Induction of neurogenesis in the adult rat subventricular zone and neostriatum following dopamine D3 receptor stimulation. *Eur. J. Neurosci.* 19, 2377–2387. doi: 10.1111/j.0953-816X.2004.03342.x

7

Regulation of Neurogenesis by Neurotrophins during Adulthood: Expected and Unexpected Roles

Marçal Vilar[1] and Helena Mira[2]**

[1] Neurodegeneration Unit, Unidad Funcional de Investigación de Enfermedades Crónicas-Instituto de Salud Carlos III, Madrid, Spain, [2] Molecular Neurobiology Unit, Unidad Funcional de Investigación de Enfermedades Crónicas-Instituto de Salud Carlos III, Madrid, Spain

The subventricular zone (SVZ) of the anterolateral ventricle and the subgranular zone (SGZ) of the hippocampal dentate gyrus are the two main regions of the adult mammalian brain in which neurogenesis is maintained throughout life. Because alterations in adult neurogenesis appear to be a common hallmark of different neurodegenerative diseases, understanding the molecular mechanisms controlling adult neurogenesis is a focus of active research. Neurotrophic factors are a family of molecules that play critical roles in the survival and differentiation of neurons during development and in the control of neural plasticity in the adult. Several neurotrophins and neurotrophin receptors have been implicated in the regulation of adult neurogenesis at different levels. Here, we review the current understanding of neurotrophin modulation of adult neurogenesis in both the SVZ and SGZ. We compile data supporting a variety of roles for neurotrophins/neurotrophin receptors in different scenarios, including both expected and unexpected functions.

Keywords: adult neurogenesis, neural stem cell, neurotrophin, p75NTR, TrkB, BDNF, NT3

Edited by:
José Luis Trejo,
Institute Cajal - Consejo Superior de Investigaciones Científicas, Spain

Reviewed by:
Stefano Farioli Vecchioli,
Consiglio Nazionale delle Ricerche, Italy
John W. Cave,
Weill Cornell Medical College, USA

****Correspondence:***
Marçal Vilar
mvilar@isciii.es;
Helena Mira
hmira@isciii.es

INTRODUCTION

Neurotrophins (NTs) are implicated in the maintenance and survival of the peripheral and central nervous systems and mediate several forms of synaptic plasticity (Chao, 2003; Ceni et al., 2014; Hempstead, 2014; Lu et al., 2014). Nerve growth factor (NGF) was the first discovered member of the family (Cohen et al., 1954), which also includes brain-derived neurotrophic factor (BDNF), neurotrophin-3 (NT3), and neurotrophin 4/5 (NT4/5) (reviewed recently in Bothwell, 2014). Neurotrophins were first identified as survival factors for developing neurons, but are pleiotropic molecules that can exert a variety of functions, including the regulation of neuronal differentiation, axonal and dendritic growth, and synaptic plasticity (Bothwell, 2014).

NTs interact with two distinct receptors, a cognate member of the Trk receptor tyrosine kinase family and the common p75 neurotrophin receptor (p75NTR), which belongs to the tumor necrosis factor receptor (TNFR) superfamily of death receptors (Friedman and Greene, 1999; Huang and Reichardt, 2003). Tropomyosin receptor kinase (Trk) receptors belong to the family of receptor tyrosine kinases (reviewed in Deinhardt and Chao, 2014) and contain an extracellular domain at which the NT binds, a single transmembrane domain, and an intracellular domain (ICD) with tyrosine kinase activity. Three different Trks have been identified in mammals: TrkA, TrkB, and TrkC. NGF is the preferred ligand for TrkA, BDNF, and NT4/5 are preferred for TrkB, and NT3 for TrkC. These specificities are not absolute, and NT3 is also a ligand for TrkA and TrkB. In addition to full length (FL) receptors, splice variants containing either deletions in the extracellular domain or intracellular truncations including the kinase domain have been described. These receptor molecules may influence ligand specificity, restrict its availability by internalization, or act as dominant-negative modulators. Splice variants of TrkB, designated T1 and T2, are expressed at high levels in the mature brain (Klein et al., 1990).

While Trk receptors bind only to mature neurotrophins, p75NTR also interacts with pro-neurotrophins, increasing the complexity of its signaling. Upon pro-NGF binding, cell death is induced by a complex consisting of p75NTR and sortilin (Hempstead, 2014). Similarly, pro-BDNF induces axon pruning of hippocampal neurons in culture (Hempstead, 2015). Although, Trk signaling is involved in survival and differentiation (Reichardt, 2006; Deinhardt and Chao, 2014), p75NTR participates in several signaling pathways (Kraemer et al., 2014) governed by the cell context and the formation of complexes with different co-receptors and ligands, such as sortilin/pro-NGF in cell death (Nykjaer et al., 2004) and Nogo/Lingo-1/NgR in axonal growth (Wang et al., 2002; Mi et al., 2004). p75NTR also undergoes shedding and receptor intramembrane proteolysis (RIP), resulting in the release of its ICD, which itself possesses signaling capabilities related to migration, proliferation, and transcriptional modulation (Jung et al., 2003; Kanning et al., 2003; Skeldal et al., 2012). Two different isoforms of p75NTR have been described, a long isoform and a short isoform (Naumann et al., 2002). These isoforms differ based on the presence or absence of the NT binding domain, respectively.

In recent years, NTs and their receptors have emerged as important regulators of adult neurogenesis. The production of new neurons persists throughout life in two regions or niches of the mammalian brain in which neurotrophins are also present: the subependymal or subventricular zone (SVZ) adjacent to the lateral ventricles, and the subgranular zone (SGZ) of the dentate gyrus in the hippocampal formation. Neurogenesis persists in these specialized areas owing to the existence of a population of neural stem cells (NSCs) that retain the capacity to proliferate and generate new neurons via a series of intermediate progenitor cells. NSCs can also give rise to glial cells. In both the SVZ and SGZ, these NSCs are largely regulated by local signals emanating from other niche cell types such as astrocytes or endothelial cells. In addition, SVZ-NSCs contact the ventricular lumen and are regulated by signals within the cerebral spinal fluid (CSF), and by signals released by ependymal cells. Neuroblasts and immature neurons born in the SVZ are exposed to signals from the rostral migratory stream (RMS) during their journey to the olfactory bulb (OB), where they terminally integrate.

Here, we review the current understanding of the role of neurotrophins and their receptors in the regulation of adult neurogenesis, as well as the underlying mechanisms. We discuss the main findings pertaining to the two main neurogenic niches of the adult brain, the SVZ and the SGZ. We also highlight unexpected findings that have expanded the traditional perspective of neurotrophin function.

EXPRESSION PATTERN OF NEUROTROPHINS AND THEIR RECEPTORS IN THE NEUROGENIC NICHES OF THE ADULT SVZ AND SGZ

The expression of NTs by local cells in the rodent SVZ niche is generally very low, although some ligands such as BDNF can be detected by immunohistochemistry (**Figure 1A**; Galvao et al., 2008). In addition, several NTs are expressed in the choroid plexus (CP), which secretes CSF components that become readily accessible to SVZ-NSCs, the so-called type B cells. The most abundantly expressed neurotrophin in the CP is NT4 (Galvao et al., 2008). NT3 is also released by CP capillaries and by endothelial cells (Delgado et al., 2014). In primates, NGF and BDNF are expressed by SVZ astrocytes while NT3 is found in ependymal cells (Tonchev, 2011). BDNF is mainly detected in the rostral migratory stream (RMS) and the OB (Maisonpierre et al., 1990; Bath et al., 2008; Galvao et al., 2008; Snapyan et al., 2009; Bagley and Belluscio, 2010). In the RMS, BDNF is synthesized by the endothelial cells of blood vessels that outline the migratory stream for new neurons (Snapyan et al., 2009). In the OB, the BDNF ligand is largely concentrated in the mitral and glomerular layers (Bergami et al., 2013). The cellular source of BDNF in the OB is yet to be clarified. Recently, Bergami et al. suggested that both local glutamatergic neurons (mitral and tufted cells) and long projecting neurons from the anterior olfactory nucleus (AON) and piriform cortex (PC) are the main sources of BDNF in the OB (Bergami et al., 2013).

The expression pattern of neurotrophin receptors in the adult mouse SVZ, as revealed by RT-PCR (Galvao et al., 2008), indicates that TrkB is the most abundant receptor, although TrkC is also present (**Figure 1A**). Despite some controversy, the prevailing view is that in both the mouse and rat SVZ truncated TrkB-T1 is expressed in ependymal cells and in type B cells (Chiaramello et al., 2007; Bath et al., 2008). This includes the BrdU-retaining cells that correspond to the slowly dividing NSCs. Type B NSCs also express TrkC, but not TrkA (Delgado et al., 2014). Maturing neuroblasts in the RMS appear to express the truncated form of TrkB, but express TrkB-FL upon entering the OB (Kirschenbaum and Goldman, 1995; Gascon et al., 2005; Bath et al., 2008; Snapyan et al., 2009; Bagley and Belluscio, 2010; Bergami et al., 2013). By contrast, p75NTR is expressed in intermediate progenitors (type C cells) of the SVZ and in neuroblasts (type A cells) of the SVZ/RMS (Galvao et al., 2008). Intriguingly, in rats a larger proportion of SVZ cells express p75NTR, although this receptor does not significantly co-localize with type B markers such as GFAP and appears to be largely confined to $EGFR^{+}$ type C progenitor cells, with some low level expression in $PSA\text{-}NCAM^{+}$ or DCX^{+} neuroblasts (Giuliani et al., 2004; Young et al., 2007). This suggests that p75NTR may play a greater role in the regulation of SVZ progenitor proliferation in rats than in mice, and that neurotrophin signaling in the two species may differ slightly. In primates, TrkA is present in SVZ astrocytes and immature neurons, TrkB is detected in astrocytes and neural progenitors, and TrkC is found in ependymal cells (Tonchev, 2011).

Neurotrophic factors and their receptors are abundantly expressed in the hippocampus, with an expression pattern that differs markedly to that of the SVZ (**Figure 1B**). For instance, NT3 is produced at very high levels in the dentate gyrus and is mainly expressed in neurons (Maisonpierre et al., 1990; Lauterborn et al., 1994; Shimazu et al., 2006). BDNF is also strongly expressed (Li et al., 2008). Both BDNF mRNA and protein expression are particularly high, with mossy fiber

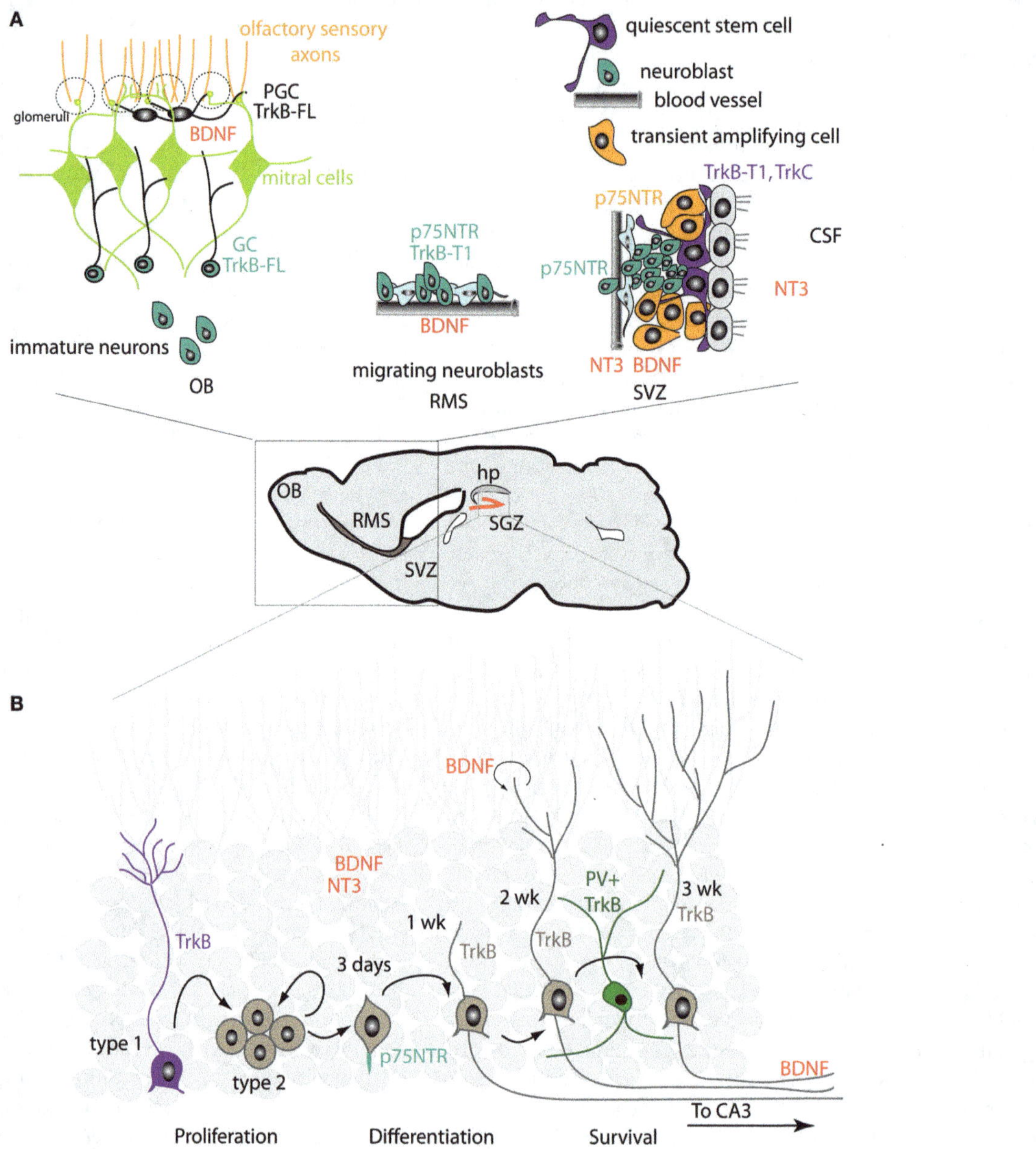

FIGURE 1 | Expression patterns of neurotrophins and their receptors in the adult SVZ-RMS-OB and SGZ. (A) *Right.* In the SVZ, NT3 is released into the CSF by the choroid plexus and is produced by the endothelial cells of blood vessels. BDNF is also present in the SVZ. Truncated TrkB-T1 is expressed in ependymal cells and in NSCs. NSCs also express TrkC. p75NTR is found in transient amplifying intermediate progenitors and in neuroblasts. *Middle.* In the RMS, BDNF is synthesized by the endothelial cells of blood vessels that outline the migratory stream. Neuroblasts express truncated TrkB-T1 and p75NTR. *Left.* In the OB, BDNF is concentrated in the mitral and glomerular layers. Immature neurons entering the OB acquire the expression of TrkB-FL, which is detected in granule cells (GC) and in periglomerular cells (PGC). **(B)** In the dentate gyrus, high levels of NT3 and BDNF are produced by mature neurons. BDNF is also produced by newly generated neurons. Mossy fiber axons of dentate granule neurons display strong BDNF immunoreactivity. TrkB is expressed in NSCs with radial morphology (Type 1 cells). Proliferating progenitors (Type 2 cells) have low TrkB levels. Young neurons and more mature granule neurons re-acquire high levels of TrkB expression. Parvalbumin (PV)-positive interneurons also express TrkB. p75NTR is expressed in newborn cells initiating axon growth, before entry of the axon fibers to the CA3 area, and is enriched at the initiation site of the axon fiber.

axons of dentate granule neurons displaying strong BDNF immunoreactivity due to anterograde transport (Conner et al., 1997). BDNF is also likely expressed in non-neuronal cells (Murer et al., 2001). In the adult macaque brain, the highest levels of BDNF are found in the hippocampus, indicating that BDNF also plays an important role in SGZ neurogenesis in non-murine species (Mori et al., 2004). TrkB appears to be broadly expressed: its expression is high in NSCs with radial morphology and low in proliferating progenitors, while young DCX$^+$ neurons and more mature granule neurons re-acquire high levels of TrkB expression (Donovan et al., 2008). By contrast, p75NTR expression is observed in a very narrow time window during the course of SGZ neurogenesis. Retroviral tracing experiments indicate that p75NTR expression is mainly confined to newborn cells between 3 and 7 days after retroviral injection (Zuccaro et al., 2014); these correspond to cells initiating the growth of the axon and dendritic processes, before axonal fibers reach the CA3 area (Zhao et al., 2006). At this stage, p75NTR is asymmetrically enriched at the initiation site of axon fibers and in proximal axon segments. In more mature neurons p75NTR expression is decreased and the asymmetric distribution of the receptor is lost (Zuccaro et al., 2014). Interestingly, p75NTR (but not TrkA) appears to be also localized in the primary cilia of dentate gyrus granule neurons, a specialized structure that acts as a sensory organelle and is involved in signal transduction (Chakravarthy et al., 2010).

FUNCTIONAL SIGNIFICANCE OF NEUROTROPHINS AND THEIR RECEPTORS IN THE SVZ

The few studies that have analyzed the effects of BDNF in the postnatal and adult SVZ have yielded mixed results. Galvao and coworkers reported that BDNF infusion reduces SVZ proliferation in both mice and rats. However, species-specific differences do exist; BDNF infusion and adenoviral vector-mediated overexpression of BDNF have no effect on OB neurogenesis in mice, or attenuate it in the long term (Galvao et al., 2008; Reumers et al., 2008), but have been shown in some studies to increase the number of new OB neurons in rats (Zigova et al., 1998; Benraiss et al., 2001; Henry et al., 2007).

Abundant data implicate BDNF in neuroblast migration along the RMS, although it remains to be established which receptor (TrkB-FL, TrkB-T1, or p75NTR) mediates this activity. In acute slice preparations, BDNF expressed by endothelial cells promotes neuronal migration along the RMS via p75NTR expressed on neuroblasts (Snapyan et al., 2009). BDNF/TrkB signaling may also contribute to the modulation of neuroblast migration (Bagley and Belluscio, 2010). However, grafting studies in which SVZ cells from TrkB knockout (TrkB-KO) and wild type (WT) mice were transplanted into the SVZ of adult WT mice suggest that TrkB is not essential at a cell-autonomous level for the migration of newly generated OB neurons (Galvao et al., 2008). In line with these observations, Bergami and colleagues observed no changes in the RMS migration of adult-born neurons from TrkB$^{lox/lox}$ mice, in which the TrkB-FL is deleted in progenitors by Cre expression (Bergami et al., 2013).

BDNF and TrkB participate in the long term survival and maturation of specific interneuron subpopulations of the OB. Berghuis et al. reported that loss of BDNF decreases the number and complexity of parvalbumin$^+$ (PV$^+$) cells in the external plexiform layer (Berghuis et al., 2006). Other authors have shown that periglomerular tyrosine hydroxylase$^+$ (TH$^+$) dopaminergic neurons are more sensitive to TrkB loss (Galvao et al., 2008; Bergami et al., 2013). TrkB deletion compromises the survival of TH$^+$ neurons, an effect that is accompanied by an increase in the number of calretinin$^+$ (CR$^+$) neurons, suggesting that TrkB regulates the balance between different classes of adult-born neurons (Bergami et al., 2013). As mentioned above, both local and long projecting neurons are sources of BDNF in the OB (Bergami et al., 2013). This may explain the existence of a BDNF expression gradient, which results in differences in BDNF availability, and the heterogeneous distribution of apoptotic TrkB-KO neurons in the OB (Bergami et al., 2013). Experiments with the mutant BDNF variant Val66Met suggest that activity-dependent BDNF release is required to ensure the survival of newly born OB neurons (Bath et al., 2008).

Using conditional knockout mice, Bergami and coworkers performed an in-depth analysis of the late role of TrkB-FL in OB neurogenesis. They elegantly showed that while newborn TrkB-FL-deficient neurons of the granule cell layer (GCL) have normal dendritic trees, the spine density of these neurons is compromised. By contrast, in newborn TH$^+$, TrkB-FL-deficient neurons of the periglomerular cell layer both dendritic arborization and spine growth are impaired, further highlighting the TrkB-dependency of this neuronal subpopulation. Notably, phospholipase C-γ signaling appears to mediate the effects of TrkB on spine growth, while Shc/PI3K signaling is involved in dendritic branching (Bergami et al., 2013).

The role of p75NTR in the SVZ remains to be established. p75NTR$^+$ cells are present in the SVZ and in the RMS in young and adult animals (Giuliani et al., 2004; Gascon et al., 2007; Young et al., 2007; Galvao et al., 2008). The Bartlett group identified a small population of precursor cells that express high levels of p75NTR and respond to BDNF (Young et al., 2007), in agreement with previous findings (Bibel et al., 2004). In p75NTR^{ExIII}-knockout animals, which lack the full-length receptor but express the short isoform, these authors observed a reduction in the number of PSA-NCAM$^+$ SVZ migrating neuroblasts and a decrease in OB size *in vivo*, suggesting a role of p75NTR in the migration and possibly survival of mature neurons in the OB (Young et al., 2007). However, these findings were subsequently challenged by those of another group (Bath et al., 2008), who failed to detect such differences. A recent study reported that p75NTR is expressed in migrating neuroblasts and responds to vasculature-secreted BDNF (Snapyan et al., 2009). Taken together, the available data suggest that p75NTR plays a dual role in OB neurogenesis, regulating proliferation in the SVZ by controlling the production of neuronal precursors (Young et al., 2007; Bath et al., 2008), and regulating migration of RMS neuroblasts en route to the OB (Snapyan et al., 2009).

In addition to neurotrophin signaling via p75NTR, amyloid peptide Aβ appears to regulate the proliferation of neural progenitors and adult neurogenesis via p75NTR (Sotthibundhu et al., 2009). Exogenous and endogenous stimulation of SVZ precursor cells by Aβ promote neurogenesis (Sotthibundhu et al., 2009). This effect is dependent on p75NTR expression by precursor cells, and can be blocked by preventing the proteolytic processing of p75NTR (Sotthibundhu et al., 2009). Overstimulation of p75NTR$^+$ neural progenitor cell division by Aβ in early life may result in premature depletion of the stem cell pool and a rapid decline in basal neurogenesis later in life (Sotthibundhu et al., 2009), as shown for instance in models of aging in which Aβ levels are increased (Diaz-Moreno et al., 2013).

Recent studies have shown that the role of neurotrophins in adult neurogenesis is even more complex than previously thought. Delgado and coworkers revealed an unprecedented role of NT3 in regulating the quiescent state of adult SVZ-NSCs (Delgado et al., 2014). They found that NT3 released by brain endothelial cells and choroid plexus capillaries is bound by NSCs, promoting their quiescence. Furthermore, by infusing NT3 into the lateral ventricle they obtained evidence suggesting that NSCs take up the neurotrophin via receptors located in their primary cilium, which acts as a sensor for ligands circulating in the CSF. The proliferative rate of NSCs was increased in young (2-month-old) Ntf3 heterozygous mice, in which NT3 expression is reduced. These mice also showed increased numbers of BrdU-retaining stem cells. A similar phenotype was observed in conditional Ntf3 knockout mice in which NT3 expression is specifically abolished in blood vessels. Interestingly, the cell fate of NSC progeny appeared not to depend on NT3 levels; the proportion of newly generated oligodendrocytes in the corpus callosum and that of newly generated neurons in the OB were similarly increased in Ntf3 heterozygous mice in response to the increase in NSC activity. In line with this observation, the authors detected increases in all specific OB interneuron subpopulations analyzed, further supporting the view that neuronal subtype identity is independent of NT3. In older (8-month-old) animals, NSCs prematurely differentiated into astrocytes, leading to NSC loss. These findings suggest that a decrease in the availability of NT3 results first in hyperproliferation, followed by premature exhaustion of the NSC pool. From a mechanistic standpoint, NT3 activates the nitric oxide synthase isoform eNOS in NSCs, resulting in production of the second messenger NO and cytostasis.

FUNCTIONAL SIGNIFICANCE OF NEUROTROPHINS AND THEIR RECEPTORS IN THE SGZ

In the dentate gyrus NT3 facilitates learning and memory, possibly by stimulating neuronal differentiation and/or the survival of newly born cells (Shimazu et al., 2006). Conditional Ntf3-knockout mice in which the gene encoding NT3 is deleted in the brain throughout development show normal proliferation in the SGZ, a reduction in the number of newly generated NeuN^{+} granule neurons, and an increase in the proportion of cells that do not express differentiation markers, pointing to a role of NT3, and perhaps also its preferred receptor TrkC, in maturation (Shimazu et al., 2006).

The p75NTR receptor also regulates hippocampal neurogenesis (Catts et al., 2008). In p75NTR^{ExIII}-knockout animals, which lack the full-length receptor but express the short p75NTR isoform, a reduction in the number of neuroblasts and newborn neurons in the dentate gyrus is paralleled by an increase in the death of newly born cells and impaired performance of hippocampus-dependent behavioral tasks (Catts et al., 2008). However, p75NTR^{ExIV}-knockout mice, in which both the long and short isoforms are deleted, show an increase in the number and complexity of DCX^{+} newborn neurons and a decrease in cell death (Poser et al., 2015). These contradictory findings may be explained by the differing levels of expression of the short isoform between the two mouse models, although a detailed study of the expression of the short isoform in the mouse hippocampus has yet to be performed. The artifactual overexpression of the p75 ICD in p75NTR^{ExIV} knockout mice (Paul et al., 2004) may also explain the different hippocampal phenotypes found in the two p75NTR-knockout strains. The analysis of adult neurogenesis in newly developed conditional mouse models, in which both the short and long p75NTR isoforms are cleanly deleted (Boskovic et al., 2014; Zuccaro et al., 2014), may shed some light on these discrepant findings. A study of p75$^{lox/lox}$ animals by Zuccaro and coworkers focused on axon growth, and demonstrated that polarized expression of p75NTR specifies the future axon in newly generated neurons of the adult SGZ (Zuccaro et al., 2014). These authors also found that the injection of lentiviruses transducing shRNA against p75NTR increases the proportion of new neurons lacking an axon, and that axogenesis in p75$^{lox/lox}$ animals is impaired by the conditional deletion of the receptor in progenitors.

The overall importance of BDNF/TrkB in adult hippocampal neurogenesis is clear. For example, neurogenesis is attenuated by BDNF knockdown in the dentate gyrus using lentiviral-mediated RNAi (Taliaz et al., 2010), but increased in response to exogenous BDNF injection (Scharfman et al., 2005). Nonetheless, there is less of a consensus as regards the participation of BDNF/TrkB in certain aspects of neurogenesis, such as the proliferation of progenitor cells and the survival of new neurons. TrkB is required for normal proliferation and neurogenesis in the SGZ, although conflicting results have been reported. Conditional deletion of TrkB in hippocampal NSCs reduces SGZ proliferation in postnatal day 15 (P15) animals and in adults, but has no effect on overall cell survival (Li et al., 2008). Animals with impaired TrkB activation (TrkB-T1-overexpressing mice) display an increase in proliferation and a reduction in survival (Lee et al., 2002; Sairanen et al., 2005). *In vitro*, BDNF promotes the proliferation of hippocampal neural progenitor cultures in a TrkB-dependent manner (Li et al., 2008).

In BDNF germline heterozygous mice, both increases (Sairanen et al., 2005) and decreases (Lee et al., 2002) in proliferation have been reported, as measured 1 day after BrdU injection. Studies using conditional knockout mice in which mature hippocampal neurons lack the BDNF gene have also been inconclusive, with some authors describing increased proliferation of SGZ progenitor cells (Chan et al., 2008) and others reporting no alteration (Choi et al., 2009). These conflicting results have not yet been explained, although it is possible that developmental and/or behavioral differences between the strains used in the aforementioned studies may contribute to the divergent findings. The functional role of BDNF in the survival of new neurons in the adult dentate gyrus is a matter of some debate. Impairment of basal levels of survival in BDNF heterozygous mice has been reported in some studies (Sairanen et al., 2005) but not in others (Rossi et al., 2006). Survival of newborn cells is also slightly attenuated in mice in which BDNF is deleted in granule neurons (Choi et al., 2009; Gao et al., 2009).

A greater consensus has been reached however regarding the role of BDNF/TrkB signaling in dendrite morphogenesis in newborn SGZ neurons (Bergami et al., 2008; Wang et al., 2015). Dendrite and spine growth is markedly altered in adult-born granule neurons of $TrkB^{lox/lox}$ mice, in which TrkB-FL is deleted in progenitors via Cre expression (Bergami et al., 2008). Moreover, TrkB-deficient neurons show impaired synaptic plasticity, and a proportion of these newly generated neurons die during the transition from immature to more mature stages. In line with these findings, a dramatic reduction in dendritic spine density has been described in the dentate gyrus of BDNF heterozygous mice (Zhu et al., 2009), and dendritic development, synaptic formation, and synaptic maturation are all impaired in postnatal-born granule neurons in BDNF conditional knockout mice (Gao et al., 2009). BDNF has also been shown to regulate late phases of neuronal differentiation, and dendritic development of adult-generated granule neurons is compromised in BDNF conditional mutants (Chan et al., 2008).

A recent study showed that dendrite growth is decreased in response to BDNF deletion in adult-born hippocampal neurons using retroviral vectors, and increased by BDNF overexpression (Wang et al., 2015). This effect appears to be largely autocrine, as BDNF deletion in newborn neurons only gives rise to dendritic abnormalities similar to those observed in conditional knockout mice in which BDNF is deleted throughout the entire forebrain. This is consistent with the full restoration of normal dendritic development in adult-born cells of BDNF conditional knockouts in which BDNF is selectively re-expressed (Wang et al., 2015). The autocrine production of the neurotrophin may depend on neuronal activity due to excitatory synaptic inputs onto the developing dendrites of the newborn neurons, or due to the earlier excitatory action of GABA released by interneurons (Wang et al., 2015). Interestingly, BDNF expression is highly complex and the protein can be translated from different mRNA species harboring either a short or a long 3′ untranslated region (3′ UTR), the latter of which targets BDNF mRNA to dendrites for local translation. BDNF translated from this long 3′ UTR mRNA in dendrites indirectly promotes the maturation of adult-born neurons, via GABAergic interneurons in the dentate gyrus (Waterhouse et al., 2012). $Bdnf^{klox/klox}$ mice, in which the long 3′ UTR is truncated, show increased progenitor proliferation and impaired differentiation and maturation of newborn hippocampal neurons. Similar results have been obtained in mice with selective deletion of TrkB in parvalbumin (PV)-expressing GABAergic interneurons. These results indicate that locally synthesized BDNF in the dendrites of granule neurons promotes differentiation and maturation of progenitor cells in the SGZ at least in part by enhancing GABA release from PV^{+} GABAergic interneurons (Waterhouse et al., 2012).

A fascinating aspect of the regulation of adult hippocampal neurogenesis by NTs is the connection between BDNF and the modulation of hippocampal neurogenesis by external stimuli, a topic that has been extensively studied in recent years (reviewed recently in Vivar et al., 2013 and Aimone et al., 2014). Adult neurogenesis in the dentate gyrus is enhanced by voluntary exercise, exposure to an enriched environment, and chronic antidepressant administration. Interestingly, many studies have shown that physical exercise increases hippocampal expression of BDNF (and NGF, but apparently not NT3; Cotman and Berchtold, 2002; Berchtold et al., 2005; Vaynman and Gomez-Pinilla, 2005; Cotman et al., 2007; Vivar et al., 2013). This increase correlates with the beneficial effects of exercise. For instance, long-term voluntary running increases BDNF levels while improving spatial memory and hippocampal neurogenesis (Marlatt et al., 2012). Eight months of forced exercise prevents the age-related impairments in both plasticity and BDNF expression in the dentate gyrus (O'Callaghan et al., 2009). Five weeks of treadmill running increases BDNF and TrkB expression, enhances NSC proliferation, and promotes the maturation and survival of immature neurons (Wu et al., 2008). TrkB ablation in adult hippocampal NSCs also blocks the effect of voluntary exercise on proliferation and neurogenesis (Li et al., 2008). Specific deletion of BDNF in mature hippocampal neurons has only a modest impact on the exercise-mediated increase in SGZ proliferation, suggesting that additional sources of BDNF are involved in this process (Choi et al., 2009). Interestingly, BDNF deletion in adult-born granule cells abolishes the increase in dendritic growth induced by running (Wang et al., 2015). This suggests that the effects of exercise on dendritic growth depend on autocrine BDNF signaling occurring in the newly generated neurons.

Environmental enrichment (EE) also increases hippocampal BDNF levels (but not NGF expression) in long term but not short term EE paradigms (Ickes et al., 2000; Kuzumaki et al., 2011). Up-regulation of BDNF in EE is caused by histone modifications of the BDNF promoter (Kuzumaki et al., 2011). As regards the role of this neurotrophin in EE, it has been reported that hippocampal neurogenesis is not increased in BDNF heterozygous mice placed in an enriched environment for 8 weeks. In the same EE setup, wild-type and NT4-knockout mice show a two-fold increase in hippocampal neurogenesis, pointing to BDNF as a central player in the EE-mediated induction of neurogenesis (Rossi et al., 2006). However, more recent studies have challenged this view. The positive effect of EE on proliferation is unaffected in a different model using mice with reduced hippocampal BDNF levels, such as those with conditional ablation of BDNF in mature hippocampal neurons (Choi et al., 2009). Moreover, conditional deletion of BDNF in mature neurons impairs dendritic development of DCX^{+} immature neurons in mice in standard housing (Chan et al., 2008; Choi et al., 2009), a defect rescued by EE (Choi et al., 2009). Altered dendritic spine density in the dentate gyrus of BDNF heterozygous mice is also partly rescued by EE (Zhu et al., 2009), suggesting that EE can modulate dendritic development even in mice with low BDNF levels. Recent findings suggest that BDNF levels are increased in EE only when running wheels are accessible to the animals, indicating that physical exercise may be the critical factor required to trigger BDNF overexpression in EE (Kobilo et al., 2011).

Antidepressants also increase BDNF/TrkB expression in the hippocampus (Nibuya et al., 1995; Russo-Neustadt et al., 2000; Sairanen et al., 2005), and their behavioral effects are mimicked by BDNF infusion (Shirayama et al., 2002). TrkB ablation in adult hippocampal NSCs blocks the increase in proliferation and neurogenesis that occurs in response to antidepressants (Li et al., 2008). Moreover, chronic antidepressant administration impairs the survival of newly generated SGZ neurons in BDNF heterozygous mice and in transgenic mice expressing the dominant negative TrkB-T1 isoform (Sairanen et al., 2005).

CONCLUDING REMARKS

In recent years a large number of studies have investigated the role of NTs in adult neurogenesis, identifying both expected and unexpected functions for this protein family of ligands and their receptors. A recurrent theme has been the prominent role of BDNF/TrkB in dendrite and spine morphogenesis, both in the OB and the dentate gyrus. Furthermore, p75NTR has been linked to progenitor proliferation and migration in the SVZ-RMS and to axon initiation in the SGZ. NT3 appears to play a very early role in the SVZ as a modulator of NSC quiescence and a late role in the dentate gyrus, where it likely regulates maturation/survival of newly generated neurons. Despite these advances, several key questions remain unanswered. For instance, the function of pro-neurotrophins and their regulation by external stimuli has been scarcely addressed. Cross-talk between NTs and other niche factors also remains largely unexplored. More studies are clearly needed to fully understand the signaling pathways operating downstream of NTs and their receptors, and to determine whether or not these pathways are altered in pathological processes. We anticipate that future research will add to and further refine current knowledge, and possibly uncover additional functions for neurotrophins in adult neurogenesis, both in health and disease.

AUTHOR CONTRIBUTIONS

All authors listed, have made substantial, direct, and intellectual contribution to the work, and approved it for publication.

ACKNOWLEDGMENTS

This work was supported by grants from the Ministerio de Economía y Competitividad, Acción Estratégica de Salud (PI12/101), and the Comunidad de Madrid (S2010/BMD-2336) to HM; and from the Ministerio de Economía y Competitividad (BFU2013-42746-P) to MV.

REFERENCES

Aimone, J. B., Li, Y., Lee, S. W., Clemenson, G. D., Deng, W., and Gage, F. H. (2014). Regulation and function of adult neurogenesis: from genes to cognition. *Physiol. Rev.* 94, 991–1026. doi: 10.1152/physrev.00004.2014

Bagley, J. A., and Belluscio, L. (2010). Dynamic imaging reveals that brain-derived neurotrophic factor can independently regulate motility and direction of neuroblasts within the rostral migratory stream. *Neuroscience* 169, 1449–1461. doi: 10.1016/j.neuroscience.2010.05.075

Bath, K. G., Mandairon, N., Jing, D., Rajagopal, R., Kapoor, R., Chen, Z. Y., et al. (2008). Variant brain-derived neurotrophic factor (Val66Met) alters adult olfactory bulb neurogenesis and spontaneous olfactory discrimination. *J. Neurosci.* 28, 2383–2393. doi: 10.1523/JNEUROSCI.4387-07.2008

Benraiss, A., Chmielnicki, E., Lerner, K., Roh, D., and Goldman, S. A. (2001). Adenoviral brain-derived neurotrophic factor induces both neostriatal and olfactory neuronal recruitment from endogenous progenitor cells in the adult forebrain. *J. Neurosci.* 21, 6718–6731.

Berchtold, N. C., Chinn, G., Chou, M., Kesslak, J. P., and Cotman, C. W. (2005). Exercise primes a molecular memory for brain-derived neurotrophic factor protein induction in the rat hippocampus. *Neuroscience* 133, 853–861. doi: 10.1016/j.neuroscience.2005.03.026

Bergami, M., Rimondini, R., Santi, S., Blum, R., Gotz, M., and Canossa, M. (2008). Deletion of TrkB in adult progenitors alters newborn neuron integration into hippocampal circuits and increases anxiety-like behavior. *Proc. Natl. Acad. Sci. U.S.A.* 105, 15570–15575. doi: 10.1073/pnas.0803702105

Bergami, M., Vignoli, B., Motori, E., Pifferi, S., Zuccaro, E., Menini, A., et al. (2013). TrkB signaling directs the incorporation of newly generated periglomerular cells in the adult olfactory bulb. *J. Neurosci.* 33, 11464–11478. doi: 10.1523/JNEUROSCI.4812-12.2013

Berghuis, P., Agerman, K., Dobszay, M. B., Minichiello, L., Harkany, T., and Ernfors, P. (2006). Brain-derived neurotrophic factor selectively regulates dendritogenesis of parvalbumin-containing interneurons in the main olfactory bulb through the PLCgamma pathway. *J. Neurobiol.* 66, 1437–1451. doi: 10.1002/neu.20319

Bibel, M., Richter, J., Schrenk, K., Tucker, K. L., Staiger, V., Korte, M., et al. (2004). Differentiation of mouse embryonic stem cells into a defined neuronal lineage. *Nat. Neurosci.* 7, 1003–1009. doi: 10.1038/nn1301

Boskovic, Z., Alfonsi, F., Rumballe, B. A., Fonseka, S., Windels, F., and Coulson, E. J. (2014). The role of p75NTR in cholinergic basal forebrain structure and function. *J. Neurosci.* 34, 13033–13038. doi: 10.1523/JNEUROSCI.2364-14.2014

Bothwell, M. (2014). NGF, BDNF, NT3, and NT4. *Handb. Exp. Pharmacol.* 220, 3–15. doi: 10.1007/978-3-642-45106-5_1

Catts, V. S., Al-Menhali, N., Burne, T. H., Colditz, M. J., and Coulson, E. J. (2008). The p75 neurotrophin receptor regulates hippocampal neurogenesis and related behaviours. *Eur. J. Neurosci.* 28, 883–892. doi: 10.1111/j.1460-9568.2008.06390.x

Ceni, C., Unsain, N., Zeinieh, M. P., and Barker, P. A. (2014). Neurotrophins in the regulation of cellular survival and death. *Handb. Exp. Pharmacol.* 220, 193–221. doi: 10.1007/978-3-642-45106-5_8

Chakravarthy, B., Gaudet, C., Menard, M., Atkinson, T., Chiarini, A., Dal Pra, I., et al. (2010). The p75 neurotrophin receptor is localized to primary cilia in adult murine hippocampal dentate gyrus granule cells. *Biochem. Biophys. Res. Commun.* 401, 458–462. doi: 10.1016/j.bbrc.2010.09.081

Chan, J. P., Cordeira, J., Calderon, G. A., Iyer, L. K., and Rios, M. (2008). Depletion of central BDNF in mice impedes terminal differentiation of new granule neurons in the adult hippocampus. *Mol. Cell. Neurosci.* 39, 372–383. doi: 10.1016/j.mcn.2008.07.017

Chao, M. V. (2003). Neurotrophins and their receptors: a convergence point for many signalling pathways. *Nat. Rev. Neurosci.* 4, 299–309. doi: 10.1038/nrn1078

Chiaramello, S., Dalmasso, G., Bezin, L., Marcel, D., Jourdan, F., Peretto, P., et al. (2007). BDNF/ TrkB interaction regulates migration of SVZ precursor cells via PI3-K and MAP-K signalling pathways. *Eur. J. Neurosci.* 26, 1780–1790. doi: 10.1111/j.1460-9568.2007.05818.x

Choi, S. H., Li, Y., Parada, L. F., and Sisodia, S. S. (2009). Regulation of hippocampal progenitor cell survival, proliferation and dendritic development by BDNF. *Mol. Neurodegener.* 4, 52. doi: 10.1186/1750-1326-4-52

Cohen, S., Levi-Montalcini, R., and Hamburger, V. (1954). A Nerve Growth-Stimulating Factor Isolated from Sarcom as 37 and 180. *Proc. Natl. Acad. Sci. U.S.A.* 40, 1014–1018. doi: 10.1073/pnas.40.10.1014

Conner, J. M., Lauterborn, J. C., Yan, Q., Gall, C. M., and Varon, S. (1997). Distribution of brain-derived neurotrophic factor (BDNF) protein and mRNA in the normal adult rat CNS: evidence for anterograde axonal transport. *J. Neurosci.* 17, 2295–2313.

Cotman, C. W., and Berchtold, N. C. (2002). Exercise: a behavioral intervention to enhance brain health and plasticity. *Trends Neurosci.* 25, 295–301. doi: 10.1016/S0166-2236(02)02143-4

Cotman, C. W., Berchtold, N. C., and Christie, L. A. (2007). Exercise builds brain health: key roles of growth factor cascades and inflammation. *Trends Neurosci.* 30, 464–472. doi: 10.1016/j.tins.2007.06.011

Deinhardt, K., and Chao, M. V. (2014). Trk receptors. *Handb. Exp. Pharmacol.* 220, 103–119. doi: 10.1007/978-3-642-45106-5_5

Delgado, A. C., Ferron, S. R., Vicente, D., Porlan, E., Perez-Villalba, A., Trujillo, C. M., et al. (2014). Endothelial NT-3 delivered by vasculature and CSF promotes quiescence of subependymal neural stem cells through nitric oxide induction. *Neuron* 83, 572–585. doi: 10.1016/j.neuron.2014.06.015

Diaz-Moreno, M., Hortiguela, R., Goncalves, A., Garcia-Carpio, I., Manich, G., Garcia-Bermudez, E., et al. (2013). Abeta increases neural stem cell activity in senescence-accelerated SAMP8 mice. *Neurobiol. Aging* 34, 2623–2638. doi: 10.1016/j.neurobiolaging.2013.05.011

Donovan, M. H., Yamaguchi, M., and Eisch, A. J. (2008). Dynamic expression of TrkB receptor protein on proliferating and maturing cells in the adult mouse dentate gyrus. *Hippocampus* 18, 435–439. doi: 10.1002/hipo.20410

Friedman, W. J., and Greene, L. A. (1999). Neurotrophin signaling via Trks and p75. *Exp. Cell Res.* 253, 131–142. doi: 10.1006/excr.1999.4705

Galvao, R. P., Garcia-Verdugo, J. M., and Alvarez-Buylla, A. (2008). Brain-derived neurotrophic factor signaling does not stimulate subventricular zone neurogenesis in adult mice and rats. *J. Neurosci.* 28, 13368–13383. doi: 10.1523/JNEUROSCI.2918-08.2008

Gao, X., Smith, G. M., and Chen, J. (2009). Impaired dendritic development and synaptic formation of postnatal-born dentate gyrus granular neurons in the absence of brain-derived neurotrophic factor signaling. *Exp. Neurol.* 215, 178–190. doi: 10.1016/j.expneurol.2008.10.009

Gascon, E., Vutskits, L., Jenny, B., Durbec, P., and Kiss, J. Z. (2007). PSA-NCAM in postnatally generated immature neurons of the olfactory bulb: a crucial role in regulating p75 expression and cell survival. *Development* 134, 1181–1190. doi: 10.1242/dev.02808

Gascon, E., Vutskits, L., Zhang, H., Barral-Moran, M. J., Kiss, P. J., Mas, C., et al. (2005). Sequential activation of p75 and TrkB is involved in dendritic development of subventricular zone-derived neuronal progenitors *in vitro*. *Eur. J. Neurosci.* 21, 69–80. doi: 10.1111/j.1460-9568.2004.03849.x

Giuliani, A., D'Intino, G., Paradisi, M., Giardino, L., and Calza, L. (2004). p75(NTR)-immunoreactivity in the subventricular zone of adult male rats: expression by cycling cells. *J. Mol. Histol.* 35, 749–758. doi: 10.1007/s10735-004-9609-2

Hempstead, B. L. (2014). Deciphering proneurotrophin actions. *Handb. Exp. Pharmacol.* 220, 17–32. doi: 10.1007/978-3-642-45106-5_2

Hempstead, B. L. (2015). Brain-derived neurotrophic factor: three ligands, many actions. *Trans. Am. Clin. Climatol. Assoc.* 126, 9–19. doi: 10.1021/bi00035a035

Henry, R. A., Hughes, S. M., and Connor, B. (2007). AAV-mediated delivery of BDNF augments neurogenesis in the normal and quinolinic acid-lesioned adult rat brain. *Eur. J. Neurosci.* 25, 3513–3525. doi: 10.1111/j.1460-9568.2007.05625.x

Huang, E. J., and Reichardt, L. F. (2003). Trk receptors: roles in neuronal signal transduction. *Annu. Rev. Biochem.* 72, 609–642. doi: 10.1146/annurev.biochem.72.121801.161629

Ickes, B. R., Pham, T. M., Sanders, L. A., Albeck, D. S., Mohammed, A. H., and Granholm, A. C. (2000). Long-term environmental enrichment leads to regional increases in neurotrophin levels in rat brain. *Exp. Neurol.* 164, 45–52. doi: 10.1006/exnr.2000.7415

Jung, K. M., Tan, S., Landman, N., Petrova, K., Murray, S., Lewis, R., et al. (2003). Regulated intramembrane proteolysis of the p75 neurotrophin receptor modulates its association with the TrkA receptor. *J. Biol. Chem.* 278, 42161–42169. doi: 10.1074/jbc.M306028200

Kanning, K. C., Hudson, M., Amieux, P. S., Wiley, J. C., Bothwell, M., and Schecterson, L. C. (2003). Proteolytic processing of the p75 neurotrophin receptor and two homologs generates C-terminal fragments with signaling capability. *J. Neurosci.* 23, 5425–5436.

Kirschenbaum, B., and Goldman, S. A. (1995). Brain-derived neurotrophic factor promotes the survival of neurons arising from the adult rat forebrain subependymal zone. *Proc. Natl. Acad. Sci. U.S.A.* 92, 210–214. doi: 10.1073/pnas.92.1.210

Klein, R., Conway, D., Parada, L. F., and Barbacid, M. (1990). The trkB tyrosine protein kinase gene codes for a second neurogenic receptor that lacks the catalytic kinase domain. *Cell* 61, 647–656. doi: 10.1016/0092-8674(90)90476-U

Kobilo, T., Liu, Q. R., Gandhi, K., Mughal, M., Shaham, Y., and van Praag, H. (2011). Running is the neurogenic and neurotrophic stimulus in environmental enrichment. *Learn. Mem.* 18, 605–609. doi: 10.1101/lm.2283011

Kraemer, B. R., Yoon, S. O., and Carter, B. D. (2014). The biological functions and signaling mechanisms of the p75 neurotrophin receptor. *Handb. Exp. Pharmacol.* 220, 121–164. doi: 10.1007/978-3-642-45106-5_6

Kuzumaki, N., Ikegami, D., Tamura, R., Hareyama, N., Imai, S., Narita, M., et al. (2011). Hippocampal epigenetic modification at the brain-derived neurotrophic factor gene induced by an enriched environment. *Hippocampus* 21, 127–132. doi: 10.1002/hipo.20775

Lauterborn, J. C., Isackson, P. J., and Gall, C. M. (1994). Cellular localization of NGF and NT-3 mRNAs in postnatal rat forebrain. *Mol. Cell. Neurosci.* 5, 46–62. doi: 10.1006/mcne.1994.1005

Lee, J., Seroogy, K. B., and Mattson, M. P. (2002). Dietary restriction enhances neurotrophin expression and neurogenesis in the hippocampus of adult mice. *J. Neurochem.* 80, 539–547. doi: 10.1046/j.0022-3042.2001.00747.x

Li, Y., Luikart, B. W., Birnbaum, S., Chen, J., Kwon, C. H., Kernie, S. G., et al. (2008). TrkB regulates hippocampal neurogenesis and governs sensitivity to antidepressive treatment. *Neuron* 59, 399–412. doi: 10.1016/j.neuron.2008.06.023

Lu, B., Nagappan, G., and Lu, Y. (2014). BDNF and synaptic plasticity, cognitive function, and dysfunction. *Handb. Exp. Pharmacol.* 220, 223–250. doi: 10.1007/978-3-642-45106-5_9

Maisonpierre, P. C., Belluscio, L., Friedman, B., Alderson, R. F., Wiegand, S. J., Furth, M. E., et al. (1990). NT-3, BDNF, and NGF in the developing rat nervous system: parallel as well as reciprocal patterns of expression. *Neuron* 5, 501–509. doi: 10.1016/0896-6273(90)90089-X

Marlatt, M. W., Potter, M. C., Lucassen, P. J., and van Praag, H. (2012). Running throughout middle-age improves memory function, hippocampal neurogenesis, and BDNF levels in female C57BL/6J mice. *Dev. Neurobiol.* 72, 943–952. doi: 10.1002/dneu.22009

Mi, S., Lee, X., Shao, Z., Thill, G., Ji, B., Relton, J., et al. (2004). LINGO-1 is a component of the Nogo-66 receptor/p75 signaling complex. *Nat. Neurosci.* 7, 221–228. doi: 10.1038/nn1188

Mori, T., Shimizu, K., and Hayashi, M. (2004). Differential expression patterns of TrkB ligands in the macaque monkey brain. *Neuroreport* 15, 2507–2511. doi: 10.1097/00001756-200411150-00015

Murer, M. G., Yan, Q., and Raisman-Vozari, R. (2001). Brain-derived neurotrophic factor in the control human brain, and in *Alzheimer's* disease and Parkinson's disease. *Prog. Neurobiol.* 63, 71–124. doi: 10.1016/S0301-0082(00)00014-9

Naumann, T., Casademunt, E., Hollerbach, E., Hofmann, J., Dechant, G., Frotscher, M., et al. (2002). Complete deletion of the neurotrophin receptor p75NTR leads to long-lasting increases in the number of basal forebrain cholinergic neurons. *J. Neurosci.* 22, 2409–2418.

Nibuya, M., Morinobu, S., and Duman, R. S. (1995). Regulation of BDNF and trkB mRNA in rat brain by chronic electroconvulsive seizure and antidepressant drug treatments. *J. Neurosci.* 15, 7539–7547.

Nykjaer, A., Lee, R., Teng, K. K., Jansen, P., Madsen, P., Nielsen, M. S., et al. (2004). Sortilin is essential for proNGF-induced neuronal cell death. *Nature* 427, 843–848. doi: 10.1038/nature02319

O'Callaghan, R. M., Griffin, E. W., and Kelly, A. M. (2009). Long-term treadmill exposure protects against age-related neurodegenerative change in the rat hippocampus. *Hippocampus* 19, 1019–1029. doi: 10.1002/hipo.20591

Paul, C. E., Vereker, E., Dickson, K. M., and Barker, P. A. (2004). A pro-apoptotic fragment of the p75 neurotrophin receptor is expressed in p75NTRExonIV null mice. *J. Neurosci.* 24, 1917–1923. doi: 10.1523/JNEUROSCI.5397-03.2004

Poser, R., Dokter, M., von Bohlen Und Halbach, V., Berger, S. M., Busch, R., Baldus, M., et al. (2015). Impact of a deletion of the full-length and short isoform of p75NTR on cholinergic innervation and the population of postmitotic doublecortin positive cells in the dentate gyrus. *Front. Neuroanat.* 9:63. doi: 10.3389/fnana.2015.00063

Reichardt, L. F. (2006). Neurotrophin-regulated signalling pathways. *Philos. Trans. R. Soc. Lond. B. Biol. Sci.* 361, 1545–1564. doi: 10.1098/rstb.2006.1894

Reumers, V., Deroose, C. M., Krylyshkina, O., Nuyts, J., Geraerts, M., Mortelmans, L., et al. (2008). Noninvasive and quantitative monitoring of adult neuronal stem cell migration in mouse brain using bioluminescence imaging. *Stem Cells* 26, 2382–2390. doi: 10.1634/stemcells.2007-1062

Rossi, C., Angelucci, A., Costantin, L., Braschi, C., Mazzantini, M., Babbini, F., et al. (2006). Brain-derived neurotrophic factor (BDNF) is required for the enhancement of hippocampal neurogenesis following environmental enrichment. *Eur. J. Neurosci.* 24, 1850–1856. doi: 10.1111/j.1460-9568.2006.05059.x

Russo-Neustadt, A. A., Beard, R. C., Huang, Y. M., and Cotman, C. W. (2000). Physical activity and antidepressant treatment potentiate the expression of specific brain-derived neurotrophic factor transcripts in the rat hippocampus. *Neuroscience* 101, 305–312. doi: 10.1016/S0306-4522(00)00349-3

Sairanen, M., Lucas, G., Ernfors, P., Castren, M., and Castren, E. (2005). Brain-derived neurotrophic factor and antidepressant drugs have different but coordinated effects on neuronal turnover, proliferation, and survival in the adult dentate gyrus. *J. Neurosci.* 25, 1089–1094. doi: 10.1523/JNEUROSCI.3741-04.2005

Scharfman, H., Goodman, J., Macleod, A., Phani, S., Antonelli, C., and Croll, S. (2005). Increased neurogenesis and the ectopic granule cells after intrahippocampal BDNF infusion in adult rats. *Exp. Neurol.* 192, 348–356. doi: 10.1016/j.expneurol.2004.11.016

Shimazu, K., Zhao, M., Sakata, K., Akbarian, S., Bates, B., Jaenisch, R., et al. (2006). NT-3 facilitates hippocampal plasticity and learning and memory by regulating neurogenesis. *Learn. Mem.* 13, 307–315. doi: 10.1101/lm.76006

Shirayama, Y., Chen, A. C., Nakagawa, S., Russell, D. S., and Duman, R. S. (2002). Brain-derived neurotrophic factor produces antidepressant effects in behavioral models of depression. *J. Neurosci.* 22, 3251–3261.

Skeldal, S., Sykes, A. M., Glerup, S., Matusica, D., Palstra, N., Autio, H., et al. (2012). Mapping of the interaction site between sortilin and the p75 neurotrophin receptor reveals a regulatory role for the sortilin intracellular domain in p75 neurotrophin receptor shedding and apoptosis. *J. Biol. Chem.* 287, 43798–43809. doi: 10.1074/jbc.M112.374710

Snapyan, M., Lemasson, M., Brill, M. S., Blais, M., Massouh, M., Ninkovic, J., et al. (2009). Vasculature guides migrating neuronal precursors in the adult mammalian forebrain via brain-derived neurotrophic factor signaling. *J. Neurosci.* 29, 4172–4188. doi: 10.1523/JNEUROSCI.4956-08.2009

Sotthibundhu, A., Li, Q. X., Thangnipon, W., and Coulson, E. J. (2009). Abeta(1-42) stimulates adult SVZ neurogenesis through the p75 neurotrophin receptor. *Neurobiol. Aging* 30, 1975–1985. doi: 10.1016/j.neurobiolaging.2008.02.004

Taliaz, D., Stall, N., Dar, D. E., and Zangen, A. (2010). Knockdown of brain-derived neurotrophic factor in specific brain sites precipitates behaviors associated with depression and reduces neurogenesis. *Mol. Psychiatry* 15, 80–92. doi: 10.1038/mp.2009.67

Tonchev, A. B. (2011). Brain ischemia, neurogenesis, and neurotrophic receptor expression in primates. *Arch. Ital. Biol.* 149, 225–231. doi: 10.4449/aib.v149i2.1368

Vaynman, S., and Gomez-Pinilla, F. (2005). License to run: exercise impacts functional plasticity in the intact and injured central nervous system by using neurotrophins. *Neurorehabil. Neural Repair* 19, 283–295. doi: 10.1177/1545968305280753

Vivar, C., Potter, M. C., and van Praag, H. (2013). All about running: synaptic plasticity, growth factors and adult hippocampal neurogenesis. *Curr. Top. Behav. Neurosci.* 15, 189–210. doi: 10.1007/7854_2012_220

Wang, K. C., Kim, J. A., Sivasankaran, R., Segal, R., and He, Z. (2002). P75 interacts with the Nogo receptor as a co-receptor for Nogo, MAG and OMgp. *Nature* 420, 74–78. doi: 10.1038/nature01176

Wang, L., Chang, X., She, L., Xu, D., Huang, W., and Poo, M. M. (2015). Autocrine action of BDNF on dendrite development of adult-born hippocampal neurons. *J. Neurosci.* 35, 8384–8393. doi: 10.1523/JNEUROSCI.4682-14.2015

Waterhouse, E. G., An, J. J., Orefice, L. L., Baydyuk, M., Liao, G. Y., Zheng, K., et al. (2012). BDNF promotes differentiation and maturation of adult-born neurons through GABAergic transmission. *J. Neurosci.* 32, 14318–14330. doi: 10.1523/JNEUROSCI.0709-12.2012

Wu, A., Ying, Z., and Gomez-Pinilla, F. (2008). Docosahexaenoic acid dietary supplementation enhances the effects of exercise on synaptic plasticity and cognition. *Neuroscience* 155, 751–759. doi: 10.1016/j.neuroscience.2008.05.061

Young, K. M., Merson, T. D., Sotthibundhu, A., Coulson, E. J., and Bartlett, P. F. (2007). p75 neurotrophin receptor expression defines a population of BDNF-responsive neurogenic precursor cells. *J. Neurosci.* 27, 5146–5155. doi: 10.1523/JNEUROSCI.0654-07.2007

Zhao, C., Teng, E. M., Summers, R. G. Jr., Ming, G. L., and Gage, F. H. (2006). Distinct morphological stages of dentate granule neuron maturation in the adult mouse hippocampus. *J. Neurosci.* 26, 3–11. doi: 10.1523/JNEUROSCI.3648-05.2006

Zhu, S. W., Codita, A., Bogdanovic, N., Hjerling-Leffler, J., Ernfors, P., Winblad, B., et al. (2009). Influence of environmental manipulation on exploratory behaviour in male BDNF knockout mice. *Behav. Brain Res.* 197, 339–346. doi: 10.1016/j.bbr.2008.09.032

Zigova, T., Pencea, V., Wiegand, S. J., and Luskin, M. B. (1998). Intraventricular administration of BDNF increases the number of newly generated neurons in the adult olfactory bulb. *Mol. Cell. Neurosci.* 11, 234–245. doi: 10.1006/mcne.1998.0684

Zuccaro, E., Bergami, M., Vignoli, B., Bony, G., Pierchala, B. A., Santi, S., et al. (2014). Polarized expression of p75(NTR) specifies axons during development and adult neurogenesis. *Cell Rep.* 7, 138–152. doi: 10.1016/j.celrep.2014.02.039

8

Sexual Stimulation Increases the Survival of New Cells in the Accessory Olfactory Bulb of the Male Rat

*Nancy M. Unda, Wendy Portillo *, Rebeca Corona and Raúl G. Paredes*

Neurobiología Conductual y Cognitiva, Instituto de Neurobiología, Universidad Nacional Autónoma de México, Juriquilla, Mexico

Edited by:
Alino Martinez-Marcos, Universidad de Castilla, Spain

Reviewed by:
Juan Nacher, University of Valencia, Spain
Fernando Martinez-Garcia, Universitat Jaume I de Castelló, Spain

****Correspondence:***
Wendy Portillo
portillo@unam.mx

Sexual behavior in rodents is modulated by the olfactory system. The olfactory bulb (OB) is a structure that undergoes continues neurogenesis in adulthood. We have previously shown that 15 days after males rats pace the sexual interaction and ejaculate 1 or 3 times, there is an increase in the density of new cells that reach the accessory olfactory bulb (AOB). The aim of the present study was to evaluate if sexual behavior in male rats increases the density of new neurons that survive 45 days after sexual behavior in the AOB and in the main OB (MOB). Male rats were randomly divided in four groups: (1) Control (Ctr), males without sexual interaction; (2) Exposed (Exp), males only exposed to a sexually receptive female; (3) No pacing (NP), males that mated in conditions in which the female paced the sexual interaction; (4) One ejaculation (1E), males that paced the sexual interaction with a receptive female and ejaculated once; and (5) Three ejaculations (3E), males that paced the sexual interaction and were allowed to ejaculate three times. All males were injected with the DNA synthesis marker 5-bromo-2-deoxyuridine (BrdU), and were tested in one of the above conditions. 45 days later they were sacrificed, and the OBs were processed to identify new cells and evaluate if they had differentiated into neurons. Our data indicate that males that ejaculated three times showed an increase in the density of new cells that survive in the posterior part of the granular cell layer of the AOB and have more new neurons that the control group. However, no significant differences were found in the percentage of new cells that differentiate into neurons. No significant increase in the density of new cells was observed in the MOB. Our data show that pacing the sexual interaction until three ejaculations increases the density of new cells and neurons in the granular layer of the AOB, confirming that sexual behavior induces long-lasting plastic changes in the OB.

Keywords: neurogenesis, sexual behavior, olfactory bulb, neuronal plasticity, male rats

INTRODUCTION

In rodents, the olfactory system regulates neuroendocrine and reproductive functions, allowing animals to recognize conspecifics and to determine gender and hormonal condition (Tirindelli et al., 2009). Two systems, the main (MOS) and the accessory olfactory system (AOS) process odorants. The odorants are detected by the olfactory neurons that extend axons to the glomeruli and synapse onto dendrites of the mitral and periglomerular cells. The dendrites of periglomerular cells form reciprocal dendrodendritic synapses with dendrites of mitral cells. Granular interneurons modulate the activity of the mitral neurons, establishing microcircuits in the olfactory bulb (Murphy et al., 2005). Mitral cells of the main olfactory bulb (MOB) send their axons through the lateral olfactory tract to central regions in the brain such as the anterior olfactory nucleus, cortical and medial-anterior amygdala (AMG), olfactory tuberculus, piriform, and entorhinal cortex (Baum and Kelliher, 2009; Sosulski et al., 2011; Baum and Cherry, 2015).

The AOS is anatomically and functionally divided into anterior and posterior regions. Superficial vomeronasal neurons that express the vomeronasal receptor 1 (V1R) project axons to the anterior subdivision of the accessory olfactory bulb (aAOB). Deeper vomeronsal neurons that express the vomeronasal receptor 2 (V2R) project to the posterior subdivision of the AOB (pAOB; Herrada and Dulac, 1997; Rodriguez et al., 1999; Tirindelli et al., 2009). Mitral cells in the AOB project, in turn, to the vomeronasal AMG, which synapses onto the bed nucleus of the stria terminalis (BNST), medial preoptic area (MPOA), and ventro medial hypothalamus (VMH), among other brain centers (Kevetter and Winans, 1981; Baum and Kelliher, 2009). Functionally, exposure to volatile components of female urine activates the aAOB and to some extent the caudal part of the pAOB in the male rat, and stimulation with volatile components of male urine activates the aAOB in male and female rats. On the other hand, non-volatile components of female urine induce activation preponderantly in the pAOB and to a lesser extent in the aAOB (Sugai et al., 2006).

The MOS and AOS play crucial roles in the expression of male sexual behavior, since sexually experienced male rats with lesions of the vomeronasal organ showed alterations in sexual behavior. After the lesion, males took longer to intromit and ejaculate because they displayed more mounts but less intromission than sham lesioned animals (Saito and Moltz, 1986; Kondo et al., 2003). Male rats with lesions of the olfactory epithelium showed a decrease in the intromission frequency and an increase in the ejaculation and mount latencies (Dhungel et al., 2011).

It is well recognized that adult neurogenesis is a mechanism of adult brain plasticity. In rodents, the olfactory bulbs (OB) continuously add new cells that are generated in the subventricular zone (SVZ) and rostral migratory stream (RMS) (Stolp and Molnár, 2015). The new cells migrate tangentially along the RMS, and in 15–20 days they arrive at the OB (Petreanu and Alvarez-Buylla, 2002; Winner et al., 2002). Around 95% of the new cells differentiate into granular neurons and integrate in the granular cell layer (GrL), and a few differentiate into periglomerular neurons that are incorporated into the glomerular cell layer (GlL; Petreanu and Alvarez-Buylla, 2002; Lledo and Saghatelyan, 2005; Bagley et al., 2007; Whitman and Greer, 2009). Between 15 and 45 days after birth, the number of granular cells declines to half; in this period sensory stimulation is critical for their survival (Petreanu and Alvarez-Buylla, 2002; Winner et al., 2002), because the new cells mature morphologically and are incorporated into existing neural circuits (Petreanu and Alvarez-Buylla, 2002). Neurogenesis is a dynamic process that depends on internal and external environmental cues (Rochefort et al., 2002; Rochefort and Lledo, 2005; Mak et al., 2007; Larsen et al., 2008; Oboti et al., 2009). Recently, it was demonstrated that sexual stimulation can modulate neurogenesis in the dentate gyrus (DG) of the hippocampus. Male rats that mated once or several times showed increased cell proliferation and survival of the new cells in the DG of the hippocampus, compared to males exposed to non-receptive females or males without sexual experience (Leuner et al., 2010). Sakamoto and coworkers (Sakamoto et al., 2011) developed a transgenic mouse using tamoxifen-treated Nestin-CreER^{T2} neuron specific enolase-diphtheria toxin fragment A (NSE-DTA) that is not able to integrate new neurons. In this mouse, when the cells reach maturity the NSE promoter becomes active and induces the expression of DTA, killing the new neurons. Male mice with this mutation show a decreased frequency and duration of mounting and produce fewer vaginal plugs than control mice (Sakamoto et al., 2011).

New cells are also involved in mate recognition. Female mice form an olfactory memory of their mating partner; when a recently mated female is exposed to an unfamiliar male, a neuroendocrine reflex is triggered that leads to pregnancy block (Bruce effect). Female mice treated with the antimitotic drug cytosine arabinose (Ara-C) to abolish neurogenesis are not able to make a memory of their sexual partner, and cohabitation with the mate starts the pregnancy block (Oboti et al., 2011). In addition, administration of Ara-C to male rats decreases the intromission frequency and copulatory efficiency (total number of intromissions/sum of intromissions and mount frequency), and the males are not able to ejaculate (Lau et al., 2011). Thus, new cells play a relevant role in sexual behavior and mate recognition memory.

We previously demonstrated that male rats that pace the sexual interaction and ejaculate one or three times showed an increase in the density of new cells that reach the GrL of the AOB 15 days after sexual stimulation and some of these cells differentiate into neurons. Interestingly, no such increase was observed in those males that mated for 1 h and ejaculated around 3 times but were not allowed to pace the sexual interaction (Portillo et al., 2012). The aim of the present study was to evaluate if one sexual behavior session in male rats increases the density of new cells that survive in the OB for 45 days after mating, and if these new cells differentiate into neurons.

METHODS

Subjects

Forty adult male *Wistar* rats (300–350 g) were used in this experiment. Sexually experienced females from the same strain were used as stimulus. The females were ovariectomized and hormonally primed with estradiol benzoate (25 μg/rat, 48 h, Sigma, St. Louis, MO, USA) and progesterone (1 mg/rat, Aldrich, St. Louis, MO, USA) both diluted in corn oil to induce sexual receptivity. All the animals had unlimited access to food and water and were maintained on a reverse 12-h:12-h light-dark cycle. Experiments were carried out in accordance with the "Reglamento de la Ley General de Salud en Materia de Investigacion para la Salud" of the Mexican Health Ministry that matches NIH guidelines for the use and care of animals and approved by the Instituto de Neurobiologia animal care committee.

Behavioral Test

Before the experiment, males were trained over 3 weeks to acquire sexual experience. They were tested once per week in 30-min sessions with a sexually receptive female. Those males that ejaculated once in each session were included in the study. All the behavioral tests were done in transparent acrylic cages (dimensions: 62 × 29 × 42 cm). The floor of the cages were covered with sawdust, which was changed between behavioral tests. After the screening tests, 40 sexually experienced males were obtained and randomly divided into five groups: (1) Control (Ctr), males that were placed in a clean cage; (2) Exposed (Exp), males only exposed to a sexually receptive female in a mating cage divided by an acrylic barrier with small holes. In this way the male could smell, see and hear the receptive female, but physical contact was not possible; (3) No pacing (NP), males that mated in conditions where the females paced the sexual interaction. Subjects were placed in a mating cage divided by a barrier with a small hole in the middle that allowed the female, but not the male, to go back and forth from the male compartment; (4) One ejaculation (1E), males that controlled the sexual interaction, mated in a mating cage without the barrier, and were allowed to ejaculate one time, and (5) Three ejaculations (3E), males that controlled the sexual interaction and were allowed to ejaculate three times. For all sexual behavior tests, females were placed in the cage 5 min before the males were introduced. The following parameters of sexual behavior were registered: number of mounts, intromissions and ejaculations; mount, intromission and ejaculation latencies, and the inter-intromission interval (ejaculation latency divided by the number of intromissions) and post-ejaculatory interval (latency of the first intromission after the ejaculation minus the ejaculation latency).

BrdU Administration

Male rats ($n = 8$ per group) were intraperitoneally injected with the DNA synthesis marker 5′-Bromo-2′-deoxyuridine (BrdU) (Sigma, dissolved in NaCl 0.9%) at three different times: the first dose was given 1 h before the behavioral test, the second dose at the end of the behavioral test and the third dose, 1 h after the end of the test. The dose of BrdU was 100 mg/Kg (total 300 mg/kg). This concentration of BrdU labels the maximal number of cells and is not toxic for the subject (Cameron and McKay, 2001). All experimental males were sacrificed 45 days after the behavioral test.

Immunohistochemistry

Animals were anesthetized with an intraperitoneal injection of pentobarbital (63 mg/rat), and transcardially perfused with 200 ml 0.1 M phosphate buffer followed by 200 ml of 4% paraformaldehyde (PFA) in phosphate buffer. Brains were post-fixed 1 h in PFA and maintained in 30% sucrose (cryoprotector) until they were processed. The MOB and AOB were cut in sagittal sections of 30 μm thickness using a microtome (Leica).

To label the density of the new cells (BrdU positive), MOB and AOB slices were processed for immunohistochemistry following the procedure previously reported (Corona et al., 2011a; Portillo et al., 2012; Arzate et al., 2013). Briefly, brain slices were washed in a solution of Tris buffer (TBS) and incubated in 2N HCl for 1 h. To block non-specific sites, the tissue was incubated for 15 min in a solution containing 10% bovine albumin and 0.3% Triton X-100 (Tx), then washed in TBS and incubated with anti-BrdU mouse antibody (1:2000; BD Bioscience) for 16 h at 4°C. After the antibody, the tissue was washed in TBS, albumin bovine (1%) and Tx (0.02%) and it was incubated in biotinylated anti-mouse IgG antibody (1:500; Vector Laboratory Burlingame, CA) for 2 h. Later, the tissue was incubated for 90 min with the avidin-biotin complex (AB) followed by incubation with 0.02% diaminobenzidine (DAB). After rinsing, sections were mounted on slides, coverslipped using permount and left to dry before being analyzed under the light microscope.

Immunofluorescence

In order to identify the neuronal phenotype of the new cells that reach the granular cell layer (GrL), double staining for BrdU, and the neuronal protein NeuN was used. Following the protocol previously described (Corona et al., 2011a; Portillo et al., 2012; Arzate et al., 2013), OB slices were incubated for 48 h at 4°C simultaneously with both primary antibodies rat anti-BrdU (1:800, AbD Serotec) and mouse anti-NeuN (1:250, MILLIPORE) and then, after washing, with secondary antibodies anti-rat IgG Alexa Fluor 488 (1:1250, Invitrogen) and anti-mouse IgG Alexa Fluor 568 (1:1250, Invitrogen), respectively. After rinsing, sections were mounted on slides and coverslipped using aqua poly/mount, a non-fluorescing aqueous mounting medium (Polysciences, Inc).

Quantification of BrdU- and BrdU-NeuN Positive Cells

To quantify the density of BrdU-positive cells in the MOB and AOB, we used the software Image Pro Plus 6.1. Photomicrographs were taken with a light microscope OLYMPUS BX60 (10X objective). The BrdU-positive cells were quantified in the glomerular (GlL), and GrL of the MOB and AOB. To quantify the density of BrdU-positive cells in the MOB three circular areas of 400 μm diameter were placed in each layer. For the AOB, three circular areas of 200 μm diameter were placed in each layer of the anterior and posterior regions. We quantified four brain slices per animal. Circular areas for analysis are indicated in **Figure 1**.

To evaluate the percentage and density of BrdU-/NeuN-positive cells, images of 20X obtained with an inverted Zeiss LSM 780 confocal were analyzed. OB sections were sequentially scanned in a Z-stack analysis with a step of 0.8-μm thickness between each scan. The percentage and density of BrdU-/NeuN-positive cells was quantified in the GrL of the aAOB and pAOB for the Ctr and the 3E groups, because in this latter group we observed an increase in the density of BrdU-positive cells. Two AOB slices for each animal were analyzed.

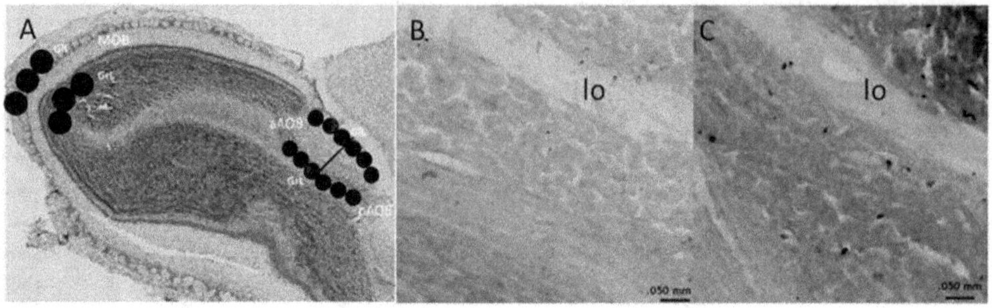

FIGURE 1 | (A) Schematic representation of the regions in which BrdU-positive cells were counted. In the MOB, cells were counted in three, 400-μm diameter circles placed in the glomerular cell layer (GlL) and granular cell layer (GrL). The AOB was divided into the anterior (aAOB) and posterior (pAOB) regions, and cells were counted in the three 200-μm circles were placed in the GlL and GrL. **(B,C)** are representative photomicrographs (10X) of the BrdU-positive cells in the GrL of the pAOB in **(B)** control and **(C)** three ejaculation groups. lo lateral olfactory tract.

TABLE 1 | Data from the sexual behavior test in the different groups: no pacing (NP), one ejaculation (1E), and three ejaculations (3E); $n = 8$ per group.

Behavioral parameters	NP	1E	3E
No. Mounts	10.78 ± 5.6	12.1 ± 4.2	11.1 ± 1.9
No. Intromissions	10.1 ± 1.8	14.3 ± 2.4	14.9 ± 1.6
No. Ejaculations	2.6 ± 0.4	1	3
Mount Lat.	177.3 ± 65.3	174.1 ± 32.4	120 ± 32
Intromission Lat.	247 ± 3	216.7 ± 41.5	209.9 ± 79.7
Ejaculation Lat.	769 ± 164.4	634 ± 150	754.8 ± 108.8
PEI	457.3 ± 45.3	413.4 ± 21.5	383.8 ± 16.6
III	75.2 ± 7.5*	41.5 ± 4	49.8 ± 4

Data were analyzed using the Kruskal-Wallis test; in case of significant differences the Tukey Post-hoc test was used. Data are expressed as the mean ± standard error. The latency (Lat) to the first mount, intromission and ejaculation, as well as the post-ejaculatory interval (PEI) and the inter-intromission interval (III) are expressed in seconds.
**Significantly different from 1E group. $P < 0.05$.*

Statistical Analysis

Data from the behavioral test were not normally distributed and therefore, they were analyzed by the Kruskal-Wallis test (K-W); in case of significant differences we used the Tukey Post hoc test. The density of BrdU-immunoreactive cells in the MOB, aAOB and pAOB was analyzed by a one-way analysis of variance (ANOVA), and the Tukey test was used as Post hoc test. The density of BrdU/NeuN positive cells was analyzed using a t-test and the percentage of BrdU/NeuN-immunoreactive cells were not normally distributed and therefore they were analyzed by a Mann-Whitney U test.

RESULTS

Sexual Behavior

Data from the sexual behavior test done when BrdU was administrated indicate that the males from the NP group show a higher inter-intromission interval than the 1E group [K-W: $\chi_{(2)}2 = 9.96, p = 0.007$]. No significant differences were found in the other parameters analyzed. **Table 1**.

BrdU-Positive Cells

AOB

Representative photomicrographs of BrdU-positive cells in the pAOB are shown in **Figure 1**. Significant differences between the groups were found in the density of BrdU-positive cells in the GrL of the pAOB ($F = 9.504, p = 0.001$). The post hoc test revealed that the males from the 3E group had significantly more new cells that survive than the Ctr, Exp, NP and 1E groups. No significant differences were found in the GlL ($F = 0.943, p = 0.452$) of the pAOB, **Figure 2B**. Similarly, no significant differences were found in the GlL ($F = 0.39, p = 0.809$) and GrL ($F = 1.302, p = 0.290$) of the aAOB, **Figure 2A**.

MOB

No differences were observed in the density of cells that survive in the GlL ($F = 0.427, p = 0.788$) or GrL ($F = 1.429, p = 0.247$) of the MOB, **Figure 2C**.

BrdU/NeuN-Positive Cells

Since we only found significant differences in the density of new cells that survive in the GrL of the AOB, we evaluated if sexual behavior increased the density and percentage of new cells that differentiate into neurons in the 3E group in comparison to the control group. In the pAOB the 3E group had more BrdU/NeuN positive cells than the Ctr group ($t = -2.8, p = 0.014$). No significant differences were found in the density of BrdU/NeuN cells in the aAOB ($t = -0.54, p = 0.6$) **Table 2**. No differences were found in the percentage of new cells that differentiate into neurons in the anterior ($T = 67, p = 0.96$) and posterior ($T = 54, p = 0.16$) GrL of the AOB (**Table 2**). Representative photomicrographies are shown in the **Figure 3**.

DISCUSSION

Our data reveal that those males that ejaculated three times pacing the sexual interaction show an increase in the density of new cells and neurons that survive in the granular cell layer (GrL) of the posterior accessory olfactory bulb (pAOB). No significant differences were found in the anterior accessory bulb (aAOB). Different kinds of socio-sexual stimulation can modulate adult

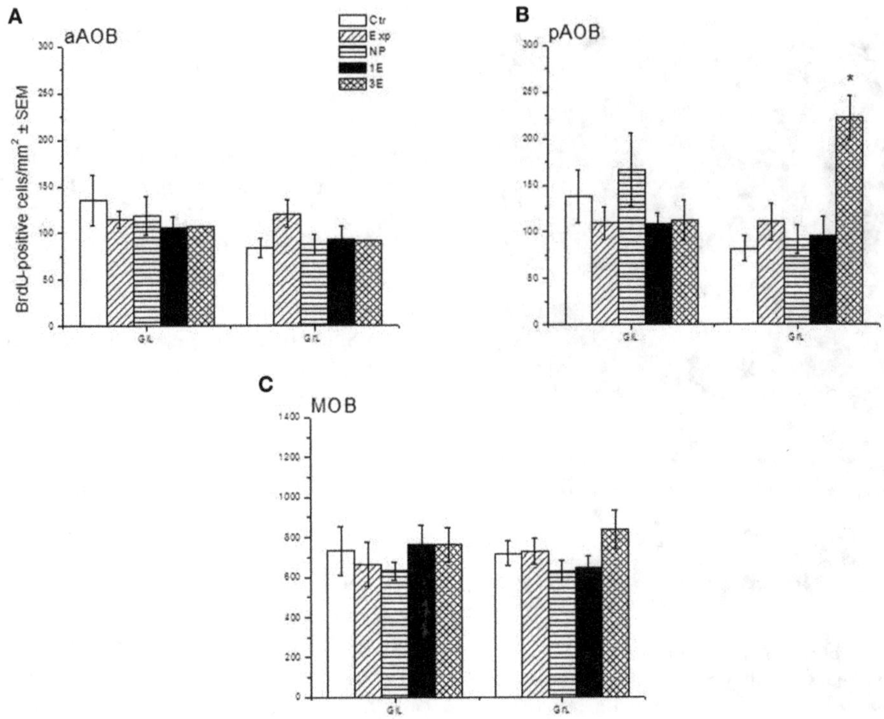

FIGURE 2 | Density of BrdU-positive cells in the sagittal plane in control (Ctr, $n = 7$), exposed (Exp, $n = 8$), non-paced (NP, $n = 8$), 1 ejaculation (1E, $n = 6$) and 3 ejaculation (3E, $n = 8$) groups. The analyzed regions were the GlL and GrL of the aAOB **(A)**, pAOB **(B)**, and MOB **(C)**. Data are expressed as the mean ± SEM. *Different from all other groups in the same layer. $P < 0.05$.

TABLE 2 | Density and percentage of BrdU/NeuN positive cells in the GrL of the AOB in control (Ctr) and three ejaculation (3E) groups.

	Density of BrdU/NeuN cells		Percentage of BrdU/NeuN cells	
	aAOB	**pAOB**	**aAOB**	**pAOB**
Ctr	5.9 ± 1.7	4.4 ± 1.9	40.11 ± 10	36.3 ± 13
3E	7 ± 1.2	13.7 ± 2.6*	47.6 ± 9.6	63.6 ± 6.7

*Different form Ctr, $P < 0.05$.

neurogenesis differentially throughout the anterior and posterior regions of the AOB. Aggressive behavior in male mice increases neurogenesis in the aAOB, and female mice exposed to male urine show an increase in the number of new cells in the pAOB (Nunez-Parra et al., 2011). Thus, the pAOB plays a relevant role in detecting sexually relevant odors, and sexual stimulation increases neurogenesis in this structure.

We previously demonstrated that neither mating nor exposure to a sexually receptive female increased the density of new cells that arrive to the MOB. In the present study we confirmed these observations, because no increase in the density of new cells that survive in the MOB were found. In male rats, mating increased the early gene activity-regulated cytoskeleton-associated protein (Arc) immunoreactivity in the granular cells of the AOB. However, sexual activity did not increase the number of Arc-positive cells in the MOB (Matsuoka et al., 2002a,b). Similarly, in male rats exposure to estrous female bedding increased the number of c-Fos (Portillo and Paredes, 2004) and Arc-positive cells in the GrL and mitral cell layer of the AOB, but not in the MOB (Matsuoka et al., 2002b). Thus, in male rats, mating and estrous female odors are not very effective in activating the MOB.

In a previous study we found that those males that pace the sexual interaction and ejaculate once showed an increase in the density of cells that arrive at the AOB 15 days after the sexual interaction (Portillo et al., 2012). However, in the present study the stimulation provided by one ejaculation was not enough to increase the density of new cells that survive in the AOB when evaluated 45 days after mating. Studies in females have shown that those female rats that paced the sexual interaction before BrdU administration and then continued mating weekly for 3 additional weeks had a significantly higher density of new cells in the granular and mitral cell layers of the AOB and the MOB, suggesting that intense sexual stimulation increases the survival of new cells in different areas of the OB (Arzate et al., 2013). Further, studies need to address if repeated mating in males that control the sexual interaction increases the density of cells in different areas of the OB.

Although males from the non-pacing group ejaculate around three times (2.6 ± 0.4), this stimulation was not able to increase the survival of the new cells in the AOB. Similar results were found in our previous studies when we demonstrated that males not allowed to pace the sexual interaction did not show an increase in the density of cells that reach the AOB 15 days after

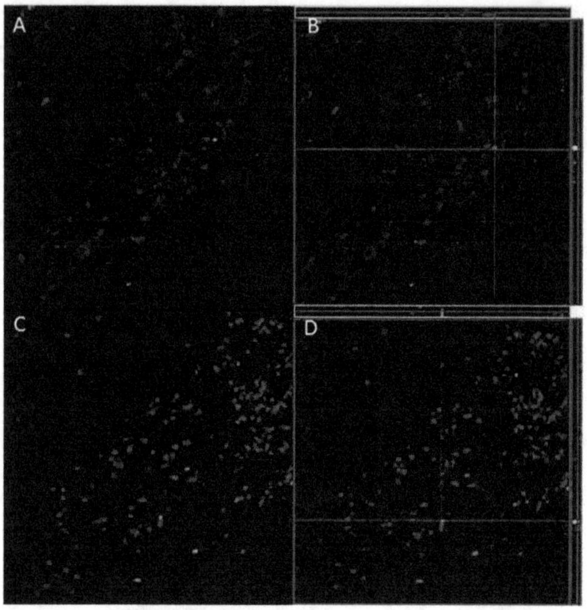

FIGURE 3 | Confocal images of cells in the GrL of the AOB, double-labeled with NeuN (red) and BrdU (green) in control (A) and 3E group (C). Projection and orthogonal plane in control **(B)** and 3E group **(D)**.

sexual behavior (Portillo et al., 2012). One of the differences between pacing and no pacing is that only when the male and female rats pace the sexual interaction, sexual behavior induce a reward state, as evaluated by the conditional place preference (CPP) paradigm (Agmo and Berenfeld, 1990; Paredes and Alonso, 1997; Camacho et al., 2009; Arzate et al., 2011; Corona et al., 2011b). It has been demonstrated that rewarding experiences such as running and intracranial self-stimulation increase the proliferation, differentiation and survival of new cells in the dentate gyrus (Takahashi et al., 2009; Garrett et al., 2012). In rodents, the rewarding properties of paced mating depend on opioids since the administration of the opioid antagonist naloxone blocks the rewarding proprieties of CPP in male and female rats that pace the sexual interaction (Agmo and Gómez, 1993; García-Horsman et al., 2008). It has been demonstrated that opioids can regulate proliferation, gliogenesis, and neurogenesis (Narita et al., 2006; Chen et al., 2008). Opioid agonists decrease proliferation in the DG of the hippocampus and increase the survival of the new cells but do not modify the differentiation linage (Pettit et al., 2012). Preliminary data from our lab indicate that the increase in the density of new cells that reach the GrL of the AOB in female rats that paced the sexual interaction is inhibited by the i.p. administration of the opioid antagonist naloxone (unpublished data). Further, studies are needed to determine if naloxone can block the increase in the number of new cells that arrive and survive in the GrL of the AOB in those males that pace the sexual interaction, to determine if the neurogenesis induced by mating is opioid dependent.

It has been shown that in male Wistar rats, the first ejaculation increases the prolactin (PRL) levels in comparison to the precopulatory values. The increase in PRL levels reaches the highest point after the second ejaculation and start to decrease after the third one (Hernandez et al., 2006). PRL increases the SVZ and OB neurogenesis *in vivo* and *in vitro* (Bridges and Grattan, 2003; Shingo et al., 2003; Larsen et al., 2008; Walker et al., 2012). In male mice, the paternal-offspring interaction increases cell proliferation in the SVZ and DG and the number of new neurons that reach the OB and DG (Mak and Weiss, 2010). Disruption of PRL signaling by the administration of a PRL-neutralizing antibody and males with targeted disruption in the PRL receptor gene showed no increase in the neurogenesis induced by the paternal-offspring interaction (Mak and Weiss, 2010). Since males that ejaculate twice show the highest levels of PRL, it is possible that the elevated levels of this hormone are involved in the increase in the survival of new cells in the AOB of males that ejaculate three times. Female rats that mate in pacing conditions show an increase in PRL levels, whereas females that mate without pacing the sexual interaction do not (McClintock and Anisko, 1982; Erskine et al., 2004). Further, research is need to evaluate if in male rats that pace the sexual interaction PRL levels increase in comparison to those males that mate without pacing the sexual interaction.

Our data show that males that ejaculated three times pacing the sexual interaction showed an increase in the density of new cells that survive in the GrL of the pAOB and they also have more new neurons that the control animals. However, no differences were found in the percentage of new cells that differentiate into neurons. Glasper and Gould (2013) found similar results; they showed that retired breeders that mate consecutively for 14 days and stay sexually inactive for another 14 days did not increase the percentage of new cells that differentiate into neurons in the DG (Glasper and Gould, 2013). On the other hand, female rats that repeatedly mate showed an increase in the percentage of new neurons that reach the AOB (Arzate et al., 2013). Further, studies are needed to determine if in the female, but not in the male rat, sexual stimulation enhances the differentiation to the neuronal linage.

To summarize, the results of the present study show that male rats that ejaculate three times in one mating session have a higher density of cells and new neurons that survive in the GrL of the AOB 45 days after mating.

AUTHOR CONTRIBUTIONS

NU, Performed the experiments and data analysis, help writing the paper; WP, Designed the study, help in writing the paper; RC, Help in the experiments; RP, Help in writing the paper and data analysis.

ACKNOWLEDGMENTS

We thank Francisco Camacho, Elsa Nidya Hernandez, Martin Garcia, Alejandra Castilla and Deisy Gasca for their excellent technical assistance and Dr. Dorothy Pless for the critical review of the manuscript. This research was supported by CONACYT 152872, 252756 (WP), 167101, Fronteras 374 (RP), and PAPITT IN203615 (WP) and IN210215 (R.P).

REFERENCES

Agmo, A., and Berenfeld, R. (1990). Reinforcing properties of ejaculation in the male rat: role of opioids and dopamine. *Behav. Neurosci.* 104, 177–182. doi: 10.1037/0735-7044.104.1.177

Agmo, A., and Gómez, M. (1993). Sexual reinforcement is blocked by infusion of naloxone into the medial preoptic area. *Behav. Neurosci.* 107, 812–818. doi: 10.1037/0735-7044.107.5.812

Arzate, D. M., Portillo, W., Corona, R., and Paredes, R. G. (2013). Repeated paced mating promotes the arrival of more newborn neurons in the main and accessory olfactory bulbs of adult female rats. *Neuroscience* 232, 151–160. doi: 10.1016/j.neuroscience.2012.12.014

Arzate, D. M., Portillo, W., Rodríguez, C., Corona, R., and Paredes, R. G. (2011). Extended paced mating tests induces conditioned place preference without affecting sexual arousal. *Horm. Behav.* 59, 674–680. doi: 10.1016/j.yhbeh.2010.08.016

Bagley, J., Larocca, G., Jimenez, D. A., and Urban, N. N. (2007). Adult neurogenesis and specific replacement of interneuron subtypes in the mouse main olfactory bulb. *BMC Neurosci.* 8:92. doi: 10.1186/1471-2202-8-92

Baum, M. J., and Cherry, J. A. (2015). Processing by the main olfactory system of chemosignals that facilitate mammalian reproduction. *Horm. Behav.* 68C, 53–64. doi: 10.1016/j.yhbeh.2014.06.003

Baum, M. J., and Kelliher, K. R. (2009). Complementary roles of the main and accessory olfactory systems in mammalian mate recognition. *Annu. Rev. Physiol.* 71, 141–160. doi: 10.1146/annurev.physiol.010908.163137

Bridges, R. S., and Grattan, D. R. (2003). Prolactin-induced neurogenesis in the maternal brain. *Trends Endocrinol. Metab.* 14, 199–201. doi: 10.1016/S1043-2760(03)00082-1

Camacho, F. J., Portillo, W., Quintero-Enríquez, O., and Paredes, R. G. (2009). Reward value of intromissions and morphine in male rats evaluated by conditioned place preference. *Physiol. Behav.* 98, 602–607. doi: 10.1016/j.physbeh.2009.09.012

Cameron, H. A., and McKay, R. D. (2001). Adult neurogenesis produces a large pool of new granule cells in the dentate gyrus. *J. Comp. Neurol.* 435, 406–417. doi: 10.1002/cne.1040

Chen, Y. L., Law, P. Y., and Loh, H. H. (2008). The other side of the opioid story: modulation of cell growth and survival signaling. *Curr. Med. Chem.* 15, 772–778. doi: 10.2174/092986708783955518

Corona, R., Camacho, F. J., García-Horsman, P., Guerrero, A., Ogando, A., and Paredes, R. G. (2011b). Different doses of estradiol benzoate induce conditioned place preference after paced mating. *Horm. Behav.* 60, 264–268. doi: 10.1016/j.yhbeh.2011.05.013

Corona, R., Larriva-Sahd, J., and Paredes, R. G. (2011a). Paced-mating increases the number of adult new born cells in the internal cellular (granular) layer of the accessory olfactory bulb. *PLoS ONE* 6:e19380. doi: 10.1371/journal.pone.0019380

Dhungel, S., Masaoka, M., Rai, D., Kondo, Y., and Sakuma, Y. (2011). Both olfactory epithelial and vomeronasal inputs are essential for activation of the medial amygdala and preoptic neurons of male rats. *Neuroscience* 199, 225–234. doi: 10.1016/j.neuroscience.2011.09.051

Erskine, M. S., Lehmann, M. L., Cameron, N. M., and Polston, E. K. (2004). Co-regulation of female sexual behavior and pregnancy induction: an exploratory synthesis. *Behav. Brain Res.* 153, 295–315. doi: 10.1016/j.bbr.2004.01.026

García-Horsman, S. P., Agmo, A., and Paredes, R. G. (2008). Infusions of naloxone into the medial preoptic area, ventromedial nucleus of the hypothalamus, and amygdala block conditioned place preference induced by paced mating behavior. *Horm. Behav.* 54, 709–716. doi: 10.1016/j.yhbeh.2008.07.011

Garrett, L., Lie, D. C., Hrabé de Angelis, M., Wurst, W., and Holter, S. M. (2012). Voluntary wheel running in mice increases the rate of neurogenesis without affecting anxiety-related behaviour in single tests. *BMC Neurosci.* 13:61. doi: 10.1186/1471-2202-13-61

Glasper, E. R., and Gould, E. (2013). Sexual experience restores age-related decline in adult neurogenesis and hippocampal function. *Hippocampus* 23, 303–312. doi: 10.1002/hipo.22090

Hernandez, M. E., Soto-Cid, A., Rojas, F., Pascual, L. I., Aranda-Abreu, G. E., Toledo, R., et al. (2006). Prostate response to prolactin in sexually active male rats. *Reprod. Biol. Endocrinol.* 4:28. doi: 10.1186/1477-7827-4-28

Herrada, G., and Dulac, C. (1997). A novel family of putative pheromone receptors in mammals with a topographically organized and sexually dimorphic distribution. *Cell* 90, 763–773. doi: 10.1016/S0092-8674(00)80536-X

Kevetter, G. A., and Winans, S. S. (1981). Connections of the corticomedial amygdala in the golden hamster. I. Efferents of the "vomeronasal amygdala." *J. Comp. Neurol.* 197, 81–98. doi: 10.1002/cne.901970107

Kondo, Y., Sudo, T., Tomihara, K., and Sakuma, Y. (2003). Activation of accessory olfactory bulb neurons during copulatory behavior after deprivation of vomeronasal inputs in male rats. *Brain Res.* 962, 232–236. doi: 10.1016/S0006-8993(02)03970-7

Larsen, C. M., Kokay, I. C., and Grattan, D. R. (2008). Male pheromones initiate prolactin-induced neurogenesis and advance maternal behavior in female mice. *Horm. Behav.* 53, 509–517. doi: 10.1016/j.yhbeh.2007.11.020

Lau, B. W., Yau, S. Y., Lee, T. M., Ching, Y. P., Tang, S. W., and So, K. F. (2011). Effect of corticosterone and paroxetine on masculine mating behavior: possible involvement of neurogenesis. *J. Sex. Med.* 8, 1390–1403. doi: 10.1111/j.1743-6109.2010.02081.x

Leuner, B., Glasper, E. R., and Gould, E. (2010). Sexual experience promotes adult neurogenesis in the hippocampus despite an initial elevation in stress hormones. *PLoS ONE* 5:e11597. doi: 10.1371/journal.pone.0011597

Lledo, P. M., and Saghatelyan, A. (2005). Integrating new neurons into the adult olfactory bulb: joining the network, life-death decisions, and the effects of sensory experience. *Trends Neurosci.* 28, 248–254. doi: 10.1016/j.tins.2005.03.005

Mak, G. K., Enwere, E. K., Gregg, C., Pakarainen, T., Poutanen, M., Huhtaniemi, I., et al. (2007). Male pheromone-stimulated neurogenesis in the adult female brain: possible role in mating behavior. *Nat. Neurosci.* 10, 1003–1011. doi: 10.1038/nn1928

Mak, G. K., and Weiss, S. (2010). Paternal recognition of adult offspring mediated by newly generated CNS neurons. *Nat. Neurosci.* 13, 753–758. doi: 10.1038/nn.2550

Matsuoka, M., Yamagata, K., Sugiura, H., Yoshida-Matsuoka, J., Norita, M., and Ichikawa, M. (2002a). Expression and regulation of the immediate-early gene product Arc in the accessory olfactory bulb after mating in male rat. *Neuroscience* 111, 251–258. doi: 10.1016/S0306-4522(01)00620-0

Matsuoka, M., Yoshida-Matsuoka, J., Sugiura, H., Yamagata, K., Ichikawa, M., and Norita, M. (2002b). Mating behavior induces differential Arc expression in the main and accessory olfactory bulbs of adult rats. *Neurosci. Lett.* 335, 111–114. doi: 10.1016/S0304-3940(02)01187-4

McClintock, M. K., and Anisko, J. J. (1982). Group mating among Norway rats I. Sex differences in the pattern and neuroendocrine consequences of copulation. *Anim. Behav.* 30, 410–425. doi: 10.1016/S0003-3472(82)80052-3

Murphy, G. J., Darcy, D. P., and Isaacson, J. S. (2005). Intraglomerular inhibition: signaling mechanisms of an olfactory microcircuit. *Nat. Neurosci.* 8, 354–364. doi: 10.1038/nn1403

Narita, M., Kuzumaki, N., Miyatake, M., Sato, F., Wachi, H., Seyama, Y., et al. (2006). Role of delta-opioid receptor function in neurogenesis and neuroprotection. *J. Neurochem.* 97, 1494–1505. doi: 10.1111/j.1471-4159.2006.03849.x

Nunez-Parra, A., Pugh, V., and Araneda, R. C. (2011). Regulation of adult neurogenesis by behavior and age in the accessory olfactory bulb. *Mol. Cell. Neurosci.* 47, 274–285. doi: 10.1016/j.mcn.2011.05.003

Oboti, L., Savalli, G., Giachino, C., De Marchis, S., Panzica, G. C., Fasolo, A., et al. (2009). Integration and sensory experience-dependent survival of newly-generated neurons in the accessory olfactory bulb of female mice. *Eur. J. Neurosci.* 29, 679–692. doi: 10.1111/j.1460-9568.2009.06614.x

Oboti, L., Schellino, R., Giachino, C., Chamero, P., Pyrski, M., Leinders-Zufall, T., et al. (2011). Newborn interneurons in the accessory olfactory bulb promote mate recognition in female mice. *Front. Neurosci.* 5:113. doi: 10.3389/fnins.2011.00113

Paredes, R. G., and Alonso, A. (1997). Sexual behavior regulated (paced) by the female induces conditioned place preference. *Behav. Neurosci.* 111, 123–128. doi: 10.1037/0735-7044.111.1.123

Petreanu, L., and Alvarez-Buylla, A. (2002). Maturation and death of adult-born olfactory bulb granule neurons: role of olfaction. *J. Neurosci.* 22, 6106–6113.

Pettit, A. S., Desroches, R., and Bennett, S. A. (2012). The opiate analgesic buprenorphine decreases proliferation of adult hippocampal neuroblasts and increases survival of their progeny. *Neuroscience* 200, 211–222. doi: 10.1016/j.neuroscience.2011.10.039

Portillo, W., and Paredes, R. G. (2004). Sexual incentive motivation, olfactory preference, and activation of the vomeronasal projection pathway by sexually relevant cues in non-copulating and naive male rats. *Horm. Behav.* 46, 330–340. doi: 10.1016/j.yhbeh.2004.03.001

Portillo, W., Unda, N., Camacho, F. J., Sánchez, M., Corona, R., Arzate, D. M., et al. (2012). Sexual activity increases the number of newborn cells in the accessory olfactory bulb of male rats. *Front. Neuroanat.* 6:25. doi: 10.3389/fnana.2012.00025

Rochefort, C., Gheusi, G., Vincent, J. D., and Lledo, P. M. (2002). Enriched odor exposure increases the number of newborn neurons in the adult olfactory bulb and improves odor memory. *J. Neurosci.* 22, 2679–2689.

Rochefort, C., and Lledo, P. M. (2005). Short-term survival of newborn neurons in the adult olfactory bulb after exposure to a complex odor environment. *Eur. J. Neurosci.* 22, 2863–2870. doi: 10.1111/j.1460-9568.2005.04486.x

Rodriguez, I., Feinstein, P., and Mombaerts, P. (1999). Variable patterns of axonal projections of sensory neurons in the mouse vomeronasal system. *Cell* 97, 199–208. doi: 10.1016/S0092-8674(00)80730-8

Saito, T. R., and Moltz, H. (1986). Copulatory behavior of sexually naive and sexually experienced male rats following removal of the vomeronasal organ. *Physiol. Behav.* 37, 507–510. doi: 10.1016/0031-9384(86)90215-5

Sakamoto, M., Imayoshi, I., Ohtsuka, T., Yamaguchi, M., Mori, K., and Kageyama, R. (2011). Continuous neurogenesis in the adult forebrain is required for innate olfactory responses. *Proc. Natl. Acad. Sci. U.S.A.* 108, 8479–8484. doi: 10.1073/pnas.1018782108

Shingo, T., Gregg, C., Enwere, E., Fujikawa, H., Hassam, R., Geary, C., et al. (2003). Pregnancy-stimulated neurogenesis in the adult female forebrain mediated by prolactin. *Science* 299, 117–120. doi: 10.1126/science.1076647

Sosulski, D. L., Bloom, M. L., Cutforth, T., Axel, R., and Datta, S. R. (2011). Distinct representations of olfactory information in different cortical centres. *Nature* 472, 213–216. doi: 10.1038/nature09868

Stolp, H. B., and Molnár, Z. (2015). Neurogenic niches in the brain: help and hindrance of the barrier systems. *Front. Neurosci.* 9:20. doi: 10.3389/fnins.2015.00020

Sugai, T., Yoshimura, H., Kato, N., and Onoda, N. (2006). Component-dependent urine responses in the rat accessory olfactory bulb. *Neuroreport* 17, 1663–1667. doi: 10.1097/01.wnr.0000239950.14954.59

Takahashi, T., Zhu, Y., Hata, T., Shimizu-Okabe, C., Suzuki, K., and Nakahara, D. (2009). Intracranial self-stimulation enhances neurogenesis in hippocampus of adult mice and rats. *Neuroscience* 158, 402–411. doi: 10.1016/j.neuroscience.2008.10.048

Tirindelli, R., Dibattista, M., Pifferi, S., and Menini, A. (2009). From pheromones to behavior. *Physiol. Rev.* 89, 921–956. doi: 10.1152/physrev.00037.2008

Walker, T. L., Vukovic, J., Koudijs, M. M., Blackmore, D. G., Mackay, E. W., Sykes, A. M., et al. (2012). Prolactin stimulates precursor cells in the adult mouse hippocampus. *PLoS ONE* 7:e44371. doi: 10.1371/journal.pone.0044371

Whitman, M. C., and Greer, C. A. (2009). Adult neurogenesis and the olfactory system. *Prog Neurobiol* 89, 162–175. doi: 10.1016/j.pneurobio.2009.07.003

Winner, B., Cooper-Kuhn, C. M., Aigner, R., Winkler, J., and Kuhn, H. G. (2002). Long-term survival and cell death of newly generated neurons in the adult rat olfactory bulb. *Eur. J. Neurosci.* 16, 1681–1689. doi: 10.1046/j.1460-9568.2002.02238.x

9

The Role of Astrocytes in the Generation, Migration, and Integration of New Neurons in the Adult Olfactory Bulb

Archana Gengatharan[1], *Rodrigo R. Bammann*[1] *and Armen Saghatelyan*[1,2*]

[1] *Cellular Neurobiology Unit, Centre de Recherche de l'Institut Universitaire en Santé Mentale de Québec, Quebec, QC, Canada,* [2] *Department of Psychiatry and Neuroscience, Université Laval, Quebec, QC, Canada*

Edited by:
Laura López-Mascaraque, Instituto Cajal-CSIC, Spain

Reviewed by:
Jose Manuel Garcia-Verdugo, University of Valencia, Spain
Felipe Ortega, Universidad Complutense de Madrid, Spain

***Correspondence:**
Armen Saghatelyan
armen.saghatelyan@fmed.ulaval.ca

In mammals, new neurons in the adult olfactory bulb originate from a pool of neural stem cells in the subventricular zone of the lateral ventricles. Adult-born cells play an important role in odor information processing by adjusting the neuronal network to changing environmental conditions. Olfactory bulb neurogenesis is supported by several non-neuronal cells. In this review, we focus on the role of astroglial cells in the generation, migration, integration, and survival of new neurons in the adult forebrain. In the subventricular zone, neural stem cells with astrocytic properties display regional and temporal specificity when generating different neuronal subtypes. Non-neurogenic astrocytes contribute to the establishment and maintenance of the neurogenic niche. Neuroblast chains migrate through the rostral migratory stream ensheathed by astrocytic processes. Astrocytes play an important regulatory role in neuroblast migration and also assist in the development of a vasculature scaffold in the migratory stream that is essential for neuroblast migration in the postnatal brain. In the olfactory bulb, astrocytes help to modulate the network through a complex release of cytokines, regulate blood flow, and provide metabolic support, which may promote the integration and survival of new neurons. Astrocytes thus play a pivotal role in various processes of adult olfactory bulb neurogenesis, and it is likely that many other functions of these glial cells will emerge in the near future.

Keywords: olfactory bulb, stem cells, astrocytes, interneurons, rostral migratory stream, blood vessels

INTRODUCTION

The olfactory bulb (OB), which plays a central role in odor information processing, has a multi-layered cellular architecture. Mitral and tufted cells are the principal neurons of the OB (Shepherd et al., 2004) and transmit information received from olfactory sensory neurons to the piriform cortex, as well as the entorhinal cortex and the amygdala (Davis, 2004; Shepherd et al., 2004). Information processing in the OB is modulated by two other groups of interneurons, that is, periglomerular cells (PG) and granule cells (GC), which form dendro-dendritic synapses with the principal neurons (Urban, 2002; Fukunaga et al., 2014). Interestingly, a substantial number of PGs and GCs are constantly renewed during adulthood. This unusual form of plasticity, which was first brought to light some fifty years ago and was confirmed by subsequent research

(Altman and Das, 1965; Altman, 1969; Luskin, 1993; Lois and Alvarez-Buylla, 1994; Doetsch et al., 1999), allows the OB circuitry to be fine-tuned in response to olfactory behaviors (Imayoshi et al., 2008; Breton-Provencher et al., 2009; Sultan et al., 2011; Alonso et al., 2012; Arruda-Carvalho et al., 2014). Many neurons arrive daily at the OB; therefore, it is necessary to tightly control the migration and neurochemical diversity of these cells, and to optimize the structure and function of the OB network by selectively controlling newborn cells survival and synaptic pruning. Astrocytes play a pivotal role in all these processes. In this review, we summarize the current knowledge of the role of astrocytes in adult OB neurogenesis and discuss possible future directions in this exciting field.

NEUROGENIC AND NON-NEUROGENIC ASTROCYTES IN THE ADULT SVZ

Neural Stem Cells

Adult neural stem cells (NSC) residing in the subventricular zone (SVZ), which are also called B1 cells, are derived from radial glial cells and have several astrocytic features. They express the glial fibrillary acidic (GFAP), glutamate aspartate transporter, and brain lipid-binding proteins (Codega et al., 2014; Fuentealba et al., 2015; Llorens-Bobadilla et al., 2015). They also present ultra structural properties of astrocytes, including a light cytoplasm, thick bundles of intermediate filaments, gap junctions, glycogen granules, and dense bodies (Jackson and Alvarez-Buylla, 2008). NSC can exist in either the quiescent or the active state. Once activated, GFAP-positive B1 cells express epidermal growth factor receptor (EGFR) and give rise to EGFR-positive transit-amplifying C cells that in turn proliferate to generate CD24-expressing migrating neuroblasts. Fluorescence-activated cell sorting (FACS) using a combination of markers such as CD24, GFAP, and EGFR has been used to purify activated stem cells, transit-amplifying C cells, and neuroblasts (Pastrana et al., 2009). Cells that express both EGFR and GFAP are activated B1 stem cells that can be eliminated by an antimitotic treatment (Pastrana et al., 2009). In contrast, GFAP-positive cells that do not express EGFR may be either quiescent stem cells or SVZ niche astrocytes. These cell populations can be further distinguished by the expression of transmembrane glycoprotein, CD133 (prominin), which is present on the primary cilia of neural progenitors (Mirzadeh et al., 2008; Beckervordersandforth et al., 2010; Codega et al., 2014). Using a combination of these markers, it has been shown that quiescent B1 stem cells do not express nestin, an intermediate filament protein considered to be a marker of NSC (Codega et al., 2014). The quiescent state of B1 cells is actively maintained by the GPCR ligands S1P and PDG_2 (Codega et al., 2014), whereas BLBP is more restricted to active NSC (Giachino et al., 2014).

Adult NSC display regional and temporal specificity in generating different types of bulbar interneurons (Merkle et al., 2007; Batista-Brito et al., 2008; Fuentealba et al., 2015). Based on viral labeling of NSC in distinct spatial SVZ sub-regions, it has been shown that dorsal NSC generate mostly superficial GC and dopaminergic tyrosine hydroxylase (TH)-positive PG, whereas ventral NSC produce deep GC and calbindin-positive PG (Merkle et al., 2007). Calretinin-positive GC and PG, as well as four new subtypes of bulbar interneurons, are mostly derived from NSC located in the anterior and anterior-ventral tip of SVZ, respectively (Merkle et al., 2007, 2014). A lineage tracing method consisting of introducing a large library of 24-base-pair oligonucleotide barcodes into the cells recently revealed that regional specification becomes evident at mouse embryonic stage E11.5, which is maintained from the embryonic to the adult stage (Fuentealba et al., 2015).

This regional heterogeneity is determined by the combinatory action of morphogens and transcriptional factors. For example, lineage tracing of the Emx1 and Gsh2 transcriptional factors, which are highly expressed in the embryonic cortex ventricular zone and the lateral ganglionic eminence, respectively, has shown that Emx1 progenitor cells reside in the adult dorsal SVZ and generate calretinin-positive superficial GC, whereas NSC derived from the Gsh2 lineage produce calbindin-positive interneurons and very low numbers of calretinin-expressing cells (Young et al., 2007). Deep GCs are derived from the Nkx2.1 domain in the ventral SVZ (Delgado and Lim, 2015), whereas four new types of interneurons derived from the anterior-ventral tip of the SVZ are generated from microdomains patterned by the Nkx6.2 and Zic family of transcriptional factors (Merkle et al., 2014). Transcriptional factor Pax6 has a dual role and is required for generating neuronal progenitors and also for directing them toward dopaminergic PG (Hack et al., 2005). In contrast, zinc finger transcription factor Sp8 is required for the specification of calretinin and gabaergic/nondopaminergic PG (Waclaw et al., 2006). NSC in the adult SVZ also generate a small number glutamatergic juxtaglomerular cells in the OB that is specified by the expression of the Neurog2 and Tbr2 transcriptional factors expressed in the subset of progenitors in the dorsal SVZ (Brill et al., 2009). All these studies have established the repertoire of transcriptional factor codes along the dorso-ventral and rostro-caudal SVZ as well as the regional specification of adult NSC in the generation of interneuronal diversity in the OB. In addition to these transcriptional factor codes, morphogens also play an important role in the regional heterogeneity of adult NSC. A study on reporter mice with labeled sonic hedgehog (Shh)-responsive cells revealed that this morphogen gradient plays a general role in the ventro-dorsal specification of NSC (Ihrie et al., 2011). Shh-responsive cells express GFAP and give rise primarily to interneurons in the deep GC layer of the OB (Ihrie et al., 2011), similar to what has been observed after viral labeling of NSC in the ventral SVZ (Merkle et al., 2007). The removal of Shh reduces the production of ventrally derived OB interneurons. Conversely, the ectopic activation of Shh by the expression of Smo2, a constitutive active receptor in dorsal NSC, generates cells that are normally produced by progenitors in the ventral SVZ (Ihrie et al., 2011). Interestingly, a transient domain of Shh in the dorsal SVZ has also been identified, but this domain produces many cells with an oligodendrocyte lineage (Tong et al., 2015). The dorsal domain of SVZ is also determined by persistent Wnt/β-catenin signaling that specify NSC to an oligodendrocyte lineage (Azim et al., 2014a,b). Indeed, live-imaging and single cell tracking of adult NSC and their progeny has revealed that oligodendrogliogenic and neurogenic NSC constitute two distinct lineages that display different responsiveness to Wnt signaling (Ortega et al., 2013).

In addition to regional heterogeneity, adult NSC also display temporal specificity. Batista-Bristo et al. used inducible genetic fate mapping of Dlx1/2 precursors to analyze the precursors of seven OB interneuron subtypes, from embryogenesis through adulthood (Batista-Brito et al., 2008). They found that the production of calbindin-positive interneurons reaches a maximum during late embryogenesis and subsequently decreases postnatally, whereas the opposite is observed for the production of calretinin-positive cells (Batista-Brito et al., 2008). Parvalbumin-positive interneurons in the external plexiform layer are produced perinatally, while Blanes cells, which are bulbar interneurons that provide feed-forward inhibition in GC (Pressler and Strowbridge, 2006), are produced during embryogenesis (Batista-Brito et al., 2008). They also showed that the production of TH-positive cells in the glomerular layer peaks during early embryogenesis and decreases thereafter. However, it has also been demonstrated that TH-positive PG are mainly produced by postnatal NSC (De Marchis et al., 2007).

The production of different subtypes of interneurons from B1 cells is thus regionally and temporally specified. Regional specification allows embryonic information to be maintained, from neuroepithelial to radial glial then to B1 cells, whereas temporal specification controls the order and subtype of the interneurons generated. The precise interplay between temporal and regional factors remains to be determined, as does how the generation of specific interneuronal subtypes is regulated by the behavioral state of animals.

Non-Neurogenic Astrocytes

NSC are found in specialized microenvironments and are exposed to a variety of factors from the cerebral spinal fluid via small apical process bearing a non-motile primary cilium. NSC also contact blood vessels via basal processes (**Figure 1**; Doetsch et al., 1999; Mirzadeh et al., 2008). Transplanting NSC/progenitor cells into the SVZ of another animal generates OB interneurons, whereas transplanting NSC into non-neurogenic zones limits their neurogenic potential (Alvarez-Buylla and Lim, 2004). These results suggest that the SVZ microenvironment plays an important role in the maintenance of the neurogenic properties of NSC.

In addition to vasculature support and factors present in the cerebrospinal fluid, non-neurogenic astrocytes in the SVZ contribute to the establishment and maintenance of the neurogenic microenvironment. Culturing dissociated perinatal or adult SVZ NSC on astrocyte monolayers has shown that direct contact between astrocytes and SVZ precursors support the proliferation of these precursors (Lim and Alvarez-Buylla, 1999). Similarly, astrocytes from the hippocampus promote the proliferation and neuronal fate of stem cells from the dentate gyrus (Song et al., 2002). This shows that GFAP-positive cells can be sub-divided into two distinct populations, that is, those that are stem cells and those that have non-neurogenic properties but that contribute to the establishment of the SVZ microenvironment.

Labeling strategies based on the use of multiple markers (Codega et al., 2014) or on split-Cre technology (Beckervordersandforth et al., 2010) have been used to discriminate between those two cell populations, as well as other SVZ cells. In the case of split-Cre technology, the coincident activity of GFAP and prominin1 promoters enables the selective labeling and manipulation of adult NSC from non-neurogenic astrocytes (Beckervordersandforth et al., 2010). A transcriptomic analysis of these cells compared to other SVZ cells and non-neurogenic astrocytes revealed enrichment in genes involved in neuronal lineage priming, cilia biogenesis/function, and Ca^{2+}-dependent pathways (Beckervordersandforth et al., 2010). Calcium waves have been observed in the SVZ, and it has been suggested that they may define the communication network between NSC and niche astrocytes (Lacar et al., 2011). In line with this, GFAP-positive cells in the SVZ express the gap junction protein connexin 43 and display functional coupling involving 50–60 cells (Lacar et al., 2011).

Morphogens such as BMP, Notch, Wnt, and Shh are also involved in the interplay between non-neurogenic astrocytes and NSC. Shh released by astrocytes stimulates adult neural progenitors to reenter the cell cycle (Jiao and Chen, 2008). GFAP-positive cells in the SVZ express Notch 1 receptors as well as its ligands (Givogri et al., 2006). Notch signaling implies cell-cell interactions and mice deficient in Dlk1, a Notch ligand delta-like homolog, present deficits in postnatal neurogenesis in the SVZ (Ferrón et al., 2011). Dlk1 is secreted by niche astrocytes, whereas its membrane-bound isoform is present in NSC and is required for the inductive effect of secreted Dlk1 on the self-renewal of NSC (Ferrón et al., 2011). BMP signaling is also active in adult NSC (Colak et al., 2008). The conditional deletion of Smad4, a transcriptional factor that mediates BMP signaling, reduces neurogenesis and leads to increased numbers of oligodendrocytes (Colak et al., 2008). BMP ligands and their receptors are expressed by niche astrocytes (Peretto et al., 2004) and ependymal cells express noggin, a BMP feedback inhibitor (Lim et al., 2000). This suggests that there is a complex multicellular interplay between niche astrocytes, ependymal cells, and NSC in the regulation of BMP signaling in the adult SVZ. Wnt canonical, β-catenin-dependent, and non-canonical planar cell polarity (PCP) pathways have been detected in the SVZ (Hirota et al., 2015). While Wnt/β-catenin controls the proliferation of NSC and type C cells, the Wnt/PCP pathway regulates the proliferation, migration, and differentiation of neuroblasts (Hirota et al., 2015). In line with this, Wnt/β-catenin signaling activity has been detected in GFAP-positive astrocytes and Mash1-positive cells using reporter mice and stabilization of β-catenin promotes NSC proliferation (Adachi et al., 2007). Niche astrocytes promote NSC expansion and proliferation via WNT7A (Moreno-Estellés et al., 2012), and the activation of canonical Wnt signaling stimulates the oligodendrogliogenic lineage in SVZ (Ortega et al., 2013). Likewise, EGF signaling affects the proliferation of NSC and type C cells (Doetsch et al., 2002; Pastrana et al., 2009) and promotes oligodendrogenesis at the expense of neurogenesis (Aguirre and Gallo, 2007; Aguirre et al., 2007). Astrocyte-derived factors such as the pro-inflammatory cytokines IL-1β and IL-6 promote NSC neuronal differentiation, whereas

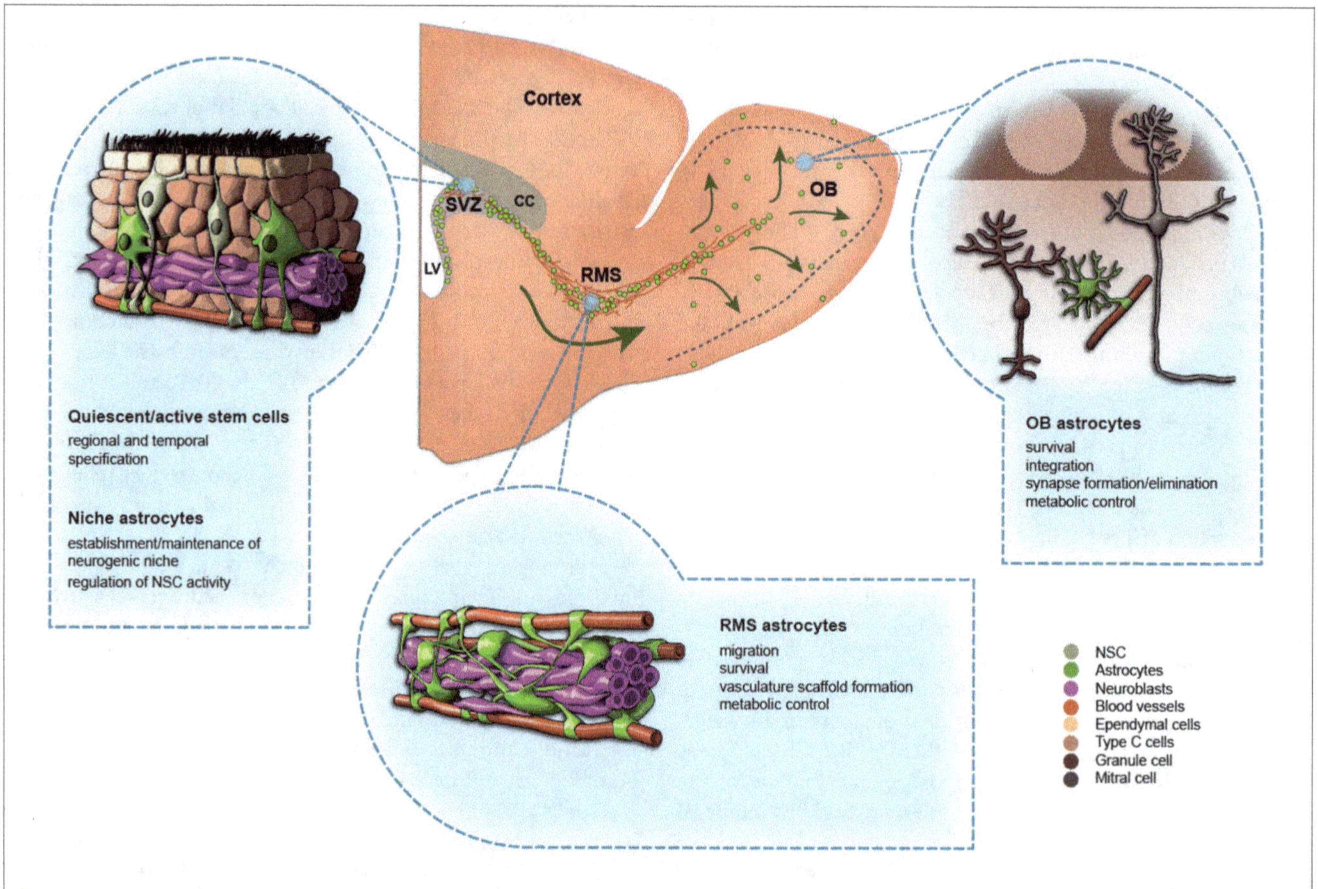

FIGURE 1 | The role of astrocytes in the adult olfactory bulb neurogenesis. A schematic drawing of the adult mouse forebrain and illustrations showing different types of astrocytes in the subventricular zone (SVZ), rostral migratory stream (RMS), and olfactory bulb (OB). The functions of each type of astrocytes are indicated.

insulin-like growth factor binding protein 6 (IGFBP6) and decorin inhibit it (Barkho et al., 2006). It has been also recently demonstrated that quiescent NSC express higher levels of tetraspanin CD9 than parenchymal astrocytes (Llorens-Bobadilla et al., 2015). Thus, while several lines of evidence show that GFAP-positive cells in the SVZ can be sub-divided into NSC and niche cells, the relationship between them remains to be investigated. The use of specific tools to selectively identify and manipulate these two populations will help to pursue this goal. Interestingly, after brain injury, a subpopulation of reactive astrocytes may acquire stem cell properties in response to Shh signaling (Sirko et al., 2013). This shows that the delimitation between neurogenic and non-neurogenic astrocytes is not fixed and may be dynamically modulated. To understand the mechanisms underlying the activation of quiescent NSC, single cell sequencing of two neurogenic regions of the adult mice (Llorens-Bobadilla et al., 2015; Shin et al., 2015) has shown that the downregulation of glycolic metabolism, Notch, and BMP signaling, combined with the concomitant upregulation of lineage-specific transcriptional factors, is required for the entrance of dormant NSC into the primed-quiescent state before they are activated (Llorens-Bobadilla et al., 2015). After an acute ischemic injury, dormant NSC enter into a pre-active state via interferon gamma signaling and are subsequently activated (Llorens-Bobadilla et al., 2015). Interestingly the downregulation of glycolic metabolism (Gascón et al., 2016) and the forced expression of neurogenic transcriptional factors (Berninger et al., 2007; Heinrich et al., 2010) have also been shown to be required for the direct reprogramming of astroglia from cortex into neurons. While it remains to be determined how similar non-neurogenic astrocytes and quiescent NSC are at the level of single cell transcriptomics and what their responses are to different microenvironmental signals, these results suggest that there are similarities in the molecular signatures of these cells.

ASTROCYTES IN THE ROSTRAL MIGRATORY STREAM

GFAP-positive astrocytes in the RMS are derived from embryonic radial glia cells (Alves et al., 2002). Some of these cells maintain stem cell properties and can generate different types of OB interneurons (Gritti et al., 2002; Merkle et al., 2007; Alonso et al., 2008). At the structural level, RMS astrocytes have elongated morphology, with their branches aligned along blood vessels and chains of migrating neuroblasts (**Figure 1**; Peretto et al., 2005; Whitman et al., 2009). Astrocytes undergo extensive reorganization in terms of their structural arrangement and expression of molecular cues postnatally (Pencea and Luskin, 2003; Peretto et al., 2005; Bozoyan et al., 2012). During early postnatal development, astrocytes are located at the borders of the RMS, where they orchestrate the proper development of the RMS (Peretto et al., 2005; Bozoyan et al., 2012). These glial cells synthesize and secrete vascular endothelial growth factor (VEGF), which controls blood vessel formation and growth (Bozoyan et al., 2012). The vasculature scaffold is, in turn, used by neuroblasts to migrate toward the OB (Snapyan et al., 2009; Whitman et al., 2009; Bozoyan et al., 2012). During postnatal development, astrocytes thus regulate the proper development of the migratory stream which takes place at the borders of the RMS. In contrast, the core of the RMS is mostly static and is devoid of proliferative and migrating cells (Pencea and Luskin, 2003; Bozoyan et al., 2012). It remains to be determined how this particular cellular organization with blood vessels, neuroblasts, and astrocytes is transferred into the center of the RMS. We have previously proposed that overall brain growth during postnatal development leads to the elongation and thinning of the RMS. This results in the collapse of the center and the maintenance of the outer border of the RMS until adulthood (Bozoyan et al., 2012).

During adulthood, astrocytes ensheath chains of neuroblasts, and several studies have shown that they play a pivotal role in neuroblast migration (Lois and Alvarez-Buylla, 1994; Snapyan et al., 2009; Kaneko et al., 2010). Neuroblasts cultured on RMS or OB astrocyte monolayers display robust migration, unlike neuroblasts cultured on cortical astrocytes. These differences are regulated by astrocyte-derived non-soluble factors (García-Marqués et al., 2010). In addition, RMS astrocytes release soluble melanoma inhibitory activity (MIA) protein, which is required for neuroblast migration (Mason et al., 2001). The disruption of the glial tube in mutant animals leads to defects in neuroblast chain migration (Chazal et al., 2000; Anton et al., 2004; Belvindrah et al., 2007; Kaneko et al., 2010). For example, neuroblast chain migration is promoted by $\beta 1$ integrin, and a deficiency in $\beta 1$ integrin leads to glial tube disorganization and ectopic migration of neuroblasts into the surrounding tissue (Belvindrah et al., 2007). Massive gliosis is observed in neural cell adhesion molecule (NCAM)-deficient mice, which lead to neuroblast migration defects. Astrocytes also express high affinity γ- aminobutyric acid (GABA) transporters whereas neuroblasts express GABA. The inhibition of GABA uptake reduces neuroblast migration (Bolteus and Bordey, 2004). The release of GABA from neuroblasts also induces Ca^{2+} fluctuations in astrocytes, leading to the insertion of high affinity TrkB receptors into the plasma membrane of astrocytes (Snapyan et al., 2009). This, in turn, traps migration promoting vasculature-derived brain derived neurotrophic factor (BDNF), which leads to the entrance of migratory cells into the stationary phase (Snapyan et al., 2009). Astrocytes also release glutamate to control the migration and survival of neuroblasts expressing NMDA receptors (Platel et al., 2010). All these studies suggest that molecular and functional modifications in astrocytes modulate neuroblast migration. Astrocytes may also undergo rapid structural changes to sustain faithful neuroblast migration. Neuroblasts secrete diffusible protein Slit1 whose receptor Robo is present on astrocytes (Kaneko et al., 2010). Astrocytes respond to the repulsive activity of neuroblast-derived Slit, leading to the formation of structurally permissive glial tunnels that enable neuronal migration (Kaneko et al., 2010).

These findings suggest that a complex tripartite interplay occurs between neuroblasts, astrocytes, and endothelial cells in the RMS. When assessing the role of specific molecular pathways in the RMS, it is thus important to consider astrocytes, neuroblasts, and blood vessels as a whole and not as "isolated" units. This will make it possible to refine our understanding of the cellular and molecular pathways that modulate the formation and maintenance of the RMS and neuronal migration. In addition, RMS astrocytes may be a heterogeneous population of cells (Peretto et al., 2005; Whitman et al., 2009; Larriva-Sahd, 2014), and further research is thus required to define the various subtypes of astroglia and their role in the RMS.

ASTROCYTES IN THE OB

Following their arrival in the OB, neuroblasts mature and establish connections in the bulbar network. This occurs initially by receiving axo-dendritic inputs and later through dendrodendritic synapses to the principal neurons (Whitman and Greer, 2007; Panzanelli et al., 2009). The OB has a high density of astrocytes (Bailey and Shipley, 1993), but their role in the maturation and integration of newborn cells remains largely unexplored. Astrocytes may have various functions in the brain network, ranging from the modulation of synaptic transmission and synaptogenesis (Piet et al., 2004; Verkhratsky and Nedergaard, 2014) to structural dynamics, transmitter uptake, and the repair of brain lesions (Correale and Farez, 2015). Interestingly, it has been shown recently that the synaptic integration of newborn hippocampal neurons is locally controlled by astrocytes (Sultan et al., 2015). Blocking vesicular release from astrocytes results in a lower spine density of newborn cells, but only on the neuronal dendrites intersecting the domains of manipulated astrocytes (Sultan et al., 2015). Since the astroglial presynaptic sheath covers the majority of synapses in the adult brain (Verkhratsky and Nedergaard, 2014), it is likely that these cells also play an important role in the formation, maintenance, and/or elimination of synapses in the adult OB.

Astrocytes may also coordinate neuronal metabolism and blood flow by controlling vasodilation and vasoconstriction in response to increased neural activity (Takano et al., 2006). This in turn may affect the survival and integration of newborn cells. Astrocytes control blood flow through the activation of glutamate receptors following intense activity of principal neurons (Takano et al., 2006) or via GABA uptake mechanisms in response to the gabaergic activity of bulbar interneurons (Doengi et al., 2009). This activation triggers an increase in intracellular calcium ions in astrocytes, releasing arachidonic acid and vasoactive metabolites (Otsu et al., 2015). This can happen in the fine processes of astrocytes independently of soma activation, which allows for fine control of blood flow (Otsu et al., 2015) and consequently the local modulation of synaptic units. Astrocytes also provide metabolic substrates from blood vessels to distant neurons through gap junctions (Rouach et al., 2008), which may modulate the morpho-functional properties of newborn neurons farther away.

Astrocytes also control the survival of adult-born neurons via the growth factor-induced release of cytokines (Khodosevich et al., 2013). Connective tissue growth factor (CTGF) is expressed by tufted cells in the OB and enhances the proapoptotic activity of astrocyte-derived transforming growth factor-beta 2 (TGF-β2) (Khodosevich et al., 2013). The release of TGF-β2 from glial cells in turn decreases the survival of PG in an activity-dependent manner (Khodosevich et al., 2013). While the role of astrocytes in the survival, integration, and synaptic maintenance of newborn cells needs to be further studied, these glial cells may modulate the structuro-functional properties of interneurons by both local and long-distance signals. They also are strategically positioned to link activity-dependent changes in blood flow and neuronal metabolism and activity.

In conclusion, astrocytes play a pivotal role in OB neurogenesis. They control the generation, migration, and survival of different subtypes of interneurons as well as the synaptic pruning of newborn cells. Although several key features of astrocytes involved in controlling bulbar neurogenesis have emerged in recent decades, more studies combining new genetic tools, functional imaging, and behavioral tests are required to decipher their role in adult neurogenesis.

AUTHOR CONTRIBUTIONS

All authors listed, have made substantial, direct and intellectual contribution to the work, and approved it for publication.

ACKNOWLEDGMENTS

This work was supported by the Canadian Institutes of Health Research (CIHR) grant to AS. We thank Mireille Massouh for preparation of illustrations. AS is a recipient of the Canada Research Chair in Postnatal Neurogenesis.

REFERENCES

Adachi, K., Mirzadeh, Z., Sakaguchi, M., Yamashita, T., Nikolcheva, T., Gotoh, Y., et al. (2007). β-catenin signaling promotes proliferation of progenitor cells in the adult mouse subventricular zone. *Stem Cells* 25, 2827–2836. doi: 10.1634/stemcells.2007-0177

Aguirre, A., Dupree, J. L., Mangin, J. M., and Gallo, V. (2007). A functional role for EGFR signaling in myelination and remyelination. *Nat. Neurosci.* 10, 990–1002. doi: 10.1038/nn1938

Aguirre, A., and Gallo, V. (2007). Reduced EGFR signaling in adult progenitors of the subventricular zone attenuates oligodendrogenesis after demyelination. *Neuron Glia Biol.* 3, 209–220. doi: 10.1017/S1740925X08000082

Alonso, M., Lepousez, G., Wagner, S., Bardy, C., Gabellec, M.-M., Torquet, N., et al. (2012). Activation of adult-born neurons facilitates learning and memory. *Nat. Neurosci.* 15, 897–904. doi: 10.1038/nn.3108

Alonso, M., Ortega-Pérez, I., Grubb, M. S., Bourgeois, J.-P., Charneau, P., and Lledo, P.-M. (2008). Turning astrocytes from the rostral migratory stream into neurons: a role for the olfactory sensory organ. *J. Neurosci.* 28, 11089–11102. doi: 10.1523/JNEUROSCI.3713-08.2008

Altman, J. (1969). Autoradiographic and histological studies of postnatal neurogenesis. IV. Cell proliferation and migration in the anterior forebrain, with special reference to persisting neurogenesis in the olfactory bulb. *J. Comp. Neurol.* 137, 433–457. doi: 10.1002/cne.901370404

Altman, J., and Das, G. D. (1965). Autoradiographic and histological evidence of postnatal hippocampal neurogenesis in rats. *J. Comp. Neurol.* 124, 319–335. doi: 10.1002/cne.901240303

Alvarez-Buylla, A., and Lim, D. A. (2004). For the long run. *Neuron* 41, 683–686. doi: 10.1016/S0896-6273(04)00111-4

Alves, J. A. J., Barone, P., Engelender, S., Fróes, M. M., and Menezes, J. R. L. (2002). Initial stages of radial glia astrocytic transformation in the early postnatal anterior subventricular zone. *J. Neurobiol.* 52, 251–265. doi: 10.1002/neu.10087

Anton, E. S., Ghashghaei, H. T., Weber, J. L., McCann, C., Fischer, T. M., Cheung, I. D., et al. (2004). Receptor tyrosine kinase ErbB4 modulates neuroblast migration and placement in the adult forebrain. *Nat. Neurosci.* 7, 1319–1328. doi: 10.1038/nn1345

Arruda-Carvalho, M., Akers, K. G., Guskjolen, A., Sakaguchi, M., Josselyn, S. A., and Frankland, P. W. (2014). Posttraining ablation of adult-generated olfactory granule cells degrades odor–reward memories. *J. Neurosci.* 34, 15793–15803. doi: 10.1523/JNEUROSCI.2336-13.2014

Azim, K., Fischer, B., Hurtado-Chong, A., Draganova, K., Cantù, C., Zemke, M., et al. (2014a). Persistent wnt/β-catenin signaling determines dorsalization of the postnatal subventricular zone and neural stem cell specification into oligodendrocytes and glutamatergic neurons. *Stem Cells* 32, 1301–1312. doi: 10.1002/stem.1639

Azim, K., Rivera, A., Raineteau, O., and Butt, A. M. (2014b). GSK3β regulates oligodendrogenesis in the dorsal microdomain of the subventricular zone via Wnt-β-catenin signaling. *Glia* 62, 778–789. doi: 10.1002/glia.22641

Bailey, M. S., and Shipley, M. T. (1993). Astrocyte subtypes in the rat olfactory bulb: morphological heterogeneity and differential laminar distribution. *J. Comp. Neurol.* 328, 501–526. doi: 10.1002/cne.903280405

Barkho, B. Z., Song, H., Aimone, J. B., Smrt, R. D., Kuwabara, T., Nakashima, K., et al. (2006). Identification of astrocyte-expressed factors that modulate neural stem/progenitor cell differentiation. *Stem Cells Dev.* 15, 407–421. doi: 10.1089/scd.2006.15.407

Batista-Brito, R., Close, J., MacHold, R., Ekker, M., and Fishell, G. (2008). The distinct temporal origins of olfactory bulb interneuron subtypes. *J. Neurosci.* 28, 3966–3975. doi: 10.1523/JNEUROSCI.5625-07.2008

Beckervordersandforth, R., Tripathi, P., Ninkovic, J., Bayam, E., Lepier, A., Stempfhuber, B., et al. (2010). *In vivo* fate mapping and expression analysis reveals molecular hallmarks of prospectively isolated adult neural stem cells. *Cell Stem Cell* 7, 744–758. doi: 10.1016/j.stem.2010.11.017

Belvindrah, R., Hankel, S., Walker, J., Patton, B. L., and Müller, U. (2007). β1 integrins control the formation of cell chains in the adult rostral migratory stream. *J. Neurosci.* 27, 2704–2717. doi: 10.1523/JNEUROSCI.2991-06.2007

Berninger, B., Costa, M. R., Koch, U., Schroeder, T., Sutor, B., Grothe, B., et al. (2007). Functional properties of neurons derived from *in vitro* reprogrammed postnatal astroglia. *J. Neurosci.* 27, 8654–8664. doi: 10.1523/JNEUROSCI.1615-07.2007

Bolteus, A. J., and Bordey, A. (2004). GABA release and uptake regulate neuronal precursor migration in the postnatal subventricular zone. *J. Neurosci.* 24, 7623–7631. doi: 10.1523/JNEUROSCI.1999-04.2004

Bozoyan, L., Khlghatyan, J., and Saghatelyan, A. (2012). Astrocytes control the development of the migration-promoting vasculature scaffold in the postnatal brain via VEGF signaling. *J. Neurosci.* 32, 1687–1704. doi: 10.1523/JNEUROSCI.5531-11.2012

Breton-Provencher, V., Lemasson, M., Peralta, M. R. III., and Saghatelyan, A. (2009). Interneurons produced in adulthood are required for the normal functioning of the olfactory bulb network and for the execution of selected olfactory behaviors. *J. Neurosci.* 29, 15245–15257. doi: 10.1523/JNEUROSCI.3606-09.2009

Brill, M. S., Ninkovic, J., Winpenny, E., Hodge, R. D., Ozen, I., Yang, R., et al. (2009). Adult generation of glutamatergic olfactory bulb interneurons. *Nat. Neurosci.* 12, 1524–1533. doi: 10.1038/nn.2416

Chazal, G., Durbec, P., Jankovski, A., Rougon, G., and Cremer, H. (2000). Consequences of neural cell adhesion molecule deficiency on cell migration in the rostral migratory stream of the mouse. *J. Neurosci.* 20, 1446–1457.

Codega, P., Silva-Vargas, V., Paul, A., Maldonado-Soto, A. R., DeLeo, A. M., Pastrana, E., et al. (2014). Prospective identification and purification of quiescent adult neural stem cells from their *in vivo* niche. *Neuron* 82, 545–559. doi: 10.1016/j.neuron.2014.02.039

Colak, D., Mori, T., Brill, M. S., Pfeifer, A., Falk, S., Deng, C., et al. (2008). Adult neurogenesis requires smad4-mediated bone morphogenic protein signaling in stem cells. *J. Neurosci.* 28, 434–446. doi: 10.1523/JNEUROSCI.4374-07.2008

Correale, J., and Farez, M. F. (2015). The role of astrocytes in multiple sclerosis progression. *Front. Neurol.* 6:180. doi: 10.3389/fneur.2015.00180

Davis, R. L. (2004). Olfactory learning. *Neuron* 44, 31–48. doi: 10.1016/j.neuron.2004.09.008

Delgado, R. N., and Lim, D. A. (2015). Embryonic Nkx2.1-expressing neural precursor cells contribute to the regional heterogeneity of adult V-SVZ neural stem cells. *Dev. Biol.* 407, 265–274. doi: 10.1016/j.ydbio.2015.09.008

De Marchis, S., Bovetti, S., Carletti, B., Hsieh, Y.-C., Garzotto, D., Peretto, P., et al. (2007). Generation of distinct types of periglomerular olfactory bulb interneurons during development and in adult mice: implication for intrinsic properties of the subventricular zone progenitor population. *J. Neurosci.* 27, 657–664. doi: 10.1523/JNEUROSCI.2870-06.2007

Doengi, M., Hirnet, D., Coulon, P., Pape, H.-C., Deitmer, J. W., and Lohr, C. (2009). GABA uptake-dependent Ca2+ signaling in developing olfactory bulb astrocytes. *Proc. Natl. Acad. Sci. U.S.A.* 106, 17570–17575. doi: 10.1073/pnas.0809513106

Doetsch, F., Caillé, I., Lim, D. A., García-Verdugo, J. M., and Alvarez-Buylla, A. (1999). Subventricular zone astrocytes are neural stem cells in the adult mammalian brain. *Cell* 97, 703–716. doi: 10.1016/S0092-8674(00)80783-7

Doetsch, F., Petreanu, L., Caille, I., Garcia-Verdugo, J.-M., and Alvarez-Buylla, A. (2002). EGF converts transit-amplifying neurogenic precursors in the adult brain into multipotent stem cells. *Neuron* 36, 1021–1034. doi: 10.1016/S0896-6273(02)01133-9

Ferrón, S. R., Charalambous, M., Radford, E., McEwen, K., Wildner, H., Hind, E., et al. (2011). Postnatal loss of Dlk1 imprinting in stem cells and niche astrocytes regulates neurogenesis. *Nature* 475, 381–385. doi: 10.1038/nature10229

Fuentealba, L. C., Rompani, S. B., Parraguez, J. I., Obernier, K., Romero, R., Cepko, C. L., et al. (2015). Embryonic origin of postnatal neural stem cells. *Cell* 161, 1644–1655. doi: 10.1016/j.cell.2015.05.041

Fukunaga, I., Herb, J. T., Kollo, M., Boyden, E. S., and Schaefer, A. T. (2014). Independent control of gamma and theta activity by distinct interneuron networks in the olfactory bulb. *Nat. Neurosci.* 17, 1208–1216. doi: 10.1038/nn.3760

García-Marqués, J., De Carlos, J. A., Greer, C. A., and López-Mascaraque, L. (2010). Different astroglia permissivity controls the migration of olfactory bulb interneuron precursors. *Glia* 58, 218–230. doi: 10.1002/glia.20918

Gascón, S., Murenu, E., Masserdotti, G., Ortega, F., Russo, G. L., Petrik, D., et al. (2016). Identification and successful negotiation of a metabolic checkpoint in direct neuronal reprogramming. *Cell Stem Cell* 18, 1–14. doi: 10.1016/j.stem.2015.12.003

Giachino, C., Basak, O., Lugert, S., Knuckles, P., Obernier, K., Fiorelli, R., et al. (2014). Molecular diversity subdivides the adult forebrain neural stem cell population. *Stem Cells* 32, 70–84. doi: 10.1002/stem.1520

Givogri, M. I., de Planell, M., Galbiati, F., Superchi, D., Gritti, A., Vescovi, A., et al. (2006). Notch signaling in astrocytes and neuroblasts of the adult subventricular zone in health and after cortical injury. *Dev. Neurosci.* 28, 81–91. doi: 10.1159/000090755

Gritti, A., Bonfanti, L., Doetsch, F., Caille, I., Alvarez-Buylla, A., Lim, D. A., et al. (2002). Multipotent neural stem cells reside into the rostral extension and olfactory bulb of adult rodents. *J. Neurosci.* 22, 437–445.

Hack, M. A., Saghatelyan, A., de Chevigny, A., Pfeifer, A., Ashery-Padan, R., Lledo, P.-M., et al. (2005). Neuronal fate determinants of adult olfactory bulb neurogenesis. *Nat. Neurosci.* 8, 865–872. doi: 10.1038/nn1479

Heinrich, C., Blum, R., Gascón, S., Masserdotti, G., Tripathi, P., Sánchez, R., et al. (2010). Directing astroglia from the cerebral cortex into subtype specific functional neurons. *PLoS Biol.* 8:e1000373. doi: 10.1371/journal.pbio.1000373

Hirota, Y., Sawada, M., Huang, S.-H., Ogino, T., Ohata, S., Kubo, A., et al. (2015). Roles of wnt signaling in the neurogenic niche of the adult mouse ventricular-subventricular zone. *Neurochem. Res.* 41, 222–230. doi: 10.1007/s11064-015-1766-z

Ihrie, R. A., Shah, J. K., Harwell, C. C., Levine, J. H., Guinto, C. D., Lezameta, M., et al. (2011). Persistent sonic hedgehog signaling in adult brain determines neural stem cell positional identity. *Neuron* 71, 250–262. doi: 10.1016/j.neuron.2011.05.018

Imayoshi, I., Sakamoto, M., Ohtsuka, T., Takao, K., Miyakawa, T., Yamaguchi, M., et al. (2008). Roles of continuous neurogenesis in the structural and functional integrity of the adult forebrain. *Nat. Neurosci.* 11, 1153–1161. doi: 10.1038/nn.2185

Jackson, E. L., and Alvarez-Buylla, A. (2008). Characterization of adult neural stem cells and their relation to brain tumors. *Cells Tissues Organs* 188, 212–224. doi: 10.1159/000114541

Jiao, J., and Chen, D. F. (2008). Induction of neurogenesis in nonconventional neurogenic regions of the adult central nervous system by niche astrocyte-produced signals. *Stem Cells* 26, 1221–1230. doi: 10.1634/stemcells.2007-0513

Kaneko, N., Marín, O., Koike, M., Hirota, Y., Uchiyama, Y., Wu, J. Y., et al. (2010). New neurons clear the path of astrocytic processes for their rapid migration in the adult brain. *Neuron* 67, 213–223. doi: 10.1016/j.neuron.2010.06.018

Khodosevich, K., Lazarini, F., von Engelhardt, J., Kaneko, H., Lledo, P.-M., and Monyer, H. (2013). Connective tissue growth factor regulates interneuron survival and information processing in the olfactory bulb. *Neuron* 79, 1136–1151. doi: 10.1016/j.neuron.2013.07.011

Lacar, B., Young, S. Z., Platel, J.-C., and Bordey, A. (2011). Gap junction-mediated calcium waves define communication networks among murine postnatal neural progenitor cells. *Eur. J. Neurosci.* 34, 1895–1905. doi: 10.1111/j.1460-9568.2011.07901.x

Larriva-Sahd, J. (2014). Structural variation and interactions among astrocytes of the rostral migratory stream and olfactory bulb: II. Golgi and electron microscopic study of the adult rat. *Neurosci. Res.* 89, 10–30. doi: 10.1016/j.neures.2014.08.011

Lim, D. A., and Alvarez-Buylla, A. (1999). Interaction between astrocytes and adult subventricular zone precursors stimulates neurogenesis. *Proc. Natl. Acad. Sci. U.S.A.* 96, 7526–7531. doi: 10.1073/pnas.96.13.7526

Lim, D. A., Tramontin, A. D., Trevejo, J. M., Herrera, D. G., García-Verdugo, J. M., and Alvarez-Buylla, A. (2000). Noggin antagonizes BMP signaling to create a niche for adult neurogenesis. *Neuron* 28, 713–726. doi: 10.1016/S0896-6273(00)00148-3

Llorens-Bobadilla, E., Zhao, S., Baser, A., Saiz-Castro, G., Zwadlo, K., and Martin-Villalba, A. (2015). Single-cell transcriptomics reveals a population of dormant neural stem cells that become activated upon brain injury. *Cell Stem Cell* 17, 329–340. doi: 10.1016/j.stem.2015.07.002

Lois, C., and Alvarez-Buylla, A. (1994). Long-distance neuronal migration in the adult mammalian brain. *Science* 264, 1145–1148. doi: 10.1126/science.8178174

Luskin, M. B. (1993). Restricted proliferation and migration of postnatally generated neurons derived from the forebrain subventricular zone. *Neuron* 11, 173–189. doi: 10.1016/0896-6273(93)90281-U

Mason, H. A., Ito, S., and Corfas, G. (2001). Extracellular signals that regulate the tangential migration of olfactory bulb neuronal precursors: inducers, inhibitors, and repellents. *J. Neurosci.* 21, 7654–7663.

Merkle, F. T., Fuentealba, L. C., Sanders, T. A., Magno, L., Kessaris, N., and Alvarez-Buylla, A. (2014). Adult neural stem cells in distinct microdomains generate previously unknown interneuron types. *Nat. Neurosci.* 17, 207–214. doi: 10.1038/nn.3610

Merkle, F. T., Mirzadeh, Z., and Alvarez-Buylla, A. (2007). Mosaic organization of neural stem cells in the adult brain. *Science* 317, 381–384. doi: 10.1126/science.1144914

Mirzadeh, Z., Merkle, F. T., Soriano-Navarro, M., García-Verdugo, J. M., and Alvarez-Buylla, A. (2008). Neural stem cells confer unique pinwheel architecture to the ventricular surface in neurogenic regions of the adult brain. *Cell Stem Cell* 3, 265–278. doi: 10.1016/j.stem.2008.07.004

Moreno-Estellés, M., Gonzalez-Gómez, P., Hortigüela, R., Díaz-Moreno, M., San Emeterio, J., Carvalho A. L., et al. (2012). Symmetric expansion of neural stem cells from the adult olfactory bulb is driven by astrocytes via WNT7A. *Stem Cells* 30, 2796–2809. doi: 10.1002/stem.1243

Ortega, F., Gascón, S., Masserdotti, G., Deshpande, A., Simon, C., Fischer, J., et al. (2013). Oligodendrogliogenic and neurogenic adult subependymal zone neural stem cells constitute distinct lineages and exhibit differential responsiveness to Wnt signalling. *Nat. Cell Biol.* 15, 602–613. doi: 10.1038/ncb2736

Otsu, Y., Couchman, K., Lyons, D. G., Collot, M., Agarwal, A., Mallet, J.-M., et al. (2015). Calcium dynamics in astrocyte processes during neurovascular coupling. *Nat. Neurosci.* 18, 210–218. doi: 10.1038/nn.3906

Panzanelli, P., Bardy, C., Nissant, A., Pallotto, M., Sassoè-Pognetto, M., Lledo, P.-M., et al. (2009). Early synapse formation in developing interneurons of the adult olfactory bulb. *J. Neurosci.* 29, 15039–15052. doi: 10.1523/JNEUROSCI.3034-09.2009

Pastrana, E., Cheng, L.-C., and Doetsch, F. (2009). Simultaneous prospective purification of adult subventricular zone neural stem cells and their progeny. *Proc. Natl. Acad. Sci. U.S.A.* 106, 6387–6392. doi: 10.1073/pnas.0810407106

Pencea, V., and Luskin, M. B. (2003). Prenatal development of the rodent rostral migratory stream. *J. Comp. Neurol.* 463, 402–418. doi: 10.1002/cne.10746

Peretto, P., Dati, C., De Marchis, S., Kim, H. H., Ukhanova, M., Fasolo, A., et al. (2004). Expression of the secreted factors noggin and bone morphogenetic proteins in the subependymal layer and olfactory bulb of the adult mouse brain. *Neuroscience* 128, 685–696. doi: 10.1016/j.neuroscience.2004.06.053

Peretto, P., Giachino, C., Aimar, P., Fasolo, A., and Bonfanti, L. (2005). Chain formation and glial tube assembly in the shift from neonatal to adult subventricular zone of the rodent forebrain. *J. Comp. Neurol.* 487, 407–427. doi: 10.1002/cne.20576

Piet, R., Vargová, L., Syková, E., Poulain, D. A., and Oliet, S. H. R. (2004). Physiological contribution of the astrocytic environment of neurons to intersynaptic crosstalk. *Proc. Natl. Acad. Sci. U.S.A.* 101, 2151–2155. doi: 10.1073/pnas.0308408100

Platel, J.-C., Dave, K. A., Gordon, V., Lacar, B., Rubio, M. E., and Bordey, A. (2010). NMDA receptors activated by subventricular zone astrocytic glutamate are critical for neuroblast survival prior to entering a synaptic network. *Neuron* 65, 859–872. doi: 10.1016/j.neuron.2010.03.009

Pressler, R. T., and Strowbridge, B. W. (2006). Blanes cells mediate persistent feedforward inhibition onto granule cells in the olfactory bulb. *Neuron* 49, 889–904. doi: 10.1016/j.neuron.2006.02.019

Rouach, N., Koulakoff, A., Abudara, V., Willecke, K., and Giaume, C. (2008). Astroglial metabolic networks sustain hippocampal synaptic transmission. *Science* 322, 1551–1555. doi: 10.1126/science.1164022

Shepherd, G. M., Chen, W. R., and Greer, C. A. (2004). "Olfactory bulb," in *The Synaptic Organization of the Brain*, ed G. M. Shepherd (New York, NY: Oxford University Press), 165–216.

Shin, J., Berg, D. A., Zhu, Y., Shin, J. Y., Song, J., Bonaguidi, M. A., et al. (2015). Single-cell RNA-seq with waterfall reveals molecular cascades underlying adult neurogenesis. *Cell Stem Cell* 17, 360–372. doi: 10.1016/j.stem.2015.07.013

Sirko, S., Behrendt, G., Johansson, P. A., Tripathi, P., Costa, M. R., Bek, S., et al. (2013). Reactive glia in the injured brain acquire stem cell properties in response to sonic hedgehog. *Cell Stem Cell* 12, 426–439. doi: 10.1016/j.stem.2013.01.019

Snapyan, M., Lemasson, M., Brill, M. S., Blais, M., Massouh, M., Ninkovic, J., et al. (2009). Vasculature guides migrating neuronal precursors in the adult mammalian forebrain via brain-derived neurotrophic factor signaling. *J. Neurosci.* 29, 4172–4188. doi: 10.1523/JNEUROSCI.4956-08.2009

Song, H., Stevens, C. F., and Gage, F. H. (2002). Astroglia induce neurogenesis from adult neural stem cells. *Nature* 417, 39–44. doi: 10.1038/417039a

Sultan, S., Li, L., Moss, J., Petrelli, F., Cassé, F., Gebara, E., et al. (2015). Synaptic integration of adult-born hippocampal neurons is locally controlled by astrocytes. *Neuron* 88, 957–972. doi: 10.1016/j.neuron.2015.10.037

Sultan, S., Rey, N., Sacquet, J., Mandairon, N., and Didier, A. (2011). Newborn neurons in the olfactory bulb selected for long-term survival through olfactory learning are prematurely suppressed when the olfactory memory is erased. *J. Neurosci.* 31, 14893–14898. doi: 10.1523/JNEUROSCI.3677-11.2011

Takano, T., Tian, G.-F., Peng, W., Lou, N., Libionka, W., Han, X., et al. (2006). Astrocyte-mediated control of cerebral blood flow. *Nat. Neurosci.* 9, 260–267. doi: 10.1038/nn1623

Tong, C. K., Fuentealba, L. C., Shah, J. K., Lindquist, R. A., Ihrie, R. A., Guinto, C. D., et al. (2015). A dorsal SHH-dependent domain in the V-SVZ produces large numbers of oligodendroglial lineage cells in the postnatal brain. *Stem Cell Rep.* 5, 461–470. doi: 10.1016/j.stemcr.2015.08.013

Urban, N. N. (2002). Lateral inhibition in the olfactory bulb and in olfaction. *Physiol. Behav.* 77, 607–612. doi: 10.1016/S0031-9384(02)00895-8

Verkhratsky, A., and Nedergaard, M. (2014). Astroglial cradle in the life of the synapse. *Philos. Trans. R. Soc. B Biol. Sci.* 369, 1654. doi: 10.1098/rstb.2013.0595

Waclaw, R. R., Allen, Z. J. II, Bell, S. M., Erdélyi, F., Szabó, G., Potter, S. S., et al. (2006). The zinc finger transcription factor sp8 regulates the generation and diversity of olfactory bulb interneurons. *Neuron* 49, 503–516. doi: 10.1016/j.neuron.2006.01.018

Whitman, M. C., Fan, W., Rela, L., Rodriguez-Gil, D. J., and Greer, C. A. (2009). Blood vessels form a migratory scaffold in the rostral migratory stream. *J. Comp. Neurol.* 516, 94–104. doi: 10.1002/cne.22093

Whitman, M. C., and Greer, C. A. (2007). Synaptic integration of adult-generated olfactory bulb granule cells: basal axodendritic centrifugal input precedes apical dendrodendritic local circuits. *J. Neurosci.* 27, 9951–9961. doi: 10.1523/JNEUROSCI.1633-07.2007

Young, K. M., Fogarty, M., Kessaris, N., and Richardson, W. D. (2007). Subventricular zone stem cells are heterogeneous with respect to their embryonic origins and neurogenic fates in the adult olfactory bulb. *J. Neurosci.* 27, 8286–8296. doi: 10.1523/JNEUROSCI.0476-07.2007

10

Molecular Mechanisms Regulating the Dendritic Development of Newborn Olfactory Bulb Interneurons in a Sensory Experience-Dependent Manner

*Sei-ichi Yoshihara, Hiroo Takahashi and Akio Tsuboi **

Laboratory for the Molecular Biology of Neural Systems, Advanced Medical Research Center, Nara Medical University, Kashihara, Japan

Inhibitory interneurons in the olfactory bulb are generated continuously throughout life in the subventricular zone and differentiate into periglomerular and granule cells. Neural circuits that undergo reorganization by newborn olfactory bulb interneurons are necessary for odor detection, odor discrimination, olfactory memory, and innate olfactory responses. Although sensory experience has been shown to regulate development in a variety of species and in various structures, including the retina, cortex, and hippocampus, little is known about how sensory experience regulates the dendritic development of newborn olfactory bulb interneurons. Recent studies revealed that the 5T4 oncofetal trophoblast glycoprotein and the neuronal Per/Arnt/Sim domain protein 4 (Npas4) transcription factor regulate dendritic branching and dendritic spine formation, respectively, in olfactory bulb interneurons. Here, we summarize the molecular mechanisms that underlie the sensory input-dependent development of newborn interneurons and the formation of functional neural circuitry in the olfactory bulb.

Keywords: adult neurogenesis, olfactory bulb interneuron, neural activity-dependent, dendritogenesis, spinogenesis, 5T4, Npas4

Edited by:
Laura López-Mascaraque, Instituto Cajal (CSIC), Spain

Reviewed by:
Harold Cremer, Centre National de La Recherche Scientifique, France
Krishna Vadodaria, Salk Institute for Biological Science, USA

****Correspondence:***
Akio Tsuboi
atsuboi@naramed-u.ac.jp

INTRODUCTION

Sensory experience is recognized as a critical factor in the development and plastic modification of neural circuits in vertebrates (Katz and Shatz, 1996; Sanes and Lichtman, 2001; Nithianantharajah and Hannan, 2006; Lepousez et al., 2013). As well as newborn hippocampal neurons (Vadodaria and Jessberger, 2013), newborn olfactory bulb (OB) interneurons are a good model for studying the postnatal modification of neural circuits by sensory inputs from the external world. Specific odorants activate olfactory sensory neurons that express the corresponding odorant receptors (Mori and Sakano, 2011; Takeuchi and Sakano, 2014). The olfactory sensory neurons project their axons to specific glomeruli in the OB and can subsequently activate a specific neural circuit locally, facilitating the dendritic development of OB interneurons via interactions with excitatory projection neurons, such as mitral and tufted cells (**Figure 1A**; Mori and Sakano, 2011; Lepousez et al., 2013; Figueres-Oñate et al., 2014; Imai, 2014). Precursors for OB interneurons are generated throughout life in the subventricular zone of the lateral ventricle, migrate along the rostral migratory stream (RMS) and differentiate into γ-aminobutyric acid (GABA)-releasing inhibitory interneurons, such as periglomerular cells (PGCs) and granule cells (GCs; **Figure 1A**; Chazal et al., 2000; Alvarez-Buylla et al., 2008; Lledo et al., 2008; Whitman and Greer, 2009; Adam and Mizrahi, 2010; Kaneko et al., 2010; Sakamoto et al., 2011; Sequerra, 2014). Neural circuits that undergo reorganization by newborn OB interneurons are assumed to be essential for odor detection, odor discrimination, olfactory memory, and innate olfactory responses (Alonso et al., 2012; Sakamoto et al., 2014; Gschwend et al., 2015). It is well known that odor-evoked neural activity affects the survival and integration of newborn OB interneurons (Petreanu and Alvarez-Buylla, 2002; Rochefort et al., 2002; Yamaguchi and Mori, 2005; Bastien-Dionne et al., 2010; Lin et al., 2010; Sawada et al., 2011). In addition, elimination of GCs via cell death is promoted by top-down inputs from the olfactory cortex to the OB during the postprandial period (Yokoyama et al., 2011; Komano-Inoue et al., 2014). Moreover, odor deprivation and odor-enriched environments suppress and facilitate, respectively, dendritogenesis and spinogenesis in newborn OB interneurons (Saghatelyan et al., 2005; Kelsch et al., 2009; Livneh et al., 2009; Breton-Provencher et al., 2014; Lepousez et al., 2014). However, molecular mechanisms regulating the sensory experience-dependent dendritogenesis and spinogenesis in OB newborn interneurons remain unknown. Recent studies revealed that the 5T4 oncofetal trophoblast glycoprotein regulates the dendritic arborization of OB GCs in a sensory input-dependent manner (Yoshihara et al., 2012), whereas the neuronal Per/Arnt/Sim domain protein 4 (Npas4) transcription factor controls the sensory input-dependent dendritic spine formation of OB GCs (Yoshihara et al., 2014).

DEVELOPMENT OF NEWBORN OB INTERNEURONS IS REGULATED BY ODOR-INDUCED NEURAL ACTIVITY

Neurogenesis arises continuously throughout life in two areas of the mouse brain, such as the subgranular zone of the dentate gyrus (Vadodaria and Gage, 2014) and the subventricular zone of the lateral ventricle (Tong and Alvarez-Buylla, 2014). In the latter, interneuronal neuroblasts migrate along the RMS to the OB (**Figure 1A**). After neuroblasts arrive at the OB, dendritogenesis and spinogenesis occur in those cells, which then differentiate into mature GABAergic inhibitory interneurons (GCs and PGCs) and incorporate into pre-existing neural circuits in the OB (Alvarez-Buylla et al., 2008; Lledo et al., 2008; Whitman and Greer, 2009; Adam and Mizrahi, 2010; Kaneko et al., 2010; Sakamoto et al., 2011; Sequerra, 2014). Previous studies showed that odor-evoked neural activity is required for the development of newborn OB interneurons at the following four steps.

(1) Proliferation of neural stem cells and migration of neuroblasts. An odor-enriched environment enhances proliferation of neural stem cells in both the RMS and subventricular zone, although chemical lesion of olfactory sensory neurons increases cell proliferation in the RMS alone (Alonso et al., 2008). When neuroblasts arrive at the OB, the direction of migration changes from rostral to radial (Hack et al., 2002; Saghatelyan et al., 2004; Belvindrah et al., 2011; Saha et al., 2012). Radial migration of neuroblasts in the OB is controlled by the secreted glycoprotein reelin (Hack et al., 2002) and the extracellular matrix glycoprotein tenascin-R (Saghatelyan et al., 2004; David et al., 2013). Because tenascin-R is produced by

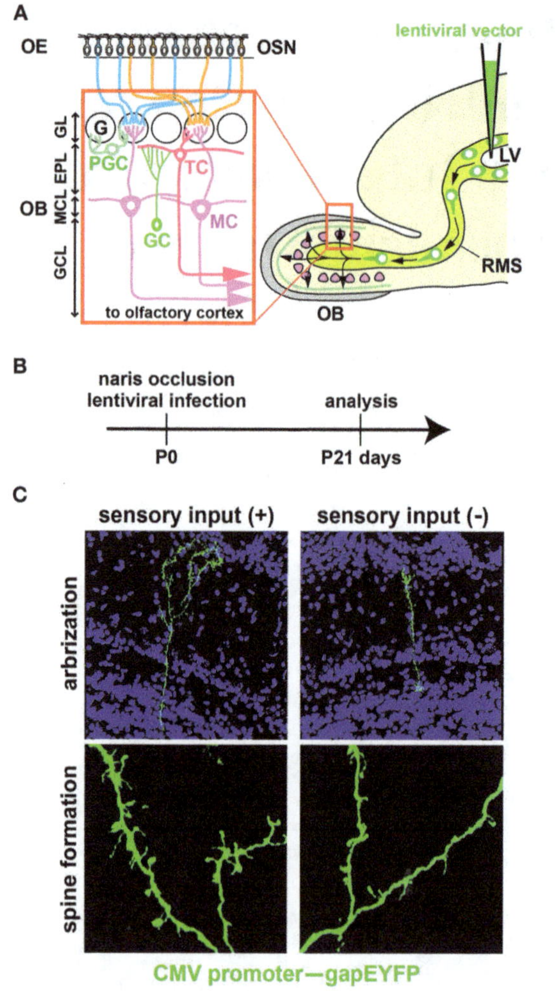

FIGURE 1 | Development of newborn OB interneurons is regulated by odor-evoked neural activity. (A) Schematic representation of the olfactory bulb neural circuitry. Olfactory bulb (OB) interneurons are generated throughout life in the subventricular zone of the lateral ventricle (LV), migrate along the rostral migratory stream (RMS), and differentiate into γ-aminobutyric acid (GABA)-releasing inhibitory interneurons such as granule cells (GCs) and periglomerular cells (PGCs) in the OB. GCs and PGCs modulate the neural activity of excitatory projection neurons, including mitral and tufted cells (MC and TC) through dendrodendritic synapses between inhibitory and excitatory neurons. EPL, external plexiform layer; G, glomerulus; GCL, granule cell layer; GL, glomerular layer; MCL, mitral cell layer; OE, olfactory epithelium; OSN, olfactory sensory neuron. **(B)** A lentiviral vector (*CMV* promoter–*gapEYFP* gene) was injected into the lateral ventricle (LV) of wild-type mice at postnatal day 0 (P0). After 3 weeks (P21), YFP^{+} interneurons can be visualized in the olfactory bulb (OB). The activity-dependent development of newborn interneurons was analyzed by injecting a lentivirus into the LV of unilaterally naris-occluded mice. **(C)** Newborn granule cells (GCs) were analyzed in the open and closed sides of the OB from P21 naris-occluded mice. GC dendrites are less branched and have lower spine density in the closed than in the open side of the OB (modified from Yoshihara et al., 2012, 2014).

pre-existing GCs and expressed in a sensory input-dependent manner, its lack decreases the radial migration of neuroblasts as well as spine development of newborn GCs (Saghatelyan et al., 2004; David et al., 2013).

(2) Differentiation, survival, and death of newborn interneurons. When immature interneurons reach a given layer in the OB, they differentiate into mature PGCs and GCs. The production levels of the GABA synthetic enzyme (glutamic acid decarboxylase 67: GAD67) and GABA in OB interneurons are regulated in an activity-dependent manner (Parrish-Aungst et al., 2011; Lau and Murthy, 2012). A PGC subtype expresses *tyrosine hydroxylase* (*TH*) gene, encoding a rate-limiting enzyme for dopamine synthesis, in an odor input-dependent manner (Bastien-Dionne et al., 2010; Bovetti et al., 2013; Lazarini et al., 2014). The *TH* expression in PGCs is controlled by transcription factors such as Er81 (Cave et al., 2010) and COUP-TFI (Bovetti et al., 2013; Zhou et al., 2015) in an activity-dependent manner, whereas the transcription factor Pax6 is upregulated in TH-positive PGCs in odor-deprived mice (Bastien-Dionne et al., 2010). In unilaterally naris-occluded mice, the apoptotic rate of newborn GCs is increased on the closed side of the OB (Rochefort et al., 2002; Yamaguchi and Mori, 2005; Bastien-Dionne et al., 2010; Lin et al., 2010; Sawada et al., 2011), whereas their survival rate is increased in odor-enriched environments (Rochefort et al., 2002; Rochefort and Lledo, 2005). The survival and death of newborn PGCs are also regulated by sensory inputs. For example, newborn PGC death is induced by the connective tissue growth factor (CTGF) secreted from external tufted cells in the OB (Khodosevich et al., 2013). In odor-stimulated glomeruli, external tufted cells secrete more CTGF protein, enhancing death of newborn PGCs through transforming growth factor-β (TGF-β) receptor signaling downstream of CTGF (Khodosevich et al., 2013). In addition, olfactory deprivation negatively affects the survival of newborn calretinin-positive PGCs (Kato et al., 2012), whereas odor enrichment increases the cell number of TH-positive PGCs (Bonzano et al., 2014).

(3) Dendritic morphogenesis of newborn interneurons. In odor deprivation, the length and branching number of GC dendrites are decreased; by contrast, they are increased in an odor-enriched environment (**Figures 1B,C**; Saghatelyan et al., 2005; Yoshihara et al., 2012). $GABA_A$ receptor mutant mice exhibit impaired dendritic branching and spine formation in OB GCs, suggesting that GABAergic synaptic transmission is important for proper dendritogenesis and spinogenesis (Pallotto et al., 2012). Furthermore, fragile X mental retardation protein (FMRP), which is an mRNA-binding protein essential for multiple aspects of neuronal mRNA metabolism, downregulates dendritic spine formation in OB GCs and is necessary for activity-dependent dendritic remodeling (Scotto-Lomassese et al., 2011).

(4) Dendritic spine formation of newborn interneurons. Through their dendritic spines, OB interneurons connect to projection neurons (mitral and tufted cells) to modulate activity (Lledo et al., 2008; Adam and Mizrahi, 2010; Imai, 2014). In odor-deprived mice, the dendritic spine formation of OB interneurons is suppressed in the distal dendritic domain and accelerated in the proximal dendritic domain; by contrast, dendritic spine formation is increased in the distal dendritic domain in odor-enriched environments (**Figure 1C**; Saghatelyan et al., 2005; Kelsch et al., 2009, 2012b; Livneh et al., 2009; Breton-Provencher et al., 2014; Lepousez et al., 2014). It is suggested that synapses of neonatal-born GCs retain a higher level of plasticity in response to changes in neural activity than those of adult-born GCs (Kelsch et al., 2012b). Odor input-dependent neural activity induces the formation and retraction of filopodia in the distal dendritic domain of GCs via NMDA receptor signaling (Kelsch et al., 2012a; Breton-Provencher et al., 2014). In OB GCs, odor-discrimination learning increases spine density in proximal dendritic domains, which receive top-down inputs from the olfactory cortex (Yokoyama et al., 2011; Komano-Inoue et al., 2014; Lepousez et al., 2014). Furthermore, corticotropin-releasing hormone (CRH) is produced in a subtype of OB interneurons at the external plexiform layer in an activity-dependent manner. When CRH is received by newly generated OB GCs, synaptogenesis in the GC dendrites is accelerated via CRH receptor signaling (Garcia et al., 2014).

5T4 GLYCOPROTEIN REGULATES DENDRITIC BRANCHING OF NEWBORN OB GRANULE CELLS IN A SENSORY INPUT-DEPENDENT MANNER

Although odor-evoked neural activity is required for proper dendritic development of OB interneurons, its regulatory mechanisms remain unexplained. DNA microarray and *in situ* hybridization screenings in the unilaterally naris-occluded OB identified the oncofetal trophoblast glycoprotein gene, *5T4*, which is expressed in a specific subtype of OB interneurons following sensory experience (Imamura et al., 2006; Yoshihara et al., 2012). 5T4 is a type I membrane protein with an extracellular domain containing seven leucine-rich repeats bordered by characteristic leucine-rich repeat N- and C-flanking regions and a cytoplasmic domain containing a PDZ interaction motif (King et al., 1999). The 5T4 protein was first identified while searching for molecules with invasive properties shared by placental trophoblasts and cancer cells (Hole and Stern, 1990). The *5T4* gene expression is upregulated in many different carcinomas, while showing only low levels in most normal tissues (Southall et al., 1990) except for high levels in the brain and ovary (King et al., 1999; Barrow et al., 2005).

In the OB, the *5T4* gene is expressed not only in a subtype of PGCs at the glomerular layer, but also in a subtype of GCs (5T4-positive GCs) at the mitral-cell and superficial-GC layers (Imamura et al., 2006; Yoshihara et al., 2012). In the odor-deprived OB, the number of 5T4-positive GCs is decreased in the mitral-cell, and superficial-GC layers, indicating that the expression of *5T4* in 5T4-positive GCs is dependent on sensory inputs (Imamura et al., 2006; Yoshihara et al., 2012). Overexpression of *5T4* in newborn GCs by injecting lentiviral vectors into the lateral ventricle gives rise to more branched dendrites than those observed in control GCs (Yoshihara et al., 2012). In addition, *5T4*-overexpressing GCs have more branched dendrites even under sensory deprivation, whereas both *5T4* knockdown and knockout (KO) significantly reduce the dendritic branching of GCs in the OB (Yoshihara et al., 2012). Thus, 5T4 protein appears to be necessary for dendritic branching in OB interneurons.

It was recently shown that 5T4 is both induced by and negatively regulates the Wnt canonical pathway, which then facilitates the response to the noncanonical pathway (**Figure 2**; Kagermeier-Schenk et al., 2011; Zhao et al., 2014). Thus, neural activity may induce the production of a canonical Wnt ligand to upregulate *5T4*, which subsequently blocks the canonical pathway and favors the noncanonical pathway in OB interneurons by inhibiting the internalization of a Wnt-coreceptor, low-density lipoprotein receptor-related protein 6 (LPR6) (Kagermeier-Schenk et al., 2011; Zhao et al., 2014). In fact, compared with the wild type, disruption of the *Wnt5a* gene, which encodes a noncanonical Wnt ligand expressed in a subtype of OB interneurons, gives rise to reduced dendritic extension in GCs (Pino et al., 2011). It is possible that Wnt5a production regulates the noncanonical planar cell polarity pathway, leading to facilitation of dendritic arborization (van Amerongen and Nusse, 2009; Hirota et al., 2012). Recently, *5T4* deletion and domain-swap experiments established that the 5T4 intracellular domain without a PDZ-binding motif is necessary and sufficient for the dendritic branching of OB GCs, but the 5T4 extracellular leucine-rich repeat domain is not necessary for dendritic branching (Yoshihara et al., 2012). However, the 5T4 extracellular domain is reportedly essential for inhibition of Wnt/β-catenin signaling (Kagermeier-Schenk et al., 2011; Zhao et al., 2014). Therefore, it is likely that 5T4 regulates dendritic branching in a Wnt signaling-independent manner. Because the 5T4 intracellular region may interact with cytoskeletal proteins to regulate the dendritic arborization of GCs, the identification of 5T4-associating proteins will enable us to understand the mechanisms regulating the dendritic development of OB interneurons in an activity-dependent manner.

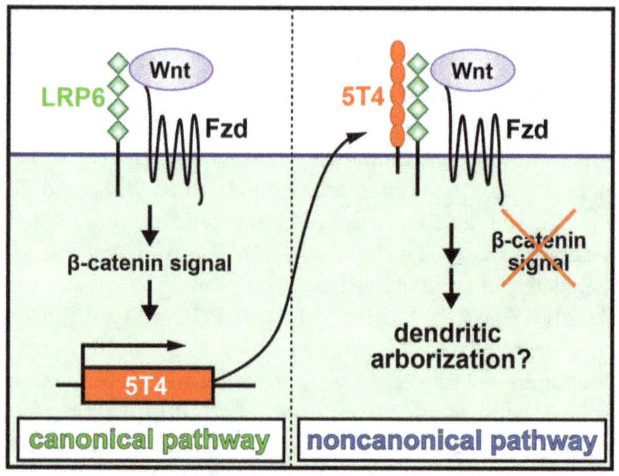

FIGURE 2 | Schematic diagram of dendritic development in newborn OB granule cells regulated by odor inputs. 5T4 leucine-rich repeat (LRR)-containing transmembrane protein is induced by and downregulates the Wnt canonical pathway. Neural activity may induce the production of a canonical Wnt ligand to upregulate *5T4*, which subsequently blocks the canonical pathway and favors the noncanonical pathway in OB interneurons by inhibiting the internalization of a Wnt-coreceptor, low-density lipoprotein receptor-related protein 6 (LPR6). This leads to facilitation of dendritic arborization in OB GCs (modified from Kagermeier-Schenk et al., 2011; Yoshihara et al., 2012).

NPAS4 TRANSCRIPTION FACTOR REGULATES DENDRITIC SPINE FORMATION OF NEWBORN OB GRANULE CELLS IN A SENSORY INPUT-DEPENDENT MANNER

Although odor-induced neural activity is required for spine formation in OB interneurons, its regulatory mechanism remains unresolved. DNA microarray and *in situ* hybridization screenings identified a transcription factor gene, *Npas4*, which is expressed in a subtype of OB GCs following sensory experience (Bepari et al., 2012; Yoshihara et al., 2014). *Npas4* is an immediate early gene induced by neural activity via a calcium-dependent signaling pathway (Lin et al., 2008; Pruunsild et al., 2011; Ramamoorthi et al., 2011; Bloodgood et al., 2013). In addition, Npas4 promotes the formation of inhibitory synapses in the developing visual system (Lin et al., 2008; Bloodgood et al., 2013) and adjusts the homeostatic inhibitory/excitatory balance in excitatory neurons to induce visual cortical plasticity (Maya-Vetencourt et al., 2012). Moreover, the Npas4 protein interacts with several promoters regulated by neural activity and mediates *brain-derived neurotrophic factor* (*BDNF*) gene expression in cortical pyramidal and hippocampal CA3 neurons (Lin et al., 2008; Pruunsild et al., 2011; Ramamoorthi et al., 2011; Bloodgood et al., 2013).

Overexpression of *Npas4* in newborn OB GCs by injecting lentiviruses into the lateral ventricle gives rise to an increase in spine density even under sensory deprivation conditions (Yoshihara et al., 2014). Furthermore, *Npas4* overexpression increases the number of puncta stained by either the postsynaptic marker gephyrin or pre-synaptic marker synaptoporin at the distal region of GC dendrites. By contrast, both *Npas4* knockdown and KO cause a significant reduction in the spine density of GC dendrites (Yoshihara et al., 2014). Thus, Npas4 is necessary and sufficient for increasing sensory input-dependent synaptogenesis in OB GCs. Interestingly, Npas4 is also required for activity-dependent spine development of adult-born GCs in the hippocampal dentate gyrus (Sim et al., 2013).

The mechanism for the Npas4 regulation of synaptogenesis in OB interneurons was explored using chromatin immunoprecipitation sequencing (ChIP-Seq) to search for Npas4 target genes in homogenized OB tissues with an Npas4 antibody associating with the promoter regions that bind Npas4. A novel target of Npas4, the oncogenic E3 ubiquitin ligase gene, *murine double minute 2* (*Mdm2*), is expressed at low levels in the wild-type OB but at higher levels in the *Npas4* KO OB (Yoshihara et al., 2014). Lateral ventricle injections of lentiviruses to either overexpress or knockdown *Mdm2* showed reduction and enhancement, respectively, in the spine density of GC dendrites compared with those in controls (Yoshihara et al., 2014), demonstrating that *Mdm2* is a *bona fide* target gene of Npas4 and that *Mdm2* expression is suppressed by Npas4 (**Figure 3**).

Mdm2 is localized at synapses, ubiquitinates and degrades postsynaptic density protein-95 (PSD-95) in rat hippocampal neurons (Colledge et al., 2003). However, according to the data of western blot analysis, the amount of PSD-95 protein is similar in wild-type and *Npas4* KO OBs (Yoshihara et al., 2014). Thus, to reveal the mechanism by which Mdm2 regulates synaptogenesis in OB interneurons, Mdm2 target proteins that are produced differentially between wild-type and *Npas4* KO OBs were searched using isobaric tags for relative and absolute quantitation (iTRAQ) proteomics (Yoshihara et al., 2014). Proteomic and cell-line analyses revealed that Mdm2 ubiquitinates and leads to the degradation of a microtubule-associated protein, doublecortin (Dcx). Dcx is generally used as a marker for immature neurons in the adult neurogenic lineage (Brown et al., 2003; Saaltink et al., 2012). Dcx regulates the migration and dendritic development of migrating neurons in the OB core region, including the RMS and the deep GC layer (Ocbina et al., 2006; Belvindrah et al., 2011). Immunohistochemical analysis of OB sections with a Dcx antibody indicates that the intensity of immunofluorescent signals in GC dendrites at the external-plexiform and GC layers are two-fold lower in the *Npas4* KO OB than in the wild-type OB (Yoshihara et al., 2014). Furthermore, overexpression and knockdown of *Dcx* achieved by injecting lentiviruses into the lateral ventricle enhance and reduce, respectively, spine density in GC dendrites (Yoshihara et al., 2014). Thus, Dcx plays an important role in increasing the dendritic spine density of OB GCs: Npas4 protein inhibits *Mdm2* expression, which prevents ubiquitination and degradation of Dcx, thereby promoting dendritic spine development in OB GCs following sensory experience (**Figure 3**).

Interestingly, two Dcx homologs, Dcx-like kinases 1 and 2 (Dclk1/Dclk2), reportedly regulate dendritic spine formation in hippocampal neurons (Shin et al., 2013). It was also recently demonstrated that Dcx is necessary for synapse formation in proper neuromuscular junction in the mouse and human (Bourgeois et al., 2015). Dcx and Dclk1/Dclk2 bind to an actin-binding protein, spinophilin, which is known to regulate spine morphology (Tsukada et al., 2003). Dcx also induces the bundling and cross-linking of microtubules and F-actin (Tsukada et al., 2005). Thus, the microtubule-binding protein Dcx family may play a crucial role in dendritic spine development of OB GCs.

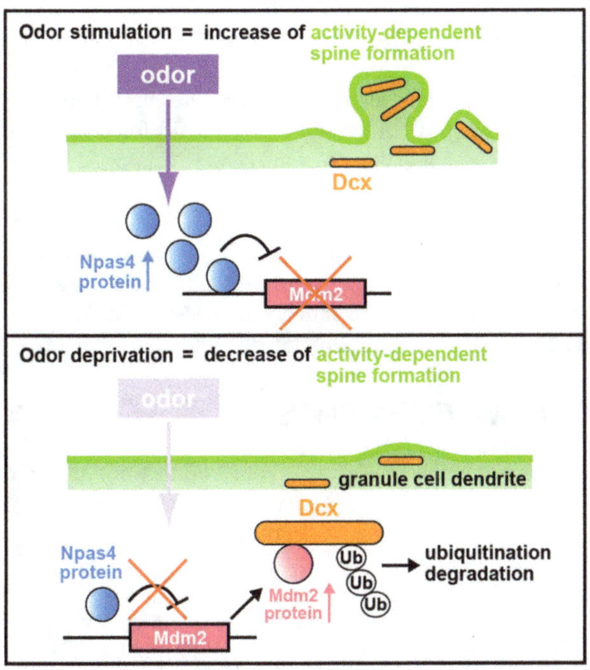

FIGURE 3 | Schematic diagram of dendritic spine formation in newborn OB granule cells regulated by odor inputs. In wild-type olfactory bulb (OB) granule cells (GCs), odor stimulation induces *Npas4* expression to suppress *Mdm2* expression. The suppression of *Mdm2* promotes the spine formation of GC dendrites mediated by doublecortin (Dcx). By contrast, odor deprivation decreases *Npas4* expression in OB GCs to upregulate the expression of *Mdm2*, leading to ubiquitination of Dcx. This results in degradation of Dcx and reduced dendritic spine density in OB GCs, as in the case of *Npas4*-knockout OB GCs (modified from Yoshihara et al., 2014).

PERSPECTIVES

In the cerebral cortex and hippocampus, neural activity regulates a program of gene transcription to affect synaptic development and plasticity (Ebert and Greenberg, 2013). Elevation of intracellular calcium levels induced by neural activity leads to activation of genes for multiple signaling molecules, including calmodulin kinase II (CaMK II), protein kinase A, cyclic AMP-responsive element-binding protein (CREB), and calcineurin (Ebert and Greenberg, 2013; Kawashima et al., 2014). CREB signaling is required for the survival, migration, and dendritic development of OB interneurons (Herold et al., 2011). Activation of the multiple signaling cascades facilitates the expression of neural activity-dependent genes, including the immediate early genes *c-fos*, *egr1*, and *Arc* (Ebert and Greenberg, 2013; Kawashima et al., 2014). A recent study found that neuronal activity induces DNA breaks in the promoters of immediate early genes and facilitates their expression (Madabhushi et al., 2015). Among the immediate early genes, c-fos and egr1 transcription factors activate genes for BDNF and Arc to regulate synaptic development (Ebert and Greenberg, 2013). In newborn OB interneurons, several immediate early genes (*c-fos*, *egr1*, and *Arc*) are expressed in a sensory input-dependent manner (Guthrie et al., 1993; Inaki et al., 2002; Busto et al., 2009; Bepari et al., 2012). Because the expression of the *5T4* gene is at a basal level in OB GCs after exiting the RMS, it is important to explore how the odor input-dependent expression is regulated by transcription factors, including those immediate early genes described above. It was recently reported that *BDNF* overexpression increases dendritic spine density of GCs (McDole et al., 2015). Therefore, future studies that identify the target genes of these immediate early genes, including *Npas4*, will allow us to understand the molecular mechanisms underlying activity-dependent development in newborn OB interneurons.

The functional significance of sensory input-dependent development in newborn OB interneurons has been explored. Olfactory experiences, such as odor-enrichment and odor-discrimination learning, regulate the maturation and survival of adult-born OB interneurons (Alonso et al., 2006; Livneh et al., 2009; Breton-Provencher et al., 2014; Lepousez et al., 2014). Newborn OB interneurons possess specific properties that are different from those of pre-existing interneurons, such as enhanced synaptic plasticity during a critical time window (Carleton et al., 2003; Panzanelli et al., 2009; Pallotto et al., 2012; Livneh et al., 2014), suggesting that these newborn interneurons uniquely contribute to odor processing. Consistent with this suggestion, odor detection and odor-discrimination learning are reportedly impaired in mice with diminished adult neurogenesis in the OB (Gheusi et al., 2000; Enwere et al., 2004; Breton-Provencher et al., 2009). However, the genetic ablation of adult-born interneurons causes deficits in innate olfactory responses, including predator avoidance and sexual behaviors (Sakamoto et al., 2011), but not in other normal olfactory abilities, such as odor detection and simple odor discrimination (Imayoshi et al., 2008; Sakamoto et al., 2011). This incongruence could be attributable to differences in the subtypes and numbers of OB interneurons that were manipulated in the individual studies. However, none of the methodologies used in these studies, including physically or genetically eliminating newborn cells, block the birth of adult-born OB interneurons in a spatially and temporally specific manner (Gheusi et al., 2000; Enwere et al., 2004; Imayoshi et al., 2008; Breton-Provencher et al., 2009; Sultan et al., 2010; Lazarini et al., 2014). A genetic activation study in which channelrhodopsin-2 was selectively expressed in newborn GCs showed that photostimulation of adult-born neurons (2 months old) facilitates difficult odor-discrimination learning and improves odor memory, whereas photostimulation of postnatal day 6-born neurons does not (Alonso et al., 2012; Gschwend et al., 2015). On the other hand, genetic inhibition of synaptic transmission in postnatal-born neurons impairs difficult odor-discrimination learning (Sakamoto et al., 2014). Because Dcx is produced in younger mature GCs, but is absent in older mature GCs (Brown et al., 2003), Npas4 may regulate dendritic spine formation in the younger but not the older mature GCs (Yoshihara et al., 2014). Interestingly, conditional KO of *Npas4* function in OB neurons impairs difficult odor-discrimination learning without affecting the ability to detect odors (Yoshihara et al., 2014), suggesting that spine development in newborn younger GCs is required in part for olfactory behaviors. By regulating the activity-dependent synaptic development of newborn OB GCs, Npas4 may play a role in shaping the functional neural circuitry involved in olfactory discrimination learning. Collectively, these studies provide important evidence that newborn OB interneurons, in which spine formation is regulated by Npas4 in a sensory experience-dependent manner, play a functional role in the OB circuitry and thus in its behavioral manifestation. Because GCs can be divided into several subtypes (Merkle et al., 2014), it is assumed that each GC subtype forms a distinct local circuit in the OB (Mori et al., 1983; Orona et al., 1983; Shepherd et al., 2004). Thus, future studies that individually manipulate the subtypes of OB interneurons in a spatially and temporally specific manner will help us to understand their functions in the OB circuitry.

AUTHOR CONTRIBUTIONS

SY, HT, and AT wrote the paper.

FUNDING

This work was supported by Grants-in-Aid for Scientific Research on (B) (AT), (C) (HT and SY), and Innovative Areas (Adaptive circuit shift) (AT) from the Ministry of Education, Culture, Sports, Science and Technology (MEXT), Japan. AT was supported by grants from the Smoking Research Foundation, Japanese Applied Enzymology Foundation, Senshin Medical Research Foundation, and Ono Medical Research Foundation, and a Nara Medical University Grant-in-Aid for Collaborative Research Projects in Japan. SY and HT were supported by grants from Takeda Science Foundation and Astellas Foundation for Research on Metabolic Disorders, Japan. SY was supported by a grant from Terumo Foundation for Life Sciences and Arts. HT was supported by grants from the Salt Science Research Foundation (no. 14C3), Mishima Kaiun Memorial Foundation, and Banyu Life Science International Foundation in Japan.

ACKNOWLEDGMENTS

We thank all members of the Tsuboi laboratory and the animal facility staff of Nara Medical University for their assistance.

REFERENCES

Adam, Y., and Mizrahi, A. (2010). Circuit formation and maintenance - perspectives from the mammalian olfactory bulb. *Curr. Opin. Neurobiol.* 20, 134–140. doi: 10.1016/j.conb.2009.11.001

Alonso, M., Lepousez, G., Wagner, S., Bardy, C., Gabellec, M. M., Torquet, N., et al. (2012). Activation of adult-born neurons facilitates learning and memory. *Nat. Neurosci.* 15, 897–904. doi: 10.1038/nn.3108

Alonso, M., Ortega-Pérez, I., Grubb, M. S., Bourgeois, J. P., Charneau, P., and Lledo, P. M. (2008). Turning astrocytes from the rostral migratory stream into neurons: a role for the olfactory sensory organ. *J. Neurosci.* 28, 11089–11102. doi: 10.1523/jneurosci.3713-08.2008

Alonso, M., Viollet, C., Gabellec, M. M., Meas-Yedid, V., Olivo-Marin, J. C., and Lledo, P. M. (2006). Olfactory discrimination learning increases the survival of adult-born neurons in the olfactory bulb. *J. Neurosci.* 26, 10508–10513. doi: 10.1523/JNEUROSCI.2633-06.2006

Alvarez-Buylla, A., Kohwi, M., Nguyen, T. M., and Merkle, F. T. (2008). The heterogeneity of adult neural stem cells and the emerging complexity of their niche. *Cold Spring Harb. Symp. Quant. Biol.* 73, 357–365. doi: 10.1101/sqb.2008.73.019

Barrow, K. M., Ward, C. M., Rutter, J., Ali, S., and Stern, P. L. (2005). Embryonic expression of murine 5T4 oncofoetal antigen is associated with morphogenetic events at implantation and in developing epithelia. *Dev. Dyn.* 233, 1535–1545. doi: 10.1002/dvdy.20482

Bastien-Dionne, P. O., David, L. S., Parent, A., and Saghatelyan, A. (2010). Role of sensory activity on chemospecific populations of interneurons in the adult olfactory bulb. *J. Comp. Neurol.* 518, 1847–1861. doi: 10.1002/cne.22307

Belvindrah, R., Nissant, A., and Lledo, P. M. (2011). Abnormal neuronal migration changes the fate of developing neurons in the postnatal olfactory bulb. *J. Neurosci.* 31, 7551–7562. doi: 10.1523/JNEUROSCI.6716-10.2011

Bepari, A. K., Watanabe, K., Yamaguchi, M., Tamamaki, N., and Takebayashi, H. (2012). Visualization of odor-induced neuronal activity by immediate early gene expression. *BMC Neurosci.* 13:140. doi: 10.1186/1471-2202-13-140

Bloodgood, B. L., Sharma, N., Browne, H. A., Trepman, A. Z., and Greenberg, M. E. (2013). The activity-dependent transcription factor NPAS4 regulates domain-specific inhibition. *Nature* 503, 121–125. doi: 10.1038/nature12743

Bonzano, S., Bovetti, S., Fasolo, A., Peretto, P., and De Marchis, S. (2014). Odour enrichment increases adult-born dopaminergic neurons in the mouse olfactory bulb. *Eur. J. Neurosci.* 40, 3450–3457. doi: 10.1111/ejn.12724

Bourgeois, F., Messéant, J., Kordeli, E., Petit, J. M., Delers, P., Bahi-Buisson, N., et al. (2015). A critical and previously unsuspected role for doublecortin at the neuromuscular junction in mouse and human. *Neuromuscul. Disord.* 25, 461–473. doi: 10.1016/j.nmd.2015.01.012

Bovetti, S., Bonzano, S., Garzotto, D., Giannelli, S. G., Iannielli, A., Armentano, M., et al. (2013). COUP-TFI controls activity-dependent tyrosine hydroxylase expression in adult dopaminergic olfactory bulb interneurons. *Development* 140, 4850–4859. doi: 10.1242/dev.089961

Breton-Provencher, V., Coté, D., and Saghatelyan, A. (2014). Activity of the principal cells of the olfactory bulb promotes a structural dynamic on the distal dendrites of immature adult-born granule cells via activation of NMDA receptors. *J. Neurosci.* 34, 1748–1759. doi: 10.1523/jneurosci.3013-13.2014

Breton-Provencher, V., Lemasson, M., Peralta, M. R. III., and Saghatelyan, A. (2009). Interneurons produced in adulthood are required for the normal functioning of the olfactory bulb network and for the execution of selected olfactory behaviors. *J. Neurosci.* 29, 15245–15257. doi: 10.1523/jneurosci.3606-09.2009

Brown, J. P., Couillard-Després, S., Cooper-Kuhn, C. M., Winkler, J., Aigner, L., and Kuhn, H. G. (2003). Transient expression of doublecortin during adult neurogenesis. *J. Comp. Neurol.* 467, 1–10. doi: 10.1002/cne.10874

Busto, G. U., Elie, J. E., Kermen, F., Garcia, S., Sacquet, J., Jourdan, F., et al. (2009). Expression of Zif268 in the granule cell layer of the adult mouse olfactory bulb is modulated by experience. *Eur. J. Neurosci.* 29, 1431–1439. doi: 10.1111/j.1460-9568.2009.06689.x

Carleton, A., Petreanu, L. T., Lansford, R., Alvarez-Buylla, A., and Lledo, P. M. (2003). Becoming a new neuron in the adult olfactory bulb. *Nat. Neurosci.* 6, 507–518. doi: 10.1038/nn1048

Cave, J. W., Akiba, Y., Banerjee, K., Bhosle, S., Berlin, R., and Baker, H. (2010). Differential regulation of dopaminergic gene expression by Er81. *J. Neurosci.* 30, 4717–4724. doi: 10.1523/JNEUROSCI.0419-10.2010

Chazal, G., Durbec, P., Jankovski, A., Rougon, G., and Cremer, H. (2000). Consequences of neural cell adhesion molecule deficiency on cell migration in the rostral migratory stream of the mouse. *J. Neurosci.* 20, 1446–1457.

Colledge, M., Snyder, E. M., Crozier, R. A., Soderling, J. A., Jin, Y., Langeberg, L. K., et al. (2003). Ubiquitination regulates PSD-95 degradation and AMPA receptor surface expression. *Neuron* 40, 595–607. doi: 10.1016/S0896-6273(03)00687-1

David, L. S., Schachner, M., and Saghatelyan, A. (2013). The extracellular matrix glycoprotein tenascin-R affects adult but not developmental neurogenesis in the olfactory bulb. *J. Neurosci.* 33, 10324–10339. doi: 10.1523/JNEUROSCI.5728-12.2013

Ebert, D. H., and Greenberg, M. E. (2013). Activity-dependent neuronal signalling and autism spectrum disorder. *Nature* 493, 327–337. doi: 10.1038/nature11860

Enwere, E., Shingo, T., Gregg, C., Fujikawa, H., Ohta, S., and Weiss, S. (2004). Aging results in reduced epidermal growth factor receptor signaling, diminished olfactory neurogenesis, and deficits in fine olfactory discrimination. *J. Neurosci.* 24, 8354–8365. doi: 10.1523/JNEUROSCI.2751-04.2004

Figueres-Oñate, M., Gutiérrez, Y., and López-Mascaraque, L. (2014). Unraveling Cajal's view of the olfactory system. *Front. Neuroanat.* 8:55. doi: 10.3389/fnana.2014.00055

Garcia, I., Quast, K. B., Huang, L., Herman, A. M., Selever, J., Deussing, J. M., et al. (2014). Local CRH signaling promotes synaptogenesis and circuit integration of adult-born neurons. *Dev. Cell* 30, 645–659. doi: 10.1016/j.devcel.2014.07.001

Gheusi, G., Cremer, H., McLean, H., Chazal, G., Vincent, J. D., and Lledo, P. M. (2000). Importance of newly generated neurons in the adult olfactory bulb for odor discrimination. *Proc. Natl. Acad. Sci. U.S.A.* 97, 1823–1828. doi: 10.1073/pnas.97.4.1823

Gschwend, O., Abraham, N. M., Lagier, S., Begnaud, F., Rodriguez, I., and Carleton, A. (2015). Neuronal pattern separation in the olfactory bulb improves odor discrimination learning. *Nat. Neurosci.* 18, 1474–1482. doi: 10.1038/nn.4089

Guthrie, K. M., Anderson, A. J., Leon, M., and Gall, C. (1993). Odor-induced increases in c-fos mRNA expression reveal an anatomical "unit" for odor processing in olfactory bulb. *Proc. Natl. Acad. Sci. U.S.A.* 90, 3329–3333. doi: 10.1073/pnas.90.8.3329

Hack, I., Bancila, M., Loulier, K., Carroll, P., and Cremer, H. (2002). Reelin is a detachment signal in tangential chain-migration during postnatal neurogenesis. *Nat. Neurosci.* 5, 939–945. doi: 10.1038/nn923

Herold, S., Jagasia, R., Merz, K., Wassmer, K., and Lie, D. C. (2011). CREB signalling regulates early survival, neuronal gene expression and morphological development in adult subventricular zone neurogenesis. *Mol. Cell. Neurosci.* 46, 79–88. doi: 10.1016/j.mcn.2010.08.008

Hirota, Y., Sawada, M., Kida, Y. S., Huang, S. H., Yamada, O., Sakaguchi, M., et al. (2012). Roles of planar cell polarity signaling in maturation of neuronal precursor cells in the postnatal mouse olfactory bulb. *Stem Cells* 30, 1726–1733. doi: 10.1002/stem.1137

Hole, N., and Stern, P. L. (1990). Isolation and characterization of 5T4, a tumour-associated antigen. *Int. J. Cancer* 45, 179–184. doi: 10.1002/ijc.2910450132

Imai, T. (2014). Construction of functional neuronal circuitry in the olfactory bulb. *Semin. Cell Dev. Biol.* 35, 180–188. doi: 10.1016/j.semcdb.2014.07.012

Imamura, F., Nagao, H., Naritsuka, H., Murata, Y., Taniguchi, H., and Mori, K. (2006). A leucine-rich repeat membrane protein, 5T4, is expressed by a subtype of granule cells with dendritic arbors in specific strata of the mouse olfactory bulb. *J. Comp. Neurol.* 495, 754–768. doi: 10.1002/cne.20896

Imayoshi, I., Sakamoto, M., Ohtsuka, T., Takao, K., Miyakawa, T., Yamaguchi, M., et al. (2008). Roles of continuous neurogenesis in the structural and functional integrity of the adult forebrain. *Nat. Neurosci.* 11, 1153–1161. doi: 10.1038/nn.2185

Inaki, K., Takahashi, Y. K., Nagayama, S., and Mori, K. (2002). Molecular-feature domains with posterodorsal-anteroventral polarity in the symmetrical sensory maps of the mouse olfactory bulb: mapping of odourant-induced Zif268 expression. *Eur. J. Neurosci.* 15, 1563–1574. doi: 10.1046/j.1460-9568.2002.01991.x

Kagermeier-Schenk, B., Wehner, D., Ozhan-Kizil, G., Yamamoto, H., Li, J., Kirchner, K., et al. (2011). The transmembrane protein Waif1/5T4 inhibits Wnt/β-catenin signaling and activates noncanonical Wnt pathways by modifying LRP6 subcellular localization. *Dev. Cell* 21, 1129–1143. doi: 10.1016/j.devcel.2011.10.015

Kaneko, N., Marín, O., Koike, M., Hirota, Y., Uchiyama, Y., Wu, J. Y., et al. (2010). New neurons clear the path of astrocytic processes for their rapid migration in the adult brain. *Neuron* 67, 213–223. doi: 10.1016/j.neuron.2010.06.018

Kato, Y., Kaneko, N., Sawada, M., Ito, K., Arakawa, S., and Murakami, S., et al. (2012). A subtype-specific critical period for neurogenesis in the postnatal development of mouse olfactory glomeruli. *PLoS ONE* 7:e48431. doi: 10.1371/journal.pone.0048431

Katz, L. C., and Shatz, C. J. (1996). Synaptic activity and the construction of cortical circuits. *Science* 274, 1133–1138. doi: 10.1126/science.274.5290.1133

Kawashima, T., Okuno, H., and Bito, H. (2014). A new era for functional labeling of neurons: activity-dependent promoters have come of age. *Front. Neural Circuits.* 8:37. doi: 10.3389/fncir.2014.00037

Kelsch, W., Li, Z., Eliava, M., Goengrich, C., and Monyer, H. (2012a). GluN2B-containing NMDA receptors promote wiring of adult-born neurons into olfactory bulb circuits. *J. Neurosci.* 32, 12603–12611. doi: 10.1523/JNEUROSCI.1459-12.2012

Kelsch, W., Lin, C. W., Mosley, C. P., and Lois, C. (2009). A critical period for activity-dependent synaptic development during olfactory bulb adult neurogenesis. *J. Neurosci.* 29, 11852–11858. doi: 10.1523/JNEUROSCI.2406-09.2009

Kelsch, W., Sim, S., and Lois, C. (2012b). Increasing heterogeneity in the organization of synaptic inputs of mature olfactory bulb neurons generated in newborn rats. *J. Comp. Neurol.* 520, 1327–1338. doi: 10.1002/cne.22799

Khodosevich, K., Lazarini, F., von Engelhardt, J., Kaneko, H., Lledo, P. M., and Monyer, H. (2013). Connective tissue growth factor regulates interneuron survival and information processing in the olfactory bulb. *Neuron* 79, 1136–1151. doi: 10.1016/j.neuron.2013.07.011

King, K. W., Sheppard, F. C., Westwater, C., Stern, P. L., and Myers, K. A. (1999). Organisation of the mouse and human 5T4 oncofoetal leucine-rich glycoprotein genes and expression in foetal and adult murine tissues. *Biochim. Biophys. Acta* 1445, 257–270. doi: 10.1016/S0167-4781(99)00055-X

Komano-Inoue, S., Manabe, H., Ota, M., Kusumoto-Yoshida, I., Yokoyama, T. K., Mori, K., et al. (2014). Top-down inputs from the olfactory cortex in the postprandial period promote elimination of granule cells in the olfactory bulb. *Eur. J. Neurosci.* 40, 2724–2733. doi: 10.1111/ejn.12679

Lau, C. G., and Murthy, V. N. (2012). Activity-dependent regulation of inhibition via GAD67. *J. Neurosci.* 32, 8521–8531. doi: 10.1523/JNEUROSCI.1245-12.2012

Lazarini, F., Gabellec, M. M., Moigneu, C., de Chaumont, F., Olivo-Marin, J. C., and Lledo, P. M. (2014). Adult neurogenesis restores dopaminergic neuronal loss in the olfactory bulb. *J. Neurosci.* 34, 14430–14442. doi: 10.1523/JNEUROSCI.5366-13.2014

Lepousez, G., Nissant, A., Bryant, A. K., Gheusi, G., Greer, C. A., and Lledo, P. M. (2014). Olfactory learning promotes input-specific synaptic plasticity in adult-born neurons. *Proc. Natl. Acad. Sci. U.S.A.* 111, 13984–13989. doi: 10.1073/pnas.1404991111

Lepousez, G., Valley, M. T., and Lledo, P. M. (2013). The impact of adult neurogenesis on olfactory bulb circuits and computations. *Annu. Rev. Physiol.* 75, 339–363. doi: 10.1146/annurev-physiol-030212-183731

Lin, C. W., Sim, S., Ainsworth, A., Okada, M., Kelsch, W., and Lois, C. (2010). Genetically increased cell-intrinsic excitability enhances neuronal integration into adult brain circuits. *Neuron* 65, 32–39. doi: 10.1016/j.neuron.2009.12.001

Lin, Y., Bloodgood, B. L., Hauser, J. L., Lapan, A. D., Koon, A. C., Kim, T. K., et al. (2008). Activity-dependent regulation of inhibitory synapse development by Npas4. *Nature* 455, 1198–1204. doi: 10.1038/nature07319

Livneh, Y., Adam, Y., and Mizrahi, A. (2014). Odor processing by adult-born neurons. *Neuron* 81, 1097–1110. doi: 10.1016/j.neuron.2014.01.007

Livneh, Y., Feinstein, N., Klein, M., and Mizrahi, A. (2009). Sensory input enhances synaptogenesis of adult-born neurons. *J. Neurosci.* 29, 86–97. doi: 10.1523/JNEUROSCI.4105-08.2009

Lledo, P. M., Merkle, F. T., and Alvarez-Buylla, A. (2008). Origin and function of olfactory bulb interneuron diversity. *Trends Neurosci.* 31, 392–400. doi: 10.1016/j.tins.2008.05.006

Madabhushi, R., Gao, F., Pfenning, A. R., Pan, L., Yamakawa, S., Seo, J., et al. (2015). Activity-induced DNA breaks govern the expression of neuronal early-response genes. *Cell* 161, 1592–1605. doi: 10.1016/j.cell.2015.05.032

Maya-Vetencourt, J. F., Tiraboschi, E., Greco, D., Restani, L., Cerri, C., Auvinen, P., et al. (2012). Experience-dependent expression of NPAS4 regulates plasticity in adult visual cortex. *J. Physiol. (Lond).* 590, 4777–4787. doi: 10.1113/jphysiol.2012.234237

McDole, B., Isgor, C., Pare, C., and Guthrie, K. (2015). BDNF over-expression increases olfactory bulb granule cell dendritic spine density *in vivo*. *Neuroscience* 304, 146–160. doi: 10.1016/j.neuroscience.2015.07.056

Merkle, F. T., Fuentealba, L. C., Sanders, T. A., Magno, L., Kessaris, N., and Alvarez-Buylla, A. (2014). Adult neural stem cells in distinct microdomains generate previously unknown interneuron types. *Nat. Neurosci.* 17, 207–214. doi: 10.1038/nn.3610

Mori, K., Kishi, K., and Ojima, H. (1983). Distribution of dendrites of mitral, displaced mitral, tufted, and granule cells in the rabbit olfactory bulb. *J. Comp. Neurol.* 219, 339–355. doi: 10.1002/cne.902190308

Mori, K., and Sakano, H. (2011). How is the olfactory map formed and interpreted in the mammalian brain? *Annu. Rev. Neurosci.* 34, 467–499. doi: 10.1146/annurev-neuro-112210-112917

Nithianantharajah, J., and Hannan, A. J. (2006). Enriched environments, experience-dependent plasticity and disorders of the nervous system. *Nat. Rev. Neurosci.* 7, 697–709. doi: 10.1038/nrn1970

Ocbina, P. J., Dizon, M. L., Shin, L., and Szele, F. G. (2006). Doublecortin is necessary for the migration of adult subventricular zone cells from neurospheres. *Mol. Cell. Neurosci.* 33, 126–135. doi: 10.1016/j.mcn.2006.06.014

Orona, E., Scott, J. W., and Rainer, E. C. (1983). Different granule cell populations innervate superficial and deep regions of the external plexiform layer in rat olfactory bulb. *J. Comp. Neurol.* 217, 227–237. doi: 10.1002/cne.902170209

Pallotto, M., Nissant, A., Fritschy, J. M., Rudolph, U., Sassoè-Pognetto, M., Panzanelli, P., et al. (2012). Early formation of GABAergic synapses governs the development of adult-born neurons in the olfactory bulb. *J. Neurosci.* 32, 9103–9115. doi: 10.1523/JNEUROSCI.0214-12.2012

Panzanelli, P., Bardy, C., Nissant, A., Pallotto, M., Sassoè-Pognetto, M., Lledo, P. M., et al. (2009). Early synapse formation in developing interneurons of the adult olfactory bulb. *J. Neurosci.* 29, 15039–15052. doi: 10.1523/JNEUROSCI.3034-09.2009

Parrish-Aungst, S., Kiyokage, E., Szabo, G., Yanagawa, Y., Shipley, M. T., and Puche, A. C. (2011). Sensory experience selectively regulates transmitter synthesis enzymes in interglomerular circuits. *Brain Res.* 1382, 70–76. doi: 10.1016/j.brainres.2011.01.068

Petreanu, L., and Alvarez-Buylla, A. (2002). Maturation and death of adult-born olfactory bulb granule neurons: role of olfaction. *J. Neurosci.* 22, 6106–6113.

Pino, D., Choe, Y., and Pleasure, S. J. (2011). Wnt5a controls neurite development in olfactory bulb interneurons. *ASN Neuro.* 3:e00059. doi: 10.1042/AN20100038

Pruunsild, P., Sepp, M., Orav, E., Koppel, I., and Timmusk, T. (2011). Identification of cis-elements and transcription factors regulating neuronal activity-dependent transcription of human BDNF gene. *J. Neurosci.* 31, 3295–3308. doi: 10.1523/JNEUROSCI.4540-10.2011

Ramamoorthi, K., Fropf, R., Belfort, G. M., Fitzmaurice, H. L., McKinney, R. M., Neve, R. L., et al. (2011). Npas4 regulates a transcriptional program in CA3 required for contextual memory formation. *Science* 334, 1669–1675. doi: 10.1126/science.1208049

Rochefort, C., Gheusi, G., Vincent, J. D., and Lledo, P. M. (2002). Enriched odor exposure increases the number of newborn neurons in the adult olfactory bulb and improves odor memory. *J. Neurosci.* 22, 2679–2689.

Rochefort, C., and Lledo, P. M. (2005). Short-term survival of newborn neurons in the adult olfactory bulb after exposure to a complex odor environment. *Eur. J. Neurosci.* 22, 2863–2870. doi: 10.1111/j.1460-9568.2005.04486.x

Saaltink, D. J., Håvik, B., Verissimo, C. S., Lucassen, P. J., and Vreugdenhil, E. (2012). Doublecortin and doublecortin-like are expressed in overlapping and non-overlapping neuronal cell population: implications for neurogenesis. *J. Comp. Neurol.* 520, 2805–2823. doi: 10.1002/cne.23144

Saghatelyan, A., de Chevigny, A., Schachner, M., and Lledo, P. M. (2004). Tenascin-R mediates activity-dependent recruitment of neuroblasts in the adult mouse forebrain. *Nat. Neurosci.* 7, 347–356. doi: 10.1038/nn1211

Saghatelyan, A., Roux, P., Migliore, M., Rochefort, C., Desmaisons, D., Charneau, P., et al. (2005). Activity-dependent adjustments of the inhibitory network in the olfactory bulb following early postnatal deprivation. *Neuron* 46, 103–116. doi: 10.1016/j.neuron.2005.02.016

Saha, B., Ypsilanti, A. R., Boutin, C., Cremer, H., and Chédotal, A. (2012). Plexin-B2 regulates the proliferation and migration of neuroblasts in the postnatal and adult subventricular zone. *J. Neurosci.* 32, 16892–16905. doi: 10.1523/JNEUROSCI.0344-12.2012

Sakamoto, M., Ieki, N., Miyoshi, G., Mochimaru, D., Miyachi, H., Imura, T., et al. (2014). Continuous postnatal neurogenesis contributes to formation of the olfactory bulb neural circuits and flexible olfactory associative learning. *J. Neurosci.* 34, 5788–5799. doi: 10.1523/JNEUROSCI.0674-14.2014

Sakamoto, M., Imayoshi, I., Ohtsuka, T., Yamaguchi, M., Mori, K., and Kageyama, R. (2011). Continuous neurogenesis in the adult forebrain is required for innate olfactory responses. *Proc. Natl. Acad. Sci. U.S.A.* 108, 8479–8484. doi: 10.1073/pnas.1018782108

Sanes, J. R., and Lichtman, J. W. (2001). Induction, assembly, maturation and maintenance of a postsynaptic apparatus. *Nat. Rev. Neurosci.* 2, 791–805. doi: 10.1038/35097557

Sawada, M., Kaneko, N., Inada, H., Wake, H., Kato, Y., Yanagawa, Y., et al. (2011). Sensory input regulates spatial and subtype-specific patterns of neuronal turnover in the adult olfactory bulb. *J. Neurosci.* 31, 11587–11596. doi: 10.1523/JNEUROSCI.0614-11.2011

Scotto-Lomassese, S., Nissant, A., Mota, T., Néant-Féry, M., Oostra, B. A., Greer, C. A., et al. (2011). Fragile X mental retardation protein regulates new neuron differentiation in the adult olfactory bulb. *J. Neurosci.* 31, 2205–2215. doi: 10.1523/JNEUROSCI.5514-10.2011

Sequerra, E. B. (2014). Subventricular zone progenitors in time and space: generating neuronal diversity. *Front. Cell. Neurosci.* 8:434. doi: 10.3389/fncel.2014.00434

Shepherd, G. M., Chen, W. R., and Greer, C. A. (2004). "Olfactory bulb," in *The Synaptic Organization of the Brain*, ed G. M. Shepherd (Oxford: Oxford University Press), 165–216.

Shin, E., Kashiwagi, Y., Kuriu, T., Iwasaki, H., Tanaka, T., Koizumi, H., et al. (2013). Doublecortin-like kinase enhances dendritic remodelling and negatively regulates synapse maturation. *Nat. Commun.* 4, 1440. doi: 10.1038/ncomms2443

Sim, S., Antolin, S., Lin, C. W., Lin, Y., and Lois, C. (2013). Increased cell-intrinsic excitability induces synaptic changes in new neurons in the adult dentate gyrus that require Npas4. *J. Neurosci.* 33, 7928–7940. doi: 10.1523/JNEUROSCI.1571-12.2013

Southall, P. J., Boxer, G. M., Bagshawe, K. D., Hole, N., Bromley, M., and Stern, P. L. (1990). Immunohistological distribution of 5T4 antigen in normal and malignant tissues. *Br. J. Cancer* 61, 89–95. doi: 10.1038/bjc.1990.20

Sultan, S., Mandairon, N., Kermen, F., Garcia, S., Sacquet, J., and Didier, A. (2010). Learning-dependent neurogenesis in the olfactory bulb determines long-term olfactory memory. *FASEB J.* 24, 2355–2363. doi: 10.1096/fj.09-151456

Takeuchi, H., and Sakano, H. (2014). Neural map formation in the mouse olfactory system. *Cell. Mol. Life Sci.* 71, 3049–3057. doi: 10.1007/s00018-014-1597-0

Tong, C. K., and Alvarez-Buylla, A. (2014). SnapShot: adult neurogenesis in the V-SVZ. *Neuron* 81, 220–220.e1. doi: 10.1016/j.neuron.2013.12.004

Tsukada, M., Prokscha, A., Oldekamp, J., and Eichele, G. (2003). Identification of neurabin II as a novel doublecortin interacting protein. *Mech. Dev.* 120, 1033–1043. doi: 10.1016/S0925-4773(03)00177-1

Tsukada, M., Prokscha, A., Ungewickell, E., and Eichele, G. (2005). Doublecortin association with actin filaments is regulated by neurabin II. *J. Biol. Chem.* 280, 11361–11368. doi: 10.1074/jbc.m405525200

Vadodaria, K. C., and Gage, F. H. (2014). SnapShot: adult hippocampal neurogenesis. *Cell* 156, 1114–1114.e1. doi: 10.1016/j.cell.2014.02.029

Vadodaria, K. C., and Jessberger, S. (2013). Maturation and integration of adult born hippocampal neurons: signal convergence onto small Rho GTPases. *Front. Synaptic Neurosci.* 5:4. doi: 10.3389/fnsyn.2013.00004

van Amerongen, R., and Nusse, R. (2009). Towards an integrated view of Wnt signaling in development. *Development* 136, 3205–3214. doi: 10.1242/dev.033910

Whitman, M. C., and Greer, C. A. (2009). Adult neurogenesis and the olfactory system. *Prog Neurobiol.* 89, 162–175. doi: 10.1016/j.pneurobio.2009.07.003

Yamaguchi, M., and Mori, K. (2005). Critical period for sensory experience-dependent survival of newly generated granule cells in the adult mouse olfactory bulb. *Proc. Natl. Acad. Sci. U.S.A.* 102, 9697–9702 doi: 10.1073/pnas.0406082102

Yokoyama, T. K., Mochimaru, D., Murata, K., Manabe, H., Kobayakawa, K., Kobayakawa, R., et al. (2011). Elimination of adult-born neurons in the olfactory bulb is promoted during the postprandial period. *Neuron* 71, 883–897. doi: 10.1016/j.neuron.2011.05.046

Yoshihara, S., Takahashi, H., Nishimura, N., Kinoshita, M., Asahina, R., Kitsuki, M., et al. (2014). Npas4 regulates Mdm2 and thus Dcx in experience-dependent olfactory bulb interneuron dendritic spine development. *Cell Rep.* 8, 843–857. doi: 10.1016/j.celrep.2014.06.056

Yoshihara, S., Takahashi, H., Nishimura, N., Naritsuka, H., Shirao, T., Hirai, H., et al. (2012). 5T4 glycoprotein regulates the sensory input-dependent development of a specific subtype of newborn interneurons in the mouse olfactory bulb. *J. Neurosci.* 32, 2217–2226. doi: 10.1523/JNEUROSCI.5907-11.2012

Zhao, Y., Malinauskas, T., Harlos, K., and Jones, E. Y. (2014). Structural insights into the inhibition of Wnt signaling by cancer antigen 5T4/Wnt-activated inhibitory factor 1. *Structure* 22, 612–620. doi: 10.1016/j.str.2014.01.009

Zhou, X., Liu, F., Tian, M., Xu, Z., Liang, Q., Wang, C., et al. (2015). Transcription factors COUP-TFI and COUP-TFII are required for the production of granule cells in the mouse olfactory bulb. *Development* 142, 1593–1605. doi: 10.1242/dev.115279

11

Neurogenesis, Neurodegeneration, Interneuron Vulnerability, and Amyloid-β in the Olfactory Bulb of APP/PS1 Mouse Model of Alzheimer's Disease

Carlos De la Rosa-Prieto, Daniel Saiz-Sanchez, Isabel Ubeda-Banon, Alicia Flores-Cuadrado and Alino Martinez-Marcos *

Neuroplasticity and Neurodegeneration Laboratory, CRIB, Ciudad Real Medical School, Universidad de Castilla-La Mancha, Ciudad Real, Spain

Edited by:
Grigori Enikolopov, Stony Brook University, USA

Reviewed by:
Armen Saghatelyan, Université Laval, Canada
Eric D. Laywell, Florida State University, USA

***Correspondence:**
Alino Martinez-Marcos
alino.martinez@uclm.es

Alzheimer's disease (AD) is the most prevalent neurodegenerative disease, mostly idiopathic and with palliative treatment. Neuropathologically, it is characterized by intracellular neurofibrillary tangles of tau protein and extracellular plaques of amyloid β peptides. The relationship between AD and neurogenesis is unknown, but two facts are particularly relevant. First, early aggregation sites of both proteinopathies include the hippocampal formation and the olfactory bulb (OB), which have been correlated to memory and olfactory deficits, respectively. These areas are well-recognized integration zones of newly-born neurons in the adult brain. Second, molecules, such as amyloid precursor protein (APP) and presenilin-1 are common to both AD etiology and neurogenic development. Adult neurogenesis in AD models has been studied in the hippocampus, but only occasionally addressed in the OB and results are contradictory. To gain insight on the relationship between adult neurogenesis and AD, this work analyzes neurogenesis, neurodegeneration, interneuron vulnerability, and amyloid-β involvement in the OB of an AD model. Control and double-transgenic mice carrying the APP and the presenilin-1 genes, which give rise amyloid β plaques have been used. BrdU-treated animals have been studied at 16, 30, 43, and 56 weeks of age. New-born cell survival (BrdU), neuronal loss (using neuronal markers NeuN and PGP9.5), differential interneuron (calbindin-, parvalbumin-, calretinin- and somatostatin-expressing populations) vulnerability, and involvement by amyloid β have been analyzed. Neurogenesis increases with aging in the granule cell layer of control animals from 16 to 43 weeks. No neuronal loss has been observed after quantifying NeuN or PGP9.5. Regarding interneuron population vulnerability: calbindin-expressing neurons remains unchanged; parvalbumin-expressing neurons trend to increase with aging in transgenic animals; calretinin-expressing neurons increase with aging in transgenic mice and decrease in control animals and neurogenesis is higher in control as compared to transgenic animals at given ages, finally; somatostatin-expressing neurons of transgenic mice decrease with aging and as compared to controls. Amyloid β aggregates with aging in the granule cell layer, which may be related to the particular involvement of somatostatin-expressing cells.

Keywords: adult neurogenesis, calbindin, calretinin, parvalbumin, somatostatin

INTRODUCTION

Alzheimer's disease (AD) is the most prevalent neurodegenerative disease and the main cause of dementia (Reiman, 2014). It is characterized by cognitive deficits and nowadays treatments are palliative. Two associated proteinopathies yield aggregates into the brain: tau protein that form intracellular neurofibrillary tangles and insoluble forms of amyloid β (Aβ) peptides that assembles into extracellular plaques (Goedert and Spillantini, 2006; Ballard et al., 2011). Neuropathological staging of these deposits show that early sites of involvement include the OB and the hippocampal formation (Ohm and Braak, 1987; Braak and Braak, 1991; Braak et al., 2006; Attems et al., 2014; Braak and Del Trecidi, 2015). These areas correlate with initial symptoms, namely olfactory (Devanand et al., 2015) and declarative memory deficits (Jahn, 2013).

Interestingly, the subventricular zone of the lateral ventricles (SVZ) and the hippocampal subgranular zone (SGZ) were described as the two main neurogenic niches giving rise to newly-born neurons migrating and integrating into the adult olfactory bulb (OB) and the dentate gyrus (DG) of the hippocampus, respectively (Altman, 1962; Altman and Das, 1965; Luskin, 1993; Lois and Alvarez-Buylla, 1994). Decades later, the functional significance of new neurons integrated into adult OB (Lepousez et al., 2013) and DG (Deng et al., 2010) is only partially known.

AD and adult neurogenesis are not only linked by common sites where early pathology occurs and newly-born neurons integrate in the preexisting circuitry, but share a number of common molecules to both processes (Kaneko and Sawamoto, 2009; Lazarov and Marr, 2010, 2013; Lazarov et al., 2010; Mu and Gage, 2011; Winner et al., 2011). Increasing evidence suggest that molecular players in Alzheimer disease, including amyloid precursor protein (APP) and presenilin 1 (PS1) and its metabolites, play a role in adult neurogenesis (Lazarov and Marr, 2010). Soluble APPα regulate neural progenitor cell proliferation. Thus, miscleavage of APP would readily influence on developmental and postnatal neurogenesis, which could contribute to cognitive deficits characterizing AD (Lazarov and Demars, 2012). On the other hand, PS1 is not only prominently expressed in the embryonic brain but is also a crucial regulator of Notch and Wnt signaling (Winner et al., 2011), key pathways in neural differentiation. In addition, polymorphisms in the apolipoprotein E (apoE, the ε4 isoform) gene show the most significant effects on relative genetic risk of AD. Experiments in transgenic mice carrying human apoE4 have shown apoptosis of neural progenitor cells after environmental enrichment suggesting that apoE4 is somewhat compromising neurogenesis (Levi and Michaelson, 2007).

Data on neurogenic rate changes in AD models are quite variable depending on the different transgenic mice, experimental conditions, and markers analyzed; and, it is not always obvious to distinguish it from changes due to physiological aging (Lazarov and Marr, 2010; Winner et al., 2011). Data in the model used in the present study (APPswe/PS1ΔE9) show reduced hippocampal neurogenesis (Verret et al., 2007; Niidome et al., 2008). This impairment in neurogenesis take place early in life long before amyloid deposition suggesting that the decrease of neurogenic rate may be a contributor factor rather than a result of neural dysfunction (Demars et al., 2010). Interestingly, the reduction in neuroblasts, as confirmed by quantitative Western blot analysis of doublecortin content, was restricted to the hippocampal but not to the OB neurogenic system (Zhang et al., 2007).

Data from different authors and our previous results indicate a differential interneuron vulnerability in postmortem tissue from Alzheimer's patients and in transgenic mice model (Fonseca and Soriano, 1995; Solodkin et al., 1996; Brady and Mufson, 1997; Leuba et al., 1998; Iritani et al., 2001; Saiz-Sanchez et al., 2010, 2012, 2013, 2015, 2016).

Therefore, the present study aims at characterizing the neurogenic process in the OB of APP/PS1 mice by analyzing the neurogenic and neurodegeneration rates and the role Aβ in the survival of new and preexisting interneuron populations.

MATERIALS AND METHODS

Experimental Animals

For this study, 20 female hemizygous double transgenic mice (B6C3-Tg-APPswe, PSEN1dD9-85Dbo/J) model of AD and 20 female non-carrier mice have been used (004462, The Jackson Laboratory, USA). These transgenic mice express a chimeric mouse/human APP (Mo/HuAPP695swe) and a mutant human presenilin 1 (PS1-dD9), each controlled by independent mouse prion protein (PrP) promoter elements (Jankowsky et al., 2001, 2004). The APPswe/PSEN1dD9 (APPxPS1) mouse model is characterized by increasing Aβ levels with aging (Jankowsky et al., 2004; Van Groen et al., 2006). Four experimental groups of five transgenic and five non-carrier animals were stablished according to survival times (16, 30, 43, and 56 weeks). The animals were housed on a standard 12/12 h light/dark cycle, at 21°C with food and water *ad libitum*. All of the animal research procedures described herein were in agreement with European (Directive 2010/63/EU) and Spanish (RD 53/2013) legislation on the protection of animals used for scientific purposes. All experiments described were approved by the Ethical Committee of Animal Research of the University of Castilla-La Mancha (grant BFU2010-15729).

Bromodeoxyuridine Administration, Perfusion, and Sectioning

BrdU (5-bromo-2′-deoxyuridine, Fluka, Madrid, Spain) administration included four i.p. doses (at 2-h intervals) of 10 mg/mL BrdU in phosphate-buffered saline (PBS, 0.15 M NaCl, 0.01 M sodium phosphate pH 7.4) totalizing a dose of 200 mg/kg in 1 day. This dose was employed following previous results in our laboratory to optimize labeling without increasing apoptosis (Martínez-Marcos et al., 2000a,b; Martinez-Marcos et al., 2005; De La Rosa-Prieto et al., 2009). Two week afterwards,

Abbreviations: Aβ, amyloid β; AD, Alzheimer's disease; APP, amyloid precursor protein; BrdU, bromodeoxyuridine; CB, calbindin; CR, calretinin; DG, dentate gyrus; ePL, external plexiform layer; GL, glomerular layer; GrL, granule cell layer; iPL, internal plexiform layer, MOB, main olfactory bulb; NeuN, Fox3-NeuN; OB, olfactory bulb; PS1, presenilin 1; PV, parvalbumin; SGZ, subgranular zone; SST, somatostatin; SVZ, subventricular zone; TG, transgenic; WT, wild type.

animals were anesthetized with a combined dose of ketamine hydrochloride (Ketolar, Parke-Davis, Madrid, Spain, 1.5 mL/kg, 75 mg/kg), and xylazine (Xilagesic, Calier, Barcelona, Spain, 0.5 mL/kg, 10 mg/kg) and perfused with saline solution followed by 4% w/v paraformaldehyde fixative in phosphate buffer (0.1 M sodium phosphate pH 7.2). Brains were postfixed in 4% w/v paraformaldehyde, cryoprotected in 30% w/v sucrose, and the olfactory bulbs frontally sectioned (50 μm) using a freezing sliding microtome (Microm HM450). Sections were consecutively collected into 96-well-plates and maintained at 4°C in preserving solution (PBS containing 20% v/v glycerol and 30% v/v ethylene glycol) for further processing.

Immunofluorescence Procedures

Six sections from rostral to caudal OB of each animal were chosen (separated 400 um) and rinsed overnight with Tris-buffered saline (TBS; 0.15 M NaCl, 0.05 M Tris, HCl pH 7.6) and blocked with 10% v/v normal donkey serum (NDS; Vector Laboratories, Burlingame, CA) in TBS for 60 min at room temperature. Sections were then incubated overnight with rabbit anti-amyloid beta (Aβ, 1:250, Cell Signaling, 2454, MA, USA), goat anti-calretinin (CR, 1:1000, Santa Cruz, sc-11644, CA, USA), monoclonal mouse anti-calbindin D-28k (CB, 1:5000, Swant, 300, Switzerland), goat anti-somatostatin (SST, 1:1000, Santa Cruz, sc-7819, CA, USA), goat anti-parvalbumin (PV,1:2000, Swant, PVG-213, Switzerland), mouse monoclonal PGP9.5 (PGP9.5 13C4/I3C4, 1:1000, abcam, ab8189, Cambridge, MA, USA), or rabbit anti-NeuN (NeuN, 1:500, abcam, ab104225, Cambridge, MA, USA) diluted in TBS with 5% v/v normal goat serum and 0.3% Triton X-100 at 4°C. Then, sections were incubated for 2 h at room temperature with Alexas 488, 555, 568, or 647 anti-multiple species (1:200 in TBS with 2% of normal goat serum and 0.2% Triton X-100; Invitrogen, Eugene, OR).

Sections were then rinsed with TBS and incubated in ice-cold paraformaldehyde 4% v/v for 15 min. Rinsed again and incubated in 2N HCL at 37° during 1 h. After rinsed several times, sections were incubated overnight with mouse anti-BrdU (BrdU,1:40, Dako, M0744, Glostrup, Denmark). Sections were subsequently incubated for 2 h at room temperature with Alexa 488, anti-mouse (1:200 in TBS with 2% of normal goat serum and 0.2% Triton X-100; Invitrogen, Eugene, OR), and counterstained using DAPI (1 μg/ml in TBS, Santa Cruz, SC-3598) for 5 min in the dark.

Analysis of Labeled Cells

The images of different fluorophores were analyzed using ImageJ and ZEN software from Zeiss using the profile and ortho tools of ZEN software. GraphPad Prism® v.6 (San Diego, CA, USA) was used for statistical analyses. Kolmogorov–Smirnov and Wald–Wolfowitz tests were carried out to analyze the normality and randomness of the sample ($P > 0.05$). Statistical comparisons were performed using an unpaired two-tailed *t*-test, or one-way or two-way ANOVA followed by Bonferroni and Tukey *post-hoc* tests to estimate the significance of differences between age groups, markers, areas, WT, and TG animals. All data are represented as mean ± SEM. Differences were regarded as statistically significant at * or $\#P < 0.05$, ** or $\#\#P < 0.01$, *** or $\#\#\#P < 0.001$, and $^{****}P < 0.0001$.

RESULTS

The aim of the present report has been to study in depth the relationship between adult neurogenesis and AD by analyzing neurogenic rate, neurodegeneration, interneuron vulnerability, and Aβ involvement in the OB of control and transgenic mice over time. The different layers of the main OB (MOB; **Figure 1A**) have been grouped for analysis: granule (GrL) and internal plexiform (iPL), mitral (ML), and external plexiform (ePL), and glomerular (GL), and nerve (NL) layers (**Figure 1B**).

Analysis of BrdU-Labeled Cells

The labeling of BrdU-positive cells was mainly concentrated in the GrL and GL of control and transgenic animals at different ages (**Figures 1C–F**). The analysis of BrdU-labeled cells over time revealed an increasing trend in the GrL with aging that was statistically significant between 16 (**Figure 1C**) and 43 (**Figure 1D**) weeks in control animals (**Figure 1G**) [Two-way ANOVA genotype vs. age: Interaction $F_{(3,\ 62)} = 1.846$; $p = 0.1482$; Age $F_{(3,\ 62)} = 3.220$; $p = 0.0287$; Genotype $F_{(1,\ 62)} = 0.0002612$; $p = 0.9872$]. This trend was not observed in the GL (**Figure 1G**) [Two-way ANOVA genotype vs. age: Interaction $F_{(3,\ 63)} = 0.5647$; $p = 0.6403$; Age $F_{(3,\ 63)} = 2.676$; $p = 0.0547$; Genotype $F_{(1,\ 63)} = 7.260$; $p = 0.0090$].

Regarding genotype comparison, no clear differences were observed in the GrL, but in the GL, the number of BrdU-labeled cells was in general lower in transgenic (**Figure 1F**) as compared to control (**Figure 1E**) animals.

Analysis of NeuN- and PGP9.5-Labeled Cells

In order to evaluate a possible neuronal loss, two neural markers have been used in the OB of control and transgenic mice: NeuN has been used to label neurons in GrL (**Figures 2A,B**) and GL (**Figures 2E,F**), and PGP9.5 in ML (**Figures 2C,D**) since not all neural populations are labeled by commercial neural markers (see Supplementary Figure 1) (Bagley et al., 2007; Bianchi et al., 2014).

Statistical analysis showed no significant changes over time and genotype or between control and transgenic animals in the GrL (**Figure 2G**) [Two-way ANOVA (genotype vs. age): Interaction $F_{(3,\ 28)} = 0.7079$; $p = 0.5554$; Age $F_{(3,\ 28)} = 0.9086$; $p = 0.4494$; Genotype $F_{(1,\ 28)} = 0.7859$; $p = 0.3829$], ML [Two-way ANOVA (genotype vs. age): Interaction $F_{(3,\ 28)} = 2.443$; $p = 0.0849$; Age $F_{(3,\ 28)} = 0.8184$; $p = 0.4946$; Genotype $F_{(1,\ 28)} = 0.2668$; $p = 0.6095$] or GL [Two-way ANOVA (genotype vs. age): Interaction $F_{(3,\ 28)} = 2.054$; $p = 0.1291$; Age $F_{(3,\ 28)} = 2.496$; $p = 0.0803$; Genotype $F_{(1,\ 28)} = 0.005049$; $p = 0.9439$].

Analysis of Interneuron Markers

Calbindin-positive neurons were mostly concentrated in the GL in both control (**Figures 3A,C**) and transgenic (**Figures 3B,D**) animals. No significant changes were observed with aging (**Figures 3A,B** vs. **Figures 3C,D**) or genotype (**Figures 3A,C** vs.

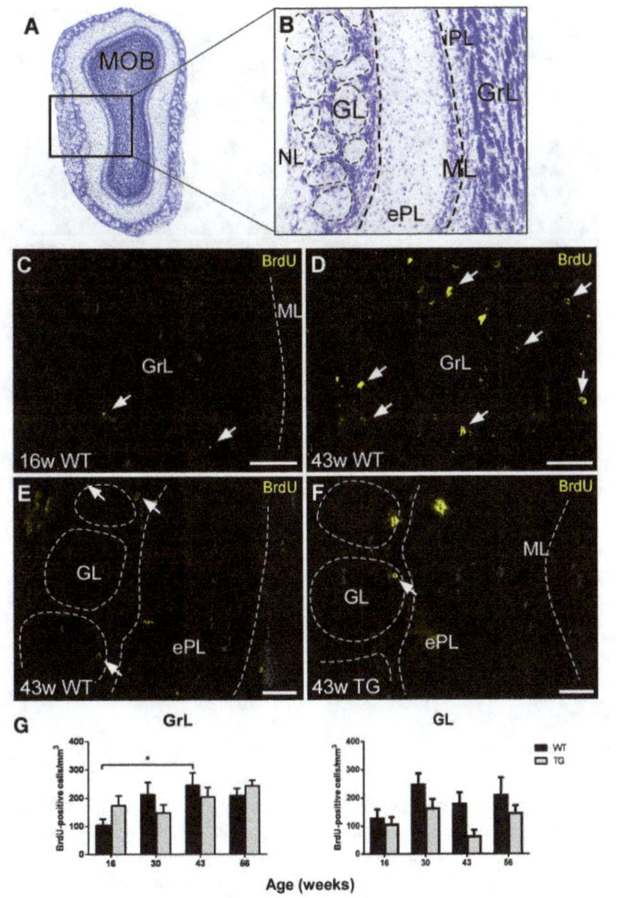

FIGURE 1 | Analysis of neurogenesis in the olfactory bulb by quantification of bromodeoxyuridine-labeled cells. (A,B) , Nissl staining of a mouse main olfactory bulb showing all cell layers where analysis has been carried out. **(C–F)**, examples of bromodeoxyuridine-positive cells at different ages, in different layers, and in wild type and transgenic animals illustrating statistical analysis. **(G)**, graphics illustrating the estimation of bromodeoxyuridine-positive cells/mm^3 in control and transgenic animals in different layers with aging. Calibration bar, 50 μm. White arrows point to labeled cells. *$P < 0.05$.

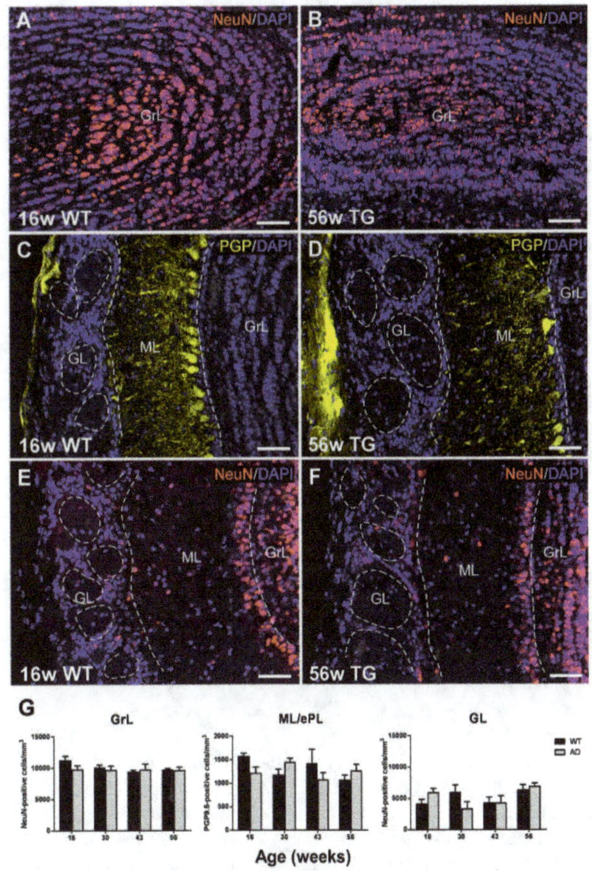

FIGURE 2 | Analysis of neurodegeneration in the olfactory bulb by quantification of NeuN- and PGP9.5-labeled cells. Confocal images showing NeuN-positive **(A,B,E,F)** and PGP9.5-positive cells **(C,D)** counterstained with DAPI. **(G)**, graphics illustrating the estimation of NeuN- and PGP9.5-positive cells/mm^3 in control and transgenic animals in the different layers with aging. Calibration bar, 50 μm.

Figures 3B,D) as demonstrated statistically (**Figure 3E**) [Two-way ANOVA (genotype vs. age): Interaction $F_{(3, 28)} = 1.679$; $p = 0.1940$; Age $F_{(3, 28)} = 1.942$; $p = 0.1457$; Genotype $F_{(1, 28)} = 0.2197$; $p = 0.6429$].

Most parvalbumin-labeled neurons appeared in the ML/ePL in control (**Figures 4A,C**) and transgenic mice (**Figures 4B,D**). The expression appear to increase from 16 (**Figures 4A,B**) to 56 (**Figures 4C,D**) in both control and transgenic animals. Statistical analysis demonstrated a significant increase from 16 to 43 and 56 weeks in transgenic animals (**Figure 4E**). No changes were significant between control and transgenic animals [Two-way ANOVA (genotype vs. age): Interaction $F_{(3, 28)} = 2.026$; $p = 0.1331$; Age $F_{(3, 28)} = 3.617$; $p = 0.0252$; Genotype $F_{(1, 28)} = 0.6551$; $p = 0.4251$].

Calretinin-expressing cells were distributed in the GrL/iPL and ML/ePL—where positive mitral cells have been included in the analysis—, but particularly in the GL/NL in both control and transgenic animals (**Figures 5A–F**). In the GrL/iPL of transgenic animals, the expression significantly increased from 30 (**Figure 5A**) to 56 (**Figure 5B**) weeks (**Figure 5G**) [Two-way ANOVA (genotype vs. age): Interaction $F_{(3, 28)} = 3.334$; $p = 0.0336$; Age $F_{(3, 28)} = 1.875$; $p = 0.1568$; Genotype $F_{(1, 28)} = 1.481$; $p = 0.2338$]. At 30 weeks, the expression in control animals was higher as compared to transgenic animals [*T*-test two tailed control vs. transgenic: $t_7 = 2.873$; $p = 0.0239$]. In the ML/ePL of control animals, the expression significantly decreased from 16 (**Figure 5C**) to 30, 43, and 56 (**Figure 5E**) weeks (**Figure 5G**); and, at 16 weeks, the expression in control animals (**Figure 5C**) was higher as compared to transgenic (**Figure 5D**) animals (**Figure 5F**) [Two-way ANOVA (genotype vs. age): Interaction $F_{(3, 28)} = 3.208$; $p = 0.0382$; Age $F_{(3, 28)} = 6.341$; $p = 0.0020$; Genotype $F_{(1, 28)} = 2.021$; $p = 0.1662$] [*T*-test two tailed control vs. transgenic: $p > 0.05$]. In the GL/NL, no significant changes with aging or genotype were detected (**Figures 5A–G**) [Two-way ANOVA (genotype vs. age): Interaction $F_{(3, 28)} = 1.031$; $p = 0.3940$; Age $F_{(3, 28)} = 0.7346$; $p = 0.5402$; Genotype $F_{(1, 28)} = 0.1791$; $p = 0.6754$].

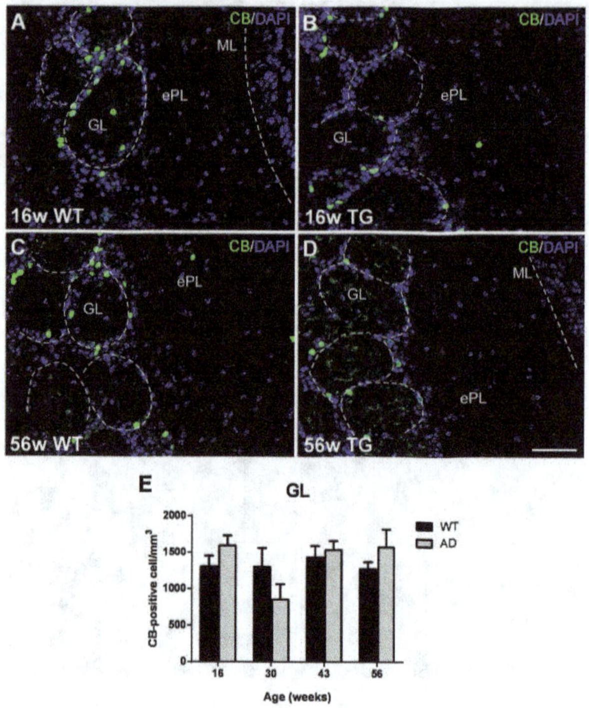

FIGURE 3 | Vulnerability analysis of calbindin-expressing cells in the olfactory bulb. (A–D), Confocal images showing calbindin-positive cells in the glomerular layer of control and transgenic animals at different ages. **(E)**, graphics illustrating the estimation of calbindin-positive cells/mm^3 in control and transgenic animals in the glomerular layer with aging. Calibration bar, 50 μm.

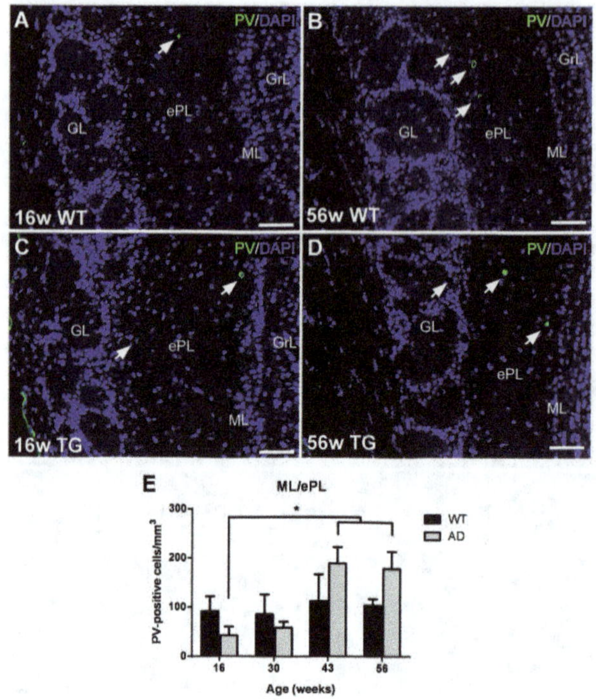

FIGURE 4 | Vulnerability analysis of parvalbumin-expressing cells in the olfactory bulb. (A–D), confocal images showing parvalbumin-positive cells in the mitral/external plexiform layer of control and transgenic animals at different ages. **(E)**, Graphics illustrating the estimation of parvalbumin-positive cells/mm^3 in control and transgenic animals in the mitral/external plexiform layer with aging. Calibration bar, 50 μm. White arrows point to labeled cells. $^*P < 0.05$.

Finally, regarding somatostatin-expression, cell bodies were mostly present in the ePL (**Figure 6A**) and only occasionally in the GrL (**Figure 6C**). Cell bodies degenerate with the disease leaving cell debris (**Figure 6A** vs. **Figure 6B** and **Figure 6C** vs. **Figure 6D**). To address, if cell bodies and/or fibers were reduced in different degree, we quantified the % of area within each region of interest occupied by somatostatin labeling (including cell bodies plus fibers) and total somatostatin positive cell bodies in the ePL. In this area, the reduction in % of area occupied by fibers and cell bodies starts early (at 30 weeks of age) and the reduction of somatostatin cell bodies is even sooner (at 16 weeks of age), suggesting that soluble pathology focuses on cell bodies (see discussion) (**Figure 6E**). Analysis of positive fibers and cells in the ePL [Two-way ANOVA (genotype vs. age): Interaction $F_{(3, 27)} = 2.308$; $p = 0.0990$; Age $F_{(3, 27)} = 0.8809$; $p = 0.4633$; Genotype $F_{(1, 27)} = 10.61$; $p = 0.0030$], GrL [Two-way ANOVA (genotype vs. age): Interaction $F_{(3, 27)} = 2.027$; $p = 0.1338$; Age $F_{(3, 27)} = 2.864$; $p = 0.0552$; Genotype $F_{(1, 27)} = 22.68$; $p < 0.0001$] and cell bodies in the ePL [Two-way ANOVA (genotype vs. age): Interaction $F_{(3, 27)} = 0.9887$; $p = 0.4129$; Age $F_{(3, 27)} = 7.861$; $p = 0.0006$; Genotype $F_{(1, 27)} = 71.01$; $p < 0.0001$] reveal significant lower expression in transgenic vs. control animals (**Figure 6E**). Further, in transgenic animals, a significant decrease with aging was observed in the expression of fibers and cells in the GrL [Two-way ANOVA (genotype vs. age): Interaction $F_{(3, 27)} = 2.027$; $p = 0.1338$; Age $F_{(3, 27)} = 2.864$; $p = 0.0552$; Genotype $F_{(1, 27)} = 22.68$; $p < 0.0001$] and in the expression of cell bodies in the ePL [Two-way ANOVA (genotype vs. age): Interaction $F_{(3, 27)} = 0.9887$; $p = 0.4129$; Age $F_{(3, 27)} = 7.861$; $p = 0.0006$; Genotype $F_{(1, 27)} = 71.01$; $p < 0.0001$] (**Figures 6E–G**).

Analysis of Aβ

As expected in the transgenic model, Aβ aggregation increased over time, but mostly restricted to the granule cell layer (**Figures 7A–E**). Percentage of area occupied by Aβ within GrL was significantly increased from 16 and 30 weeks vs. 43 and 56 weeks and from 43 to 56 weeks (**Figure 7F**) [One way ANOVA age: $F_{(3, 13)} = 91.87$, $p < 0.0001$].

Co-localization of Aβ, Interneuron Markers, and BrdU

Since analysis of interneuron vulnerability revealed that calretinin-positive and, particularly, somatostatin-positive cells were decreased in transgenic animals, additional colocalization experiments were carried out to provide qualitative observations (see Supplementary Figure 2). Examples of somatostatin-positive cells with a dystrophic appearance (Supplementary Figure 2A) were placed in Aβ plaques (Supplementary Figure 2B) surrounded by Aβ aggregates (Supplementary Figure 2C).

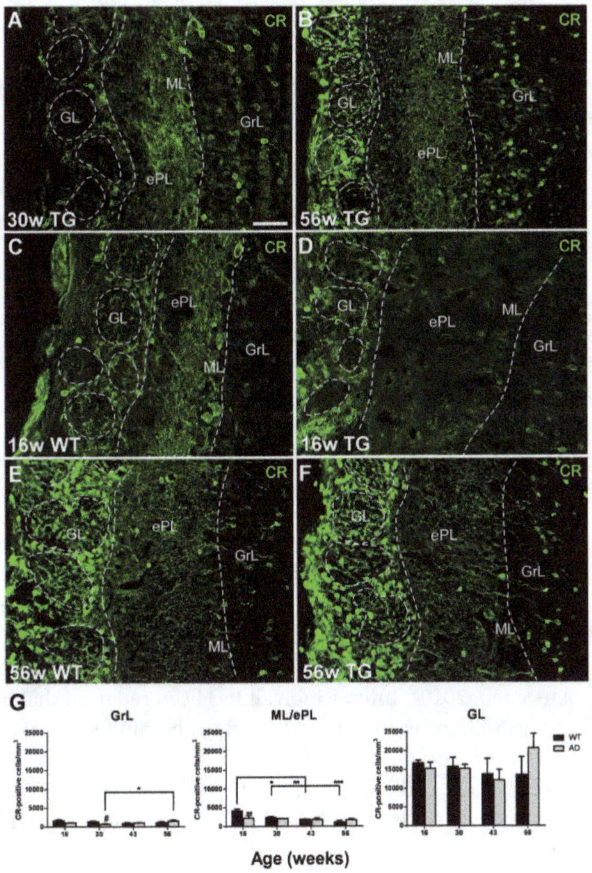

FIGURE 5 | Vulnerability analysis of calretinin-expressing cells in the olfactory bulb. (A–F), confocal images showing calretinin-positive cells in the different layers of control and transgenic animals at distinct ages. **(G)**, graphics illustrating the estimation of calretinin-positive cells/mm^3 in control and transgenic animals in the different layers with aging. Calibration bar, 50 μm. $^*P < 0.05$, $^{**}P < 0.01$, $^{***}P < 0.001$.

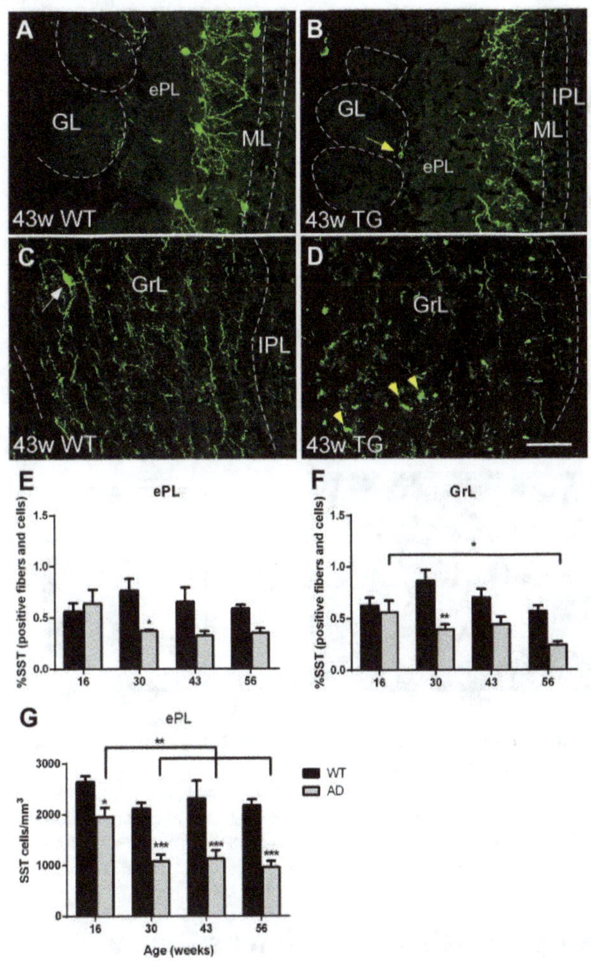

FIGURE 6 | Vulnerability analysis of somatostatin-expressing cells and fibers in the olfactory bulb. (A–D), Confocal images showing somatostatin-positive cells and fibers in the different layers of control and transgenic animals at distinct ages. **(E–G)**, graphics illustrating both % of area occupied by somatostatin cell bodies and fibers within ePL and GrL and the estimation of total somatostatin-positive in the ePL (cells/mm3) in control and transgenic animals. Calibration bar, 50 μm. White arrows point to labeled cells. Yellow arrow point to labeled periglomerular cell and yellow arrowheads to cell debries. $^*P < 0.05$, $^{**}P < 0.01$, $^{***}P < 0.001$.

Calretinin-positive cells (Supplementary Figure 2D) were also located in Aβ plaques (Supplementary Figures 2E,F).

The low rate of BrdU-labeled cells coexpressing interneuron markers prevented to carry out quantitative analysis. Only a small percentage of them were observed co-expressing somatostatin or calretinin (Supplementary Figure 3) and amyloid β (see Supplementary Figure 4).

DISCUSSION

In the present report, neurogenesis, neurodegeneration, interneuron vulnerability, and amyloid β involvement has been investigated in the OB of mouse model of AD and control animals over time. The main results include: neurogenesis increases with aging in the granule cell layer of control animals from 16 to 43 weeks. No neurodegeneration changes have been observed after quantifying NeuN or PGP9.5. Calbindin-expressing neurons remains unchanged. Parvalbumin-expressing neurons trend to increase with aging in transgenic animals. Calretinin-expressing neurons increase with aging in transgenic mice in the GrL and decrease in control animals in the ML and it is higher in control as compared to transgenic animals at given ages. Somatostatin-expressing neurons of transgenic mice decrease with aging and abruptly as compared to controls. Amyloid β aggregates with aging in the granule cell layer, which may be related to the particular involvement of somatostatin-expressing cells.

Therefore, neurogenesis in transgenic animals, in contrast to control animals, do not increase with aging. Regarding interneuron vulnerability, calbindin expression is not altered, parvalbumin expression is increased, calretinin increases in transgenic and decreases in control animals and somatostatin is strongly reduced with aging and in transgenic animals as compared to controls. This evidences differential vulnerability among interneuron pupulations which may be related to Aβ pathology.

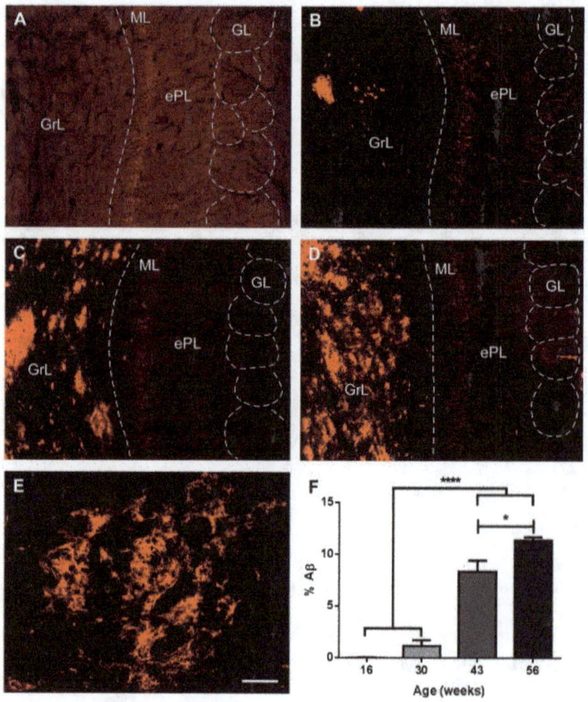

FIGURE 7 | Amyloid β aggregation over time in the olfactory bulb of transgenic animals. (A–D), %Aβ aggregates in transgenic mice at 16, 30, 43, and 56 weeks, respectively. **(E)**, high power of a plaque. **(F)**, graphics illustrating % of area occupied by Aβ, virtually restricted to the granule cell layer. Calibration bar for **(A–D)**, 80 μm, for E, 20 μm. *$P < 0.05$, ****$P < 0.0001$.

Neurogenesis in Alzheimer's Disease

Fifty years after the first seminal report of neurogenesis in the adult brain (Altman and Das, 1965), the specific role of new-born cells integrated in the DG (Kempermann et al., 2015) or OB (Lepousez et al., 2015) is not fully understood. Growing interest has focused on therapeutic opportunities, particularly regarding neurodegenerative diseases, in particular Huntington's, Parkinson's, and Alzheimer's diseases (Kaneko and Sawamoto, 2009; Lazarov et al., 2010; Winner et al., 2011; Winner and Winkler, 2015).

In the case of AD, there is a number of molecules implicated in its etiology that also play a key role in adult neurogenesis such as ApoE, PS1, APP, and its metabolites (Lazarov and Marr, 2010; Mu and Gage, 2011). In particular, it has been demonstrated that soluble APPα regulates neural progenitor cell proliferation and that miscleavage of APP could greatly influence in developmental and postnatal neurogenesis, which could contribute to symptomatic cognitive deficits in AD (Lazarov and Demars, 2012).

Data on neurogenic rates are quite variable depending on species, age, environment, and disease. Neurogenesis occurs in postnatal and adult rodents and postnatal humans (Lazarov and Marr, 2013) but, in adult humans, there is substantial hippocampal and striatal neurogenesis and it is no detectable in the OB (Bergmann et al., 2015). There is a general agreement regarding reduction of neurogenesis with aging (Hamilton et al., 2013), which contrast with our present results in control animals. In the granule cell layer, it has been described a decreasing number of new-born cell with aging (Petrenau and Alvarez-Buylla, 2002; Winner et al., 2002), which does not match our results. It is interesting to note that previous reports show non-significant peaks at 20 (Petrenau and Alvarez-Buylla, 2002) and 24 weeks (Winner et al., 2002) and ours results a significant peak at 43 weeks. Likely these discrepancies are due methodological differences regarding the method used: BrdU vs. [^{3}H]-thymidine or BrdU administration in 1 day vs. 4 consecutive days. In diseased brains, however, data are highly variable depending on the pathology analyzed. Even in AD, data are controversial depending on model used, experimental conditions, markers or area studied (Lazarov and Marr, 2010; Winner et al., 2011).

Reports in the double APP/PS1 transgenic model show a reduced hippocampal neurogenesis. Niidome and colleagues describe no reduction of proliferating cells in the SVZ, but a significant decrease in the SGZ (Niidome et al., 2008). Verret and colleagues report that, although hippocampal proliferation was unaffected, survival of newborn cells 4 weeks later was dramatically diminished (Verret et al., 2007). Conversely, Demars and colleagues, conclude that this neurogenesis impairment occurs early in life long before amyloid deposition (Demars et al., 2010). Interestingly, it has been reported that the reduction in neuroblasts was restricted to the hippocampal but not to the OB neurogenic system (Zhang et al., 2007). In fact, our results (**Figure 1**) show no significant reduction in the number of BrdU-labeled cells in the glomerular layer in APP/PS1 model.

Amyloid β Proteinopathy and Interneuron Population Involvement

Alzheimer disease is a neurodegenerative disease and as such, neuronal loss is expected. It is difficult, however, to distinguish neurodegenerative changes that accompany normal aging (Attems et al., 2015) from those that characterize AD. In the hippocampus, for instance, a significant cell loss was reported in CA1 in Alzheimer's patients, whereas there was almost no neuron loss in the normal aging group (West et al., 1994). In the OB, it has been reported that the total number of cells and the number of mitral cells were the same for controls and patients, but the volume of the bulb and the number of cells in the anterior olfactory nucleus was reduced up to 75% in younger patients (Ter Laak et al., 1994). Our results on the number of NeuN- and PGP9.5-positive cells in the different layers of the bulb reveal no neuronal loss with aging in both control and transgenic mice suggesting that volume reduction must be due to neuropil reorganization and shrinkage.

Amyloid β aggregation in the OB has been described as an early event in the neuropathology of AD (Ohm and Braak, 1987; Jellinger and Attems, 2005; Attems et al., 2012, 2014). In APP/PS1 mouse model, Aβ aggregation has been reported in the olfactory cortex (Saiz-Sanchez et al., 2012) as well as in the OB and anterior olfactory nucleus (Saiz-Sanchez et al., 2013). The present data are in agreement with these reports showing an accumulative aggregation of Aβ plaques in the OB, but restricted to the granule cell layer.

It has been described that the different interneuron populations show differential expression and vulnerability in the disease as compared to controls in given areas (Iritani et al., 2001; Saiz-Sanchez et al., 2016) and not in others (Leuba et al., 1998). In human tissue, it has been reported a 50% reduction in somatostatin expression in the anterior olfactory nucleus matching a high co-localization with Aβ (Saiz-Sanchez et al., 2010). In the piriform cortex, somatostatin and calretinin expression was reduced showing high co-localization with Aβ, whereas parvalbumin expression was increased (Saiz-Sanchez et al., 2015) in agreement with our present results. It is interesting to note that not only Aβ aggregates, but soluble Aβ—not detected with the used antibody—is particularly toxic for neurons. Other authors describes that calretinin-positive cells are resistant to neurodegeneration in the human temporal cortex (Fonseca and Soriano, 1995)—which matches the light increase described herein—and other authors reports differential vulnerability of parvalbumin-positive cells depending on the hippocampal field (Brady and Mufson, 1997) or entorhinal cortex (Solodkin et al., 1996; Mikkonen et al., 1999). In the olfactory cortex of APP/PS1 model, similar results were found being somatostatin and calretinin expression severely reduced and calbindin and parvalbumin expression later and only moderately reduced (Saiz-Sanchez et al., 2012). It is interesting to note that previous reports in our laboratory (Saiz-Sanchez et al., 2012, 2013) studied groups up to 8 months of age, whereas in the present report these observations were extended up to 56 weeks. Therefore, present data are in agreement with previous reports and enlarge previous descriptions reveling, for instance, a late increase of parvalbumin expression that could constitute a compensatory mechanism of some calcium binding protein expressing interneuron populations. In the OB, previous results were similar (Saiz-Sanchez et al., 2013) and in agreement with present data were calretinin- and, particularly somatostatin-, expression was reduced in transgenic as compared to control animals.

Regarding Alzheimer's etiology, it has been described that decreased somatostatin expression may predispose to Aβ accumulation. This finding has raised the possibility that somatostatin receptor agonists may be of therapeutic value in AD (Hama and Saido, 2005; Iwata et al., 2005; Saito et al., 2005; Saido and Iwata, 2006). The present results further support the idea that somatostatin expressing neurons are early and preferentially involved by Aβ pathology in AD and that this could be on its etiology.

AUTHOR CONTRIBUTIONS

CD experiments and analysis. DS, IU, AF analysis and quantification. AM coordination and writing.

ACKNOWLEDGMENTS

This study was supported by the Spanish Ministry of Science and Innovation-FEDER: grant BFU2010-15729; Spanish Ministry of Economy and Competitiveness-FEDER: grant SAF2014-52300-R; Autonomous Government of Castilla-La Mancha-FEDER: grant PEIC-2014-006-P.

REFERENCES

Altman, J. (1962). Are new neurons formed in the brains of adult mammals? *Science* 135, 1127–1128. doi: 10.1126/science.135.3509.1127

Altman, J., and Das, G. D. (1965). Autoradiographic and histological evidence of postnatal hippocampal neurogenesis in rats. *J. Comp. Neurol.* 124, 319–335. doi: 10.1002/cne.901240303

Attems, J., Thomas, A., and Jellinger, K. (2012). Correlations between cortical and subcortical tau pathology. *Neuropathol. Appl. Neurobiol.* 38, 582–590. doi: 10.1111/j.1365-2990.2011.01244.x

Attems, J., Walker, L., and Jellinger, K. A. (2014). Olfactory bulb involvement in neurodegenerative diseases. *Acta Neuropathol.* 127, 459–475. doi: 10.1007/s00401-014-1261-7

Attems, J., Walker, L., and Jellinger, K. A. (2015). Olfaction and aging: a mini-review. *Gerontology* 61, 485–490. doi: 10.1159/000381619

Bagley, J., Larocca, G., Jimenez, D. A., and Urban, N. N. (2007). Adult neurogenesis and specific replacement of interneuron subtypes in the mouse main olfactory bulb. *BMC Neurosci.* 8:92. doi: 10.1186/1471-2202-8-92

Ballard, C., Gauthier, S., Corbett, A., Brayne, C., Aarsland, D., and Jones, E. (2011). Alzheimer's disease. *Lancet* 377, 1019–1031. doi: 10.1016/S0140-6736(10)61349-9

Bergmann, O., Spalding, K. L., and Frisen, J. (2015). Adult Neurogenesis in Humans. *Cold Spring Harb. Perspect. Biol.* 7:a018994. doi: 10.1101/cshperspect.a018994

Bianchi, P., Bettini, S., Guidi, S., Ciani, E., Trazzi, S., Stagni, F., et al. (2014). Age-related impairment of olfactory bulb neurogenesis in the Ts65Dn mouse model of Down syndrome. *Exp. Neurol.* 251, 1–11. doi: 10.1016/j.expneurol.2013.10.018

Braak, H., Alafuzoff, I., Arzberger, T., Kretzschmar, H., and Del Tredici, K. (2006). Staging of Alzheimer disease-associated neurofibrillary pathology using paraffin sections and immunocytochemistry. *Acta Neuropathol.* 112, 389–404. doi: 10.1007/s00401-006-0127-z

Braak, H., and Braak, E. (1991). Neuropathological stageing of Alzheimer-related changes. *Acta Neuropathol.* 82, 239–259. doi: 10.1007/BF00308809

Braak, H., and Del Trecidi, K. (2015). Neuroanatomy and pathology of sporadic Alzheimer's disease. *Adv. Anat. Embryol. Cell Biol.* 215, 1–162. doi: 10.1007/978-3-319-12679-1_1

Brady, D. R., and Mufson, E. J. (1997). Parvalbumin-immunoreactive neurons in the hippocampal formation of Alzheimer's diseased brain. *Neuroscience* 80, 1113–1125. doi: 10.1016/S0306-4522(97)00068-7

De La Rosa-Prieto, C., Saiz-Sanchez, D., Ubeda-Bañon, I., Argandoña-Palacios, L., Garcia-Muñozguren, S., and Martinez-Marcos, A. (2009). Fate of marginal neuroblasts in the vomeronasal epithelium of adult mice. *J. Comp. Neurol.* 517, 723–736. doi: 10.1002/cne.22188

Demars, M., Hu, Y. S., Gadadhar, A., and Lazarov, O. (2010). Impaired neurogenesis is an early event in the etiology of familial Alzheimer's disease in transgenic mice. *J. Neurosci. Res.* 88, 2103–2117. doi: 10.1002/jnr.22387

Deng, W., Aimone, J. B., and Gage, F. H. (2010). New neurons and new memories: how does adult hippocampal neurogenesis affect learning and memory? *Nat. Rev. Neurosci.* 11, 339–350. doi: 10.1038/nrn2822

Devanand, D. P., Lee, S., Manly, J., Andrews, H., Schupf, N., Doty, R. L., et al. (2015). Olfactory deficits predict cognitive decline and Alzheimer dementia in an urban community. *Neurology* 84, 182–189. doi: 10.1212/WNL.0000000000001132

Fonseca, M., and Soriano, E. (1995). Calretinin-immunoreactive neurons in the normal human temporal cortex and in Alzheimer's disease. *Brain Res.* 691, 83–91. doi: 10.1016/0006-8993(95)00622-W

Goedert, M., and Spillantini, M. G. (2006). A century of Alzheimer's disease. *Science* 314, 777–781. doi: 10.1126/science.1132814

Hama, E., and Saido, T. C. (2005). Etiology of sporadic Alzheimer's disease: somatostatin, neprilysin, and amyloid beta peptide. *Med. Hypotheses* 65, 498–500. doi: 10.1016/j.mehy.2005.02.045

Hamilton, L. K., Joppé, S. E., M Cochard, L., and Fernandes, K. J. (2013). Aging and neurogenesis in the adult forebrain: what we have learned and where we should go from here. *Eur. J. Neurosci.* 37, 1978–1986. doi: 10.1111/ejn.12207

Iritani, S., Niizato, K., and Emson, P. C. (2001). Relationship of calbindin D28K-immunoreactive cells and neuropathological changes in the hippocampal formation of Alzheimer's disease. *Neuropathology* 21, 162–167. doi: 10.1046/j.1440-1789.2001.00393.x

Iwata, N., Higuchi, M., and Saido, T. C. (2005). Metabolism of amyloid-beta peptide and Alzheimer's disease. *Pharmacol. Ther.* 108, 129–148. doi: 10.1016/j.pharmthera.2005.03.010

Jahn, H. (2013). Memory loss in Alzheimer's disease. *Dialogues Clin. Neurosci.* 15, 445–454.

Jankowsky, J. L., Slunt, H. H., Gonzales, V., Jenkins, N. A., Copeland, N. G., and Borchelt, D. R. (2004). APP processing and amyloid deposition in mice haplo-insufficient for presenilin 1. *Neurobiol. Aging* 25, 885–892. doi: 10.1016/j.neurobiolaging.2003.09.008

Jankowsky, J. L., Slunt, H. H., Ratovitski, T., Jenkins, N. A., Copeland, N. G., and Borchelt, D. R. (2001). Co-expression of multiple transgenes in mouse CNS: a comparison of strategies. *Biomol. Eng.* 17, 157–165. doi: 10.1016/S1389-0344(01)00067-3

Jellinger, K. A., and Attems, J. (2005). Alzheimer pathology in the olfactory bulb. *Neuropathol. Appl. Neurobiol.* 31, 203. doi: 10.1111/j.1365-2990.2004.00619.x

Kaneko, N., and Sawamoto, K. (2009). Adult neurogenesis and its alteration under pathological conditions. *Neurosci. Res.* 63, 155–164. doi: 10.1016/j.neures.2008.12.001

Kempermann, G., Song, H., and Gage, F. H. (2015). Neurogenesis in the adult hippocampus. *Cold Spring Harb. Perspect. Med.* 5:a018812. doi: 10.1101/cshperspect.a018812

Lazarov, O., and Demars, M. P. (2012). All in the family: how the APPs regulate neurogenesis. *Front. Neurosci.* 6:81. doi: 10.3389/fnins.2012.00081

Lazarov, O., and Marr, R. A. (2010). Neurogenesis and Alzheimer's disease: at the crossroads. *Exp. Neurol.* 223, 267–281. doi: 10.1016/j.expneurol.2009.08.009

Lazarov, O., and Marr, R. A. (2013). Of mice and men: neurogenesis, cognition and Alzheimer's disease. *Front. Aging Neurosci.* 5:43. doi: 10.3389/fnagi.2013.00043

Lazarov, O., Mattson, M. P., Peterson, D. A., Pimplikar, S. W., and Van Praag, H. (2010). When neurogenesis encounters aging and disease. *Trends Neurosci.* 33, 569–579. doi: 10.1016/j.tins.2010.09.003

Lepousez, G., Nissant, A., and Lledo, P. M. (2015). Adult neurogenesis and the future of the rejuvenating brain circuits. *Neuron* 86, 387–401. doi: 10.1016/j.neuron.2015.01.002

Lepousez, G., Valley, M. T., and Lledo, P. M. (2013). The impact of adult neurogenesis on olfactory bulb circuits and computations. *Annu. Rev. Physiol.* 75, 339–363. doi: 10.1146/annurev-physiol-030212-183731

Leuba, G., Kraftsik, R., and Saini, K. (1998). Quantitative distribution of parvalbumin, calretinin, and calbindin D-28k immunoreactive neurons in the visual cortex of normal and Alzheimer cases. *Exp. Neurol.* 152, 278–291. doi: 10.1006/exnr.1998.6838

Levi, O., and Michaelson, D. M. (2007). Environmental enrichment stimulates neurogenesis in apolipoprotein E3 and neuronal apoptosis in apolipoprotein E4 transgenic mice. *J. Neurochem.* 100, 202–210. doi: 10.1111/j.1471-4159.2006.04189.x

Lois, C., and Alvarez-Buylla, A. (1994). Long-distance neuronal migration in the adult mammalian brain. *Science* 264, 1145–1148. doi: 10.1126/science.8178174

Luskin, M. B. (1993). Restricted proliferation and migration of postnatally generated neurons derived from the forebrain subventricular zone. *Neuron* 11, 173–189. doi: 10.1016/0896-6273(93)90281-U

Martinez-Marcos, A., Jia, C., Quan, W., and Halpern, M. (2005). Neurogenesis, migration, and apoptosis in the vomeronasal epithelium of adult mice. *J. Neurobiol.* 63, 173–187. doi: 10.1002/neu.20128

Martínez-Marcos, A., Ubeda-Bañón, I., Deng, L., and Halpern, M. (2000a). Neurogenesis in the vomeronasal epithelium of adult rats: evidence for different mechanisms for growth and neuronal turnover. *J. Neurobiol.* 44, 423–435. doi: 10.1002/1097-4695(20000915)44:43.0.CO;2-H

Martínez-Marcos, A., Ubeda-Bañón, I., and Halpern, M. (2000b). Cell turnover in the vomeronasal epithelium: evidence for differential migration and maturation of subclasses of vomeronasal neurons in the adult opossum. *J. Neurobiol.* 43, 50–63. doi: 10.1002/(SICI)1097-4695(200004)43:13.0.CO;2-N

Mikkonen, M., Alafuzoff, I., Tapiola, T., Soininen, H., and Miettinen, R. (1999). Subfield- and layer-specific changes in parvalbumin, calretinin and calbindin-D28K immunoreactivity in the entorhinal cortex in Alzheimer's disease. *Neuroscience* 92, 515–532. doi: 10.1016/S0306-4522(99)00047-0

Mu, Y., and Gage, F. H. (2011). Adult hippocampal neurogenesis and its role in Alzheimer's disease. *Mol. Neurodegener.* 6:85. doi: 10.1186/1750-1326-6-85

Niidome, T., Taniuchi, N., Akaike, A., Kihara, T., and Sugimoto, H. (2008). Differential regulation of neurogenesis in two neurogenic regions of APPswe/PS1dE9 transgenic mice. *Neuroreport* 19, 1361–1364. doi: 10.1097/WNR.0b013e32830e6dd6

Ohm, T. G., and Braak, H. (1987). Olfactory bulb changes in Alzheimer's disease. *Acta Neuropathol.* 73, 365–369. doi: 10.1007/BF00688261

Petrenau, L., and Alvarez-Buylla, A. (2002). Maturation and death of adult-born olfactory bulb granule neurons: role on olfaction. *J. Neurosci.* 22, 6106–6113.

Reiman, E. M. (2014). Alzheimer's disease and other dementias: advances in 2013. *Lancet Neurol.* 13, 3–5. doi: 10.1016/S1474-4422(13)70257-6

Saido, T. C., and Iwata, N. (2006). Metabolism of amyloid beta peptide and pathogenesis of Alzheimer's disease. Towards presymptomatic diagnosis, prevention and therapy. *Neurosci. Res.* 54, 235–253. doi: 10.1016/j.neures.2005.12.015

Saito, T., Iwata, N., Tsubuki, S., Takaki, Y., Takano, J., Huang, S. M., et al. (2005). Somatostatin regulates brain amyloid beta peptide Abeta42 through modulation of proteolytic degradation. *Nat. Med.* 11, 434–439. doi: 10.1038/nm1206

Saiz-Sanchez, D., De La Rosa-Prieto, C., Ubeda-Bañon, I., and Martinez-Marcos, A. (2013). Interneurons and beta-amyloid in the olfactory bulb, anterior olfactory nucleus and olfactory tubercle in APPxPS1 transgenic mice model of Alzheimer's disease. *Anat. Rec. (Hoboken).* 296, 1413–1423. doi: 10.1002/ar.22750

Saiz-Sanchez, D., De La Rosa-Prieto, C., Ubeda-Banon, I., and Martinez-Marcos, A. (2015). Interneurons, tau and amyloid-beta in the piriform cortex in Alzheimer's disease. *Brain Struct. Funct.* 220, 2011–2025. doi: 10.1007/s00429-014-0771-3

Saiz-Sanchez, D., Flores-Cuadrado, A., Ubeda-Bañon, I., De La Rosa-Prieto, C., and Martinez-Marcos, A. (2016). Interneurons in the human olfactory system in Alzheimer's disease. *Exp. Neurol.* 276, 13–21. doi: 10.1016/j.expneurol.2015.11.009

Saiz-Sanchez, D., Ubeda-Bañon, I., De La Rosa-Prieto, C., Argandoña-Palacios, L., Garcia-Muñozguren, S., Insausti, R., et al. (2010). Somatostatin, tau, and beta-amyloid within the anterior olfactory nucleus in Alzheimer disease. *Exp. Neurol.* 223, 347–350. doi: 10.1016/j.expneurol.2009.06.010

Saiz-Sanchez, D., Ubeda-Banon, I., De La Rosa-Prieto, C., and Martinez-Marcos, A. (2012). Differential expression of interneuron populations and correlation with amyloid-beta deposition in the olfactory cortex of an AbetaPP/PS1 transgenic mouse model of Alzheimer's disease. *J. Alzheimers. Dis.* 31, 113–129. doi: 10.3233/JAD-2012-111889

Solodkin, A., Veldhuizen, S. D., and Van Hoesen, G. W. (1996). Contingent vulnerability of entorhinal parvalbumin-containing neurons in Alzheimer's disease. *J. Neurosci.* 16, 3311–3321.

Ter Laak, H. J., Renkawek, K., and Van Workum, F. P. (1994). The olfactory bulb in Alzheimer disease: a morphologic study of neuron loss, tangles, and senile plaques in relation to olfaction. *Alzheimer Dis. Assoc. Disord.* 8, 38–48. doi: 10.1097/00002093-199408010-00007

Van Groen, T., Kiliaan, A. J., and Kadish, I. (2006). Deposition of mouse amyloid beta in human APP/PS1 double and single AD model transgenic mice. *Neurobiol. Dis.* 23, 653–662. doi: 10.1016/j.nbd.2006.05.010

Verret, L., Jankowsky, J. L., Xu, G. M., Borchelt, D. R., and Rampon, C. (2007). Alzheimer's-type amyloidosis in transgenic mice impairs survival of newborn neurons derived from adult hippocampal neurogenesis. *J. Neurosci.* 27, 6771–6780. doi: 10.1523/JNEUROSCI.5564-06.2007

West, M. J., Coleman, P. D., Flood, D. G., and Troncoso, J. C. (1994). Differences in the pattern of hippocampal neuronal loss in normal ageing and Alzheimer's disease. *Lancet* 344, 769–772. doi: 10.1016/S0140-6736(94)92338-8

Winner, B., Cooper-Kuhn, C. M., Aigner, R., Winkler, J., and Kuhn, H. G. (2002). Long-term survival and cell death of newly generated neurons in the adult rat olfactory bulb. *Eur. J. Neurosci.* 16, 1681–1689. doi: 10.1046/j.1460-9568.2002.02238.x

Winner, B., Kohl, Z., and Gage, F. H. (2011). Neurodegenerative disease and adult neurogenesis. *Eur. J. Neurosci.* 33, 1139–1151. doi: 10.1111/j.1460-9568.2011.07613.x

Winner, B., and Winkler, J. (2015). Adult neurogenesis in neurodegenerative diseases. *Cold Spring Harb. Perspect. Biol.* 7:a021287. doi: 10.1101/cshperspect.a021287

Zhang, C., Mcneil, E., Dressler, L., and Siman, R. (2007). Long-lasting impairment in hippocampal neurogenesis associated with amyloid deposition in a knock-in mouse model of familial Alzheimer's disease. *Exp. Neurol.* 204, 77–87. doi: 10.1016/j.expneurol.2006.09.018

12

Environmental Enrichment, Age, and PPARα Interact to Regulate Proliferation in Neurogenic Niches

Margarita Pérez-Martín[1†], Patricia Rivera[2†], Eduardo Blanco[2,3†], Clara Lorefice[1,2], Juan Decara[2], Francisco J. Pavón[2], Antonia Serrano[2], Fernando Rodríguez de Fonseca[2] and Juan Suárez[2]*

[1] Departamento de Biología Celular, Genética y Fisiología, Instituto de Investigación Biomédica de Málaga, Universidad de Málaga, Málaga, Spain, [2] UGC Salud Mental, Instituto de Investigación Biomédica de Málaga, Universidad de Málaga-Hospital Universitario Regional de Málaga, Málaga, Spain, [3] Departament de Pedagogia i Psicologia, Facultat d'Educació, Psicologia i Treball Social, Universitat de Lleida, Lleida, Spain

Edited by:
José Luis Trejo, Cajal Institute-CSIC, Spain

Reviewed by:
Francis G. Szele, University of Oxford, UK
Djoher Nora Abrous, Institut des Neurosciences de Bordeaux, France
María Llorens-Martín, Consejo Superior de Investigaciones Científicas, Spain

***Correspondence:**
Juan Suárez
juan.suarez@ibima.eu;
fernando.rodriguez@ibima.eu

[†] First co-authors.

Peroxisome proliferator-activated receptor alpha (PPARα) ligands have been shown to modulate recovery after brain insults such as ischemia and irradiation by enhancing neurogenesis. In the present study, we investigated the effect of the genetic deletion of PPARα receptors on the proliferative rate of neural precursor cells (NPC) in the adult brain. The study was performed in aged *Pparα*$^{-/-}$ mice exposed to nutritional (treats) and environmental (games) enrichments for 20 days. We performed immunohistochemical analyses of cells containing the replicating cell DNA marker 5-bromo-2′-deoxyuridine (BrdU+) and the immature neuronal marker doublecortin (Dcx+) in the main neurogenic zones of the adult brain: subgranular zone of dentate gyrus (SGZ), subventricular zone of lateral ventricles (SVZ), and/or hypothalamus. Results indicated a reduction in the number of BrdU+ cells in the neurogenic zones analyzed as well as Dcx+ cells in the SGZ during aging (2, 6, and 18 months). *Pparα* deficiency alleviated the age-related reduction of NPC proliferation (BrdU+ cells) in the SVZ of the 18-months-old mice. While no genotype effect on NPC proliferation was detected in the SGZ during aging, an accentuated reduction in the number of Dcx+ cells was observed in the SGZ of the 6-months-old *Pparα*$^{-/-}$ mice. Exposing the 18-months-old mice to nutritional and environmental enrichments reversed the *Pparα*$^{-/-}$-induced impairment of NPC proliferation in the neurogenic zones analyzed. The enriched environment did not modify the number of SGZ Dcx+ cells in the 18 months old *Pparα*$^{-/-}$ mice. These results identify PPARα receptors as a potential target to counteract the naturally observed decline in adult NPC proliferation associated with aging and impoverished environments.

Keywords: aging, environment, PPARα, subventricular zone, hippocampus, neurogenesis

---

Abbreviations: 3v, third ventricle; ARC, arcuate nucleus of hypothalamus; BrdU, 5-bromo-2′-deoxyuridine; Dcx, doublecortin; EE, enriched environment; gcl, granular cell layer; lv, lateral ventricle; ml, molecular layer; NPC, neural proliferative cells; pcl, polymorphic cell layer; *Pparα*$^{-/-}$, homozygous knockout in peroxisome proliferator-activated receptor alpha; SE, standard environment; SGZ, subgranular zone of dentate gyrus; Str, striatum; SVZ, subventricular zone of the lateral ventricles; VMH, ventromedial nucleus of hypothalamus; WT, wild-type.

INTRODUCTION

Neural progenitor/proliferative cells (NPC) are derived from embryonic radial-glial cells that have the ability to divide, self-renew and generate functional differentiated cells (neurons and glia) during the entire life of the animal (Doetsch, 2003b). NPC are localized in discrete regions of the adult mammalian brain called stem cells niches, such as the subventricular zone (SVZ) lining the walls of the lateral ventricles and the subgranular zone (SGZ) of the hippocampal dentate gyrus, which are capable of promoting neurogenesis and gliogenesis (Doetsch et al., 1999; Doetsch, 2003a; Lie et al., 2004; Albayram et al., 2011). In the last decade, several studies evidenced the hypothalamus as a novel neurogenic zone in the adult brain, especially after insults (Rivera et al., 2011; Robins et al., 2013; Maggi et al., 2014; Lin and Iacovitti, 2015; Lin et al., 2015).

It is well-known that NPC proliferation and neuronal differentiation are regulated by intrinsic (growth factors, neurotransmitters, hormones) and external (environment, caloric intake, drugs) factors, as well as by epigenetic mechanisms that intermediate in between the environment and the genome (Alvarez-Buylla and Lim, 2004; Arias-Carrion et al., 2007; Montalban-Loro et al., 2015). A critical factor affecting the rate of adult neurogenesis is age (Drapeau et al., 2003; Aizawa et al., 2009; Coras et al., 2010; Ngwenya et al., 2015). In adult rodents, hippocampal neurogenesis persists throughout the lifespan but suffers from progressive age-associated declines (Kuhn et al., 1996; McDonald and Wojtowicz, 2005). This fact is relevant since aging is also associated with an increased risk for cerebral insults, even in healthy subjects. Multiple studies have linked the age-induced decline of NPC and neurogenesis with neurodegenerative diseases and cognitive performance (Van Praag et al., 2005; Paillard, 2015). However, others reports have suggested that such a relationship does not exist (Bizon and Gallagher, 2003; Merrill et al., 2003). Several factors have a positive influence on cerebral decline associated with normal aging. In this line, environmental enrichment, including nutrition and physical activity, may improve brain function in normal animals and in animals with brain-related disorders, such as Alzheimer and other aging-related cerebral diseases, which, in part, are likely mediated through the enhancement of neurogenesis (Fan et al., 2007; Zhao et al., 2015; Garthe et al., 2016).

Peroxisome proliferator-activated receptors (PPARs) belong to a nuclear receptor superfamily capable of regulating physiological responses associated with inflammatory responses, energy metabolism, and cell proliferation, differentiation, migration and survival (Rosen and Spiegelman, 2001; Smith et al., 2003; Fidaleo et al., 2014). It has been reported that PPARα and its endogenous ligands (eicosanoids, leukotrienes, and endocannabinoid-like molecules such as oleoylethanolamide or OEA) support a role in neuroprotection against oxidative stress, which is target for neurodegenerative diseases and contribute to normal brain aging (Nunomura et al., 2012; Zolezzi et al., 2013; Fidaleo et al., 2014). PPARα is expressed in neuronal, astroglial, and ependymal cells and may be relevant in glutamatergic, dopaminergic, and cholinergic neurotransmission (Zhou and Waxman, 1998; Avshalumov and Rice, 2002; Melis et al., 2013). For instance, PPARα activity modulates acetylcholine release and ameliorates cognitive and memory decline associated with aging (Hajjar et al., 2012). OEA-PPARα interaction facilitates memory consolidation through noradrenergic activity (Campolongo et al., 2009), modulates satiety responses through hypothalamic neurons (Romano et al., 2013), and regulates motivational responses for alcohol through the peripheral nervous system (Bilbao et al., 2015). Interestingly, the involvement of PPARα in cell proliferation and apoptosis (Roberts et al., 2002; Cimini et al., 2007; Cimini and Ceru, 2008) as well as neural cell differentiation and maturation has been demonstrated (Cristiano et al., 2005; Bento-Abreu et al., 2007; Fandel et al., 2013). PPARα activation (for instance, through the elevation of the PPARα endogenous ligands in the brain) preserves hippocampal neurogenesis and inhibits microglial activity (Ramanan et al., 2009; Rivera et al., 2015a).

Although, PPARα may be a potential therapeutic target in neurodegenerative, neuroinflammatory and neurocognitive alterations related to Alzheimer and Parkinson's diseases (Plaza-Zabala et al., 2010; Scuderi et al., 2012; Fidaleo et al., 2014; González-Aparicio et al., 2014), the involvement of PPARα in age-related decline and environmental enrichment-induced enhancement of adult neurogenesis is still uncertain. The present study designed an experimental approach to investigate the potential role of PPARα in adult NPC proliferation by focusing on the impact of sustained external stimulation through food and play. Immunohistochemistry were performed to analyze cells that contained the replicating cell DNA marker 5-bromo-2′-deoxyuridine (BrdU+) in the main neurogenic zones (SVZ, SGZ, and hypothalamus), as well as cells expressing the immature neuronal factor doublecortin (Dcx+) in the SGZ. This study was performed in adult aged mice lacking *Pparα* gene expression (*Pparα*$^{-/-}$) that were previously exposed to nutritional (treats) and environmental (games) enrichments for 20 days.

MATERIALS AND METHODS

Ethics Statement

The protocols and procedures were approved by the Ethics Committee of Malaga University (CEUMA: 2014-0001-A) and performed in compliance with European animal research laws [European Communities Council Directives2010/63/UE, 90/219/CEE, Regulation (EC) No 1946/2003] and Spanish National and Regional Guidelines for Animal Experimentation and Use of Genetically Modified Organisms (Real Decreto 53/2013, Ley 32/2007, and Ley 9/2003, Real Decreto 178/2004, Decreto 320/2010). All efforts were made to minimize animal suffering and reduce the number of animals used.

Animals

Adult wild-type (WT) and *Pparα*$^{-/-}$ (KO) male mice (The Jackson Laboratories, Bar Harbor, ME, USA) derived from intercrosses between heterozygous *Pparα*$^{+/-}$ mice on a C57Bl/6 background were jointly housed in cages and maintained in standard conditions at 20 ± 2°C room temperature with 40 ± 5% relative humidity and a 12-h light/dark cycle with a dawn/dusk effect (Animal House, University of Málaga). Standard rodent chow (Prolab RMH 2500, 2.9 kcal/g) and water were available *ad libitum*.

Aging

The SVZ, SGZ and hypothalamus of the WT and *Pparα*$^{-/-}$ mice at ages of 2, 6, and 18 months old were analyzed. Six experimental groups were obtained depending on the age and genotype ($n = 6$ mice per group): WT 2 months group, WT 6 months group, WT 18 months group, *Pparα*$^{-/-}$ (KO) 2 months group, *Pparα*$^{-/-}$ (KO) 6 months group, and *Pparα*$^{-/-}$ (KO) 18 months group.

Environmental Enrichment

A new batch of WT and *Pparα*$^{-/-}$ mice at 18 months old ($n = 10$ animals per genotype) were randomly selected to perform the environmental enrichment experiments. Thus, half of the mice from each genotype ($n = 5$) were housed in an enriched environment (EE) or standard environment (SE) cages for 20 days (**Figure 1**). We designed two EE configurations (a and b, see **Figure 1A**), which consisted of two large cages (59.5 × 38 × 20 cm) with different set of objects and games such as ramps, floor platforms, tunnels, and toys. WT and *Pparα*$^{-/-}$ mice were changed to a or b environmental configurations every 2 days, up to 20 days, to avoid habituation induced by prolonged contextual (spatial) stimulation. Nutritional enrichment was also performed by adding different treats such as fruits, crackers, and cheese in cycles of 6 days for 20 days (**Figure 1B**). The control WT and *Pparα*$^{-/-}$ mice were housed in standard environment cages (equal cage dimension but no objects inside) and fed with the standard chow but without nutritional enrichment (treats). Four experimental groups were obtained depending on the genotype and environment ($n = 5$ mice per group): WT SE group, WT EE group, *Pparα*$^{-/-}$ (KO) SE group, and *Pparα*$^{-/-}$ (KO) EE group.

BrdU Administration

5′-bromo-2′-deoxyuridine (BrdU, cat. no. B5002, Sigma, St. Louis, MO, USA) was dissolved at 15 mg/mL in sterile 0.9% NaCl solution. BrdU was i.p. administered at a dose of 50 mg/kg body weight once per day for 3 consecutive days (day 17–19) and twice at the last EE-day (day 20, 4 h between injections). The animals were killed 12 h after the last injection of BrdU was administered.

Brain Collection

All animals were intraperitoneally (i.p.) anesthetized (sodium pentobarbital, 50 mg/kg body weight) and transcardially perfused

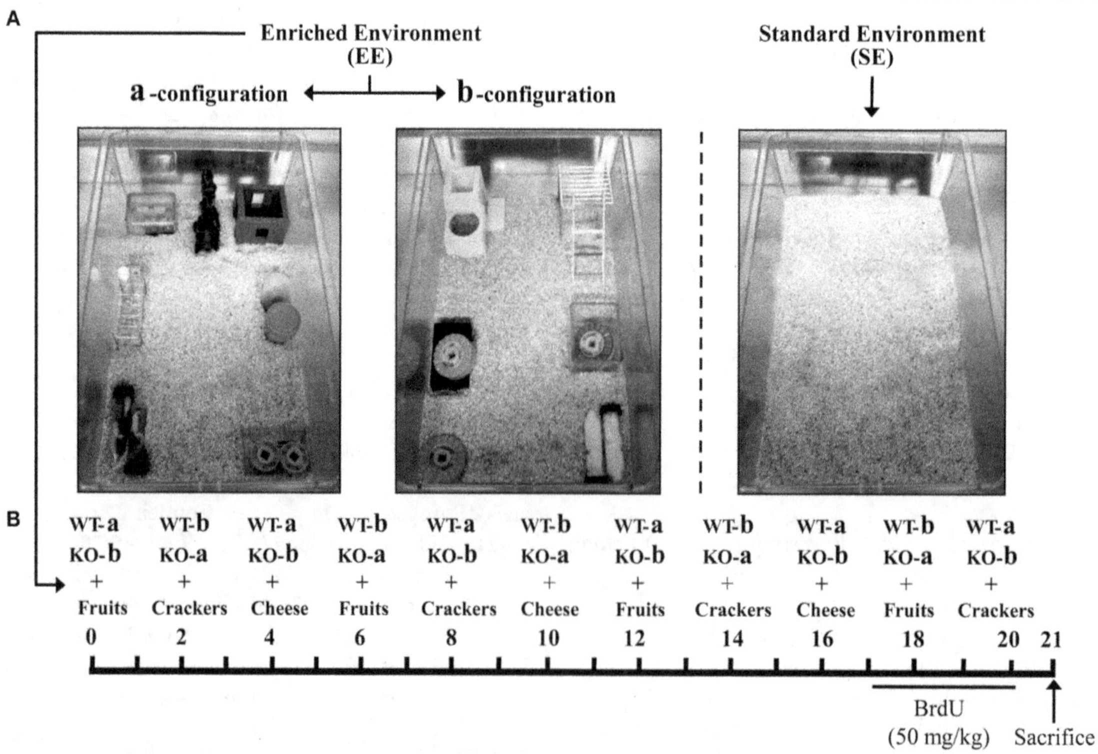

FIGURE 1 | (A) Housing conditions of the wild-type (WT) and *Pparα*$^{-/-}$ (KO) mice. The photographs illustrated the different set of environmental configurations: two enriched environmental configurations (a and b) consisting of a contextual stimulation with ramps, floor platforms, tunnels and toys, and a standard environment (a standard housing cage). **(B)** Schematic diagram showing the experiment design. The mice from each genotype were randomly assigned to the standard environment (SE) or the nutritional and environmental enrichment (EE) for 20 days. The mice rotated between the enriched configurations a and b every 2 days. Nutritional enrichment consisted of the administration of different treats such as fruits, crackers, and cheese in cycles of 6 days. The last 4 days previous to sacrifice, all animals were injected with BrdU (50 mg/kg).

with 4% formaldehyde in 0.1 M phosphate buffer (PB). The brains were dissected out and kept in the same fixative solution overnight at 4°C. The brains were then cryoprotected and cut into 30-μm-thick coronal sections by using a sliding microtome (Leica VT1000S). Sections were divided in eight parallel series until use for immunohistochemistry.

Immunohistochemistry

Free-floating coronal sections from −1.58 to −2.46 mm Bregma levels (hippocampus and hypothalamus) and 1.42 to −0.10 mm Bregma levels (striatum) from one of the five parallel series obtained from each mouse brain were selected for each immunohistochemistry (Paxinos and Franklin, 2004). Sections were first washed several times with PBS to remove sodium azide. Then, sections were incubated in a solution of 3% hydrogen peroxide and 10% methanol in PB 0.1 M for 45 min at room temperature in darkness to inactivate endogenous peroxidase. After three washes in PBS for 10 min, DNA was denatured by exposing sections to HCl 2 N for 15 min at 37°C, followed by two washes in borate buffer 0.15 M to neutralize pH. After three additional washes in PBS for 10 min, sections were incubated in a blocking solution containing 0.3% albumin, 0.3% triton X-100 and 0.05% sodium azide in PBS for 45 min. Sections were incubated overnight in the primary antibody rat anti-BrdU (1:500; Accurate Chemical & Scientific, Westbury, NY, USA, cat. no. OBT0030G) at 4°C. For doublecortin immunohistochemistry, selected sections at hippocampal levels were firstly incubated in a solution of 3% hydrogen peroxide and 10% methanol in PB 0.1 M for 10 min, secondly incubated in a blocking solution containing 5% horse serum, 0.3% triton X-100 and 0.05% sodium azide in PBS for 1 h, and finally incubated overnight in the primary antibody goat anti-doublecortin (1:500; Santa Cruz Biotechnology, cat. no. sc-8066) at room temperature. The following day the sections were incubated in the biotinylated donkey anti-rat IgG (H+L) antibody (1:500, Novex; cat. no. A18743) or the biotinylated horse anti-goat IgG antibody (1:1000, Vector; cat. no. BA-9500) for 90 min. The sections were then incubated in ExtrAvidin peroxidase (Sigma, St. Louis, MO) diluted 1:2000 in darkness at room temperature for 1 h. Finally, immunolabeling was revealed with 0.05% diaminobenzidine (DAB; Sigma) and 0.03% H_2O_2 in PBS.

Quantification of BrdU and Doublecortin-Immunoreactive Cells

The average density of positive cells per animal was quantified. Thus, the estimation of the number of cells per section (30 μm deep) and area (mm^2) in both hemispheres was calculated according to the following formula: $Na = \sum(Q\text{-})/\sum(a_{str})$, where $\sum Q$- is the total number of positive cells counted per animal and a_{str} is the area of the structure analyzed. Each structure analyzed consisted of ~6 coronal sections, which resulted in one of every five equidistant sections (one representative section for each 180 μm) according to the rostro-caudal extent. To outline the area of study, the region of interest was drawn in each structure, whose identification was performed at Bregma −1.58 to −2.46 mm in hippocampal and hypothalamic levels, and at Bregma 1.42 to −0.10 mm in striatal levels according to a mouse brain atlas and cytoarchitectonic criteria (Paxinos and Franklin, 2004). Thus, the BrdU-immunoreactive (-ir) nuclei and doublecortin-ir cells that came into focus were manually counted in the subgranular zone (SGZ) of the dentate gyrus and/or the subventricular zone (SVZ) of the lateral ventricles. Regarding the hypothalamus, counting was performed in the ventromedial (VMH) and arcuate (ARC) nuclei of the hypothalamus and median eminence. Quantification were performed using a standard optical microscope with the 40X objective (Nikon Instruments Europe B.V., Amstelveen, The Netherlands) coupled to the NIS-Elements Imaging Software 3.00 (Nikon). The data were expressed as the number of positive cells per area (mm^2).

Statistical Analysis

Statistical analysis of the results was performed using the computer program GraphPad Prism version 5.04 (GraphPad Software Inc., San Diego, CA, USA). Data were represented as the mean ± s.e.m. for five-six determinations depending on the experimental group. Statistical analysis was performed using two-way ANOVA followed by Bonferroni *post hoc* test for multiple comparisons. $P < 0.05$ was considered to be significant.

RESULTS

Effect of Age and Genotype on SVZ, SGZ, and Hypothalamic Cell Proliferation

Typical clustering of newborn cells containing nuclear BrdU labeling was observed in the SVZ of the lateral ventricles extending from the ventral to the dorsolateral ventricular peak and into the rostral migratory stream following a transversal view of the adult mouse brain (**Figure 2**). This arrangement of the SVZ BrdU+ cells was more evident in the younger mice that the older ones. Scattered BrdU+ cells were found in the SGZ of the dentate gyrus as well as in a hypothalamic area, by the wall of the third ventricle, including the hypothalamic ventromedial and arcuate nuclei, and the median eminence. Qualitatively, we observed a less number of cells containing BrdU in the three neurogenic niches during the ages analyzed (**Figure 2**).

Two-way ANOVA showed an age effect (2, 6, and 18 months) on the three neurogenic areas [SVZ: $F_{(2,\ 19)} = 12.98$; $P < 0.001$; SGZ: $F_{(2,\ 19)} = 41.73$, $P < 0.001$; hypothalamus: $F_{(2,\ 19)} = 5.51$; $P < 0.05$; **Figure 2**]. Interestingly, a genotype effect (WT and KO) was found in the number of BrdU+ cells in the SVZ [$F_{(1,\ 19)} = 6.45$, $P < 0.05$], but not in the SGZ or hypothalamus. No interaction between age and genotype was detected, that is, PPARα deficiency did not produce a different effect on cell proliferation during aging.

After performing the Bonferroni analysis, we found a decreased number of BrdU+ cells in the SVZ of the lateral ventricles of the 18 months old WT mice compared to that of the 2 and 6 months old WT mice ($^{**\#\#}P < 0.01$; (**Figures 2A,D–F**). The number of BrdU+ cells was lower in the SVZ of the 18 months old KO mice than that of the 6 months old KO mice ($^{\$}P < 0.05$), but in increased compared to those of the 18 months old WT mice ($^{\&}P < 0.05$; (**Figures 2A,F–I**). In the SGZ of the dentate gyrus, the number of BrdU+ cells decreased in the 6 and 18 months old WT mice ($^{***}P < 0.01$ and $^{***}P < 0.001$,

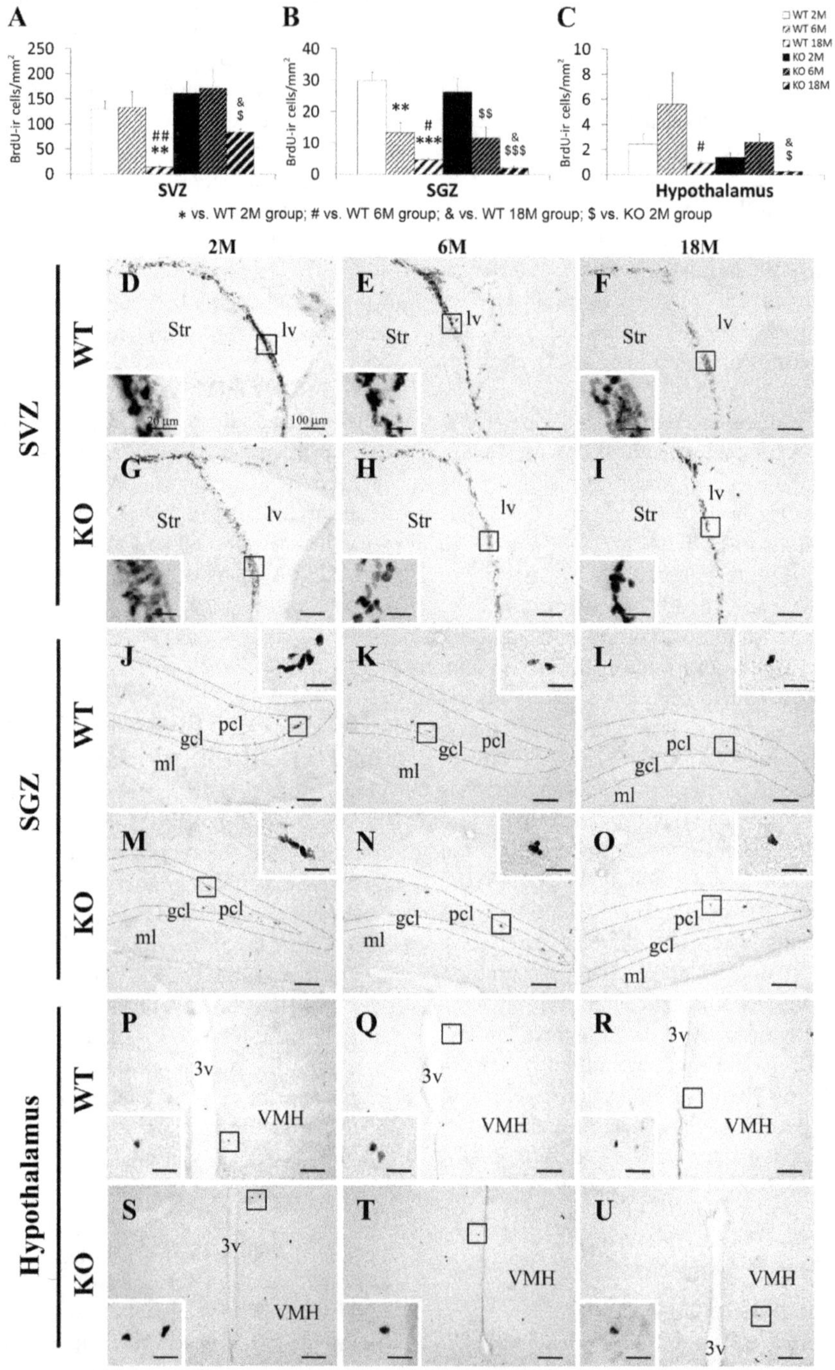

FIGURE 2 | Effect of age (2, 6, and 18 months) on the number of cells that contained BrdU in the SVZ (A), SGZ (B), and hypothalamus (C) of WT and *Ppar*$\alpha^{-/-}$ (KO) mice. The data were expressed as the media of the number of BrdU+ cells per area (mm^2) + s.e.m ($N = 6$). Bonferroni's test: $^{**}P < 0.01$, $^{***}p < 0.001$ vs. WT 2M group; $^{\#}P < 0.05$, $^{\#\#}P < 0.01$ vs. WT 6M group; $^{\&}P < 0.05$ vs. WT 18M group; $^{\$}P < 0.05$, $^{\$\$}P < 0.01$, $^{\$\$\$}P < 0.001$ vs. KO 2M group. **(D–U)** Representative photomicrographs showing low and high (insets) magnification views of the typical clustering of newborn cells containing the BrdU labeling in the SGZ, SVZ, and hypothalamus of 2, 6, and 18 months old WT and KO mice. Scale bars (100 µm and 20 µm for insets) are included in each image.

respectively) and the 6 and 18 months old KO mice ($^{\$\$}P < 0.01$ and $^{\$\$\$}P < 0.001$, respectively) compared to the respective 2 months old WT and KO mice (**Figures 2B,J–O**). The number of BrdU+ cells in the SGZ of the 18 months old WT mice was also decreased when it was compared to that of the 6 months old WT mice ($^{\#}P < 0.05$; **Figures 2B,K,L**). The number of BrdU+ cells in the SGZ of the 18 months old KO mice was decreased when it was compared to that of the 18 months old WT mice

($^{\&}P < 0.05$; **Figures 2B,L,O**). A decrease of BrdU+ cells was also found in the hypothalamus of the 18 months old WT and KO mice compared to the respective 6 months old WT and KO mice ($^{\$}P < 0.05$; **Figures 2C,Q,R,T,U**). The number of BrdU+ cells in the hypothalamus of the 18 months old KO mice showed a decrease when it was compared to that of the 18 months old WT mice ($^{\&}P < 0.05$; **Figures 2C,R,U**).

Effect of Environmental Enrichment and Genotype on SVZ, SGZ, and Hypothalamic Cell Proliferation in 18 Months Old Mice

Scattered clustering of newborn cells containing nuclear BrdU labeling was observed in the SVZ of the 18 months old mice (**Figure 3**). Qualitatively, this arrangement of the SVZ BrdU+ cells was more prominent in the mice lacking PPARα receptors. The BrdU+ cells found in the SGZ and the hypothalamus of the older mice was very scarce. Qualitatively, we also observed a higher number of BrdU+ cells in the SGZ and the hypothalamus of the 18 months old mice exposed to the enriched environment (**Figure 3**).

Two-way ANOVA showed an environmental enrichment effect on the number of BrdU+ cells in the SGZ [$F_{(1, 21)} = 5.62$; $P < 0.05$] and the hypothalamus [$F_{(1, 21)} = 7.2$; $P < 0.05$], but not in the SVZ (**Figure 3**). A genotype effect (WT and KO) on the number of BrdU+ cells was found in the SVZ [$F_{(1, 21)} = 48.34$; $P < 0.001$] and the SGZ [$F_{(1, 21)} = 7.72$; $P < 0.05$], but not in the hypothalamus. Interaction between environmental enrichment and genotype was detected in SVZ cell proliferation [$F_{(1, 21)} = 7.47$; $P < 0.05$] and hypothalamic cell proliferation [$F_{(1, 21)} = 4.32$; $P < 0.05$], that is, PPARα deficiency produced a different effect on SVZ and hypothalamic cell proliferation in an environment dependent-manner.

A Bonferroni analysis showed that the number of BrdU+ cells increased in the SVZ, but decreased in the SGZ and the hypothalamus of the KO mice compared to the WT ones when they were housed in a standard environment ($^{*/***}P < 0.05/0.001$; (**Figures 3A–C,D,F,H,J,L,N**). The number of BrdU+ cells was also increased in the SVZ of the KO mice compared to the WT ones when they were housed in an enriched environment for 20 days ($^{\$\$}P < 0.01$; (**Figures 3A,E,G**). The number of BrdU+ cells in the SVZ of the KO mice housed in an enriched environment decreased compared to those of the respective standard environment KO group ($^{\#}P < 0.05$; (**Figures 3A,F,G**). In contrast, an increase in the number of BrdU+ cells was found in the SGZ of the WT and KO mice (**Figures 3B,H–K**) and the hypothalamus of the KO mice (**Figures 3C,N,O**) housed in an enriched environment ($^{*/\#}P < 0.05$).

Effect of Age, Genotype, and Environmental Enrichment on SGZ Cells Expressing Doublecortin

We analyzed the number of Dcx+ cells in the SGZ of the WT and KO mice with 2, 6, and 18 months old, and with or without environmental enrichment (**Figure 4**). The presence of the Dcx+ cells in the SGZ was more evident in the younger mice that the older mice. Numerous cells expressing Dcx presented a cell body with a pyramidal shape and a main fiber that crossed the granular cell layer (**Figures 4B,E**).

Two-way ANOVA showed an age effect (2, 6, and 18 months) on the number of Dcx+ cells [$F_{(2, 12)} = 10.27$, $P = 0.0025$]. No genotype effect was observed, but interaction (age vs. genotype) was found when both 6 and 18 months old mice were only considered in the analysis [$F_{(2, 8)} = 6.03$, $P = 0.0396$]. This result suggested that PPARα produced a different effect on the number of SGZ Dcx+ cell from 6 months old onward in a genotype-dependent manner. Two-way ANOVA did not show an interaction and an environmental enrichment or genotype effect on the number of Dcx+ cells in the SGZ of the 18-months-old mice, suggesting that PPARα deficiency did not produce a different effect on the number of SGZ Dcx+ cells in an environment dependent-manner.

After performing the Bonferroni analysis, we found a decreased number of Dcx+ cells in the SGZ of the 6 and 18 months old WT mice compared to that of the 2 months old WT mice ($^{*}P < 0.05$) as well as a decreased number of Dcx+ cells in the SGZ of the 18 months old WT mice compared to that of the 6 months old WT mice ($^{\#}P < 0.05$; **Figures 4A–D**). The number of Dcx+ cells was also lower in the SGZ of the 6 and 18 months old KO mice than that of the 2 months old KO mice ($^{\$\$}P < 0.01$; (**Figures 4A,E–G**). Interestingly, the number of Dcx+ cells decreased in the SGZ of the 6 months old KO mice compared to that of the respective 6 months old WT mice ($^{\$}P < 0.05$; (**Figures 4A,C,F**). The Bonferroni analysis also indicated that the number of Dcx+ cells increased in the SGZ of the 18 months old WT mice when they were housed in a enriched environment compared to the WT ones with standard environment ($^{*}P < 0.05$; (**Figures 4H,I,J**). No change was observed in the 18 months old KO mice with enriched environment (**Figures 4H,K,L**).

DISCUSSION

In the present study we propose that PPARα may play a differential modulatory role in the maintenance of the adult cell proliferation depending on the neurogenic niche, the age and the environment under our experimental conditions. Our results are consistent with the well-known neurogenesis decline through the mouse lifespan (McDonald and Wojtowicz, 2005; Ngwenya et al., 2015). However, the absence of PPARα alleviated the age-related reduction of NPC proliferation (BrdU+ cells) in the SVZ of the 18 months old mice, while no genotype effect was detected regarding this fact in the SGZ and hypothalamus (**Figure 5A**). Interestingly, an accentuated reduction in the number of Dcx+ cells was observed in the SGZ of the 6 months old *Pparα*$^{-/-}$ mice. An enriched environment involving different contextual stimulation consisting of objects (ramps, floor platforms, tunnels, and toys) and treats (fruits, crackers, and cheese) for 20 days in aged mice lacking PPARα counteracted the accentuated decrease of NPC proliferation in the SGZ and the hypothalamus, and reestablished the cell proliferation reduction that was observed in the SVZ of older wild-type mice (**Figure 5B**). The enriched environment likely increased both cell proliferation and

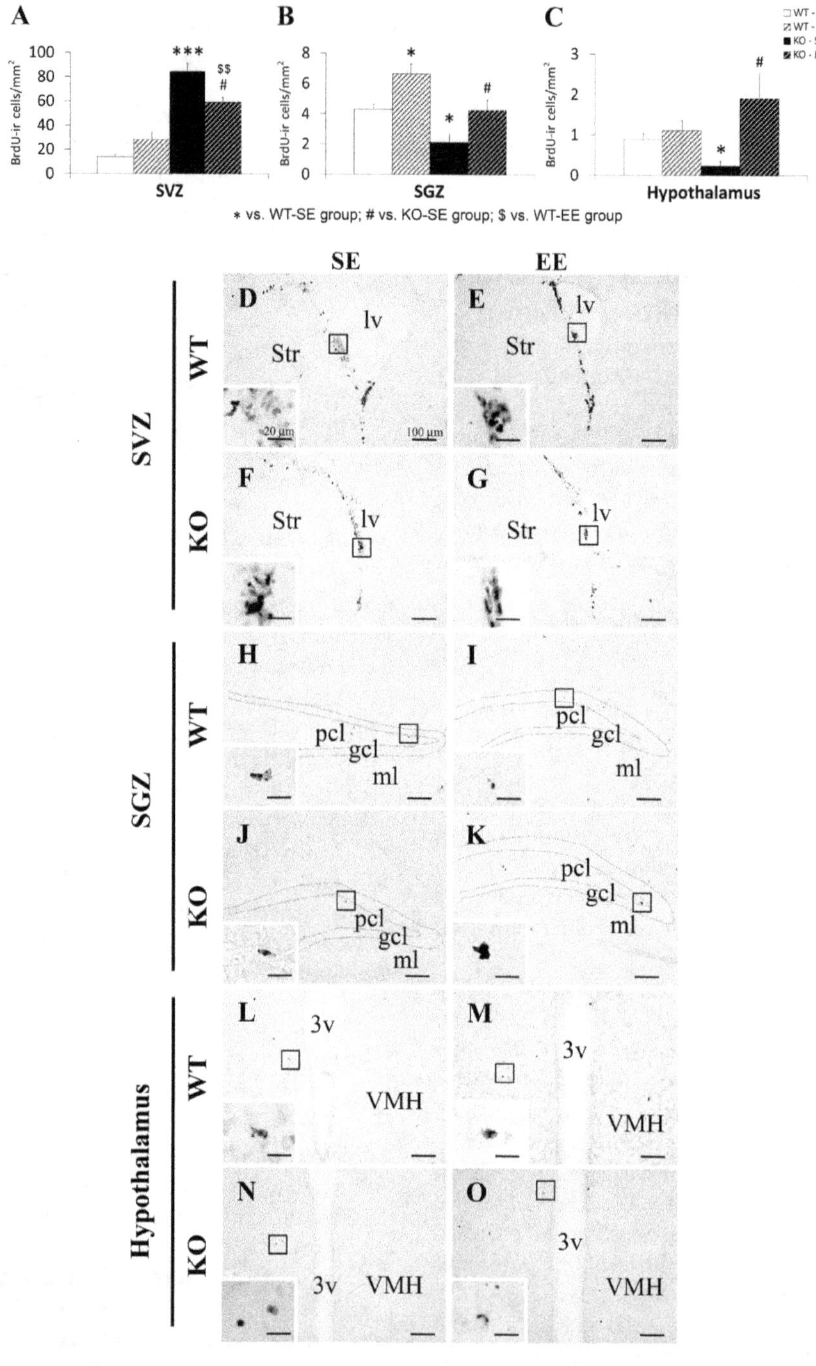

FIGURE 3 | Effect of environment (SE and EE) on the number of cells that contained BrdU in the SVZ (A), SGZ (B) and hypothalamus (C) of WT and *Pparα*$^{-/-}$ (KO) mice. The data were expressed as the media of the number of BrdU+ cells per area (mm^2) + s.e.m (N =5). Bonferroni's test: $^{*}P < 0.05$, $^{***}P < 0.001$ vs. WT-SE group; $^{\#}P < 0.05$ vs. KO-SE group; $^{\$\$}P < 0.01$ vs. WT-EE group. **(D–O)** Representative photomicrographs showing low and high (insets) magnification views of the typical clustering of newborn cells containing the BrdU labeling in the SGZ, SVZ and hypothalamus of WT or KO mice in a standard (SE) or enriched (EE) environment. Scale bars (100 and 20 μm for insets) are included in each image.

maturation in the hippocampus of the 18 months old WT mice, as the number of BrdU+ cells and Dcx+ cells was elevated in the SGZ. However, the enriched environment did not increase the very low number of the SGZ Dcx+ cells in the 18 months old *Pparα*$^{-/-}$ mice, as could be expected. In summary, the SGZ of the older *Pparα*$^{-/-}$ mice exposed to environmental enrichment showed an increase in cell proliferation but no change was found in the number of immature neurons expressing doublecortin. These results in the SGZ suggest an anticipation of the age-dependent neurogenesis decline as a similar low number of

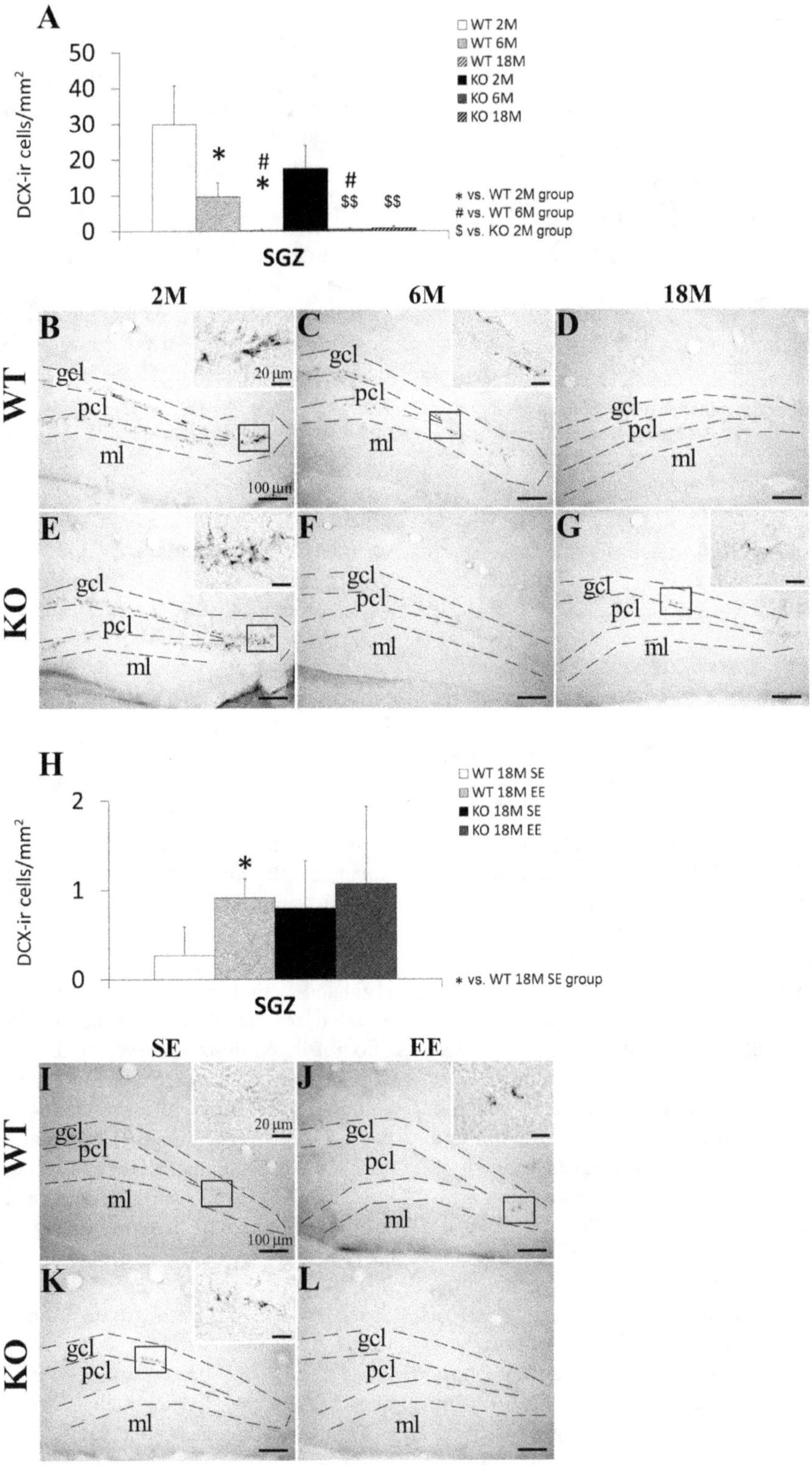

FIGURE 4 | Effect of age (2, 6, and 18 months) (A–G) and enriched environment (H–L) on the number of cells expressing doublecortin (Dcx) in the SGZ of WT and *Pparα*$^{-/-}$ (KO) mice. The data were expressed as the media of the number of Dcx+ cells per area (mm^2) + s.e.m (N =5). Bonferroni's test: $^*P < 0.05$ vs. WT 2M group or WT 18M SE group; $^\#P < 0.05$ vs. WT 6M group; $^{\$\$}P < 0.01$ vs. KO 2M group. **(B–G)** Representative photomicrographs showing low and high (insets) magnification views of the Dcx+ cells in the SGZ of 2, 6, and 18 months old WT and KO mice. **(I–L)** Representative microphotographs showing low and high (insets) magnification views of the Dcx+ cells in the SGZ of 18 months old WT and KO mice in a standard (SE) or enriched (EE) environment. Scale bars (100 µm and 40 µm for insets) are included in each image.

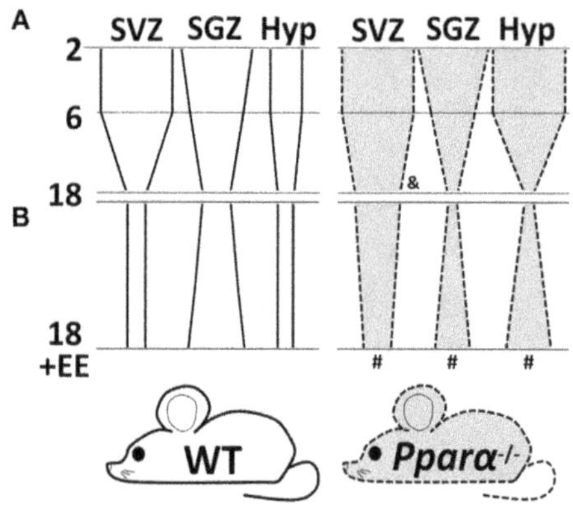

FIGURE 5 | A schematic diagram summarizing the changes of cell proliferation (BrdU+ cells) in the SVZ, SGZ and hypothalamus of wild-type (continuous lines and white background) and Pparα-/- (dashed lines and gray background) mice during aging (A) and after an exposure to an nutritional and environmental enrichment for 20 days (B). Symbols indicate significant changes of cell proliferation between genotypes (WT vs. Pparα$^{-/-}$) in the 18 months old mice (&) and between environments (SE vs. EE) in the 18 months old Pparα$^{-/-}$ mice (#).

Dcx+ cells was observed in the 6 and 18 months old *Pparα*$^{-/-}$ mice compared to the progressive cell number decline in the respective wild-type mice. A putative impaired neurogenesis in the hippocampus of the older *Pparα*$^{-/-}$ mice may be of great therapeutic relevance regarding the positive correlation between cognitive dysfunctions and hippocampal neurogenesis decline during aging (Drapeau et al., 2003; Aizawa et al., 2009; Coras et al., 2010). Further studies will be needed to elucidate the specific role of PPARα signaling system (including endogenous activators, such as OEA, and their synthesizing and degrading enzymes) in cell proliferation and neuronal maturation in the hippocampal SGZ of the adult brain during aging.

PPARα and theirs endogenous ligands such as OEA are involved in the modulation of antioxidant responses, neurotransmission, neuroinflammation, and neurogenesis, which can confer protective roles in models of neurodegenerative and neurocognitive diseases (Heneka et al., 2007; Aleshin and Reiser, 2013; Fidaleo et al., 2014). This nuclear receptor is highly expressed in neuronal populations of certain brain areas such as the hippocampus (Moreno et al., 2004; Rivera et al., 2014), which are particularly implicated in the modulation of learning and memory consolidation. An interesting study aimed at correlating PPARα activation and the expression of brain-derived neurotrophic factor (BDNF) in hippocampal neurons demonstrated an improved learning and memory in an animal model of Alzheimer disease via PPARα (Roy et al., 2015). Overall, PPARα activation by endogenous (OEA and palmitoylethanolamide) and/or exogenous (fenofibrate) agonists shows a neuroprotective role by increasing brain cell proliferation and improving neuronal survival associated with spatial long-term memory after different cerebral insults such as whole-brain irradiation, cerebral ischemia, and Alzheimer disease (Ramanan et al., 2009; Scuderi et al., 2012; Yang et al., 2015). In this sense, it is appropriate to evaluate whether PPARα regulates the NPC proliferation decline throughout adulthood. Interestingly, we demonstrate that PPARα likely acts as a differential, homeostatic modulator of aging-induced cell proliferation decline in the principal neurogenic niches of the adult brain. As we have found differences in the rate of NPC proliferation in the SVZ of the older mice lacking PPARα (18 months old), in contrast with the younger mice (2 months), the participation of this receptor in neurogenesis may be directly related to aging. Further studies will be needed to assess the protective role of PPARα associated with improved neurogenesis and better memory performance among the elderly.

Environmental factors can provide profound influences on brain development and functioning during lifespan. It is well-documented the beneficial effects of enriching environments with physical, social and sensory stimuli on neurogenesis, neuronal sprouting, learning, and memory, suggesting an important therapeutic approach in the prevention and/or recovery of neurodegenerative diseases (Mohammed et al., 2002; Kuzumaki et al., 2011; Garthe et al., 2016). Enriched inputs are able to modulate brain plasticity during all stages of life as a consequence of a variety of responses triggered by neurotrophic and neurogenic factors (Pérez-Martín et al., 2005; García-Segura et al., 2007; Arevalo et al., 2015). Regarding the influence of the environment in the old age, a recent study demonstrated that an enriched environment counteracted the decrease of BDNF levels in the hippocampus of molarless mice, which was in turn associated with the amelioration of proliferation, survival and differentiation of newborn cells in the SGZ and the improvement of hippocampus-dependent spatial memory (Kondo et al., 2015). A previous study indicated that the growth hormone may provide a protective role in old animals as its administration ameliorated neuronal loss associated with aging (Azcoitia et al., 2005). In agreement with this study, chronic IGF-1 treatment reduced spatial learning impairment and up-regulated neural proliferation in the SGZ of aged female rats exposed to prenatal stress (Darnaudéry et al., 2006). To go further into the hypothesis, we evaluated the beneficial effects of an enriched environment involving different sets of objects and games (ramps, floor platforms, tunnels and toys) accompanied by nutritional enrichment (fruits, crackers and cheese) for 20 days in old aged mice lacking PPARα that showed impaired effects on NPC proliferation. In agreement with this premise, our results indicated that the enriched environment counteracted the PPARα deficiency-induced reduction of cell proliferation in the SGZ and the hypothalamus of older mice. Surprisingly, PPARα deficiency increased cell proliferation in the SVZ of the older mice. These results should be interpreted regarding a specific vulnerability of *Pparα*$^{-/-}$ mice associated with senescence and deficiency of PPARα-mediated neuroprotection. Both facts probably resulted in a poor survival of new neurons in those brain regions, such as olfactory bulb and striatum, which are tangentially and radially targeted by the NPC of the SVZ. Thus, it is consistent that vulnerability associated with old age and PPARα deficiency could be the major inducer of striatal neurogenesis. Previous studies established that inflammation accompanying an ischemic insult triggers a marked increase of NPC in the SVZ and leads to the recruitment of formed neuroblasts to repair the damaged striatum (Arvidsson et al., 2002; Thored et al., 2006; Chapman et al., 2015; Lin et al., 2015). Our data evidenced that *Pparα*$^{-/-}$ mice housed in enriched environment for 20 days showed a partial recovery toward the basal rate of NPC proliferation that characterizes the SVZ of the older wild-type mice. The enriched environment including contextual stimulation (objects and games) and nutritional treats likely contributes to neuroprotection, which can, in turn, enhance survival of the new-born neurons and, as a consequence, the restoration of the NPC proliferative rate to control levels in the SVZ. We hypothesize that this process is closely regulated by neurotrophic factors (e.g., IGF-1 and estradiol; García-Segura et al., 2007; Arevalo et al., 2015). Future studies will be designed to elucidate the regulation of the main neurotrophic factors (BDNF, IGF-1, estradiol) by PPARα activation along the elderly.

It should be highlighted the discrepancies of the effects of the enriched environment on NPC proliferation in the SVZ, SGZ, and hypothalamus of the *Pparα*$^{-/-}$ mice. A similar discrepancy regarding the different neurogenic zone of the adult rodent brain was also described in previous studies when neurogenesis was evaluated after different insults such as the exposure to cocaine, alcohol, or a very high fat diet (Rivera et al., 2011, 2015a,b; Blanco-Calvo et al., 2014). In previous studies, we described that adult male rats with a prolonged intake of a high fat diet and treated with the CB1 receptor antagonist AM251 or mice with a repeated administration of cocaine and treated with the CB1 and CB2 receptor antagonists Rimonabant and AM630, respectively, showed an increased neural proliferation in the SGZ, but a decreased neural proliferation in the SVZ (Rivera et al., 2011; Blanco-Calvo et al., 2014). In two recent studies from our group, we described that the reduction of neural proliferation in the SVZ and SGZ after the inhibition of the fatty acid amide hydrolase (FAAH) by the repeated administration of URB597, and the increase of neural proliferation in the SVZ and SGZ after CB2 receptor stimulation in alcohol-exposed rats were not observed in the hypothalamus (Rivera et al., 2015a,b).

As a conclusion, the present study indicates that PPARα deficiency differentially alters the age-induced decline of NPC proliferation in relevant neurogenic niches (SVZ, SGZ, and hypothalamus) of the adult mouse brain. These data suggest a potential modulatory role for PPARα in the age-induced neurogenesis decline. This modulation is brain area dependent. While, in the SVZ, the absence of PPARα promotes more proliferation at older ages, in the SGZ the absence of this receptor may lead to maintain a deficiency in neurogenesis. These results suggest that PPARα in the SVZ likely acts as a neuroprotective factor. The exposition to nutritional and environmental enrichments of the older mice (18 months old) reversed the *Pparα*$^{-/-}$-induced impairment of NPC proliferation in the three neurogenic zones analyzed, but no change was found in hippocampal neuronal maturation. In the SVZ the enhanced cell proliferation is not further potentiated by environmental enrichment, whereas EE boosts cell proliferation in the SGZ and hypothalamus of the *Pparα*$^{-/-}$ animal. Further studies with PPARα activators such as OEA are needed to investigate whether this role can be of therapeutic value for behavioral impairment associated with aging.

AUTHOR CONTRIBUTIONS

All authors had full access to all data in the study and take responsibility for the integrity of the data and the accuracy of the data analyses. Study concept and design: MP, PR, EB, FR, and JS. Acquisition of data: PR, EB, CL, and JD. Analysis and interpretation of data: MP, PR, EB, FR, and JS. Drafting of the manuscript: MP, FR, and JS. Critical revision of the manuscript for important intellectual content, obtained funding and study supervision: FP, AS, FR, and JS.

ACKNOWLEDGMENTS

Grant sponsor: 7th Framework Programme of European Union. Grant number: HEALTH-F2-2008-223713, REPROBESITY to FR. Grant sponsor: Instituto de Salud Carlos III (ISCIII), Ministerio de Economía y Competitividad (MINECO), UE-ERDF. Grant numbers: PI13/02261 to FR. and CP12/03109 to JS. Grant sponsor: Red de Trastornos Adictivos, ISCIII, MINECO. Grant number: RD12/0028/0001 to FR. Grant sponsor: Plan Nacional Sobre Drogas, Ministerio de Sanidad y Consumo. Grant number: PNSD2010/143 and PNSD2015/047 to JS. Grant sponsor: Fundació La Marató de TV3. Grant number: 386/C/2011. Grant sponsor: Consejería de Economía, Innovación y Ciencia, Junta de Andalucía, UE/ERDF. Grant numbers: PI45403 and CTS-8221 to FR. Grant sponsor: Consejería de Salud, Junta de Andalucía, UE/ERDF. Grant number: SAS111224 to FR. JS, FP and AS hold "Miguel Servet" research contracts from the National System of Health, ISCIII (grant numbers: CP12/03109, CP14/00212 and CP14/00173, respectively).

REFERENCES

Aizawa, K., Ageyama, N., Yokoyama, C., and Hisatsune, T. (2009). Age-dependent alteration in hippocampal neurogenesis correlates with learning performance of macaque monkeys. *Exp. Anim.* 58, 403–407. doi: 10.1538/expanim.58.403

Albayram, O., Alferink, J., Pitsch, J., Piyanova, A., Neitzert, K., Poppensieker, K., et al. (2011). Role of CB1 cannabinoid receptors on GABAergic neurons in brain aging. *Proc. Natl. Acad. Sci. U.S.A.* 108, 11256–11261. doi: 10.1073/pnas.1016442108

Aleshin, S., and Reiser, G. (2013). Role of the peroxisome proliferator-activated receptors (PPAR)-alpha, beta/delta and gamma triad in regulation of reactive oxygen species signaling in brain. *Biol. Chem.* 394, 1553–1570. doi: 10.1515/hsz-2013-0215

Alvarez-Buylla, A., and Lim, D. A. (2004). For the long run: maintaining germinal niches in the adult brain. *Neuron* 41, 683–686. doi: 10.1016/S0896-6273(04)00111-4

Arevalo, M. A., Azcoitia, I., Gonzalez-Burgos, I., and Garcia-Segura, L. M. (2015). Signaling mechanisms mediating the regulation of synaptic plasticity and memory by estradiol. *Horm. Behav.* 74, 19–27. doi: 10.1016/j.yhbeh.2015.04.016

Arias-Carrion, O., Olivares-Bunuelos, T., and Drucker-Colin, R. (2007). [Neurogenesis in the adult brain]. *Rev. Neurol.* 44, 541–550.

Arvidsson, A., Collin, T., Kirik, D., Kokaia, Z., and Lindvall, O. (2002). Neuronal replacement from endogenous precursors in the adult brain after stroke. *Nat. Med.* 8, 963–970. doi: 10.1038/nm747

Avshalumov, M. V., and Rice, M. E. (2002). NMDA receptor activation mediates hydrogen peroxide-induced pathophysiology in rat hippocampal slices. *J. Neurophysiol.* 87, 2896–2903. doi: 10.1152/jn.01011.2001

Azcoitia, I., Perez-Martin, M., Salazar, V., Castillo, C., Ariznavarreta, C., Garcia-Segura, L. M., et al. (2005). Growth hormone prevents neuronal loss in the aged rat hippocampus. *Neurobiol. Aging* 26, 697–703. doi: 10.1016/j.neurobiolaging.2004.06.007

Bento-Abreu, A., Tabernero, A., and Medina, J. M. (2007). Peroxisome proliferator-activated receptor-alpha is required for the neurotrophic effect of oleic acid in neurons. *J. Neurochem.* 103, 871–881. doi: 10.1111/j.1471-4159.2007.04807.x

Bilbao, A., Serrano, A., Cippitelli, A., Pavón, F. J., Giuffrida, A., Suárez, J., et al. (2015). Role of the satiety factor oleoylethanolamide in alcoholism. *Addict. Biol.* doi: 10.1111/adb.12276. [Epub ahead of print].

Bizon, J. L., and Gallagher, M. (2003). Production of new cells in the rat dentate gyrus over the lifespan: relation to cognitive decline. *Eur. J. Neurosci.* 18, 215–219. doi: 10.1046/j.1460-9568.2003.02733.x

Blanco-Calvo, E., Rivera, P., Arrabal, S., Vargas, A., Pavón, F. J., Serrano, A., et al. (2014). Pharmacological blockade of either cannabinoid CB1 or CB2 receptors prevents both cocaine-induced conditioned locomotion and cocaine-induced reduction of cell proliferation in the hippocampus of adult male rat. *Front. Integr. Neurosci.* 7:106. doi: 10.3389/fnint.2013.00106

Campolongo, P., Roozendaal, B., Trezza, V., Cuomo, V., Astarita, G., Fu, J., et al. (2009). Fat-induced satiety factor oleoylethanolamide enhances memory consolidation. *Proc. Natl. Acad. Sci. U.S.A.* 106, 8027–8031. doi: 10.1073/pnas.0903038106

Chapman, K. Z., Ge, R., Monni, E., Tatarishvili, J., Ahlenius, H., Arvidsson, A., et al. (2015). Inflammation without neuronal death triggers striatal neurogenesis comparable to stroke. *Neurobiol. Dis.* 83, 1–15. doi: 10.1016/j.nbd.2015.08.013

Cimini, A., and Ceru, M. P. (2008). Emerging roles of peroxisome proliferator-activated receptors (PPARs) in the regulation of neural stem cells proliferation and differentiation. *Stem Cell Rev.* 4, 293–303. doi: 10.1007/s12015-008-9024-2

Cimini, A., Cristiano, L., Benedetti, E., D'Angelo, B., and Ceru, M. P. (2007). PPARs expression in adult mouse neural stem cells: modulation of PPARs during astroglial differentiaton of NSC. *PPAR Res.* 2007:48242. doi: 10.1155/2007/48242

Coras, R., Siebzehnrubl, F. A., Pauli, E., Huttner, H. B., Njunting, M., Kobow, K., et al. (2010). Low proliferation and differentiation capacities of adult hippocampal stem cells correlate with memory dysfunction in humans. *Brain* 133, 3359–3372. doi: 10.1093/brain/awq215

Cristiano, L., Cimini, A., Moreno, S., Ragnelli, A. M., and Paola Ceru, M. (2005). Peroxisome proliferator-activated receptors (PPARs) and related transcription factors in differentiating astrocyte cultures. *Neuroscience* 131, 577–587. doi: 10.1016/j.neuroscience.2004.11.008

Darnaudéry, M., Perez-Martin, M., Bélizaire, G., Maccari, S., and Garcia-Segura, L. M. (2006). Insulin-like growth factor 1 reduces age-related disorders induced by prenatal stress in female rats. *Neurobiol. Aging* 27, 119–127. doi: 10.1016/j.neurobiolaging.2005.01.008

Doetsch, F. (2003a). The glial identity of neural stem cells. *Nat. Neurosci.* 6, 1127–1134. doi: 10.1038/nn1144

Doetsch, F. (2003b). A niche for adult neural stem cells. *Curr. Opin. Genet. Dev.* 13, 543–550. doi: 10.1016/j.gde.2003.08.012

Doetsch, F., Garcia-Verdugo, J. M., and Alvarez-Buylla, A. (1999). Regeneration of a germinal layer in the adult mammalian brain. *Proc. Natl. Acad. Sci. U.S.A.* 96, 11619–11624. doi: 10.1073/pnas.96.20.11619

Drapeau, E., Mayo, W., Aurousseau, C., Le Moal, M., Piazza, P. V., and Abrous, D. N. (2003). Spatial memory performances of aged rats in the water maze predict levels of hippocampal neurogenesis. *Proc. Natl. Acad. Sci. U.S.A.* 100, 14385–14390. doi: 10.1073/pnas.2334169100

Fan, Y., Liu, Z., Weinstein, P. R., Fike, J. R., and Liu, J. (2007). Environmental enrichment enhances neurogenesis and improves functional outcome after cranial irradiation. *Eur. J. Neurosci.* 25, 38–46. doi: 10.1111/j.1460-9568.2006.05269.x

Fandel, D., Wasmuht, D., Avila-Martin, G., Taylor, J. S., Galan-Arriero, I., and Mey, J. (2013). Spinal cord injury induced changes of nuclear receptors PPARalpha and LXRbeta and modulation with oleic acid/albumin treatment. *Brain Res.* 1535, 89–105. doi: 10.1016/j.brainres.2013.08.022

Fidaleo, M., Fanelli, F., Ceru, M. P., and Moreno, S. (2014). Neuroprotective properties of peroxisome proliferator-activated receptor alpha (PPARalpha) and its lipid ligands. *Curr. Med. Chem.* 21, 2803–2821. doi: 10.2174/0929867321666140303143455

García-Segura, L. M., Diz-Chaves, Y., Perez-Martin, M., and Darnaudéry, M. (2007). Estradiol, insulin-like growth factor-I and brain aging. *Psychoneuroendocrinology* 32(Suppl. 1), S57–S61. doi: 10.1016/j.psyneuen.2007.03.001

Garthe, A., Roeder, I., and Kempermann, G. (2016). Mice in an enriched environment learn more flexibly because of adult hippocampal neurogenesis. *Hippocampus* 26, 261–271. doi: 10.1002/hipo.22520

González-Aparicio, R., Blanco, E., Serrano, A., Pavon, F. J., Parsons, L. H., Maldonado, R., et al. (2014). The systemic administration of oleoylethanolamide exerts neuroprotection of the nigrostriatal system in experimental Parkinsonism. *Int. J. Neuropsychopharmacol.* 17, 455–468. doi: 10.1017/S1461145713001259

Hajjar, T., Meng, G. Y., Rajion, M. A., Vidyadaran, S., Othman, F., Farjam, A. S., et al. (2012). Omega 3 polyunsaturated fatty acid improves spatial learning and hippocampal peroxisome proliferator activated receptors (PPARalpha and PPARgamma) gene expression in rats. *BMC Neurosci.* 13:109. doi: 10.1186/1471-2202-13-109

Heneka, M. T., Landreth, G. E., and Hull, M. (2007). Drug insight: effects mediated by peroxisome proliferator-activated receptor-gamma in CNS disorders. *Nat. Clin. Pract. Neurol.* 3, 496–504. doi: 10.1038/ncpneuro0586

Kondo, H., Kurahashi, M., Mori, D., Iinuma, M., Tamura, Y., Mizutani, K., et al. (2015). Hippocampus-dependent spatial memory impairment due to molar tooth loss is ameliorated by an enriched environment. *Arch. Oral Biol.* 61, 1–7. doi: 10.1016/j.archoralbio.2015.10.006

Kuhn, H. G., Dickinson-Anson, H., and Gage, F. H. (1996). Neurogenesis in the dentate gyrus of the adult rat: age-related decrease of neuronal progenitor proliferation. *J. Neurosci.* 16, 2027–2033.

Kuzumaki, N., Ikegami, D., Tamura, R., Hareyama, N., Imai, S., Narita, M., et al. (2011). Hippocampal epigenetic modification at the brain-derived neurotrophic factor gene induced by an enriched environment. *Hippocampus* 21, 127–132. doi: 10.1002/hipo.20775

Lie, D. C., Song, H., Colamarino, S. A., Ming, G. L., and Gage, F. H. (2004). Neurogenesis in the adult brain: new strategies for central nervous system diseases. *Annu. Rev. Pharmacol. Toxicol.* 44, 399–421. doi: 10.1146/annurev.pharmtox.44.101802.121631

Lin, R., Cai, J., Nathan, C., Wei, X., Schleidt, S., Rosenwasser, R., et al. (2015). Neurogenesis is enhanced by stroke in multiple new stem cell niches along the ventricular system at sites of high BBB permeability. *Neurobiol. Dis.* 74, 229–239. doi: 10.1016/j.nbd.2014.11.016

Lin, R., and Iacovitti, L. (2015). Classic and novel stem cell niches in brain homeostasis and repair. *Brain Res.* 1628(Pt B), 327–342. doi: 10.1016/j.brainres.2015.04.029

Maggi, R., Zasso, J., and Conti, L. (2014). Neurodevelopmental origin and adult neurogenesis of the neuroendocrine hypothalamus. *Front. Cell. Neurosci.* 8:440. doi: 10.3389/fncel.2014.00440

McDonald, H. Y., and Wojtowicz, J. M. (2005). Dynamics of neurogenesis in the dentate gyrus of adult rats. *Neurosci. Lett.* 385, 70–75. doi: 10.1016/j.neulet.2005.05.022

Melis, M., Carta, G., Pistis, M., and Banni, S. (2013). Physiological role of peroxisome proliferator-activated receptors type alpha on dopamine systems. *CNS Neurol. Disord. Drug Targets* 12, 70–77. doi: 10.2174/1871527311312010012

Merrill, D. A., Karim, R., Darraq, M., Chiba, A. A., and Tuszynski, M. H. (2003). Hippocampal cell genesis does not correlate with spatial learning ability in aged rats. *J. Comp. Neurol.* 459, 201–207. doi: 10.1002/cne.10616

Mohammed, A. H., Zhu, S. W., Darmopil, S., Hjerling-Leffler, J., Ernfors, P., Winblad, B., et al. (2002). Environmental enrichment and the brain. *Prog. Brain Res.* 138, 109–133. doi: 10.1016/S0079-6123(02)38074-9

Montalban-Loro, R., Domingo-Muelas, A., Bizy, A., and Ferron, S. R. (2015). Epigenetic regulation of stemness maintenance in the neurogenic niches. *World J. Stem Cells* 7, 700–710. doi: 10.4252/wjsc.v7.i4.700

Moreno, S., Farioli-Vecchioli, S., and Ceru, M. P. (2004). Immunolocalization of peroxisome proliferator-activated receptors and retinoid X receptors in the adult rat CNS. *Neuroscience* 123, 131–145. doi: 10.1016/j.neuroscience.2003.08.064

Ngwenya, L. B., Heyworth, N. C., Shwe, Y., Moore, T. L., and Rosene, D. L. (2015). Age-related changes in dentate gyrus cell numbers, neurogenesis, and associations with cognitive impairments in the rhesus monkey. *Front. Syst. Neurosci.* 9:102. doi: 10.3389/fnsys.2015.00102

Nunomura, A., Moreira, P. I., Castellani, R. J., Lee, H. G., Zhu, X., Smith, M. A., et al. (2012). Oxidative damage to RNA in aging and neurodegenerative disorders. *Neurotoxicol. Res.* 22, 231–248. doi: 10.1007/s12640-012-9331-x

Paillard, T. (2015). Preventive effects of regular physical exercise against cognitive decline and the risk of dementia with age advancement. *Sports Med. Open* 1:4. doi: 10.1186/s40798-015-0016-x

Paxinos, G., and Franklin, K. B. J. (2004). *The Mouse Brain in Stereotaxic Coordinates, Compact, 2nd Edn.* Boston, MA: Elsevier Academic Press.

Pérez-Martín, M., Salazar, V., Castillo, C., Ariznavarreta, C., Azcoitia, I., Garcia-Segura, L. M., et al. (2005). Estradiol and soy extract increase the production of new cells in the dentate gyrus of old rats. *Exp. Gerontol.* 40, 450–453. doi: 10.1016/j.exger.2005.03.003

Plaza-Zabala, A., Berrendero, F., Suarez, J., Bermudez-Silva, F. J., Fernandez-Espejo, E., Serrano, A., et al. (2010). Effects of the endogenous PPAR-alpha agonist, oleoylethanolamide on MDMA-induced cognitive deficits in mice. *Synapse* 64, 379–389. doi: 10.1002/syn.20733

Ramanan, S., Kooshki, M., Zhao, W., Hsu, F. C., Riddle, D. R., and Robbins, M. E. (2009). The PPARalpha agonist fenofibrate preserves hippocampal neurogenesis and inhibits microglial activation after whole-brain irradiation. *Int. J. Radiat. Oncol. Biol. Phys.* 75, 870–877. doi: 10.1016/j.ijrobp.2009.06.059

Rivera, P., Arrabal, S., Vargas, A., Blanco, E., Serrano, A., Pavon, F. J., et al. (2014). Localization of peroxisome proliferator-activated receptor alpha (PPARalpha) and N-acyl phosphatidylethanolamine phospholipase D (NAPE-PLD) in cells expressing the Ca(2+)-binding proteins calbindin, calretinin, and parvalbumin in the adult rat hippocampus. *Front. Neuroanat.* 8:12. doi: 10.3389/fnana.2014.00012

Rivera, P., Bindila, L., Pastor, A., Perez-Martin, M., Pavon, F. J., Serrano, A., et al. (2015a). Pharmacological blockade of the fatty acid amide hydrolase (FAAH) alters neural proliferation, apoptosis and gliosis in the rat hippocampus, hypothalamus and striatum in a negative energy context. *Front. Cell. Neurosci.* 9:98. doi: 10.3389/fncel.2015.00098

Rivera, P., Blanco, E., Bindila, L., Alen, F., Vargas, A., Rubio, L., et al. (2015b). Pharmacological activation of CB2 receptors counteracts the deleterious effect of ethanol on cell proliferation in the main neurogenic zones of the adult rat brain. *Front. Cell. Neurosci.* 9:379. doi: 10.3389/fncel.2015.00379

Rivera, P., Romero-Zerbo, Y., Pavon, F. J., Serrano, A., Lopez-Avalos, M. D., Cifuentes, M., et al. (2011). Obesity-dependent cannabinoid modulation of proliferation in adult neurogenic regions. *Eur. J. Neurosci.* 33, 1577–1586. doi: 10.1111/j.1460-9568.2011.07650.x

Roberts, R. A., Chevalier, S., Hasmall, S. C., James, N. H., Cosulich, S. C., and Macdonald, N. (2002). PPAR alpha and the regulation of cell division and apoptosis. *Toxicology* 181–182,167–170. doi: 10.1016/S0300-483X(02)00275-5

Robins, S. C., Stewart, I., McNay, D. E., Taylor, V., Giachino, C., Goetz, M., et al. (2013). alpha-Tanycytes of the adult hypothalamic third ventricle include distinct populations of FGF-responsive neural progenitors. *Nat. Commun.* 4:2049. doi: 10.1038/ncomms3049

Romano, A., Cassano, T., Tempesta, B., Cianci, S., Dipasquale, P., Coccurello, R., et al. (2013). The satiety signal oleoylethanolamide stimulates oxytocin neurosecretion from rat hypothalamic neurons. *Peptides* 49, 21–26. doi: 10.1016/j.peptides.2013.08.006

Rosen, E. D., and Spiegelman, B. M. (2001). PPARgamma: a nuclear regulator of metabolism, differentiation, and cell growth. *J. Biol. Chem.* 276, 37731–37734. doi: 10.1074/jbc.R100034200

Roy, A., Jana, M., Kundu, M., Corbett, G. T., Rangaswamy, S. B., Mishra, R. K., et al. (2015). HMG-CoA reductase inhibitors bind to PPARalpha to upregulate neurotrophin expression in the brain and improve memory in mice. *Cell Metab.* 22, 253–265. doi: 10.1016/j.cmet.2015.05.022

Scuderi, C., Valenza, M., Stecca, C., Esposito, G., Carratu, M. R., and Steardo, L. (2012). Palmitoylethanolamide exerts neuroprotective effects in mixed neuroglial cultures and organotypic hippocampal slices via peroxisome proliferator-activated receptor-alpha. *J. Neuroinflammation* 9:49. doi: 10.1186/1742-2094-9-21

Smith, S. A., Monteith, G. R., Holman, N. A., Robinson, J. A., May, F. J., and Roberts-Thomson, S. J. (2003). Effects of peroxisome proliferator-activated receptor gamma ligands ciglitazone and 15-deoxy-delta 12,14-prostaglandin J2 on rat cultured cerebellar granule neuronal viability. *J. Neurosci. Res.* 72, 747–755. doi: 10.1002/jnr.10613

Thored, P., Arvidsson, A., Cacci, E., Ahlenius, H., Kallur, T., Darsalia, V., et al. (2006). Persistent production of neurons from adult brain stem cells during recovery after stroke. *Stem Cells* 24, 739–747. doi: 10.1634/stemcells.2005-0281

Van Praag, H., Shubert, T., Zhao, C., and Gage, F. H. (2005). Exercise enhances learning and hippocampal neurogenesis in aged mice. *J. Neurosci.* 25, 8680–8685. doi: 10.1523/JNEUROSCI.1731-05.2005

Yang, L. C., Guo, H., Zhou, H., Suo, D. Q., Li, W. J., Zhou, Y., et al. (2015). Chronic oleoylethanolamide treatment improves spatial cognitive deficits through enhancing hippocampal neurogenesis after transient focal cerebral ischemia. *Biochem. Pharmacol.* 94, 270–281. doi: 10.1016/j.bcp.2015.02.012

Zhao, Y., Chen, K., and Shen, X. (2015). Environmental Enrichment Attenuated Sevoflurane-Induced Neurotoxicity through the PPAR-gamma Signaling Pathway. *Biomed Res. Int.* 2015:107149. doi: 10.1155/2015/107149

Zhou, Y. C., and Waxman, D. J. (1998). Activation of peroxisome proliferator-activated receptors by chlorinated hydrocarbons and endogenous steroids. *Environ. Health Perspect.* 106(Suppl. 4), 983–988.

Zolezzi, J. M., Silva-Alvarez, C., Ordenes, D., Godoy, J. A., Carvajal, F. J., Santos, M. J., et al. (2013). Peroxisome proliferator-activated receptor (PPAR) gamma and PPARalpha agonists modulate mitochondrial fusion-fission dynamics: relevance to reactive oxygen species (ROS)-related neurodegenerative disorders? *PLoS ONE* 8:e64019. doi: 10.1371/journal.pone.0064019

13

Mechanisms and Functional Significance of Stroke-Induced Neurogenesis

*Quentin Marlier, Sebastien Verteneuil, Renaud Vandenbosch and Brigitte Malgrange **

GIGA-Neurosciences, University of Liege, C.H.U. Sart Tilman, Liege, Belgium

Edited by:
Laura López-Mascaraque, Cajal Institute, Spain

Reviewed by:
Stefano Farioli Vecchioli, Consiglio Nazionale delle Ricerche, Italy
John W. Cave, Weill Cornell Medical College, USA

***Correspondence:**
Brigitte Malgrange
bmalgrange@ulg.ac.be

Stroke affects one in every six people worldwide, and is the leading cause of adult disability. After stroke, some limited spontaneous recovery occurs, the mechanisms of which remain largely unknown. Multiple, parallel approaches are being investigated to develop neuroprotective, reparative and regenerative strategies for the treatment of stroke. For years, clinical studies have tried to use exogenous cell therapy as a means of brain repair, with varying success. Since the rediscovery of adult neurogenesis and the identification of adult neural stem cells in the late nineties, one promising field of investigation is focused upon triggering and stimulating this self-repair system to replace the neurons lost following brain injury. For instance, it is has been demonstrated that the adult brain has the capacity to produce large numbers of new neurons in response to stroke. The purpose of this review is to provide an updated overview of stroke-induced adult neurogenesis, from a cellular and molecular perspective, to its impact on brain repair and functional recovery.

Keywords: stroke, neurogenesis, niches, stem cells, therapy

INTRODUCTION

Stroke is the second leading cause of death, the most common cause of adult-acquired disability and affects one in every six people worldwide (Moskowitz et al., 2010). The number of people who survive a stroke is increasing, and with an aging population, the incidence and prevalence of stroke are predicted to rise even more (Sun et al., 2012). Despite years of research, effective treatments remain elusive. Currently, the only proven therapy for acute ischemic stroke is systemic thrombolysis with recombinant tissue plasminogen activator (rtPA). To be effective, rtPA must be administered within a maximum of 4.5 h after the symptoms first start. This short timeframe and potential adverse effects have limited the use of rtPA to 3–5% of stroke patients (Ruan et al., 2015). Grafting stem cells represents a compelling alternative and offers both a wide array and an unlimited supply of cells. Indeed, the transplantation of neural stem cells (NSCs), mesenchymal stem cells (MSCs), embryonic stem cells (ESCs), or induced pluripotent stem cells (iPSCs) could be used to replace neuronal loss after stroke (Kalladka and Muir, 2014). However, exogenous stem cell therapy has both technical and ethical issues. For instance, cell survival and migration rely heavily on the timing and mode of delivery (Li et al., 2010; Darsalia et al., 2011). Moreover, surgical procedure and toxicity (as cancer induction) increase the complexity of transplanted cell therapies (Kawai et al., 2010; Ben-David and Benvenisty, 2011). Finally, some ethical issues may arise from the use of fetal/embryonic cells.

Despite the fact that the central nervous system (CNS) has a limited repair capacity (Nakagomi et al., 2011), some degree of spontaneous recovery from brain ischemia invariably occurs (Yu et al., 2014). This repair process involves neurogenesis, angiogenesis, and axonal sprouting and synaptogenesis. Here we concentrate on the events that are associated with the production of new neurons and not the mechanisms that involve the reorganization of connectivity among surviving neurons, which is reviewed elsewhere (Jones and Adkins, 2015).

Recent experimental findings have raised the possibility that functional improvement after stroke may be induced through neuronal replacement by endogenous NSCs. Indeed, the original dogma that no new neurons are formed after birth has been definitively overturned during the past few decades. The discovery of the thymidine analog bromodeoxyuridine (BrdU)—that incorporates into DNA in S-phase and can be detected by immunohistochemistry—has allowed researchers to conclusively demonstrate the generation of new neurons in the brain of all adult mammals including humans (Eriksson et al., 1998; Gage, 2000). This production of new neurons in the adult brain—so-called adult neurogenesis—takes place in areas called neurogenic niches. The subventricular zone (SVZ) of the lateral ventricle and the subgranular zone (SGZ) of the dentate gyrus (DG) are the two main neurogenic niches containing adult NSCs that proliferate, divide and differentiate into mature neurons. Recently, new evidence have highlighted that adult neurogenesis could also takes place in other brain areas, along the ventricular system, mostly in pathological conditions (Lin and Iacovitti, 2015).

The capacity to produce new neurons in the adult brain and the ability of the ischemia-injured adult brain to partially recover suggest a possible relationship between adult neurogenesis and stroke recovery. Indeed, many studies have shown an increase in cell proliferation in the rodent SVZ following ischemic injury (Thored et al., 2006), and evidence for stroke-induced neurogenesis in the human brain has also been reported (Jin et al., 2006). In addition, endogenous brain repair is not limited to neurogenic niches. Recent studies have shown that glial cells surrounding the infarct core can be reactivated following ischemia. Indeed, pericytes, oligodendrocyte precursors, and astrocytes are all able to differentiate into neurons following brain injury (Robel et al., 2011; Heinrich et al., 2014; Nakagomi et al., 2015; Torper et al., 2015). Moreover, surviving neurons may reorganize their connections in a manner that supports some degree of spontaneous improvement. Therefore, a promising field of investigation is focused on triggering and stimulating this self-repair system to replace dead neurons following an ischemic attack.

STROKE PATHOPHYSIOLOGY

Stroke, also known as cerebrovascular accident, results from a transient or permanent reduction in cerebral blood flow that is restricted to the territory of a major brain artery (Woodruff et al., 2011). The two main types of stroke are hemorrhagic stroke (15%) due to bleeding and ischemic stroke (85%) due to lack of blood flow. The three main mechanisms causing ischemic stroke are thrombosis, embolism and global ischemia (Hossmann, 2012). In all of these cases, decreased or absent circulating blood deprives neurons of their necessary substrates, leading irrevocably to cell death. Although different brain regions have varying thresholds for ischemic cell damage, and certain populations of neurons are selectively more resistant to ischemia, neurons are by far the most sensitive cells, ahead of oligodendrocytes, astrocytes, and vascular cells (Woodruff et al., 2011). Despite the fact that neurological dysfunction occurs within seconds to minutes after decreased perfusion, the evolution of ischemic injury continues for several hours and even days (Moskowitz et al., 2010), leading to massive neuronal death and corresponding patient disabilities.

Acute occlusion of a major brain artery leads to spatially and temporally stereotyped events, including morphological damage that evolves over a prolonged period and which depends on the topography, severity and duration of ischemia (Hossmann, 2012). Two specific areas of damage can be defined. The first area is the rapidly formed "ischemic core," which corresponds to the irreversibly damaged tissue close to the occluded artery (Yuan, 2009). It is characterized by a $<20\%$ of baseline blood flow levels, below the energy metabolism threshold (Lo, 2008). In this area, neurons are deprived of their two main supplies: glucose and oxygen. Without these two factors, neurons are unable to produce the ATP needed to maintain ionic gradients. This energy deficit also induces the activation of voltage-gated calcium (Ca^{2+}) channels. As a consequence, an increase in intracellular Ca^{2+} concentration is observed, leading to the activation of phospholipases and proteases, which degrade membranes and proteins essential for cell integrity. Moreover, this massive accumulation of Ca^{2+} is passively followed by water, causing intracellular edema and cell swelling (Iadecola and Anrather, 2011). Unless blood flow is quickly restored, necrotic and irreversible cell death will consequently occur within minutes or a few hours. The second area is the "ischemic penumbra," a region of moderately perfused tissue surrounding the ischemic core, where oxygen is still present to irrigate neurons thanks to collateral arteries. In this area, the reduction of blood flow is not sufficient to cause energy failure and disrupt ionic gradients. Consequently, neurons remain viable but are stressed and vulnerable. Excessive extracellular accumulation of glutamate is a major factor contributing to cell death in the ischemic penumbra zone. The resulting overactivation of glutamate receptor channels of the N-methyl-D-aspartate (NMDA) subtype leads to cytoplasmic accumulation of Ca^{2+}, which activates Ca^{2+}-dependent enzymes, including calpains and caspases, and finally leads to apoptotic cell death (Iadecola and Anrather, 2011). Moreover, during ischemia, mitochondria generate reactive oxygen species (ROS), which modulate signal transduction cascades that tip the balance between pro-death and pro-survival pathways, or act directly as executioners of cell death (Moskowitz et al., 2010). The importance of cell death in the ischemic penumbra area depends upon residual cerebral blood flow (CBF). If CBF is not re-established rapidly, the neurons will die after a few hours or days. The ischemic penumbra represents a salvageable brain area, in which neuronal activity is suppressed but the tissue is potentially viable (Moskowitz et al., 2010). Therefore, early reperfusion is the major target of most therapeutic and experimental interventions in an attempt to reestablish sufficient CBF and rescue cells in the penumbra.

In addition to the above-mentioned histological features, focal ischemia leads to a robust inflammatory response that begins within a few hours. Early on, the production of cytokines by vascular cells and perivascular microglia exposed to ischemic insult contribute to the inflammatory response. Indeed, activated microglia produce toxic metabolites such as ROS and nitric oxide (NO), as well as pro-inflammatory mediators such as IL-6, matrix metalloproteinases (MMPs) and toll-like receptors, which contribute to extend brain injury (Schilling et al., 2003; del Zoppo et al., 2007; Okun et al., 2009). Although activated microglia and vascular cells appear detrimental to cell survival and recovery at the beginning of the insult, chronically activated microglia may, however, secrete beneficial factors that enhance tissue repair (Moskowitz et al., 2010). Reactive astrocytes also have a biphasic role regarding the inflammatory response to stroke. They can extend ischemic lesions by producing pro-inflammatory cytokines (del Zoppo et al., 2000), but also possess a neuroprotective role, through the release of erythropoietin, which leads to the phosphorylation and subsequent inactivation of the pro-apoptotic protein BAD (Ruscher et al., 2002; Prass et al., 2003). This could be of importance regarding spontaneous recovery and regulation of stroke-induced neurogenesis, as discussed below.

THERAPEUTIC STRATEGIES FOR STROKE

The development of therapeutic strategies aimed at overcoming neuronal loss, especially by avoiding delayed neuronal death in penumbra or by replacing dead cells in the ischemic core, is essential. Despite significant improvements after systemic thrombolysis using rtPA, only a small number of patients have timely access to this therapy. As an alternative, the most encouraging approach is stem cell therapy, by using exogenous stem cell grafts or stimulating endogenous stem cell proliferation and differentiation into cells of interest.

Exogenous Stem Cells

Cell replacement for stroke requires the regeneration of multiple functionally specialized cell types, including different kind of neurons, glial and endothelial cells, to restore the entire neurovascular unit (Kalladka and Muir, 2014). Grafting cells into the CNS represents a promising avenue for cell replacement therapies. Grafted cells could potentially differentiate into specific cell subtypes and functionally integrate into the host circuitry in order to repopulate damaged areas. Different sources of stem cells have been proposed to treat stroke and include NSCs, ESCs, iPSCs, and MSCs (**Table 1**).

NSCs are self-renewing, multipotent cells with the ability to proliferate and give rise to neurons, astrocytes and oligodendrocytes, *in vitro* and *in vivo*. They can be derived from ESCs or iPSCs, but also directly from adult stem cells located and isolated from different tissues, such as skin or blood (Anderson, 2001; Morrison, 2001). Recently, transplantation of NSCs from the adult murine brain in ischemic rats led to cell migration to ischemic regions and significant behavioral improvements compared to non-transplanted animals, although many cells died early after transplantation (Chu et al., 2005; Jiang et al., 2006; Zhang and Chopp, 2009; Darsalia et al., 2011; Song et al., 2011). Cell survival and behavior is strongly influenced by the timing and mode of their delivery. For example, intraparenchymal transplantation decreases sensorimotor dysfunctions and motor deficits, while intracerebroventricular injection does not result in any improvement (Smith et al., 2012). Moreover, upon intravenous transplantation of adult mouse NSCs after stroke, only a few percent of cells survive in the brain (Bacigaluppi et al., 2009). Importantly, exogenous stem cell therapy could enhance the endogenous self-repair system. Indeed, transplanted human NSCs, by releasing several factors such as vascular endothelial growth factor (VEGF), neurotrophins or fibroblast growth factor-2 (FGF-2), are highly effective in stimulating endogenous neurogenesis in rats when cells are delivered directly into the ischemic brain parenchyma (Sun et al., 2003; Türeyen et al., 2005; Drago et al., 2013). Finally, this improved endogenous neurogenesis is accompanied by modulation of the inflammatory response. Transplantation of adult NSCs induces a down-regulation of pro-inflammatory mediators, such as interferon-γ (IFN-γ), tumor necrosis factor alpha (TNF-α) and interleukin-1β (IL-1β) in ischemic mice brains (Bacigaluppi et al., 2009). This drastically decreases the microglia driven inflammatory response (Oki et al., 2012) and therefore host-driven repair (Martino and Pluchino, 2006; Martino et al., 2011; Kokaia et al., 2012).

ESCs are pluripotent cells derived from the inner cell mass of blastocysts. The major advantage of ESCs is that a large number of cells can be expanded in culture and differentiated in any neuronal subtype. However, major ethical (embryos destruction) and scientific (immune-compatibility, teratoma formation) issues must be overcome before using them in clinical practice (Ben-David and Benvenisty, 2011). The recently discovered human iPSCs avoid the ethical issues of ESCs by generating autologous patient-specific cells. Unfortunately, iPSCs share the tumorigenicity characteristics found in ESCs (Ben-David and Benvenisty, 2011). Indeed, when iPSCs are delivered through intracerebroventricular (ICV) injection into an ischemic rat brain, large teratomas form, and there is little behavioral improvement compared with PBS-implanted controls rats (Kawai et al., 2010). However, new neuroblasts and mature neurons have been observed in the ischemic area, revealing a direct differentiation of iPSCs (Kawai et al., 2010). Following *in vitro* pre-differentiation of iPSCs into neuroepithelial-like stem cells, no tumors were found and improvements in function, a reduced infarct size and differentiated neuronal cells were reported (Jiang et al., 2011; Oki et al., 2012; Yuan et al., 2013; Eckert et al., 2015). These data indicate that iPSCs are another source of stem cells—beside adult NSCs—able to improve stroke recovery.

Among the different stem cell types that are candidates for grafting after stroke, MSCs represent the most promising candidates. Transplantation experiments with MSCs derived from different species (rats, mice, rabbit, or human) and using different routes of administration have been performed (Chen

TABLE 1 | Summary of exogenous stem cells types and their role in stroke recovery.

	NSC	ESC	iPSC	MSC
Origin	• ESC • iPSC • Skin or blood adult stem cells	• Blastocyst inner cell mass	• Autologous patient-specific cells	• Bone marrow stromal cells
Mode of administration	• ST • IV • IA • ICV	• ST	• ST	• IV • ST
Behavior	• Proliferate, migrate and differentiate into neurons • Stimulate endogenous stem cell proliferation • Modulate inflammation response	• Differentiate into neurons	• Differentiate into neurons	• Migrate into ischemic area • Modulate inflammatory response
Therapeutic outcome	• Promote functional recovery	• Promote functional recovery	• Little functional impact	• Promote functional recovery
Advantages	• Standardized isolation • Good survival	• Culture expansion	• No ethical, moral and legal issues	• Facility to acquire • No ethical issue
Limitations	• Dependence of timing and mode of delivery • Reproducibility	• Ethical issues • Toxicity • Reproducibility	• Toxicity • Reproducibility	• Poor differentiation • Reproducibility
References	Anderson, 2001; Chu et al., 2005; Jiang et al., 2006; Martino and Pluchino, 2006; Bacigaluppi et al., 2009; Zhang and Chopp, 2009; Barkho and Zhao, 2011; Darsalia et al., 2011; Martino et al., 2011; Song et al., 2011; Hassani et al., 2012; Kokaia et al., 2012; Oki et al., 2012; Jensen et al., 2013; Mine et al., 2013; Hermann et al., 2014; Tang et al., 2014	Bühnemann et al., 2006; Daadi et al., 2008; Ben-David and Benvenisty, 2011	Kawai et al., 2010; Ben-David and Benvenisty, 2011; Jiang et al., 2011; Oki et al., 2012; Jensen et al., 2013	Li et al., 2000; Chen et al., 2001a,b; Chen et al., 2008; Kang et al., 2003; Kurozumi et al., 2005; Honma et al., 2006; Horita et al., 2006; Cui et al., 2007; Andrews et al., 2008; Koh et al., 2008; Bao et al., 2011, 2013; Gutiérrez-Fernández et al., 2011; Braun et al., 2012; Ruan et al., 2013; Wang et al., 2014; Lee et al., 2015

ESC, embryonic stem cells; IA, intra-arterial; ICV, intracerebroventricular; iPSC, induce-pluripotent stem cells; IV, intravenous; MSC, mesenchymal stem cells; NSC, neural stem cells; ST, stereotaxic.

et al., 2001a,b; Horita et al., 2006; Cui et al., 2007; Gutiérrez-Fernández et al., 2011; Braun et al., 2012; Ruan et al., 2013). Stereotaxic (ST) transplantation of adult MSCs directly into the adult brain significantly reduces the functional deficit associated with stroke (Li et al., 2000; Kang et al., 2003; Horita et al., 2006). Moreover, significant reductions in infarct volume, as well as improvements in functional outcomes have also been observed following intravenous (IV) delivery of MSCs in a rodent model of stroke (Kurozumi et al., 2005; Honma et al., 2006; Koh et al., 2008). The mechanisms underlying the beneficial effects of MSCs are multifactorial. MSCs secrete numerous growth factors and cytokines that are neurotrophic, enhance revascularization and exhibit immunomodulatory properties as well as enhancing host neurotrophic factor expression, host neurogenesis and cell replacement (Kurozumi et al., 2005; Andrews et al., 2008; Bao et al., 2011, 2013). However, the contribution of grafted cells to the replacement of lost neurons is still unclear (Chen et al., 2001a,b). The efficacy of MSC grafts is largely time-dependent. Indeed, earlier MSC transplantations are associated with better functional recovery after stroke (Lee et al., 2015). This may be linked to the decreased inflammatory processes and the secretion of trophic factors by MSCs that reduce cellular apoptosis in the early period of stroke (Wang et al., 2014).

Altogether, stem cell graft experiments have highlighted promising potential strategies regarding stroke recovery, by either directly replacing lost neurons or more importantly, by helping endogenous proliferation and modulating inflammation.

Endogenous Stem Cells

Even without any treatment, some degree of spontaneous recovery occurs after brain injury. Recent findings have shed light on the possibility that therapeutic outcomes after stroke may originate from endogenous NSCs residing in the adult brain, such as in the SVZ and the SGZ. Adult neurogenesis occurring in these areas could participate in the replacement of neurons lost following ischemia. Importantly, stroke induces cell proliferation in these specific areas, but also in other parts of the brain. These new neurogenic zones could potentially represent a "reservoir" of endogenous cells able to increase their proliferation after ischemic injury in order to repopulate damaged parenchyma. However, not much is known about the mechanisms underlying stroke-induced neurogenesis, in terms of cellular origin, molecular regulation or functional integration.

Localization

A basal rate of proliferation is present in the SVZ, SGZ and hypothalamus of the healthy adult mammalian brain. Therefore, the first experiments performed regarding stroke-induced neurogenesis have tried to determine from which part of the brain stroke-activated endogenous stem cells may come from.

Classical neurogenic niches: SGZ&SVZ

If endogenous stroke-induced neurogenesis occurs, the two most likely areas where it may happen are the two classical neurogenic niches SGZ and SVZ. In the hippocampus, NSCs—also named type-1 radial glia-like cells—are found in the SGZ, at the interface of the hilus and the granular cell layer (GCL). These cells divide slowly and give rise to type-2 cells or transit-amplifying progenitors, which divide actively to generate type-3 cells or neuroblasts. Neuroblasts exit the cell cycle and migrate a short distance into the GCL where they differentiate into immature postmitotic neurons. Around 50% of the immature neurons produced will die, and only a few newborn granule cells will be stably integrated into the synaptic network of the DG (Genin et al., 2014). This adult hippocampal neurogenesis is likely implicated in cognitive processes such as learning, memory, and cognition. Experimental models of cerebral ischemia are categorized as global or focal. In models of global ischemia, in which CBF is reduced throughout most of the brain, a 10-fold increase in SGZ progenitor proliferation has been demonstrated in many species, such as gerbils, rats, mice, monkeys as well as humans (Imai et al., 2007; Wiltrout et al., 2007). Focal ischemia models, which are more frequently used, consist of a temporary occlusion of the middle cerebral artery (MCAO) that produces infarcts in the ipsilateral area of the cerebral cortex and striatum (Ginsberg and Busto, 1989). In these models, studies have also reported a significantly enhanced proliferation of NSCs and progenitors in the SGZ (Yagita et al., 2001; Sharp et al., 2002; Wiltrout et al., 2007). Generally, the increased proliferation starts bilaterally at 3–4 days post-ischemia (Lichtenwalner and Parent, 2006), peaks at 7–10 days and returns to control levels by 3–5 weeks (Arvidsson et al., 2002; Takasawa et al., 2002; Dempsey et al., 2003; Zhu et al., 2003). One week after the ischemic episode, a 2–3-fold increase of cell production is observed in the DG as compared to the basal level seen in control animals. Over 60% of these cells express Calbindin—a calcium-binding protein normally expressed in mature granule neurons—5 weeks after the ischemia (Kee et al., 2001). Altogether, these data indicate that SGZ is likely to be one source of the endogenous stem cells responding to stroke.

The SVZ lies adjacent to the lateral ventricles along the lateral wall. It is composed of different types of NSCs classified by their self-renewal and differentiation capacities. Radial glial NSCs—the so-called type B cells—extend an apical ending that is exposed to the ventricle and possess a long basal process ending on blood vessels (Mirzadeh et al., 2010). These cells are surrounded by multiple ependymal cells (type E cells) forming pinwheel structures on the ventricle surface (Mirzadeh et al., 2008). Type B cells divide slowly to generate transit-amplifying type C cells, which proliferate actively and further differentiate into neuroblasts also named type A cells. Finally, these cells form chains and migrate over long distances toward the olfactory bulb (OB), via the rostral migratory stream (RMS). In the OB, neuroblasts migrate radially and differentiate into granule cells or periglomerular interneurons (Carleton et al., 2003).

There are numerous studies demonstrating that stroke stimulates SVZ NSCs proliferation and neurogenesis (Arvidsson et al., 2002; Kokaia and Lindvall, 2003; Thored et al., 2006). Some have demonstrated a post-MCAO activation of SVZ NSCs in rats (Jin et al., 2001; Zhang et al., 2001, 2004, 2007; Li et al., 2002; Parent et al., 2002), mice (Carlén et al., 2009; Zhang et al., 2014) and even monkeys (Tonchev et al., 2005) with an increase in proliferation markers that peaks at day 14 post-stroke. Beside this increased proliferation, it has been shown that these SVZ NSCs are migrating, differentiating and integrating into the lesion site tissue in rodent MCAO models (Zhang et al., 2001; Parent et al., 2002; Yamashita et al., 2006; Magnusson et al., 2014). Indeed, many BrdU+/NeuN+ cells were found in the post-ischemic striatum brain (Arvidsson et al., 2002) and a fluorescent tracing of SVZ proliferating cells showed that these cells directly migrate from the SVZ to the striatum in the post-ischemic rat brain (Jin et al., 2003). Ischemia may induce these newly generated neural precursors of the SVZ to revoke their normal migratory pattern, and instead to migrate toward the injured areas of the brain and aid in spontaneous recovery (Thored et al., 2006). Moreover, besides stroke-induced NSCs proliferation, non-proliferative type E cells have been shown to also be able to generate neuroblasts and astrocytes following ischemic injury (Carlén et al., 2009).

Novel neurogenic niches

Recent evidence suggests that, in addition to the canonical SGZ and SVZ, other stem cell niches are present in the adult brain. Indeed, the presence of adult NSCs has been proven in rodent hypothalamus (Kokoeva et al., 2005; Xu et al., 2005; Migaud et al., 2010; Pérez-Martín et al., 2010; Pierce and Xu, 2010) and also in the striatum of rats (Dayer et al., 2005), mice (Shapiro et al., 2009), rabbits (Luzzati et al., 2006), and monkeys (Bédard et al., 2006). Evidence for adult neurogenesis has also been shown in certain neocortical areas of the adult rat (Dayer et al., 2005), mouse (Shapiro et al., 2009) and monkey brain (Bernier et al., 2002). Finally, amygdala neurogenesis has been demonstrated in mice (Shapiro et al., 2009), rabbits (Luzzati et al., 2006), and monkeys (Bernier et al., 2002) as well as brainstem neurogenesis in rat (Bauer et al., 2005).

Hypothalamus. The most described new stem cell niche is the hypothalamus. Proliferating cells found in the hypothalamus can be divided in two groups. The first one is located in the lateral wall of the third ventricle at the level of paraventricular, ventromedial and arcuate nuclei (Hypothalamic Ventricular Zone, HVZ, **Figure 1**). The second group, formed

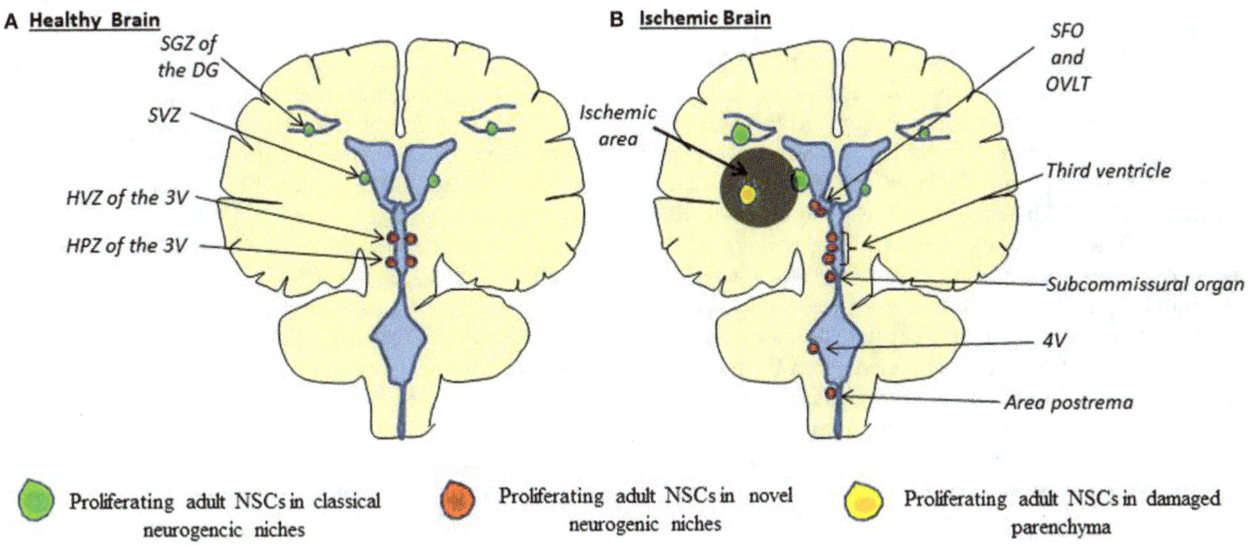

FIGURE 1 | Cellular origin of stroke-induced neurogenesis. (A) In the healthy brain, adult neural stem cells are found to proliferate in the SGZ of the DG, in the SVZ along the lateral ventricle (green) and the HVZ and HPZ along the third ventricle (red). **(B)** In the ischemic brain, proliferating adult neural stem cells are found along the third ventricle, the fourth ventricle (4V) and the CVOs (SFO, OVLT, Subcommissural organ, area postrema) (Red) as well as directly in the ischemic parenchyma (orange), besides classical neurogenic niches (Lin and Iacovitti, 2015). HVZ, hypothalamic ventricular zone; HPZ, hypothalamic proliferating zone; CVOs, Circumventricular organs; SFO, subfornical organ; OVLT, organum vasculosum of the lamina terminalis.

by tanycytes—a specialized ependymal cell type—is located at the bottom of the third ventricle in median eminence region and called the hypothalamic proliferating zone (HPZ). Physiologically, hypothalamic neurogenesis seems to play a role in energy balance; however, the rate of proliferation is much less than in the two canonical neurogenic niches (Rojczyk-Golebiewska et al., 2014). Nevertheless, tanycytes that form the rat and human HVZ express classical markers of neural precursor cells such as nestin (Wei et al., 2002) and doublecortin-like protein, a microtubule-associated protein highly homologous to doublecortin (DCX), a marker of neuroblasts and immature neurons, in the adult mouse brain (Saaltink et al., 2012). Importantly, proliferation of NSCs is enhanced on the ischemia ipsilateral side along the third ventricle (Lin et al., 2015).

Ventricular system: windows of the brain. Besides the SVZ and the median eminence, recent studies suggest that NSCs are also present at other circumventricular brain regions, particularly the sensory "circumventricular organs" (CVOs; Bennett et al., 2009; Furube et al., 2015). The sensory CVOs are the organum vasculosum of the lamina terminalis (OVLT), the subfornical organ (SFO), the pineal gland (PG), the subcommissural organ (SCO), and the area postrema (AP). The sensory CVOs, located outside the blood-brain barrier, are involved in the maintenance of a wide variety of sensory homeostatic and inflammatory pathways in the brain (Joly et al., 2007; Price et al., 2008). *In vivo* studies have revealed that CVOs cells proliferate and undergo constitutive neurogenesis and gliogenesis (Bennett et al., 2009). In addition to CVOs, proliferating cells are also found along the fourth ventricle (4V) (Lin et al., 2015). Consistent with these findings, neurospheres have been generated *in vitro* from isolated CVO and 4V cells (Bauer et al., 2005; Charrier et al., 2006; Itokazu et al., 2006).

Adult CVOs stem cells residing in a subventricular location incorporate BrdU and express the proliferation marker Ki67, as well as stem cells markers such as nestin and Sox2, as is the case in the SVZ (Bennett et al., 2009). Moreover, these cells are able to generate new neurons *in vivo*. Indeed, some proliferating cells found in CVOs were also positive for TUC-4 (TOAD (Turned On After Division)/Ulip/CRMP-4), a very early neuronal marker, and the mature neuronal marker NeuN (109). More importantly, in response to stroke in rats, an increased proliferation of NSCs in the CVOs as well as along the 4V has been observed. Similarly, proliferating cells are also observed in CVOs after stroke in humans (Sanin et al., 2013). CVO and 4V cells—like classical NSCs—are able to differentiate into oligodendrocytes, astrocytes, and neurons following stroke (Lin and Iacovitti, 2015) even if a shift toward neurogenesis was observed (Bennett et al., 2009). Interestingly, some newborn cells coming from novel neurogenic niches have been observed in a chain formation potentially migrating away from these novel niches to the infarct core (Lin et al., 2015). Taken together, the CVO reservoir of stem cells may serve as a further source of NSCs in humans for recovery after stroke.

Non-neurogenic niches

The increased proliferation and migration of endogenous stem cells in the neurogenic niches contributes to stroke-induced neurogenesis, and provides a clear link between stroke and neurogenesis. However, not only neurogenic niches must be taken into account regarding stroke-induced neurogenesis. Accumulating evidence suggests that ischemic injury induces the generation of new neurons from activated NSCs directly in the cerebral cortex (Magavi et al., 2000; Jiang et al., 2001; Jin et al., 2006; Yang et al., 2007). These ischemia-induced NSCs generate nestin-positive neurospheres *in vitro*. Following stroke, these nestin-positive cells develop in the ischemic subpial region, in proximity to blood vessels, and spread into the cortex through cortical layer 1 (Ohira et al., 2010; Nakagomi et al., 2011). These progenitor cells may originate from microvascular pericytes, as they express pericyte markers such as platelet-derived growth factor receptor β (PDGFRβ) and NG2 (Nakagomi et al., 2015). Indeed, new evidence has highlighted the multipotential differentiation capacity of vascular pericytes (PCs). PCs extracted from ischemic regions from the mouse or human brain and cultured under oxygen/glucose deprivation have developed stem cell-like features, presumably through reprogramming (Nakagomi et al., 2015). Moreover, cells from the adult human cerebral cortex that express PC markers, such as PDGFRβ and NG2, have been reprogrammed into neuronal cells by retrovirus-mediated co-expression of Sox2 and Mash1 (Karow et al., 2012). These induced-neuronal cells acquire the ability to fire repetitive action potentials and serve as synaptic targets for pre-existing neurons, indicating their capacity to integrate into neural networks. Taken together, these data show that PCs constitute a promising source of NSCs that can be activated following stroke and aid the replacement of dead neurons.

Besides PCs, recent studies have shown that under certain conditions, adult striatal parenchymal NG2-positive glial cells—i.e., oligodendrocytes precursors cells (OPCs)—are also able to generate neuronal progeny. Genetic fate mapping of individual DCX-positive cells present in the damaged parenchyma has revealed that some are of $NG2^+$-glial origin. Furthermore, overexpression of Sox2 is sufficient to induce the conversion of genetically fate-mapped $NG2^+$ glia into DCX+ cells in the adult mouse cerebral cortex following stab wound injury *in vivo* (Heinrich et al., 2014). Finally, it has also been demonstrated *in situ* in the brain that striatal $NG2^+$ cells, transfected with Ascl1, Lmx1a and Nurr1, can be reprogammed into functional neurons that integrate into the local circuitry (Torper et al., 2015).

Unexpectedly, reactive astrocytes generated following stroke also appear to be an important source of endogenous cells that aid recovery. Although parenchymal astrocytes do not divide in the healthy brain and do not form neurospheres *in vitro*, the behavior of these cells drastically changes following brain injury. Following stroke, two types of reactive astrocytes have been identified: 1/reactive elongated astrocytes, which incorporate BrdU and express progenitor markers such as SOX2 and brain lipid binding protein (BLBP), and 2/stellate astrocytes that derive from resident cortical astrocytes (Wanner et al., 2013). A proportion of these reactive astrocytes has the potential to self-renew and is multipotent *in vitro* (Lang et al., 2004). Moreover, in addition to the conversion of local parenchymal astrocytes, it has been shown that a subpopulation of reactive the astrocytes generated following stroke is SVZ-derived and contributes to the astrocyte scar (Benner et al., 2013).

The ability of reactive astrocytes to generate neurons also depends on their location. Genetic and viral lineage tracing studies have reported the generation of neurons from reactive striatal astrocytes following MCAO (Magnusson et al., 2014; Duan et al., 2015). Conversely, there is a lack of evidence for a direct *in vivo* neurogenic potential of these reactive astrocytes in the cortex, probably due to anti-neurogenic influence. Nevertheless, a latent neurogenic program is present in cortical astrocytes. Indeed, a recent study has shown that SVZ-derived NSCs are able to give rise to reactive astrocytes at the stroke site and can be converted to neurons *in vivo* following overexpression of Ascl1 (Faiz et al., 2015).

The capacity for parenchymal cells—as pericytes, NG2-positive OPCs and reactive astrocytes—to give rise to neurons following stroke opens new perspectives for their use as a repair tool for brain regeneration.

Molecular Cues

Spontaneous recovery following stroke may come 1/from the capacity of endogenous stem cells to proliferate into neurogenic niches, migrate toward the damaged parenchyma, and differentiate into neurons or 2/from parenchymal cells that proliferate, dedifferentiate into neuronal cells and survive to replace dead neurons. Understanding the molecular mechanisms regulating these processes is necessary to improve brain recovery. If neurogenic niches are a potent reservoir of NSCs that are activated following stroke, how these cells are instructed to proliferate and migrate long distances, far from the ischemic parenchyma, remains an open question (**Figure 2**).

Neurogenic niches

Proliferation. The initial response of NSCs following stroke is to increase proliferation, a process that is regulated by different environmental and molecular cues. Indeed, following stroke, the neurovascular unit combines with astrocytes, microglia and others mediators to create a favorable environment for NSCs proliferation in the neurogenic niches.

- *Neurovascular regulation*

Stroke induces dramatic changes in the vasculature (Sawada et al., 2014) and increases angiogenesis, defined as the formation of new capillaries from pre-existing vessels, suggesting a link between stroke-induced neurogenesis and blood vessels (Ruan et al., 2015). Following MCAO, reactive angiogenesis remodels the disrupted blood vessel network in the injured striatum, during a period of several days to 2 weeks after ischemia (Thored et al., 2007). Angiogenesis is found in the penumbra of the brain infarcted region in both animal models of stroke and in patients, and a positive correlation exists between survival and the density of new microvessels (Krupinski et al., 1994; Hayashi et al., 2003; Ruan et al., 2015).

This neo-angiogenesis leads to vasculature and blood flow changes. As a consequence, the levels of metabolic and gas molecules are either increased (ATP) (Suyama et al., 2012), or decreased (NO and O_2) (Matarredona et al., 2005; Panchision, 2009) around the blood vessels, and this regulates the proliferation of adjacent NSCs (Lacar et al., 2012). Moreover, fluid dynamics can also regulate the active transport of blood-derived factors, such as insulin growth factor- 1

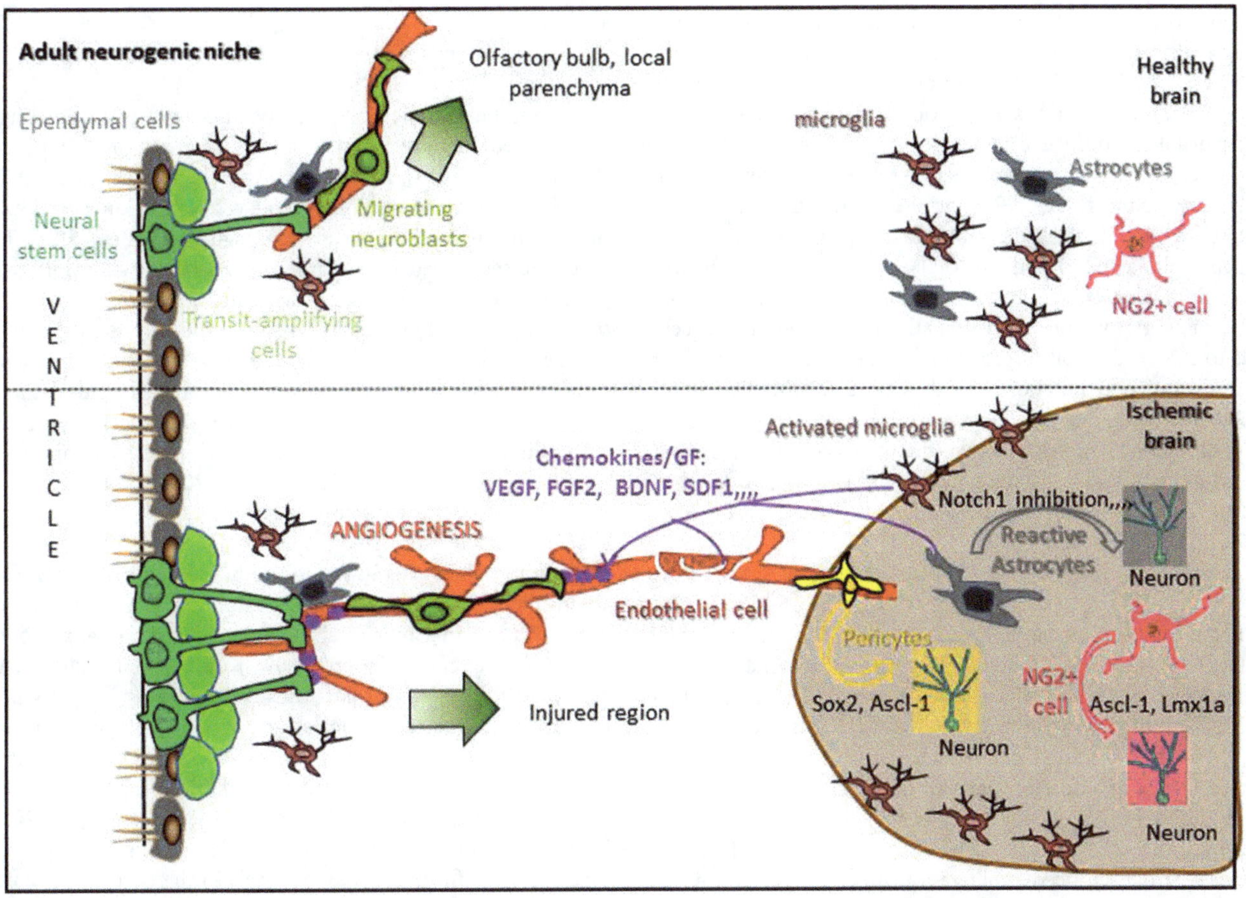

FIGURE 2 | Regulation of stroke-induced neurogenesis in a standard neurogenic niche. In the healthy brain, adult neural stem cells (Dark green) present in neurogenic niches contact blood vessels, proliferate and give rise to neuroblasts migrating from the SVZ to the olfactory bulb or from an other neurogenic niche to the local parenchyma (upper panel). Following stroke, reactive astrocytes, activated microglia, and endothelial cells release chemokines and growth factors able to reach neurogenic niches, increasing NSCs proliferation and attracting migrating neuroblasts to the ischemic area. Moreover, reactive astrocytes, NG2+ cells and pericytes are able to dedifferentiate into neurons inside the damaged parenchyma (lower panel; Hermann et al., 2014; Sawada et al., 2014).

(IGF-1), to control adult SVZ neurogenesis (Nishijima et al., 2010). Consistent with the important role of angiogenesis in the regulation of stroke-induced NSC proliferation, blocking post-ischemic angiogenesis results in a 10-fold reduction in neuroblasts in the peri-infarct cortex 7 days after stroke (Ohab et al., 2006). Finally, angiogenesis leads to changes in the expression of growth factors, chemokines and metalloproteinases that can induce NSCs proliferation. Indeed, activated endothelial cells in the ischemic area secrete VEGF, which promotes NSCs proliferation and neuronal differentiation (Jin et al., 2002; Shen et al., 2004). In response to the ischemic injury, endothelial cells also secrete BDNF, erythropoietin, IGF-1, and FGF-2, which have been shown to significantly increase progenitor cell proliferation in both the SVZ and SGZ (Wiltrout et al., 2007). Interestingly, in the SVZ, NSCs are able to promote angiogenesis by secreting several angiogenic factors such as VEGFR2, Angiopoietin-1 and FGF-2 (Liu et al., 2007). This provides another strong piece of evidence that links stroke-induced neurogenesis and angiogenesis.

Besides angiogenesis, an important feature of neurogenic niches regarding stroke-induced proliferation is their location. Indeed, the majority of endogenous NSCs are directly or indirectly in contact with the CSF and other critical factors. In the SVZ, type B cells have direct access to the lumen of the ventricles, and CVO stem cells are directly located along the 3V and 4V. In contrast, the SGZ has no direct contact with the ventricle, but the hippocampal sulcus (the groove between the DG and CA1 field) could serve as a potential point of access to CSF factors. Another common feature of neurogenic niches is the rich network of blood vessels that surround and communicate with stem cells. In the SVZ, type B cells extend basal processes that terminate directly on endothelial cells (**Figure 2**). Importantly, these vessels lack the astrocyte endfeet and endothelial tight junctions that are found elsewhere in the brain, resulting in a highly permeable blood brain barrier (BBB) at the niche site (Shen et al., 2008; Tavazoie et al., 2008). CVOs are often called the "windows of the brain." As a result, NSCs have access to both local endothelial cell-derived factors and systemic factors present in the blood stream, including circulating cytokines, chemokines and growth factors that all participate in adult neurogenesis (Goldberg and Hirschi, 2009; Lin and Iacovitti, 2015). Indeed, in physiological conditions, capillaries in the SVZ are known to be permeable to diffusible molecules released from endothelial cells, such as VEGF and pigment epithelium-derived factor (PEDF), which regulate NSCs proliferation (Jin et al., 2002; Andreu-Agulló et al., 2009). Moreover, adult NSCs express integrins (alpha6 beta1 and alphaVB8), which serve as receptors for laminin and TGFβ present within the vascular basement membranes. Activation of these pathways in endothelial cells leads to the production of growth factors that are necessary for NSC survival and function (Shen et al., 2008; Mobley et al., 2009). Moreover, growth factors, or reagents that stimulate their expression, increase stroke-induced SVZ neurogenesis, and conversely stroke-induced neurogenesis is impaired when growth factors concentrations are decreased (Chen et al., 2005; Tsai et al., 2006; Yan et al., 2006).

- *Other regulators*

In neurogenic niches, microglia are abundant and in close contact with adult NSCs. Microglia activated after ischemic brain injury are also able to produce chemokines and cytokines that aid NSCs proliferation (Gonzalez-Perez et al., 2010; Yenari et al., 2010). Notably, activated microglia are able to secrete IGF-1 to promote NSCs proliferation in both of the classical neurogenic niches (Hwang et al., 2004; Thored et al., 2009). Consistent with this, inhibition of microglial activation after cerebral ischemia decreases stroke-induced proliferation in the SVZ (Kim et al., 2009).

Finally, other potential mediators of stroke-induced proliferation neurogenesis—mainly in the classical neurogenic niches—have been described. These include Notch signaling (Wang et al., 2009), retinoic acid (Plane et al., 2008), bone morphogenetic protein (Chou et al., 2006), tumor necrosis factor-alpha (Iosif et al., 2008), and sonic hedgehog (Sims et al., 2009). Besides chemokines and soluble factors, other regulators of SVZ and DG stem cell proliferation have been described, such as microRNA (Liu et al., 2013), exercise (Luo et al., 2007), and electroacupuncture (Kim et al., 2014).

Migration. Following NSCs proliferation, the next step following stroke is the production of new neurons in the injured region. Indeed stroke can induce long-distance cell migrations of newly born immature neurons to the peri-infarct cortical area (Tsai et al., 2006; Yamashita et al., 2006). Studies have shown that following BrdU or GFP lentiviral injections into the SVZ at the time of stroke, labeled cells are detected in peri-infarct cortex at 7 and 14 days post stroke, whereas injections of BrdU directly into the cortex results in only a few BrdU+/DCX+ cells. Several critical regulators of newborn cells following stroke have been identified over the years.

- *Vascular regulation*

Similar to the regulation of stroke-induced NSCs proliferation, the vascular environment is also a key feature regarding the migration of newborn cells following stroke.

- *Scaffold cues*

During embryonic development and early postnatal stages, coordinated neurogenesis and angiogenesis are important (Sawada et al., 2014). Indeed, at the neonatal stage, SVZ-derived newborn cells migrate along blood vessels not only to the OB but also to the cerebral cortex (Le Magueresse et al., 2012). This blood vessel-guided cell migration toward the cerebral cortex gradually decreases during postnatal development, probably due to a decrease in blood vessel density in the corpus callosum (Le Magueresse et al., 2012). Following stroke, this developmental cell migration toward the cortex is reactivated, and chains of neuroblats migrate in the direction of the damaged parenchyma, along the blood vessels away from both the classical and novel niches (Pencea et al., 2001; Sawada et al., 2014; Lin et al., 2015).

Post-stroke neuroblast migration toward the injured region shares characteristic features with physiological neuroblast migration within the RMS. In both cases, neuroblasts form chain-like cell aggregates (Arvidsson et al., 2002; Parent et al., 2002; Yamashita et al., 2006) and migrate along blood vessels (Zhang and Chopp, 2009; Kojima et al., 2010; Saha et al., 2013). After stroke, during the blood vessel-guided migration, newborn neuroblasts are frequently associated with thin astrocytic processes (Jin et al., 2003; Thored et al., 2006; Yamashita et al., 2006; Kojima et al., 2010), which directly contact vascular endothelial cells (Le Magueresse et al., 2012), forming a neurovascular niche. Double labeling for BrdU and PECAM-1 confirms that blood vessels in the peri-infarct cortex contain newly born vascular endothelial cells (Lacar et al., 2012). Moreover, inhibiting angiogenesis decreases the number of new neurons in injured regions (Taguchi et al., 2004; Ohab et al., 2006; Cayre et al., 2013), suggesting that newly generated blood vessels play a role in neuronal regeneration. Since new neurons migrate along both pre-existing and newly generated blood vessels after MCAO, both old and new blood vessels appear to act as a migratory scaffold for new neuroblasts moving toward injured regions (Kojima et al., 2010; Grade et al., 2013). Thus, remodeling the blood vessel network in injured regions and regulating the direction of new neuron migration could improve the efficiency of blood vessel-guided neuronal migration and neuronal regeneration.

- *Guidance cues*

Besides their role as scaffolds, endothelial cells are also able to secrete several factors that regulate the migration of neuroblasts, both in normal and pathological conditions. During adult neurogenesis, stromal-derived factor-1α (SDF-1α), a CXC chemokine, is secreted by vascular endothelial cells and enhances the motility of neuroblasts, which express its receptor CXR4, toward the RMS (Kokovay et al., 2010). Similarly, following stroke, endothelial cells and reactive astrocytes upregulate SDF-1 (Ohab et al., 2006; Thored et al., 2006), which guides neuroblast migration toward the peri-infarct region (Robin et al., 2006). Administration of SDF-1 improves behavioral recovery during the period in which immature neurons migrate (Ohab et al.,

2006), whereas blockade of CXRC4 with the specific antagonist AMD3100 alters the migration of new neurons *in vitro* and *in vivo* (Robin et al., 2006; Thored et al., 2006; Kojima et al., 2010).

- *Astrocytes/microglia*

Activated astrocytic and microglial populations in the core and the penumbra produce several factors, including cytokines and chemokines, which may act as putative chemoattractants for proliferating progenitors. For example, the expression of monocyte chemoattractant protein-1 (MCP-1), a CC chemokine, is induced in activated microglia and astrocytes after MCAO, while migrating neuroblasts express the MCP-1 receptor CCR2 (Cayre et al., 2013). Furthermore, MCP-1 and CCR2 KO mice display a significant decrease in the number of migrating neuroblasts from the ipsilateral SVZ to the ischemic striatum (Yan et al., 2007).

- *Other regulators*

Matrix metalloproteinases (MMPs) are expressed by endothelial cells following stroke, and digest the extracellular matrix to enable migrating newborn cells to penetrate the damaged parenchyma. MMPs have been implicated in guiding neuroblast migration from the neurogenic region to the ischemic boundary (Grade et al., 2013). MMP9 is upregulated in the infarcted cortex and co-localizes with DCX+ and BrdU+ cells migrating from SVZ. Moreover, blocking the activation of MMPs severely diminishes striatal migration (Lee et al., 2006; Barkho et al., 2008).

Non-neurogenic niches

As discussed above, neurogenesis also occurs in the damaged parenchyma. However, it seems that an anti-neurogenic environment prevents reactive astrocytes from becoming neurons. A more complete understanding of the molecular mechanisms that determine gliogenesis vs. neurogenesis is important to increase the number of newborn neurons in the injured area. Notably, the oligodendrocyte transcription factor OLIG2 and the neurogenic paired-box protein PAX6 are both potent regulators of stroke-induced neurogenesis. Stereotaxic retroviral injection of either a dominant negative form of Olig2, or a PAX6 overexpression construct, in the lateral striatum of MCAO rat brains results in a significant increase in the number of DCX-expressing immature neurons (Kronenberg et al., 2010; Robel et al., 2011). In addition, inhibition of Notch signaling—a strong anti-neurogenic pathway—triggers astrocytes in the striatum and the medial cortex to enter a neurogenic program, even in physiological conditions (Magnusson et al., 2014). Moreover, TNF-α or noggin—a bone morphogenetic protein (BMP) inhibitor—can modulate the latent neurogenic capacity of parenchymal astrocytes (Michelucci et al., 2015). Therefore, modulating the fate of endogenous parenchymal astrocytes represents an interesting target to induce neurogenesis after stroke.

Functional Impact

Several recent studies have shed light on the essential role of stroke-induced neurogenesis on functional recovery. Consistent with the neuroprotective role of NSCs, targeted depletion of both DCX- or Nestin-expressing cells in the SVZ has been linked to worsened stroke lesion size and motor impairment (Wang et al., 2012; Sun et al., 2013). On the contrary, manipulations aimed at increasing neurogenesis have been shown to improve functional outcomes (Leker et al., 2007). In endothelin-induced stroked rats, a combined treatment of fluoxetine, simvastatin and ascorbic acid produces a significant increase in neurogenesis, which is coupled to a strong functional recovery (Corbett et al., 2015). In ischemic mice brains, post-stroke chronic metformin treatment has been shown to enhance angiogenesis, neurogenesis and improve functional recovery following MCAO (Jin et al., 2014). These studies establish a clear link between stroke-induced neurogenesis and functional recovery. However, it is not yet understood why spontaneous endogenous neurogenesis does not lead to a complete recovery. Many milestones have to be reached in order to obtain functional recovery following stroke. Appropriate differentiation, long-term production and survival of stroke-induced newborn neurons, as well as the inflammatory response, are all potential restrictive characteristics regarding stroke recovery.

Differentiation and integration of newborn neurons

In order to contribute to functional recovery, nascent neurons, coming from non-neurogenic regions or neurogenic niches, must mature both morphologically and functionally. Early work showed that newly generated cells in the damaged striatum express markers of medium-size spiny neurons like DARPP-32, representing 95% of neurons within the striatum (Arvidsson et al., 2002; Parent et al., 2002). More recently, newborn cells, following focal cerebral ischemia, have also been shown to express appropriate neurotransmitter synthesizing enzymes such as glutamic acid decarboxylase (GAD67) and choline acetyl-transferase (ChAT). Moreover, these neurons exhibit electrophysiological activity and functional synapses (Hou et al., 2008). These data suggest that stroke-induced newborn GABAergic and cholinergic neurons can integrate into the striatal neural networks. However, if about 90–95% of striatal neurons are GABAergic medium-size spiny projection neurons, 5–10% of the remaining neurons are local interneurons that are classically divided into parvalbumin+ (PV+), calretinin+ (CR+), somatostatin+ (SOM+), and choline acetyltransferase+ (ChAT+) neurons (Marin et al., 2000). Immunostainings performed against these different markers, coupled with BrdU labeling, have shown that SVZ neuroblasts can produce CR-expressing newborn cells in the damaged striatum (Liu et al., 2009). Finally, another study has shown that newly born immature neurons differentiate into mature PV-expressing neurons, replacing more than 20% of PV+ interneurons lost after ischemia (Teramoto et al., 2003). Taken together, these data indicate that proliferating neuroblasts that migrate into the damaged striatum following stroke are able to differentiate into a variety of functional neuronal cells.

Long-term survival/production of newborn neurons

The long-term survival of newly-formed neurons following stroke is also crucial for a successful functional recovery.

Although recent work indicates that new neurons persist for at least 3–4 months after stroke (Thored et al., 2006; Leker et al., 2007), survival of newly generated cells is inefficient (Turnley et al., 2014). Only 10% of the initial number of neuroblasts that migrate to the peri-infarct cortex express mature neuronal markers (Gu et al., 2000; Dempsey et al., 2003), while 6 weeks after ischemia, one third of DCX+/BrdU+ cells express mature neuronal markers (Thored et al., 2006). Moreover, many of these DCX+ cells co-expressing cPARP, a substrate of active caspases, which suggests there is widespread apoptosis within the DCX+ cell population (Thored et al., 2006). Taken together, these data indicate that only a small proportion of cells survive long enough to integrate into the damaged parenchyma. This may be linked to an inappropriate inflammatory response in the ischemic area that is deleterious for newborn neuron survival. In support of this, treatment with indomethacin, a non-steroidal anti-inflammatory agent, suppresses inflammation and microglial activation, and stimulates the accumulation of newborn neurons in the injured striatum following MCAO in adult rats (Hoehn et al., 2005). Moreover, up-regulation of TNFα expression following stroke has been shown to decrease SVZ progenitor proliferation, whereas blockade of TNF receptor-1 signaling has been demonstrated to increase stroke-induced SVZ cell proliferation and neuroblast formation (Iosif et al., 2008).

Initial studies suggested that increased SVZ neurogenesis is transient, as progressive recovery of certain behavioral deficits does not continue beyond 1 month. However, BrdU injections have shown a similar proportion of DCX+/BrdU+ at either at 2 or 8 weeks post-ischemia (Thored et al., 2006). Moreover, the migration of SVZ neuroblasts to the injured striatum may persist for up to 1 year after ischemia (Thored et al., 2007), suggesting that the SVZ may serve as a constant reservoir of new neurons offering a long-term window for therapeutic manipulations.

CONCLUSION

Besides rtPA treatment, there is an urgent need to develop new treatments for stroke that are aimed at ultimately replacing dead neurons. While exogenous stem cell therapy presents interesting outcomes, increasing endogenous neurogenesis constitutes the most promising therapeutic strategy. Indeed, the presence of multiple pools of endogenous adult neuroblasts that are able to proliferate, migrate and differentiate, offers multiple possibilities for interventions. These strategies require that the as yet unknown molecular mechanisms that instruct stem cells to differentiate into specific neuronal cell types will also work in the brain of the affected individual. For maximum functional recovery, transplantation should probably be combined with a stimulation of neurogenesis from endogenous NSCs.

However, several critical questions have to be addressed before clinical trials can begin. Optimization of the timing and treatment is required, along with the identification of factors that give the most favorable survival and function of new cells, irrespective of their exogenous or endogenous origin. In addition, the heterogeneity among stroke patients constitutes an important challenge. The use of clinically relevant experimental animal models is essential, since numerous successful preclinical trials have failed to confirm their efficacy upon translation to humans. Moreover, inflammation is increasingly recognized as a key factor in stroke, but whether it is detrimental or beneficial depends on the severity and stage of the ischemia. It appears that an inflammatory response during the early stages of stroke potentiate ischemic injury, while late inflammation appears to be important for recovery and repair. Future work should focus on elucidating how the immune system moves from these damaging to protective/restorative responses. Consequently, a nuanced modulation of inflammation may lead to improved exogenous and endogenous potentiality regarding stroke recovery.

Elucidating the molecular mechanisms that regulate endogenous neurogenesis in stroke can be extended to other neurodegenerative diseases. Indeed, despite different triggering events, a common feature of neurodegenerative disease is neuronal cell death and immune responses.

ACKNOWLEDGMENTS

The authors thank S. Freeman for critical reading of the manuscript. RV and BM are Postdoctoral researcher and Senior Research Associate from the Belgian National Funds for Scientific Research (FRS-FNRS), respectively. BM is funded by grants from the FRS-FNRS, the Fonds Léon Fredericq, the Fondation Médicale Reine Elisabeth, and the Belgian Science Policy (IAP-VII network P7/07).

REFERENCES

Anderson, D. J. (2001). Stem cells and pattern formation in the nervous system: the possible versus the actual. *Neuron* 30, 19–35. doi: 10.1016/S0896-6273(01)00260-4

Andreu-Agulló, C., Morante-Redolat, J. M., Delgado, A. C., and Fariñas, I. (2009). Vascular niche factor PEDF modulates Notch-dependent stemness in the adult subependymal zone. *Nat. Neurosci.* 12, 1514–1523. doi: 10.1038/nn.2437

Andrews, E. M., Tsai, S. Y., Johnson, S. C., Farrer, J. R., Wagner, J. P., Kopen, G. C., et al. (2008). Human adult bone marrow-derived somatic cell therapy results in functional recovery and axonal plasticity following stroke in the rat. *Exp. Neurol.* 211, 588–592. doi: 10.1016/j.expneurol.2008.02.027

Arvidsson, A., Collin, T., Kirik, D., Kokaia, Z., and Lindvall, O. (2002). Neuronal replacement from endogenous precursors in the adult brain after stroke. *Nat. Med.* 8, 963–970. doi: 10.1038/nm747

Bacigaluppi, M., Pluchino, S., Peruzzotti-Jametti, L., Kilic, E., Kilic, U., Salani, G., et al. (2009). Delayed post-ischaemic neuroprotection following systemic neural stem cell transplantation involves multiple mechanisms. *Brain* 132, 2239–2251. doi: 10.1093/brain/awp174

Bao, X., Wei, J., Feng, M., Lu, S., Li, G., Dou, W., et al. (2011). Transplantation of human bone marrow-derived mesenchymal stem cells promotes behavioral recovery and endogenous neurogenesis after cerebral ischemia in rats. *Brain Res.* 1367, 103–113. doi: 10.1016/j.brainres.2010.10.063

Bao, X. J., Liu, F. Y., Lu, S., Han, Q., Feng, M., Wei, J. J., et al. (2013). Transplantation of Flk-1+ human bone marrow-derived mesenchymal stem cells promotes behavioral recovery and anti-inflammatory and angiogenesis effects in an intracerebral hemorrhage rat model. *Int. J. Mol. Med.* 31, 1087–1096. doi: 10.3892/ijmm.2013.1290

Barkho, B. Z., Munoz, A. E., Li, X., Li, L., Cunningham, L. A., and Zhao, X. (2008). Endogenous matrix metalloproteinase (MMP)-3 and MMP-9 promote the differentiation and migration of adult neural progenitor cells in response to chemokines. *Stem Cells* 26, 3139–3149. doi: 10.1634/stemcells.2008-0519

Barkho, B. Z., and Zhao, X. (2011). Adult neural stem cells: response to stroke injury and potential for therapeutic applications. *Curr. Stem Cell Res. Ther.* 6, 327–338. doi: 10.2174/157488811797904362

Bauer, S., Hay, M., Amilhon, B., Jean, A., and Moyse, E. (2005). *In vivo* neurogenesis in the dorsal vagal complex of the adult rat brainstem. *Neuroscience* 130, 75–90. doi: 10.1016/j.neuroscience.2004.08.047

Bédard, A., Gravel, C., and Parent, A. (2006). Chemical characterization of newly generated neurons in the striatum of adult primates. *Exp. Brain Res.* 170, 501–512. doi: 10.1007/s00221-005-0233-5

Ben-David, U., and Benvenisty, N. (2011). The tumorigenicity of human embryonic and induced pluripotent stem cells. *Nat. Rev. Cancer* 11, 268–277. doi: 10.1038/nrc3034

Benner, E. J., Luciano, D., Jo, R., Abdi, K., Paez-Gonzalez, P., Sheng, H., et al. (2013). Protective astrogenesis from the SVZ niche after injury is controlled by Notch modulator Thbs4. *Nature* 497, 369–373. doi: 10.1038/nature12069

Bennett, L., Yang, M., Enikolopov, G., and Iacovitti, L. (2009). Circumventricular organs: a novel site of neural stem cells in the adult brain. *Mol. Cell. Neurosci.* 41, 337–347. doi: 10.1016/j.mcn.2009.04.007

Bernier, P. J., Bedard, A., Vinet, J., Levesque, M., and Parent, A. (2002). Newly generated neurons in the amygdala and adjoining cortex of adult primates. *Proc. Natl. Acad. Sci. U.S.A.* 99, 11464–11469. doi: 10.1073/pnas.172403999

Braun, R. G., Andrews, E. M., and Kartje, G. L. (2012). Kinematic analysis of motor recovery with human adult bone marrow-derived somatic cell therapy in a rat model of stroke. *Neurorehabil. Neural Repair* 26, 898–906. doi: 10.1177/1545968312446004

Bühnemann, C., Scholz, A., Bernreuther, C., Malik, C. Y., Braun, H., Schachner, M., et al. (2006). Neuronal differentiation of transplanted embryonic stem cell-derived precursors in stroke lesions of adult rats. *Brain* 129, 3238–3248. doi: 10.1093/brain/awl261

Carlén, M., Meletis, K., Göritz, C., Darsalia, V., Evergren, E., Tanigaki, K., et al. (2009). Forebrain ependymal cells are Notch-dependent and generate neuroblasts and astrocytes after stroke. *Nat. Neurosci.* 12, 259–267. doi: 10.1038/nn.2268

Carleton, A., Petreanu, L. T., Lansford, R., Alvarez-Buylla, A., and Lledo, P. M. (2003). Becoming a new neuron in the adult olfactory bulb. *Nat. Neurosci.* 6, 507–518. doi: 10.1038/nn1048

Cayre, M., Courtès, S., Martineau, F., Giordano, M., Arnaud, K., Zamaron, A., et al. (2013). Netrin 1 contributes to vascular remodeling in the subventricular zone and promotes progenitor emigration after demyelination. *Development* 140, 3107–3117. doi: 10.1242/dev.092999

Charrier, C., Coronas, V., Fombonne, J., Roger, M., Jean, A., Krantic, S., et al. (2006). Characterization of neural stem cells in the dorsal vagal complex of adult rat by *in vivo* proliferation labeling and *in vitro* neurosphere assay. *Neuroscience* 138, 5–16. doi: 10.1016/j.neuroscience.2005.10.046

Chen, J., Li, Y., Wang, L., Lu, M., Zhang, X., and Chopp, M. (2001a). Therapeutic benefit of intracerebral transplantation of bone marrow stromal cells after cerebral ischemia in rats. *J. Neurol. Sci.* 189, 49–57. doi: 10.1016/S0022-510X(01)00557-3

Chen, J., Li, Y., Wang, L., Zhang, Z., Lu, D., Lu, M., et al. (2001b). Therapeutic benefit of intravenous administration of bone marrow stromal cells after cerebral ischemia in rats. *Stroke* 32, 1005–1011. doi: 10.1161/01.STR.32.4.1005s

Chen, J., Zacharek, A., Zhang, C., Jiang, H., Li, Y., Roberts, C., et al. (2005). Endothelial nitric oxide synthase regulates brain-derived neurotrophic factor expression and neurogenesis after stroke in mice. *J. Neurosci.* 25, 2366–2375. doi: 10.1523/JNEUROSCI.5071-04.2005

Chen, Z. Z., Jiang, X. D., Zhang, L. L., Shang, J. H., Du, M. X., Xu, G., et al. (2008). Beneficial effect of autologous transplantation of bone marrow stromal cells and endothelial progenitor cells on cerebral ischemia in rabbits. *Neurosci. Lett.* 445, 36–41. doi: 10.1016/j.neulet.2008.08.039

Chou, J., Harvey, B. K., Chang, C. F., Shen, H., Morales, M., and Wang, Y. (2006). Neuroregenerative effects of BMP7 after stroke in rats. *J. Neurol. Sci.* 240, 21–29. doi: 10.1016/j.jns.2005.08.015

Chu, K., Park, K. I., Lee, S. T., Jung, K. H., Ko, S. Y., Kang, L., et al. (2005). Combined treatment of vascular endothelial growth factor and human neural stem cells in experimental focal cerebral ischemia. *Neurosci. Res.* 53, 384–390. doi: 10.1016/j.neures.2005.08.010

Corbett, A. M., Sieber, S., Wyatt, N., Lizzi, J., Flannery, T., Sibbit, B., et al. (2015). Increasing neurogenesis with fluoxetine, simvastatin and ascorbic acid leads to functional recovery in ischemic stroke. *Recent Pat. Drug Deliv. Formul.* 9, 158–166. doi: 10.2174/1872211309666150122102846

Cui, X., Chen, J., Zacharek, A., Li, Y., Roberts, C., Kapke, A., et al. (2007). Nitric oxide donor upregulation of stromal cell-derived factor-1/chemokine (CXC motif) receptor 4 enhances bone marrow stromal cell migration into ischemic brain after stroke. *Stem Cells* 25, 2777–2785. doi: 10.1634/stemcells.2007-0169

Daadi, M. M., Maag, A. L., and Steinberg, G. K. (2008). Adherent self-renewable human embryonic stem cell-derived neural stem cell line: functional engraftment in experimental stroke model. *PLoS ONE* 3:e1644. doi: 10.1371/journal.pone.0001644

Darsalia, V., Allison, S. J., Cusulin, C., Monni, E., Kuzdas, D., Kallur, T., et al. (2011). Cell number and timing of transplantation determine survival of human neural stem cell grafts in stroke-damaged rat brain. *J. Cereb. Blood Flow Metab.* 31, 235–242. doi: 10.1038/jcbfm.2010.81

Dayer, A. G., Cleaver, K. M., Abouantoun, T., and Cameron, H. A. (2005). New GABAergic interneurons in the adult neocortex and striatum are generated from different precursors. *J. Cell Biol.* 168, 415–427. doi: 10.1083/jcb.2004 07053

del Zoppo, G., Ginis, I., Hallenbeck, J. M., Iadecola, C., Wang, X., and Feuerstein, G. Z. (2000). Inflammation and stroke: putative role for cytokines, adhesion molecules and iNOS in brain response to ischemia. *Brain Pathol.* 10, 95–112. doi: 10.1111/j.1750-3639.2000.tb00247.x

del Zoppo, G. J., Milner, R., Mabuchi, T., Hung, S., Wang, X., Berg, G. I., et al. (2007). Microglial activation and matrix protease generation during focal cerebral ischemia. *Stroke* 38, 646–651. doi: 10.1161/01.STR.0000254477.34231.cb

Dempsey, R. J., Sailor, K. A., Bowen, K. K., Türeyen, K., and Vemuganti, R. (2003). Stroke-induced progenitor cell proliferation in adult spontaneously hypertensive rat brain: effect of exogenous IGF-1 and GDNF. *J. Neurochem.* 87, 586–597. doi: 10.1046/j.1471-4159.2003.02022.x

Drago, D., Cossetti, C., Iraci, N., Gaude, E., Musco, G., Bachi, A., et al. (2013). The stem cell secretome and its role in brain repair. *Biochimie* 95, 2271–2285. doi: 10.1016/j.biochi.2013.06.020

Duan, C. L., Liu, C. W., Shen, S. W., Yu, Z., Mo, J. L., Chen, X. H., et al. (2015). Striatal astrocytes transdifferentiate into functional mature neurons following ischemic brain injury. *Glia* 63, 1660–1670. doi: 10.1002/glia.22837

Eckert, A., Huang, L., Gonzalez, R., Kim, H. S., Hamblin, M. H., and Lee, J. P. (2015). Bystander Effect fuels human induced pluripotent stem cell-derived neural stem cells to quickly attenuate early stage neurological deficits after stroke. *Stem Cells Transl. Med.* 4, 841–851. doi: 10.5966/sctm.2014-0184

Eriksson, P. S., Perfilieva, E., Björk-Eriksson, T., Alborn, A. M., Nordborg, C., Peterson, D. A., et al. (1998). Neurogenesis in the adult human hippocampus. *Nat. Med.* 4, 1313–1317. doi: 10.1038/3305

Faiz, M., Sachewsky, N., Gascón, S., Bang, K. W. A., Morshead, C. M., and Nagy, A. (2015). Adult neural stem cells from the subventricular zone give rise to reactive astrocytes in the cortex after stroke. *Cell Stem Cell* 17, 1–11. doi: 10.1016/j.stem.2015.08.002

Furube, E., Morita, M., and Miyata, S. (2015). Characterization of neural stem cells and their progeny in the sensory circumventricular organs of adult mouse. *Cell Tissue Res.* 362, 347–365. doi: 10.1007/s00441-015-2201-0

Gage, F. H. (2000). Mammalian neural stem cells. *Science* 287, 1433–1438. doi: 10.1126/science.287.5457.1433

Genin, E. C., Caron, N., Vandenbosch, R., Nguyen, L., and Malgrange, B. (2014). Concise review: forkhead pathway in the control of adult neurogenesis. *Stem Cells* 32, 1398–1407. doi: 10.1002/stem.1673

Ginsberg, M. D., and Busto, R. (1989). Rodent models of cerebral ischemia. *Stroke* 20, 1627–1642. doi: 10.1161/01.STR.20.12.1627

Goldberg, J. S., and Hirschi, K. K. (2009). Diverse roles of the vasculature within the neural stem cell niche. *Regen. Med.* 4, 879–897. doi: 10.2217/rme.09.61

Gonzalez-Perez, O., Quiñones-Hinojosa, A., and Garcia-Verdugo, J. M. (2010). Immunological control of adult neural stem cells. *J. Stem Cells* 5, 23–31.

Grade, S., Weng, Y. C., Snapyan, M., Kriz, J., Malva, J. O., and Saghatelyan, A. (2013). Brain-derived neurotrophic factor promotes vasculature-associated migration of neuronal precursors toward the ischemic striatum. *PLoS ONE* 8:e55039. doi: 10.1371/journal.pone.0055039

Gu, W., Brännström, T., and Wester, P. (2000). Cortical neurogenesis in adult rats after reversible photothrombotic stroke. *J. Cereb. Blood Flow Metab.* 20, 1166–1173. doi: 10.1097/00004647-200008000-00002

Gutiérrez-Fernández, M., Rodríguez-Frutos, B., Alvarez-Grech, J., Vallejo-Cremades, M. T., Expósito-Alcaide, M., Merino, J., et al. (2011). Functional recovery after hematic administration of allogenic mesenchymal stem cells in acute ischemic stroke in rats. *Neuroscience* 175, 394–405. doi: 10.1016/j.neuroscience.2010.11.054

Hassani, Z., O'Reilly, J., Pearse, Y., Stroemer, P., Tang, E., Sinden, J., et al. (2012). Human neural progenitor cell engraftment increases neurogenesis and microglial recruitment in the brain of rats with stroke. *PLoS ONE* 7:e50444. doi: 10.1371/journal.pone.0050444

Hayashi, T., Noshita, N., Sugawara, T., and Chan, P. H. (2003). Temporal profile of angiogenesis and expression of related genes in the brain after ischemia. *J. Cereb. Blood Flow Metab.* 23, 166–180. doi: 10.1097/00004647-200302000-00004

Heinrich, C., Bergami, M., Gascón, S., Lepier, A., Viganò, F., Dimou, L., et al. (2014). Sox2-mediated conversion of NG2 glia into induced neurons in the injured adult cerebral cortex. *Stem Cell Rep.* 3, 1000–1014. doi: 10.1016/j.stemcr.2014.10.007

Hermann, D. M., Peruzzotti-Jametti, L., Schlechter, J., Bernstock, J. D., Doeppner, T. R., and Pluchino, S. (2014). Neural precursor cells in the ischemic brain - integration, cellular crosstalk, and consequences for stroke recovery. *Front. Cell. Neurosci.* 8:291. doi: 10.3389/fncel.2014.00291

Hoehn, B. D., Palmer, T. D., and Steinberg, G. K. (2005). Neurogenesis in rats after focal cerebral ischemia is enhanced by indomethacin. *Stroke* 36, 2718–2724. doi: 10.1161/01.STR.0000190020.30282.cc

Honma, T., Honmou, O., Iihoshi, S., Harada, K., Houkin, K., Hamada, H., et al. (2006). Intravenous infusion of immortalized human mesenchymal stem cells protects against injury in a cerebral ischemia model in adult rat. *Exp. Neurol.* 199, 56–66. doi: 10.1016/j.expneurol.2005.05.004

Horita, Y., Honmou, O., Harada, K., Houkin, K., Hamada, H., and Kocsis, J. D. (2006). Intravenous administration of glial cell line-derived neurotrophic factor gene-modified human mesenchymal stem cells protects against injury in a cerebral ischemia model in the adult rat. *J. Neurosci. Res.* 84, 1495–1504. doi: 10.1002/jnr.21056

Hossmann, K. A. (2012). The two pathophysiologies of focal brain ischemia: implications for translational stroke research. *J. Cereb. Blood Flow Metab.* 32, 1310–1316. doi: 10.1038/jcbfm.2011.186

Hou, S. W., Wang, Y. Q., Xu, M., Shen, D. H., Wang, J. J., Huang, F., et al. (2008). Functional integration of newly generated neurons into striatum after cerebral ischemia in the adult rat brain. *Stroke* 39, 2837–2844. doi: 10.1161/STROKEAHA.107.510982

Hwang, I. K., Yoo, K. Y., Park, S. K., An, S. J., Lee, J. Y., Choi, S. Y., et al. (2004). Expression and changes of endogenous insulin-like growth factor-1 in neurons and glia in the gerbil hippocampus and dentate gyrus after ischemic insult. *Neurochem. Int.* 45, 149–156. doi: 10.1016/j.neuint.2003.10.006

Iadecola, C., and Anrather, J. (2011). The immunology of stroke: from mechanisms to translation. *Nat. Med.* 17, 796–808. doi: 10.1038/nm.2399

Imai, F., Suzuki, H., Oda, J., Ninomiya, T., Ono, K., Sano, H., et al. (2007). Neuroprotective effect of exogenous microglia in global brain ischemia. *J. Cereb. Blood Flow Metab.* 27, 488–500. doi: 10.1038/sj.jcbfm.9600362

Iosif, R. E., Ahlenius, H., Ekdahl, C. T., Darsalia, V., Thored, P., Jovinge, S., et al. (2008). Suppression of stroke-induced progenitor proliferation in adult subventricular zone by tumor necrosis factor receptor 1. *J. Cereb. Blood Flow Metab.* 28, 1574–1587. doi: 10.1038/jcbfm.2008.47

Itokazu, Y., Kitada, M., Dezawa, M., Mizoguchi, A., Matsumoto, N., Shimizu, A., et al. (2006). Choroid plexus ependymal cells host neural progenitor cells in the rat. *Glia* 53, 32–42. doi: 10.1002/glia.20255

Jensen, M. B., Yan, H., Krishnaney-Davison, R., Al Sawaf, A., and Zhang, S. C. (2013). Survival and differentiation of transplanted neural stem cells derived from human induced pluripotent stem cells in a rat stroke model. *J. Stroke Cerebrovasc. Dis.* 22, 304–308. doi: 10.1016/j.jstrokecerebrovasdis.2011.09.008

Jiang, M., Lv, L., Ji, H., Yang, X., Zhu, W., Cai, L., et al. (2011). Induction of pluripotent stem cells transplantation therapy for ischemic stroke. *Mol. Cell. Biochem.* 354, 67–75. doi: 10.1007/s11010-011-0806-5

Jiang, Q., Ewing, J. R., Zhang, Z. G., Zhang, R. L., Hu, J., Divine, G. W., et al. (2001). Magnetization transfer MRI: application to treatment of middle cerebral artery occlusion in rat. *J. Magn. Reson. Imaging* 13, 178–184. doi: 10.1002/1522-2586(200102)13:2<178::AID-JMRI1027>3.0.CO;2-D

Jiang, Q., Zhang, Z. G., Ding, G. L., Silver, B., Zhang, L., Meng, H., et al. (2006). MRI detects white matter reorganization after neural progenitor cell treatment of stroke. *Neuroimage* 32, 1080–1089. doi: 10.1016/j.neuroimage.2006.05.025

Jin, K., Minami, M., Lan, J. Q., Mao, X. O., Batteur, S., Simon, R. P., et al. (2001). Neurogenesis in dentate subgranular zone and rostral subventricular zone after focal cerebral ischemia in the rat. *Proc. Natl. Acad. Sci. U.S.A.* 98, 4710–4715. doi: 10.1073/pnas.081011098

Jin, K., Sun, Y., Xie, L., Peel, A., Mao, X. O., Batteur, S., et al. (2003). Directed migration of neuronal precursors into the ischemic cerebral cortex and striatum. *Mol. Cell. Neurosci.* 24, 171–189. doi: 10.1016/S1044-7431(03)00159-3

Jin, K., Wang, X., Xie, L., Mao, X. O., Zhu, W., Wang, Y., et al. (2006). Evidence for stroke-induced neurogenesis in the human brain. *Proc. Natl. Acad. Sci. U.S.A.* 103, 13198–13202. doi: 10.1073/pnas.0603512103

Jin, K., Zhu, Y., Sun, Y., Mao, X. O., Xie, L., and Greenberg, D. A. (2002). Vascular endothelial growth factor (VEGF) stimulates neurogenesis *in vitro* and *in vivo*. *Proc. Natl. Acad. Sci. U.S.A.* 99, 11946–11950. doi: 10.1073/pnas.182296499

Jin, Q., Cheng, J., Liu, Y., Wu, J., Wang, X., Wei, S., et al. (2014). Improvement of functional recovery by chronic metformin treatment is associated with enhanced alternative activation of microglia/macrophages and increased angiogenesis and neurogenesis following experimental stroke. *Brain Behav. Immun.* 40, 131–142. doi: 10.1016/j.bbi.2014.03.003

Joly, J. S., Osório, J., Alunni, A., Auger, H., Kano, S., and Rétaux, S. (2007). Windows of the brain: towards a developmental biology of circumventricular and other neurohemal organs. *Semin. Cell Dev. Biol.* 18, 512–524. doi: 10.1016/j.semcdb.2007.06.001

Jones, T. A., and Adkins, D. L. (2015). Motor system reorganization after stroke: stimulating and training toward perfection. *Physiology* 30, 358–370. doi: 10.1152/physiol.00014.2015

Kalladka, D., and Muir, K. W. (2014). Brain repair: cell therapy in stroke. *Stem Cells Cloning* 7, 31–44. doi: 10.2147/SCCAA.S38003

Kang, S. K., Lee, D. H., Bae, Y. C., Kim, H. K., Baik, S. Y., and Jung, J. S. (2003). Improvement of neurological deficits by intracerebral transplantation of human adipose tissue-derived stromal cells after cerebral ischemia in rats. *Exp. Neurol.* 183, 355–366. doi: 10.1016/S0014-4886(03)00089-X

Karow, M., Sánchez, R., Schichor, C., Masserdotti, G., Ortega, F., Heinrich, C., et al. (2012). Reprogramming of pericyte-derived cells of the adult human brain into induced neuronal cells. *Cell Stem Cell* 11, 471–476. doi: 10.1016/j.stem.2012.07.007

Kawai, H., Yamashita, T., Ohta, Y., Deguchi, K., Nagotani, S., Zhang, X., et al. (2010). Tridermal tumorigenesis of induced pluripotent stem cells transplanted in ischemic brain. *J. Cereb. Blood Flow Metab.* 30, 1487–1493. doi: 10.1038/jcbfm.2010.32

Kee, N. J., Preston, E., and Wojtowicz, J. M. (2001). Enhanced neurogenesis after transient global ischemia in the dentate gyrus of the rat. *Exp. Brain Res.* 136, 313–320. doi: 10.1007/s002210000591

Kim, B. J., Kim, M. J., Park, J. M., Lee, S. H., Kim, Y. J., Ryu, S., et al. (2009). Reduced neurogenesis after suppressed inflammation by minocycline in transient cerebral ischemia in rat. *J. Neurol. Sci.* 279, 70–75. doi: 10.1016/j.jns.2008.12.025

Kim, Y. R., Kim, H. N., Ahn, S. M., Choi, Y. H., Shin, H. K., and Choi, B. T. (2014). Electroacupuncture promotes post-stroke functional recovery via enhancing endogenous neurogenesis in mouse focal cerebral ischemia. *PLoS ONE* 9:e90000. doi: 10.1371/journal.pone.0090000

Koh, S. H., Kim, K. S., Choi, M. R., Jung, K. H., Park, K. S., Chai, Y. G., et al. (2008). Implantation of human umbilical cord-derived mesenchymal stem cells as a neuroprotective therapy for ischemic stroke in rats. *Brain Res.* 1229, 233–248. doi: 10.1016/j.brainres.2008.06.087

Kojima, T., Hirota, Y., Ema, M., Takahashi, S., Miyoshi, I., Okano, H., et al. (2010). Subventricular zone-derived neural progenitor cells migrate along a blood vessel scaffold toward the post-stroke striatum. *Stem Cells* 28, 545–554. doi: 10.1002/stem.306

Kokaia, Z., and Lindvall, O. (2003). Neurogenesis after ischaemic brain insults. *Curr. Opin. Neurobiol.* 13, 127–132. doi: 10.1016/S0959-4388(03)00017-5

Kokaia, Z., Martino, G., Schwartz, M., and Lindvall, O. (2012). Cross-talk between neural stem cells and immune cells: the key to better brain repair? *Nat. Neurosci.* 15, 1078–1087. doi: 10.1038/nn.3163

Kokoeva, M. V., Yin, H., and Flier, J. S. (2005). Neurogenesis in the hypothalamus of adult mice: potential role in energy balance. *Science* 310, 679–683. doi: 10.1126/science.1115360

Kokovay, E., Goderie, S., Wang, Y., Lotz, S., Lin, G., Sun, Y., et al. (2010). Adult SVZ lineage cells home to and leave the vascular niche via differential responses to SDF1/CXCR4 signaling. *Cell Stem Cell* 7, 163–173. doi: 10.1016/j.stem.2010.05.019

Kronenberg, G., Gertz, K., Cheung, G., Buffo, A., Kettenmann, H., Götz, M., et al. (2010). Modulation of fate determinants Olig2 and Pax6 in resident glia evokes spiking neuroblasts in a model of mild brain ischemia. *Stroke* 41, 2944–2949. doi: 10.1161/STROKEAHA.110.583039

Krupinski, J., Kaluza, J., Kumar, P., Kumar, S., and Wang, J. M. (1994). Role of angiogenesis in patients with cerebral ischemic stroke. *Stroke* 25, 1794–1798. doi: 10.1161/01.STR.25.9.1794

Kurozumi, K., Nakamura, K., Tamiya, T., Kawano, Y., Ishii, K., Kobune, M., et al. (2005). Mesenchymal stem cells that produce neurotrophic factors reduce ischemic damage in the rat middle cerebral artery occlusion model. *Mol. Ther.* 11, 96–104. doi: 10.1016/j.ymthe.2004.09.020

Lacar, B., Herman, P., Platel, J. C., Kubera, C., Hyder, F., and Bordey, A. (2012). Neural progenitor cells regulate capillary blood flow in the postnatal subventricular zone. *J. Neurosci.* 32, 16435–16448. doi: 10.1523/JNEUROSCI.1457-12.2012

Lang, B., Liu, H. L., Liu, R., Feng, G. D., Jiao, X. Y., and Ju, G. (2004). Astrocytes in injured adult rat spinal cord may acquire the potential of neural stem cells. *Neuroscience* 128, 775–783. doi: 10.1016/j.neuroscience.2004.06.033

Lee, S. H., Jin, K. S., Bang, O. Y., Kim, B. J., Park, S. J., Lee, N. H., et al. (2015). Differential migration of mesenchymal stem cells to ischemic regions after middle cerebral artery occlusion in rats. *PLoS ONE* 10:e0134920. doi: 10.1371/journal.pone.0134920

Lee, S. R., Kim, H. Y., Rogowska, J., Zhao, B. Q., Bhide, P., Parent, J. M., et al. (2006). Involvement of matrix metalloproteinase in neuroblast cell migration from the subventricular zone after stroke. *J. Neurosci.* 26, 3491–3495. doi: 10.1523/JNEUROSCI.4085-05.2006

Leker, R. R., Soldner, F., Velasco, I., Gavin, D. K., Androutsellis-Theotokis, A., and McKay, R. D. (2007). Long-lasting regeneration after ischemia in the cerebral cortex. *Stroke* 38, 153–161. doi: 10.1161/01.STR.0000252156.65953.a9

Le Magueresse, C., Alfonso, J., Bark, C., Eliava, M., Khrulev, S., and Monyer, H. (2012). Subventricular zone-derived neuroblasts use vasculature as a scaffold to migrate radially to the cortex in neonatal mice. *Cereb. Cortex* 22, 2285–2296. doi: 10.1093/cercor/bhr302

Li, L., Jiang, Q., Ding, G., Zhang, L., Zhang, Z. G., Li, Q., et al. (2010). Effects of administration route on migration and distribution of neural progenitor cells transplanted into rats with focal cerebral ischemia, an MRI study. *J. Cereb. Blood Flow Metab.* 30, 653–662. doi: 10.1038/jcbfm.2009.238

Li, Y., Chen, J., and Chopp, M. (2002). Cell proliferation and differentiation from ependymal, subependymal and choroid plexus cells in response to stroke in rats. *J. Neurol. Sci.* 193, 137–146. doi: 10.1016/S0022-510X(01)00657-8

Li, Y., Chopp, M., Chen, J., Wang, L., Gautam, S. C., Xu, Y. X., et al. (2000). Intrastriatal transplantation of bone marrow nonhematopoietic cells improves functional recovery after stroke in adult mice. *J. Cereb. Blood Flow Metab.* 20, 1311–1319. doi: 10.1097/00004647-200009000-00006

Lichtenwalner, R. J., and Parent, J. M. (2006). Adult neurogenesis and the ischemic forebrain. *J. Cereb. Blood Flow Metab.* 26, 1–20. doi: 10.1038/sj.jcbfm.9600170

Lin, R., Cai, J., Nathan, C., Wei, X., Schleidt, S., Rosenwasser, R., et al. (2015). Neurogenesis is enhanced by stroke in multiple new stem cell niches along the ventricular system at sites of high BBB permeability. *Neurobiol. Dis.* 74, 229–239. doi: 10.1016/j.nbd.2014.11.016

Lin, R., and Iacovitti, L. (2015). Classic and novel stem cell niches in brain homeostasis and repair. *Brain Res.* doi: 10.1016/j.brainres.2015.04.029. [Epub ahead of print].

Liu, F., You, Y., Li, X., Ma, T., Nie, Y., Wei, B., et al. (2009). Brain injury does not alter the intrinsic differentiation potential of adult neuroblasts. *J. Neurosci.* 29, 5075–5087. doi: 10.1523/JNEUROSCI.0201-09.2009

Liu, X. S., Chopp, M., Zhang, R. L., and Zhang, Z. G. (2013). MicroRNAs in cerebral ischemia-induced neurogenesis. *J. Neuropathol. Exp. Neurol.* 72, 718–722. doi: 10.1097/NEN.0b013e31829e4963

Liu, X. S., Zhang, Z. G., Zhang, R. L., Gregg, S., Morris, D. C., Wang, Y., et al. (2007). Stroke induces gene profile changes associated with neurogenesis and angiogenesis in adult subventricular zone progenitor cells. *J. Cereb. Blood Flow Metab.* 27, 564–574. doi: 10.1038/sj.jcbfm.9600371

Lo, E. H. (2008). A new penumbra: transitioning from injury into repair after stroke. *Nat. Med.* 14, 497–500. doi: 10.1038/nm1735

Luo, C. X., Jiang, J., Zhou, Q. G., Zhu, X. J., Wang, W., Zhang, Z. J., et al. (2007). Voluntary exercise-induced neurogenesis in the postischemic dentate gyrus is associated with spatial memory recovery from stroke. *J. Neurosci. Res.* 85, 1637–1646. doi: 10.1002/jnr.21317

Luzzati, F., De Marchis, S., Fasolo, A., and Peretto, P. (2006). Neurogenesis in the caudate nucleus of the adult rabbit. *J. Neurosci.* 26, 609–621. doi: 10.1523/JNEUROSCI.4371-05.2006

Magavi, S. S., Leavitt, B. R., and Macklis, J. D. (2000). Induction of neurogenesis in the neocortex of adult mice. *Nature* 405, 951–955. doi: 10.1038/35016083

Magnusson, J. P., Göritz, C., Tatarishvili, J., Dias, D. O., Smith, E. M., Lindvall, O., et al. (2014). A latent neurogenic program in astrocytes regulated by Notch signaling in the mouse. *Science* 346, 237–241. doi: 10.1126/science.346.6206.237

Marin, O., Anderson, S. A., and Rubenstein, J. L. (2000). Origin and molecular specification of striatal interneurons. *J. Neurosci.* 20, 6063–6076.

Martino, G., and Pluchino, S. (2006). The therapeutic potential of neural stem cells. *Nat. Rev. Neurosci.* 7, 395–406. doi: 10.1038/nrn1908

Martino, G., Pluchino, S., Bonfanti, L., and Schwartz, M. (2011). Brain regeneration in physiology and pathology: the immune signature driving therapeutic plasticity of neural stem cells. *Physiol. Rev.* 91, 1281–1304. doi: 10.1152/physrev.00032.2010

Matarredona, E. R., Murillo-Carretero, M., Moreno-López, B., and Estrada, C. (2005). Role of nitric oxide in subventricular zone neurogenesis. *Brain Res. Brain Res. Rev.* 49, 355–366. doi: 10.1016/j.brainresrev.2005.01.001

Michelucci, A., Bithell, A., Burney, M. J., Johnston, C. E., Wong, K. Y., Teng, S. W., et al. (2015). The neurogenic potential of astrocytes is regulated by inflammatory signals. *Mol. Neurobiol.* doi: 10.1007/s12035-015-9296-x. [Epub ahead of print].

Migaud, M., Batailler, M., Segura, S., Duittoz, A., Franceschini, I., and Pillon, D. (2010). Emerging new sites for adult neurogenesis in the mammalian brain: a comparative study between the hypothalamus and the classical neurogenic zones. *Eur. J. Neurosci.* 32, 2042–2052. doi: 10.1111/j.1460-9568.2010.07521.x

Mine, Y., Tatarishvili, J., Oki, K., Monni, E., Kokaia, Z., and Lindvall, O. (2013). Grafted human neural stem cells enhance several steps of endogenous neurogenesis and improve behavioral recovery after middle cerebral artery occlusion in rats. *Neurobiol. Dis.* 52, 191–203. doi: 10.1016/j.nbd.2012.12.006

Mirzadeh, Z., Han, Y. G., Soriano-Navarro, M., García-Verdugo, J. M., and Alvarez-Buylla, A. (2010). Cilia organize ependymal planar polarity. *J. Neurosci.* 30, 2600–2610. doi: 10.1523/JNEUROSCI.3744-09.2010

Mirzadeh, Z., Merkle, F. T., Soriano-Navarro, M., Garcia-Verdugo, J. M., and Alvarez-Buylla, A. (2008). Neural stem cells confer unique pinwheel architecture to the ventricular surface in neurogenic regions of the adult brain. *Cell Stem Cell* 3, 265–278. doi: 10.1016/j.stem.2008.07.004

Mobley, A. K., Tchaicha, J. H., Shin, J., Hossain, M. G., and McCarty, J. H. (2009). Beta8 integrin regulates neurogenesis and neurovascular homeostasis in the adult brain. *J. Cell Sci.* 122, 1842–1851. doi: 10.1242/jcs.043257

Morrison, S. J. (2001). Neuronal potential and lineage determination by neural stem cells. *Curr. Opin. Cell Biol.* 13, 666–672. doi: 10.1016/S0955-0674(00)00269-6

Moskowitz, M. A., Lo, E. H., and Iadecola, C. (2010). The science of stroke: mechanisms in search of treatments. *Neuron* 67, 181–198. doi: 10.1016/j.neuron.2010.07.002

Nakagomi, T., Kubo, S., Nakano-Doi, A., Sakuma, R., Lu, S., Narita, A., et al. (2015). Brain vascular pericytes following ischemia have multipotential stem cell activity to differentiate into neural and vascular lineage cells. *Stem Cells* 33, 1962–1974. doi: 10.1002/stem.1977

Nakagomi, T., Molnár, Z., Nakano-Doi, A., Taguchi, A., Saino, O., Kubo, S., et al. (2011). Ischemia-induced neural stem/progenitor cells in the pia mater following cortical infarction. *Stem Cells Dev.* 20, 2037–2051. doi: 10.1089/scd.2011.0279

Nishijima, T., Piriz, J., Duflot, S., Fernandez, A. M., Gaitan, G., Gomez-Pinedo, U., et al. (2010). Neuronal activity drives localized blood-brain-barrier transport of serum insulin-like growth factor-I into the CNS. *Neuron* 67, 834–846. doi: 10.1016/j.neuron.2010.08.007

Ohab, J. J., Fleming, S., Blesch, A., and Carmichael, S. T. (2006). A neurovascular niche for neurogenesis after stroke. *J. Neurosci.* 26, 13007–13016. doi: 10.1523/JNEUROSCI.4323-06.2006

Ohira, K., Furuta, T., Hioki, H., Nakamura, K. C., Kuramoto, E., Tanaka, Y., et al. (2010). Ischemia-induced neurogenesis of neocortical layer 1 progenitor cells. *Nat. Neurosci.* 13, 173–179. doi: 10.1038/nn.2473

Oki, K., Tatarishvili, J., Wood, J., Koch, P., Wattananit, S., Mine, Y., et al. (2012). Human-induced pluripotent stem cells form functional neurons and improve recovery after grafting in stroke-damaged brain. *Stem Cells* 30, 1120–1133. doi: 10.1002/stem.1104

Okun, E., Griffioen, K. J., Lathia, J. D., Tang, S. C., Mattson, M. P., and Arumugam, T. V. (2009). Toll-like receptors in neurodegeneration. *Brain Res. Rev.* 59, 278–292. doi: 10.1016/j.brainresrev.2008.09.001

Panchision, D. M. (2009). The role of oxygen in regulating neural stem cells in development and disease. *J. Cell. Physiol.* 220, 562–568. doi: 10.1002/jcp.21812

Parent, J. M., Vexler, Z. S., Gong, C., Derugin, N., and Ferriero, D. M. (2002). Rat forebrain neurogenesis and striatal neuron replacement after focal stroke. *Ann. Neurol.* 52, 802–813. doi: 10.1002/ana.10393

Pencea, V., Bingaman, K. D., Wiegand, S. J., and Luskin, M. B. (2001). Infusion of brain-derived neurotrophic factor into the lateral ventricle of the adult rat leads to new neurons in the parenchyma of the striatum, septum, thalamus, and hypothalamus. *J. Neurosci.* 21, 6706–6717.

Pérez-Martín, M., Cifuentes, M., Grondona, J. M., López-Avalos, M. D., Gómez-Pinedo, U., García-Verdugo, J. M., et al. (2010). IGF-I stimulates neurogenesis in the hypothalamus of adult rats. *Eur. J. Neurosci.* 31, 1533–1548. doi: 10.1111/j.1460-9568.2010.07220.x

Pierce, A. A., and Xu, A. W. (2010). De novo neurogenesis in adult hypothalamus as a compensatory mechanism to regulate energy balance. *J. Neurosci.* 30, 723–730. doi: 10.1523/JNEUROSCI.2479-09.2010

Plane, J. M., Whitney, J. T., Schallert, T., and Parent, J. M. (2008). Retinoic acid and environmental enrichment alter subventricular zone and striatal neurogenesis after stroke. *Exp. Neurol.* 214, 125–134. doi: 10.1016/j.expneurol.2008.08.006

Prass, K., Scharff, A., Ruscher, K., Löwl, D., Muselmann, C., Victorov, I., et al. (2003). Hypoxia-induced stroke tolerance in the mouse is mediated by erythropoietin. *Stroke* 34, 1981–1986. doi: 10.1161/01.STR.0000080381.76409.B2

Price, C. J., Hoyda, T. D., and Ferguson, A. V. (2008). The area postrema: a brain monitor and integrator of systemic autonomic state. *Neuroscientist* 14, 182–194. doi: 10.1177/1073858407311100

Robel, S., Berninger, B., and Götz, M. (2011). The stem cell potential of glia: lessons from reactive gliosis. *Nat. Rev. Neurosci.* 12, 88–104. doi: 10.1038/nrn2978

Robin, A. M., Zhang, Z. G., Wang, L., Zhang, R. L., Katakowski, M., Zhang, L., et al. (2006). Stromal cell-derived factor 1alpha mediates neural progenitor cell motility after focal cerebral ischemia. *J. Cereb. Blood Flow Metab.* 26, 125–134. doi: 10.1038/sj.jcbfm.9600172

Rojczyk-Golebiewska, E., Palasz, A., and Wiaderkiewicz, R. (2014). Hypothalamic subependymal niche: a novel site of the adult neurogenesis. *Cell. Mol. Neurobiol.* 34, 631–642. doi: 10.1007/s10571-014-0058-5

Ruan, G. P., Han, Y. B., Wang, T. H., Xing, Z. G., Zhu, X. B., Yao, X., et al. (2013). Comparative study among three different methods of bone marrow mesenchymal stem cell transplantation following cerebral infarction in rats. *Neurol. Res.* 35, 212–220. doi: 10.1179/1743132812Y.0000000152

Ruan, L., Wang, B., ZhuGe, Q., and Jin, K. (2015). Coupling of neurogenesis and angiogenesis after ischemic stroke. *Brain Res.* 1623, 166–173. doi: 10.1016/j.brainres.2015.02.042

Ruscher, K., Freyer, D., Karsch, M., Isaev, N., Megow, D., Sawitzki, B., et al. (2002). Erythropoietin is a paracrine mediator of ischemic tolerance in the brain: evidence from an *in vitro* model. *J. Neurosci.* 22, 10291–10301.

Saaltink, D. J., Håvik, B., Verissimo, C. S., Lucassen, P. J., and Vreugdenhil, E. (2012). Doublecortin and doublecortin-like are expressed in overlapping and non-overlapping neuronal cell population: implications for neurogenesis. *J. Comp. Neurol.* 520, 2805–2823. doi: 10.1002/cne.23144

Saha, B., Peron, S., Murray, K., Jaber, M., and Gaillard, A. (2013). Cortical lesion stimulates adult subventricular zone neural progenitor cell proliferation and migration to the site of injury. *Stem Cell Res.* 11, 965–977. doi: 10.1016/j.scr.2013.06.006

Sanin, V., Heeß, C., Kretzschmar, H. A., and Schüller, U. (2013). Recruitment of neural precursor cells from circumventricular organs of patients with cerebral ischaemia. *Neuropathol. Appl. Neurobiol.* 39, 510–518. doi: 10.1111/j.1365-2990.2012.01301.x

Sawada, M., Matsumoto, M., and Sawamoto, K. (2014). Vascular regulation of adult neurogenesis under physiological and pathological conditions. *Front. Neurosci.* 8:53. doi: 10.3389/fnins.2014.00053

Schilling, M., Besselmann, M., Leonhard, C., Mueller, M., Ringelstein, E. B., and Kiefer, R. (2003). Microglial activation precedes and predominates over macrophage infiltration in transient focal cerebral ischemia: a study in green fluorescent protein transgenic bone marrow chimeric mice. *Exp. Neurol.* 183, 25–33. doi: 10.1016/S0014-4886(03)00082-7

Shapiro, L. A., Ng, K., Zhou, Q. Y., and Ribak, C. E. (2009). Subventricular zone-derived, newly generated neurons populate several olfactory and limbic forebrain regions. *Epilepsy Behav.* 14(Suppl. 1), 74–80. doi: 10.1016/j.yebeh.2008.09.011

Sharp, F. R., Liu, J., and Bernabeu, R. (2002). Neurogenesis following brain ischemia. *Brain Res. Dev. Brain Res.* 134, 23–30. doi: 10.1016/S0165-3806(01)00286-3

Shen, Q., Goderie, S. K., Jin, L., Karanth, N., Sun, Y., Abramova, N., et al. (2004). Endothelial cells stimulate self-renewal and expand neurogenesis of neural stem cells. *Science* 304, 1338–1340. doi: 10.1126/science.1095505

Shen, Q., Wang, Y., Kokovay, E., Lin, G., Chuang, S. M., Goderie, S. K., et al. (2008). Adult SVZ stem cells lie in a vascular niche: a quantitative analysis of niche cell-cell interactions. *Cell Stem Cell* 3, 289–300. doi: 10.1016/j.stem.2008.07.026

Sims, J. R., Lee, S. W., Topalkara, K., Qiu, J., Xu, J., Zhou, Z., et al. (2009). Sonic hedgehog regulates ischemia/hypoxia-induced neural progenitor proliferation. *Stroke* 40, 3618–3626. doi: 10.1161/STROKEAHA.109.561951

Smith, E. J., Stroemer, R. P., Gorenkova, N., Nakajima, M., Crum, W. R., Tang, E., et al. (2012). Implantation site and lesion topology determine efficacy of a human neural stem cell line in a rat model of chronic stroke. *Stem Cells* 30, 785–796. doi: 10.1002/stem.1024

Song, M., Kim, Y. J., Kim, Y. H., Roh, J., Kim, S. U., and Yoon, B. W. (2011). Effects of duplicate administration of human neural stem cell after focal cerebral ischemia in the rat. *Int. J. Neurosci.* 121, 457–461. doi: 10.3109/00207454.2011.576792

Sun, C., Sun, H., Wu, S., Lee, C. C., Akamatsu, Y., Wang, R. K., et al. (2013). Conditional ablation of neuroprogenitor cells in adult mice impedes recovery of poststroke cognitive function and reduces synaptic connectivity in the perforant pathway. *J. Neurosci.* 33, 17314–17325. doi: 10.1523/JNEUROSCI.2129-13.2013

Sun, F., Wang, X., Mao, X., Xie, L., and Jin, K. (2012). Ablation of neurogenesis attenuates recovery of motor function after focal cerebral ischemia in middle-aged mice. *PLoS ONE* 7:e46326. doi: 10.1371/journal.pone.0046326

Sun, Y., Jin, K., Xie, L., Childs, J., Mao, X. O., Logvinova, A., et al. (2003). VEGF-induced neuroprotection, neurogenesis, and angiogenesis after focal cerebral ischemia. *J. Clin. Invest.* 111, 1843–1851. doi: 10.1172/JCI200317977

Suyama, S., Sunabori, T., Kanki, H., Sawamoto, K., Gachet, C., Koizumi, S., et al. (2012). Purinergic signaling promotes proliferation of adult mouse subventricular zone cells. *J. Neurosci.* 32, 9238–9247. doi: 10.1523/JNEUROSCI.4001-11.2012

Taguchi, A., Soma, T., Tanaka, H., Kanda, T., Nishimura, H., Yoshikawa, H., et al. (2004). Administration of CD34+ cells after stroke enhances neurogenesis via angiogenesis in a mouse model. *J. Clin. Invest.* 114, 330–338. doi: 10.1172/JCI200420622

Takasawa, K., Kitagawa, K., Yagita, Y., Sasaki, T., Tanaka, S., Matsushita, K., et al. (2002). Increased proliferation of neural progenitor cells but reduced survival of newborn cells in the contralateral hippocampus after focal cerebral ischemia in rats. *J. Cereb. Blood Flow Metab.* 22, 299–307. doi: 10.1097/00004647-200203000-00007

Tang, Y., Wang, J., Lin, X., Wang, L., Shao, B., Jin, K., et al. (2014). Neural stem cell protects aged rat brain from ischemia-reperfusion injury through neurogenesis and angiogenesis. *J. Cereb. Blood Flow Metab.* 34, 1138–1147. doi: 10.1038/jcbfm.2014.61

Tavazoie, M., Van der Veken, L., Silva-Vargas, V., Louissaint, M., Colonna, L., Zaidi, B., et al. (2008). A specialized vascular niche for adult neural stem cells. *Cell Stem Cell* 3, 279–288. doi: 10.1016/j.stem.2008.07.025

Teramoto, T., Qiu, J., Plumier, J. C., and Moskowitz, M. A. (2003). EGF amplifies the replacement of parvalbumin-expressing striatal interneurons after ischemia. *J. Clin. Invest.* 111, 1125–1132. doi: 10.1172/JCI200317170

Thored, P., Arvidsson, A., Cacci, E., Ahlenius, H., Kallur, T., Darsalia, V., et al. (2006). Persistent production of neurons from adult brain stem cells during recovery after stroke. *Stem Cells* 24, 739–747. doi: 10.1634/stemcells.2005-0281

Thored, P., Heldmann, U., Gomes-Leal, W., Gisler, R., Darsalia, V., Taneera, J., et al. (2009). Long-term accumulation of microglia with proneurogenic phenotype concomitant with persistent neurogenesis in adult subventricular zone after stroke. *Glia* 57, 835–849. doi: 10.1002/glia.20810

Thored, P., Wood, J., Arvidsson, A., Cammenga, J., Kokaia, Z., and Lindvall, O. (2007). Long-term neuroblast migration along blood vessels in an area with transient angiogenesis and increased vascularization after stroke. *Stroke* 38, 3032–3039. doi: 10.1161/STROKEAHA.107.488445

Tonchev, A. B., Yamashima, T., Sawamoto, K., and Okano, H. (2005). Enhanced proliferation of progenitor cells in the subventricular zone and limited neuronal production in the striatum and neocortex of adult macaque monkeys after global cerebral ischemia. *J. Neurosci. Res.* 81, 776–788. doi: 10.1002/jnr.20604

Torper, O., Ottosson, D. R., Pereira, M., Lau, S., Cardoso, T., Grealish, S., et al. (2015). *In vivo* reprogramming of striatal NG2 glia into functional neurons that integrate into local host circuitry. *Cell Rep.* 12, 474–481. doi: 10.1016/j.celrep.2015.06.040

Tsai, P. T., Ohab, J. J., Kertesz, N., Groszer, M., Matter, C., Gao, J., et al. (2006). A critical role of erythropoietin receptor in neurogenesis and post-stroke recovery. *J. Neurosci.* 26, 1269–1274. doi: 10.1523/JNEUROSCI.4480-05.2006

Türeyen, K., Vemuganti, R., Bowen, K. K., Sailor, K. A., and Dempsey, R. J. (2005). EGF and FGF-2 infusion increases post-ischemic neural progenitor cell proliferation in the adult rat brain. *Neurosurgery* 57, 1254–1263. doi: 10.1227/01.neu.0000186040.96929.8a

Turnley, A. M., Basrai, H. S., and Christie, K. J. (2014). Is integration and survival of newborn neurons the bottleneck for effective neural repair by endogenous neural precursor cells? *Front. Neurosci.* 8:29. doi: 10.3389/fnins.2014.00029

Wang, L., Chopp, M., Zhang, R. L., Zhang, L., Letourneau, Y., Feng, Y. F., et al. (2009). The Notch pathway mediates expansion of a progenitor pool and neuronal differentiation in adult neural progenitor cells after stroke. *Neuroscience* 158, 1356–1363. doi: 10.1016/j.neuroscience.2008.10.064

Wang, X., Mao, X., Xie, L., Sun, F., Greenberg, D. A., and Jin, K. (2012). Conditional depletion of neurogenesis inhibits long-term recovery after experimental stroke in mice. *PLoS ONE* 7:e38932. doi: 10.1371/journal.pone.0038932

Wang, Y., Chen, X., Cao, W., and Shi, Y. (2014). Plasticity of mesenchymal stem cells in immunomodulation: pathological and therapeutic implications. *Nat. Immunol.* 15, 1009–1016. doi: 10.1038/ni.3002

Wanner, I. B., Anderson, M. A., Song, B., Levine, J., Fernandez, A., Gray-Thompson, Z., et al. (2013). Glial scar borders are formed by newly proliferated, elongated astrocytes that interact to corral inflammatory and fibrotic cells via STAT3-dependent mechanisms after spinal cord injury. *J. Neurosci.* 33, 12870–12886. doi: 10.1523/JNEUROSCI.2121-13.2013

Wei, L. C., Shi, M., Chen, L. W., Cao, R., Zhang, P., and Chan, Y. S. (2002). Nestin-containing cells express glial fibrillary acidic protein in the proliferative regions of central nervous system of postnatal developing and adult mice. *Brain Res. Dev. Brain Res.* 139, 9–17. doi: 10.1016/S0165-3806(02)00509-6

Wiltrout, C., Lang, B., Yan, Y., Dempsey, R. J., and Vemuganti, R. (2007). Repairing brain after stroke: a review on post-ischemic neurogenesis. *Neurochem. Int.* 50, 1028–1041. doi: 10.1016/j.neuint.2007.04.011

Woodruff, T. M., Thundyil, J., Tang, S. C., Sobey, C. G., Taylor, S. M., and Arumugam, T. V. (2011). Pathophysiology, treatment, and animal and cellular models of human ischemic stroke. *Mol. Neurodegener.* 6:11. doi: 10.1186/1750-1326-6-11

Xu, Y., Tamamaki, N., Noda, T., Kimura, K., Itokazu, Y., Matsumoto, N., et al. (2005). Neurogenesis in the ependymal layer of the adult rat 3rd ventricle. *Exp. Neurol.* 192, 251–264. doi: 10.1016/j.expneurol.2004.12.021

Yagita, Y., Kitagawa, K., Ohtsuki, T., Takasawa, K.-i., Miyata, T., Okano, H., et al. (2001). Neurogenesis by progenitor cells in the ischemic adult rat hippocampus. *Stroke* 32, 1890–1896. doi: 10.1161/01.STR.32.8.1890

Yamashita, T., Ninomiya, M., Hernandez Acosta, P., Garcia-Verdugo, J. M., Sunabori, T., Sakaguchi, M., et al. (2006). Subventricular zone-derived neuroblasts migrate and differentiate into mature neurons in the post-stroke adult striatum. *J. Neurosci.* 26, 6627–6636. doi: 10.1523/JNEUROSCI.0149-06.2006

Yan, Y. P., Sailor, K. A., Lang, B. T., Park, S. W., Vemuganti, R., and Dempsey, R. J. (2007). Monocyte chemoattractant protein-1 plays a critical role in neuroblast migration after focal cerebral ischemia. *J. Cereb. Blood Flow Metab.* 27, 1213–1224. doi: 10.1038/sj.jcbfm.9600432

Yan, Y. P., Sailor, K. A., Vemuganti, R., and Dempsey, R. J. (2006). Insulin-like growth factor-1 is an endogenous mediator of focal ischemia-induced neural progenitor proliferation. *Eur. J. Neurosci.* 24, 45–54. doi: 10.1111/j.1460-9568.2006.04872.x

Yang, Z., Covey, M. V., Bitel, C. L., Ni, L., Jonakait, G. M., and Levison, S. W. (2007). Sustained neocortical neurogenesis after neonatal hypoxic/ischemic injury. *Ann. Neurol.* 61, 199–208. doi: 10.1002/ana.21068

Yenari, M. A., Kauppinen, T. M., and Swanson, R. A. (2010). Microglial activation in stroke: therapeutic targets. *Neurotherapeutics* 7, 378–391. doi: 10.1016/j.nurt.2010.07.005

Yu, T. S., Washington, P. M., and Kernie, S. G. (2014). Injury-induced neurogenesis: mechanisms and relevance. *Neuroscientist.* doi: 10.1177/1073858414563616. [Epub ahead of print].

Yuan, J. (2009). Neuroprotective strategies targeting apoptotic and necrotic cell death for stroke. *Apoptosis* 14, 469–477. doi: 10.1007/s10495-008-0304-8

Yuan, T., Liao, W., Feng, N. H., Lou, Y. L., Niu, X., Zhang, A. J., et al. (2013). Human induced pluripotent stem cell-derived neural stem cells survive, migrate, differentiate, and improve neurologic function in a rat model of middle cerebral artery occlusion. *Stem Cell Res. Ther.* 4, 73. doi: 10.1186/scrt224

Zhang, R., Zhang, Z., Zhang, C., Zhang, L., Robin, A., Wang, Y., et al. (2004). Stroke transiently increases subventricular zone cell division from asymmetric to symmetric and increases neuronal differentiation in the adult rat. *J. Neurosci.* 24, 5810–5815. doi: 10.1523/JNEUROSCI.1109-04.2004

Zhang, R. L., Chopp, M., Roberts, C., Liu, X., Wei, M., Nejad-Davarani, S. P., et al. (2014). Stroke increases neural stem cells and angiogenesis in the neurogenic niche of the adult mouse. *PLoS ONE* 9:e113972. doi: 10.1371/journal.pone.0113972

Zhang, R. L., LeTourneau, Y., Gregg, S. R., Wang, Y., Toh, Y., Robin, A. M., et al. (2007). Neuroblast division during migration toward the ischemic striatum: a study of dynamic migratory and proliferative characteristics of neuroblasts from the subventricular zone. *J. Neurosci.* 27, 3157–3162. doi: 10.1523/JNEUROSCI.4969-06.2007

Zhang, R. L., Zhang, Z. G., Zhang, L., and Chopp, M. (2001). Proliferation and differentiation of progenitor cells in the cortex and the subventricular zone in the adult rat after focal cerebral ischemia. *Neuroscience* 105, 33–41. doi: 10.1016/S0306-4522(01)00117-8

Zhang, Z. G., and Chopp, M. (2009). Neurorestorative therapies for stroke: underlying mechanisms and translation to the clinic. *Lancet Neurol.* 8, 491–500. doi: 10.1016/S1474-4422(09)70061-4

Zhu, D. Y., Liu, S. H., Sun, H. S., and Lu, Y. M. (2003). Expression of inducible nitric oxide synthase after focal cerebral ischemia stimulates neurogenesis in the adult rodent dentate gyrus. *J. Neurosci.* 23, 223–229.

14

Adult Born Olfactory Bulb Dopaminergic Interneurons: Molecular Determinants and Experience-Dependent Plasticity

Sara Bonzano [1,2], *Serena Bovetti* [3], *Claudio Gendusa* [1], *Paolo Peretto* [1,2] *and Silvia De Marchis* [1,2]*

[1] *Department of Life Sciences and Systems Biology, University of Turin, Torino, Italy,* [2] *Neuroscience Institute Cavalieri Ottolenghi, University of Turin, Orbassano, Italy,* [3] *Department of Neuroscience and Brain Technologies, Istituto Italiano di Tecnologia, Genova, Italy*

Edited by:
Alino Martinez-Marcos, Universidad de Castilla, Spain

Reviewed by:
Umberto Di Porzio, National Research Council, Italy
Harold Cremer, Centre National de La Recherche Scientifique, France

***Correspondence:**
Silvia De Marchis
silvia.demarchis@unito.it

The olfactory bulb (OB) is a highly plastic brain region involved in the early processing of olfactory information. A remarkably feature of the OB circuits in rodents is the constitutive integration of new neurons that takes place during adulthood. Newborn cells in the adult OB are mostly inhibitory interneurons belonging to chemically, morphologically and functionally heterogeneous types. Although there is general agreement that adult neurogenesis in the OB plays a key role in sensory information processing and olfaction-related plasticity, the contribution of each interneuron subtype to such functions is far to be elucidated. Here, we focus on the dopaminergic (DA) interneurons: we highlight recent findings about their morphological features and then describe the molecular factors required for the specification/differentiation and maintenance of the DA phenotype in adult born neurons. We also discuss dynamic changes of the DA interneuron population related to age, environmental stimuli and lesions, and their possible functional implications.

Keywords: olfactory bulb, dopaminergic neurons, tyrosine hydroxylase, adult neurogenesis, COUP-TFI, juxtaglomerular neurons, odor enrichment, odor deprivation

INTRODUCTION

In mammals, dopaminergic (DA) neurons are classified in distinct neuronal cell groups (from A8 to A16) based on their substantial diversity (Björklund and Dunnett, 2007). DA neurons in the olfactory bulb (OB) belong to the A16 group and represent the major DA system in the forebrain (Cave and Baker, 2009). Olfactory DA cells are reliably identified by the expression of tyrosine hydroxylase (TH), the rate-limiting enzyme of catecholamine biosynthesis, since they represent the only catecholaminergic cell type found in the OB (Cave and Baker, 2009). TH-positive cells are mostly localized in the OB glomerular cell layer (GL; **Figure 1A**), where they account for nearly 10% of all juxtaglomerular cells (JGCs; Parrish-Aungst et al., 2007). TH-positive JGCs express glutamic acid decarboxylase (GAD), the rate-limiting enzyme for GABA biosynthesis, and co-release dopamine and GABA on their post-synaptic targets (Liu et al., 2013). Their electrophysiological properties have been extensively characterized (Pignatelli et al., 2005, 2009, 2013; Borin et al., 2014). TH-positive cells establish synaptic contacts with the afferent olfactory receptor neuron terminals and/or with external tufted cells and form extensive

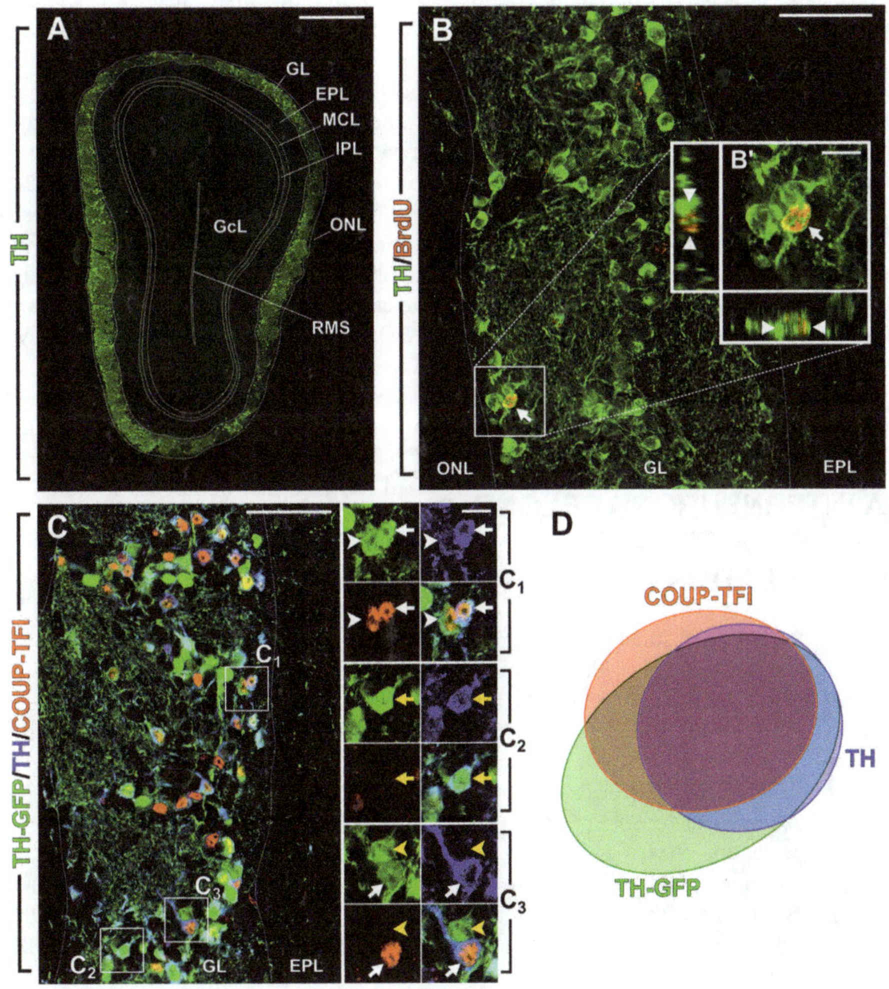

FIGURE 1 | Olfactory bulb dopaminergic interneurons. New image from previously published experiments (Bovetti et al., 2013; Bonzano et al., 2014). **(A)** Photomicrograph showing a coronal section of the olfactory bulb (OB) in a 2-month-old wild-type mouse. DA cells immunopositive for TH (green) are mostly confined within the OB glomerular layer (GL). **(B)** BrdU-positive adult born DA cell (arrow) in a representative confocal image of the OB GL double-stained for BrdU (red) and TH (green) in a mouse that received BrdU at 2 months of age and analyzed 42 days after. B′ shows higher magnification and re-slicing of the BrdU/TH double positive cell. **(C)** Multiple labeling of the OB GL in a 2-month-old TH-GFP transgenic mouse line (Sawamoto et al., 2001). GFP (green) is expressed under the control of TH promoter; TH-immunopositive cells are shown in blue and COUP-TFI immunopositive nuclei in red. C1 shows higher magnification of a cell that is triple labeled for GFP/TH/COUP-TFI (white arrow) and a cell that is double labeled for GFP and COUP-TFI (white arrowhead). C2 shows higher magnification of a cell that is double labeled for GFP and TH (yellow arrow). C3 shows a cell that is triple labeled for GFP/TH/COUP-TFI (white arrow) and a cell that is GFP-positive only (yellow arrowhead). **(D)** Venn diagram showing the overlap of the labeling for TH-GFP, TH and COUP-TFI immunoreactivity based on our previously published data (Bovetti et al., 2013). A fraction of TH-GFP positive cells is negative for both TH and COUP-TFI. As previously reported these cells are likely immature DA neurons not expressing yet TH protein (Pignatelli et al., 2009). There is a high overlap between TH-GFP/TH/COUP-TFI labeling indicating that COUP-TFI expression is tightly associated with the DA phenotype. Scale bar in A = 500 μm. Scale bar in B and C = 50 μm. Scale bar in inset B′=10 μm. Scale bar in inset C1 = 10 μm and refers to C2 and C3. ONL, olfactory nerve layer; GL, glomerular layer; EPL, external plexiform layer; MCL, mitral cell layer; IPL, internal plexiform layer; GcL, granule cell layer; RMS, rostral migratory stream of the OB.

interglomerular connections (Kiyokage et al., 2010; Kosaka and Kosaka, 2011), participating to the early steps in odor information processing that occur in the input layer of the OB. Accordingly, a recent study demonstrated a key function for DA cells in implementing gain control and reducing correlation of odor representations in the main output neurons (i.e., mitral/tufted cells) (Banerjee et al., 2015). In line with a central role for DA cells in the encoding of odor stimuli, several studies support the impact of the DA system in fundamental features of odor-driven behaviors (Kruzich and Grandy, 2004; Pavlis et al., 2006; Tillerson et al., 2006; Wei et al., 2006; Serguera et al., 2008; Lazarini et al., 2014). Moreover, olfactory dysfunction is associated to pathological states affecting the DA system, such as in Parkinson disease (Doty, 2012). Although olfactory dysfunction in PD patients could also involve OB DA cells, recent data in rodents indicate this is mostly attributable to depletion in the DA nigro-olfactory projection system (Höglinger et al., 2015).

Olfactory DA neurons have attracted significant attention over the years, because they are involved in substantial activity-dependent plasticity, regulating the level of TH expression and dopamine release according to the sensory input (Nadi et al., 1981; Baker et al., 1983, 1984; Cummings et al., 1997). Moreover, DA cells are constantly generated throughout life and recent reports pointed to a specific integration of this juxtaglomerular cell population in the GL circuits in an activity-dependent manner (Sawada et al., 2011; Bonzano et al., 2014). Because of their continuous generation throughout life, DA cells are also regarded as a potential target to exploit adult neurogenesis for dopamine system repair in the brain (see Cave et al., 2014). Here we focused on emerging aspects related to DA cells heterogeneity, molecular determinants of adult born DA neurons, their plasticity and function in the OB.

OLFACTORY DA INTERNEURONS BELONG TO TWO MAIN MORPHOLOGICALLY DISTINCT CELL POPULATIONS

The view that DA cells in the OB consist of distinct types emerged many years ago from the immunohistochemical identification of two different categories of TH-positive neurons in the rat and mouse OB (Halász et al., 1981; Baker et al., 1983; McLean and Shipley, 1988). Based on their soma size and location, TH-positive cells were initially classified either as small periglomerular cells (PG, soma diameter about 5–10 μm), positioned in the GL and representing the large majority of olfactory DA cells, or large external tufted cells (ET, soma diameter about 10–15 μm), positioned mostly at the boundary between the GL and the external plexiform layer (EPL) and rarely found within the EPL. Interestingly, DA cells belonging to the larger type are born earlier during development than the smaller ones (McLean and Shipley, 1988), possibly from local OB progenitors in the E13.5 mouse embryo (Vergaño-Vera et al., 2006), before precursors from the main germinal niches for OB interneurons (i.e., LGE, pallium, and septum) start to populate the OB and differentiate into multiple interneuron subtypes (Bovetti et al., 2007; Alvarez-Buylla et al., 2008). Furthermore, Kosaka and Kosaka (2009) showed that adult subventricular zone (SVZ) progenitors do not contribute to the generation of the larger type of DA cells, indicating this population does not undergo the neuronal turnover typical of most GL interneurons, including small-medium sized DA cells (Bovetti et al., 2009).

Morphometric investigation of TH-positive neuronal projection in the GL has successively revealed that DA cells extend processes into multiple glomeruli (Kosaka and Kosaka, 2008; Kiyokage et al., 2010), suggesting that they should be more appropriately classified as short-axon (SA) cells instead of PG and ET cells, whose processes are mostly confined to one single glomerulus (Pinching and Powell, 1971; Kiyokage et al., 2010). Importantly, Kiyokage et al. (2010) described two distinct types of SA TH-positive cells, oligoglomerular and polyglomerular, based on their process extension and average number of contacted glomeruli. The vast majority of DA cells falls within the first category (i.e., oligoglomerular), having processes spanning a relatively short region of the GL and contacting in average nearly 6 glomeruli. Polyglomerular cells show more extensive projections, contact in average nearly 40 glomeruli and are likely to correspond to the large DA cells previously described to establish long-range interglomerular connections by Kosaka and Kosaka (2008). An additional feature that allows differentiating distinct types of olfactory DA cells is the presence/absence of an axon. Both *in vivo* (Kosaka and Kosaka, 2011) and *in vitro* (Chand et al., 2015) studies clearly indicated that larger DA cells possess an axon initial segment (AIS), reminiscent of an axonal process, while the other, smaller in size do not.

Overall, most evidences point to the existence of two main morphologically and possibly functionally separate populations of olfactory DA cells, of which only one (i.e., small/medium-sized DA neurons) undergoes continuous neurogenesis during adulthood (**Figure 1B**).

MOLECULAR DETERMINANTS OF THE DA PHENOTYPE IN THE ADULT OLFACTORY BULB

The generation of OB interneuron subtypes has been demonstrated to depend on a transcriptional code that is regulated in a spatio-temporal manner (Bovetti et al., 2007; Alvarez-Buylla et al., 2008). Distinct progenitor lineages differentially contribute to the generation of TH-positive cells during development or in adult mice. By means of genetic fate mapping Kohwi et al. demonstrated that while in neonates OB TH-positive cells only marginally (4%) derive from Emx1-expressing pallial progenitors, in adult age 42% of TH-positive OB interneurons are derived from this lineage (Kohwi et al., 2007). A prominent pallial origin of postnatal/adult DA interneurons is further supported by data obtained through adenoviral-mediated labeling of regionally restricted radial glial stem cells, showing that TH-positive neurons largely derive from progenitors located in the dorsal portion of the SVZ (Merkle et al., 2007). Several transcription factors (TFs), namely Pax6, Dlx2, Id2, Klf7, ER81, Sall3, Nurr1, and Meis2 (Saino-Saito et al., 2004, 2007; Hack et al., 2005; Kohwi et al., 2005; Brill et al., 2008; Havrda et al., 2008; Cave et al., 2010; Caiazzo et al., 2011; Heng et al., 2012; Agoston et al., 2014; Vergaño-Vera et al., 2015) have been shown to be required for proper differentiation of olfactory DA neurons. Here we will limit the review to those TFs whose function in the control of olfactory DA fate has been directly demonstrated in adult born neurons (**Table 1**). Among these, Pax6 and Dlx2 play a major role (Hack et al., 2005; Kohwi et al., 2005; Brill et al., 2008; de Chevigny et al., 2012). The use of retroviral-mediated overexpression of Dlx2 in neuronal precursors along the rostral migratory stream (RMS) provided data supporting a cell-autonomous role for this TF in promoting specification of adult born neurons toward DA fate (Brill et al., 2008). Similar results, implying increased generation of DA interneurons, were previously described by over-expressing the TF Pax6 in adult neuronal precursors

TABLE 1 | Transcription factors involved in the control of adult born olfactory DA fate specification and maintenance.

TF	% of JGC type among TF+ cells	% of TF+ among TH+ cells	Experimental strategies		Phenotype	References
			Type of approach	Cellular/area targets		
Pax6	TH 78% CR 2% CB 10%	95%	- RV stereotaxic injection (overexpression)	RMS/SVZ (adult born)	Increase in adult born TH+ cells (14/21/90 dpi)	Hack et al., 2005
			-RV stereotaxic injection (loss of function)	RMS (adult born)	Decrease in adult born TH+ cells (21 dpi)	Hack et al., 2005
			-Transplantation of dLGE Pax6-deficient E16.5 progenitors	Recipient: wt adult SVZ	Decrease in TH+ cells among grafted cells (40 dpt)	Kohwi et al., 2005
			-Conditional KO (Dat-Cre* Pax6fl/fl)	Unspecific to adulthood (mature DA cells)	Decrease in TH+ cells; Decrease in DA cell survival	Ninkovic et al., 2010
			-Pax6+/Sey^{Dey}	Unspecific to adulthood	Decrease in adult born TH+ cells; decrease in DA cell survival (15–60 dpBrdU)	Curto et al., 2014
			-Pax6-ORF-GFP plasmid electroporation - Ectopic Pax6 expression in lateral SVZ	Postnatal lateral SVZ	Increase in TH+ cells (15 dpe)	de Chevigny et al., 2012
Dlx2	TH unknown CR none CB unknown	Virtually all	-RV stereotaxic injection (overexpression)	RMS (adult born)	Increase in TH+ cells paralleled by decreased CR+ cells (21–56dpi)	Brill et al., 2008
Meis2	Unknown exactly	89%	–	–	–	Allen et al., 2007
		94%	-RV stereotaxic injection (loss of function)	RMS (adult born)	Loss of adult born TH+ cells (21/60 dpi)	Agoston et al., 2014
COUP-TFI	TH 70% CR 1% CB 2%	80%	-LV stereotaxic injection (loss of function)	RMS (adult born)	Decrease in adult born TH+ cells (60 dpi); no changes at 30 dpi	Bovetti et al., 2013
			Conditional KO (Emx1-Cre*COUP-TFIfl/fl)	Unspecific to adulthood	Decrease in TH+ cell population; decrease in the % of TH+ on BrdU adult born OB INs (42dpBrdU); no changes in DA cell survival	Bovetti et al., 2013; Zhou et al., 2015

TH, tyrosine hydroxylase; TF, transcription factor; CR, calretinin; CB, calbindin; dpi, day(s) post injection; dpBrdU, day(s) post BrdU injection(s); dpe, day(s) post electroporation; dpt, day(s) post transplantation; RV, Retroviral vector; LV, Lentiviral vector; RMS, Rostral Migratory Stream; SVZ, Sub Ventricular Zone; dLGE, dorsal Lateral Ganglionic Eminence.

migrating along the RMS (Hack et al., 2005). In addition, by increasing Pax6 protein level in the lateral wall, where normally Pax6 protein is absent due to post-transcriptional inhibition by mir-7a, the acquisition of the DA phenotype in the OB is favored (de Chevigny et al., 2012). Moreover, the effect of Dlx2 overexpression is totally abrogated in the absence of Pax6 and functional direct interaction/cooperation between Dlx2 and Pax6 is needed to instruct DA fate in adult mice (Brill et al., 2008). A critical co-factor for Pax6 and Dxl2 function in exploiting DA fate commitment in adult born OB interneurons has been recently identified in Meis2, a member of the three amino acid loop extension class of atypical homeodomain-containing transcription factors (Agoston et al., 2014). Meis2, together with Pax6 and Dlx2, is needed to determine the differentiation toward a DA phenotype over the CR one by directly interacting with TH regulatory sequences (Agoston et al., 2014). Besides the instructive role for Pax6 in DA fate commitment in OB interneuron precursors, Pax6 is also critically involved in OB DA cell maintenance. Indeed, by conditionally deleting Pax6 in mature DA cells Ninkovic et al. (2010) identified Pax6 as a positive controller of mature DA cell survival through the positive regulation of crystallin αA in the adult OB.

Recently, we have identified a distinct, yet central, role in the maintenance of the DA phenotype of adult born OB interneurons for the orphan nuclear receptor COUP-TFI (Bovetti et al., 2013). Among juxtaglomerular interneurons in the adult mouse OB, COUP-TFI expression is exclusively found in DA cells, with nearly 80% of mature TH-positive cells (**Figures 1C,D**) and 90% of Pax6-positive cells double positive for COUP-TFI. Interestingly, the expression of COUP-TFI is mostly confined to DA cells generated during late postnatal/adult life, and is regulated by the sensory input. Indeed, odor deprivation through naris occlusion induces COUP-TFI down-regulation jointly with TH down-regulation in olfactory DA cells. Moreover, we observed a net impairment in TH expression in fully mature cells following ablation of COUP-TFI function in either a) DA interneuron progenitors by means of conditional COUP-TFI deletion in the Emx1-lineage or b) post-mitotic adult born neurons by lentiviral-mediated approach *in vivo* (Bovetti et al., 2013). These findings strongly indicate a role for COUP-TFI in TH expression regulation, as also recently confirmed by another study (Zhou et al., 2015). Importantly, COUP-TFI ablation on DA cells does not affect the acquisition and maturation of the DA phenotype, but impairs immediate early gene expression (i.e., egr-1; Bovetti et al., 2013). Overall, these data, together with the apparent lack of consensus binding sites for COUP-TFI on the TH promoter, strongly indicate that COUP-TFI regulates TH expression in OB cells through an activity-dependent mechanism involving immediate early gene induction and strongly argue for a maintenance rather than establishment function of COUP-TFI in the DA commitment. Thus, besides the role of TFs such as Pax6, Meis2, and Dlx2 that are directly involved in OB DA fate determination within adult SVZ neural stem cell/precursors, COUP-TFI must be part of a distinct transcription factor program that is central for the maintenance of the DA cell identity over time.

EXPERIENCE-DEPENDENT PLASTICITY OF OLFACTORY DA NEURONS: A DUAL MECHANISM INVOLVING TH-EXPRESSION REGULATION AND ADULT NEUROGENESIS

Several lines of evidence support the notion that olfactory DA neurons are unique among OB neurons, being particularly susceptible to sensory stimuli. A first level of experience-dependent plasticity of DA cells consists in the regulation of TH expression and consequently dopamine production/release, according to the sensory input. Indeed, TH expression in DA cells is strongly and reversibly down-regulated in animals subjected to odor deprivation by either chemical or surgical sensory deafferentation of the OB (Nadi et al., 1981; Kawano and Margolis, 1982; Baker et al., 1983), or naris occlusion (Baker et al., 1993). This effect does not seem to be restricted to a specific DA cell population (see above; Baker et al., 1983) and applies to both pre-existing and adult generated neurons (Bovetti et al., 2009; Bastien-Dionne et al., 2010). In parallel to TH down-regulation, odor deprivation also induces down-regulation of GAD67, which is selectively co-expressed by DA cells, but not of GAD65, which is mainly expressed by other juxtaglomerular cell types (Parrish-Aungst et al., 2011). Although the view that olfactory DA neurons are exposed to modulation of their transmitter phenotype by the olfactory input has long been recognized (Baker et al., 1983, 1984; McLean and Shipley, 1988), the molecular mechanisms underlying this phenomenon are just beginning to emerge. A direct link among the expression of immediate early genes, increased neuronal activity and TH expression in the GL has been previously hypothesized (Jin et al., 1996). As reported above, we recently identified a role for DA cell responsiveness to sensory stimuli for COUP-TFI, whose depletion in adult generated DA cells induces both reduced immediate early gene and TH expression (Bovetti et al., 2013). Moreover, recent studies highlighted the involvement of epigenetic regulatory mechanisms in the activity-dependent modulation of the neurotransmitter phenotype in OB interneurons (Banerjee et al., 2013).

Besides TH expression regulation, sensory activity can significantly impact on the composition of the DA population through modulation of adult neurogenesis. Indeed, manipulation of the sensory input by either odor deprivation or enrichment elicits, respectively, decreased or increased survival of adult generated juxtaglomerular interneurons (Bovetti et al., 2009), as previously demonstrated for granule cells (Rochefort et al., 2002; Mandairon et al., 2006). Increasing evidence points to DA cells as a selective cellular target for sensory-dependent modulation of adult neurogenesis in the GL of the OB. Using a paradigm of naris occlusion in adult mice, Sawada et al. (2011) found that among different neurochemical types of juxtaglomerular cells, TH-positive DA cells were the only one to show increased apoptosis. Interestingly, mice in which the naris was reopened showed increased integration of new DA cells after a 4 weeks recovery phase that compensate for the selective loss of DA cells due to previous deprivation. A restorative role of adult neurogenesis has been also demonstrated in another experimental paradigm in which a selective DA neuronal loss, induced by local treatment with 6-hydroxydopamine (6-OHDA) in the dorsal OB, was followed by a full recovery of DA cells (Lazarini et al., 2014). Regulation of DA cell generation in adulthood is not limited to restorative conditions but occurs also in basal physiological condition and in response to sensory enrichment. Interestingly, a net and selective increase in the glomerular DA population with age has been reported in a long term two-photon imaging study *in vivo* (Adam and Mizrahi, 2011). Although the meaning of these age-dependent changes in the DA population is unknown, these data reinforce the idea that a certain plasticity of the DA population is required for OB circuit functions. In a recent study from our group (Bonzano et al., 2014), a paradigm of prolonged (2 months) olfactory enrichment with different aromatic fragrances, which has been previously shown to affect OB neurogenesis (Rochefort et al., 2002; Bovetti et al., 2009) and olfactory memory (Rochefort et al., 2002), resulted in a selective increase in the TH-positive DA population, due to increased neurogenesis, without changes in calretinin (CR)- and calbindin (CB)-positive neurons (Bonzano et al., 2014). These results further support that adult neurogenesis does not reflect a simple turnover of the whole GL interneuron population, but it can finely modulate specific OB neuron subpopulations (i.e., DA cells) with particular functions in odor processing.

CONCLUSION AND FUTURE PERSPECTIVE

In the adult OB, DA cells are unique in term of their plasticity in response to sensory inputs. Although their involvement in mechanisms underlying the adaptation of the olfactory system to changes in sensory experience is well established, many aspects remain still unknown. The heterogeneity of DA cell population in term of morphology, connections (Kosaka and Kosaka, 2008; Kiyokage et al., 2010; Chand et al., 2015), origin (McLean and Shipley, 1988; Vergaño-Vera et al., 2006; De Marchis et al., 2007; Kohwi et al., 2007; Merkle et al., 2007) and renewal (Kosaka and Kosaka, 2009) further complicate the understanding of DA cell role in odor coding, processing and plasticity. New molecular and optical approaches able to selectively target adult born DA interneurons will hopefully bring new insights in unraveling their role in olfactory physiology. The precise *in vivo* readout of cell activity now possible exploiting the last generation of calcium and voltage indicators (Akemann et al., 2010; Chen et al., 2013; Gong et al., 2015), combined with the capability to selectively manipulate cell activity through optogenetic and chemogenetic tools (Boyden et al., 2005; Deisseroth et al., 2006; Liu et al., 2013; Sternson and Roth, 2014), are the straightforward direction toward the complete dissection of glomerular network function and adult born DA cell role in activity-dependent plasticity. Nonetheless, new molecular and genetic tools may contribute to further clarify and reach a final consensus on olfactory DA cell classification.

AUTHOR CONTRIBUTIONS

All authors listed, have made substantial, direct, and intellectual contribution to the work, and approved its final version for publication.

REFERENCES

Adam, Y., and Mizrahi, A. (2011). Long-term imaging reveals dynamic changes in the neuronal composition of the glomerular layer. *J. Neurosci.* 31, 7967–7973. doi: 10.1523/JNEUROSCI.0782-11.2011

Agoston, Z., Heine, P., Brill, M. S., Grebbin, B. M., Hau, A.-C., Kallenborn-Gerhardt, W., et al. (2014). Meis2 is a Pax6 co-factor in neurogenesis and dopaminergic periglomerular fate specification in the adult olfactory bulb. *Development* 141, 28–38. doi: 10.1242/dev.097295

Akemann, W., Mutoh, H., Perron, A., Rossier, J., and Knöpfel, T. (2010). Imaging brain electric signals with genetically targeted voltage-sensitive fluorescent proteins. *Nat. Methods* 7, 643–649. doi: 10.1038/nmeth.1479

Allen, Z. J., Waclaw, R. R., Colbert, M. C., and Campbell, K. (2007). Molecular identity of olfactory bulb interneurons: transcriptional codes of periglomerular neuron subtypes. *J. Mol. Histol.* 38, 517–525. doi: 10.1007/s10735-007-9115-4

Alvarez-Buylla, A., Kohwi, M., Nguyen, T. M., and Merkle, F. T. (2008). The heterogeneity of adult neural stem cells and the emerging complexity of their niche. *Cold Spring Harb. Symp. Quant. Biol.* 73, 357–365. doi: 10.1101/sqb.2008.73.019

Baker, H., Kawano, T., Albert, V., Joh, T. H., Reis, D. J., and Margolis, F. L. (1984). Olfactory bulb dopamine neurons survive deafferentation-induced loss of tyrosine hydroxylase. *Neuroscience* 11, 605–615. doi: 10.1016/0306-4522(84)90047-2

Baker, H., Kawano, T., Margolis, F. L., and Joh, T. H. (1983). Transneuronal regulation of tyrosine hydroxylase expression in olfactory bulb of mouse and rat. *J. Neurosci.* 3, 69–78.

Baker, H., Morel, K., Stone, D. M., and Maruniak, J. A. (1993). Adult naris closure profoundly reduces tyrosine hydroxylase expression in mouse olfactory bulb. *Brain Res.* 614, 109–116. doi: 10.1016/0006-8993(93)91023-L

Banerjee, A., Marbach, F., Anselmi, F., Koh, M. S., Davis, M. B., Garcia da Silva, P., et al. (2015). An interglomerular circuit gates glomerular output and implements gain control in the mouse olfactory bulb. *Neuron* 87, 193–207. doi: 10.1016/j.neuron.2015.06.019

Banerjee, K., Akiba, Y., Baker, H., and Cave, J. W. (2013). Epigenetic control of neurotransmitter expression in olfactory bulb interneurons. *Int. J. Dev. Neurosci.* 31, 415–423. doi: 10.1016/j.ijdevneu.2012.11.009

Bastien-Dionne, P. O., David, L. S., Parent, A., and Saghatelyan, A. (2010). Role of sensory activity on chemospecific populations of interneurons in the adult olfactory bulb. *J. Comp. Neurol.* 518, 1847–1861. doi: 10.1002/cne.22307

Björklund, A., and Dunnett, S. B. (2007). Dopamine neuron systems in the brain: an update. *Trends Neurosci.* 30, 194–202. doi: 10.1016/j.tins.2007.03.006

Bonzano, S., Bovetti, S., Fasolo, A., Peretto, P., and De Marchis, S. (2014). Odour enrichment increases adult-born dopaminergic neurons in the mouse olfactory bulb. *Eur. J. Neurosci.* 40, 3450–3457. doi: 10.1111/ejn.12724

Borin, M., Fogli Iseppe, A., Pignatelli, A., and Belluzzi, O. (2014). Inward rectifier potassium (Kir) current in dopaminergic periglomerular neurons of the mouse olfactory bulb. *Front. Cell. Neurosci.* 8:223. doi: 10.3389/fncel.2014.00223

Bovetti, S., Bonzano, S., Garzotto, D., Giannelli, S. G., Iannielli, A., Armentano, M., et al. (2013). COUP-TFI controls activity-dependent tyrosine hydroxylase expression in adult dopaminergic olfactory bulb interneurons. *Development* 140, 4850–4859. doi: 10.1242/dev.089961

Bovetti, S., Peretto, P., Fasolo, A., and De Marchis, S. (2007). Spatio-temporal specification of olfactory bulb interneurons. *J. Mol. Histol.* 38, 563–569. doi: 10.1007/s10735-007-9111-8

Bovetti, S., Veyrac, A., Peretto, P., Fasolo, A., and De Marchis, S. (2009). Olfactory enrichment influences adult neurogenesis modulating GAD67 and plasticity-related molecules expression in newborn cells of the olfactory bulb. *PLoS ONE* 4:e6359. doi: 10.1371/journal.pone.0006359

Boyden, E. S., Zhang, F., Bamberg, E., Nagel, G., and Deisseroth, K. (2005). Millisecond-timescale, genetically targeted optical control of neural activity. *Nat. Neurosci.* 8, 1263–1268. doi: 10.1038/nn1525

Brill, M. S., Snapyan, M., Wohlfrom, H., Ninkovic, J., Jawerka, M., Mastick, G. S., et al. (2008). A Dlx2- and Pax6-Dependent transcriptional code for periglomerular neuron specification in the adult olfactory bulb. *J. Neurosci.* 28, 6439–6452. doi: 10.1523/JNEUROSCI.0700-08.2008

Caiazzo, M., Colucci-D'Amato, L., Volpicelli, F., Speranza, L., Petrone, C., Pastore, L., et al. (2011). Kruppel-like factor 7 is required for olfactory bulb dopaminergic neuron development. *Exp. Cell Res.* 317, 464–473. doi: 10.1016/j.yexcr.2010.11.006

Cave, J. W., Akiba, Y., Banerjee, K., Bhosle, S., Berlin, R., and Baker, H. (2010). Differential regulation of dopaminergic gene expression by Er81. *J. Neurosci.* 30, 4717–4724. doi: 10.1523/JNEUROSCI.0419-10.2010

Cave, J. W., and Baker, H. (2009). Dopamine systems in the forebrain. *Adv. Exp. Med. Biol.* 651, 15–35. doi: 10.1007/978-1-4419-0322-8_2

Cave, J. W., Wang, M., and Baker, H. (2014). Adult subventricular zone neural stem cells as a potential source of dopaminergic replacement neurons. *Front. Neurosci.* 8:16. doi: 10.3389/fnins.2014.00016

Chand, A. N., Galliano, E., Chesters, R. A., and Grubb, M. S. (2015). A distinct subtype of dopaminergic interneuron displays inverted structural plasticity at the axon initial segment. *J. Neurosci.* 35, 1573–1590. doi: 10.1523/JNEUROSCI.3515-14.2015

Chen, T.-W., Wardill, T. J., Sun, Y., Pulver, S. R., Renninger, S. L., Baohan, A., et al. (2013). Ultrasensitive fluorescent proteins for imaging neuronal activity. *Nature* 499, 295–300. doi: 10.1038/nature12354

Cummings, D. M., Henning, H. E., and Brunjes, P. C. (1997). Olfactory bulb recovery after early sensory deprivation. *J. Neurosci.* 17, 7433–7440.

Curto, G. G., Nieto-Estévez, V., Hurtado-Chong, A., Valero, J., Gómez, C., Alonso, J. R., et al. (2014). Pax6 is essential for the maintenance and multi-lineage differentiation of neural stem cells, and for neuronal incorporation into the adult olfactory bulb. *Stem Cells Dev.* 23, 1–61. doi: 10.1089/scd.2014.0058

de Chevigny, A., Coré, N., Follert, P., Gaudin, M., Barbry, P., Béclin, C., et al. (2012). miR-7a regulation of Pax6 controls spatial origin of forebrain dopaminergic neurons. *Nat. Neurosci.* 15, 1120–1126. doi: 10.1038/nn.3142

Deisseroth, K., Feng, G., Majewska, A. K., Miesenbock, G., Ting, A., and Schnitzer, M. J. (2006). Next-generation optical technologies for illuminating genetically targeted brain circuits. *J. Neurosci.* 26, 10380–10386. doi: 10.1523/JNEUROSCI.3863-06.2006

De Marchis, S., Bovetti, S., Carletti, B., Hsieh, Y.-C., Garzotto, D., Peretto, P., et al. (2007). Generation of distinct types of periglomerular olfactory bulb interneurons during development and in adult mice: implication for intrinsic properties of the subventricular zone progenitor population. *J. Neurosci.* 27, 657–664. doi: 10.1523/JNEUROSCI.2870-06.2007

Doty, R. L. (2012). Olfactory dysfunction in Parkinson disease. *Nat. Rev. Neurol.* 8, 329–339. doi: 10.1038/nrneurol.2012.80

Gong, Y., Huang, C., Li, J. Z., Grewe, B. F., Zhang, Y., Eismann, S., et al. (2015). High-speed recording of neural spikes in awake mice and flies with a fluorescent voltage sensor. *Sciencexpress* 350, 1–11. doi: 10.1126/science.aab0810

Hack, M. A., Saghatelyan, A., de Chevigny, A., Pfeifer, A., Ashery-Padan, R., Lledo, P.-M., et al. (2005). Neuronal fate determinants of adult olfactory bulb neurogenesis. *Nat. Neurosci.* 8, 865–872. doi: 10.1038/nn1479

Halász, N., Johansson, O., Hökfelt, T., Ljungdahl, A., and Goldstein, M. (1981). Immunohistochemical identification of two types of dopamine neuron in the rat olfactory bulb as seen by serial sectioning. *J. Neurocytol.* 10, 251–259. doi: 10.1007/BF01257970

Havrda, M. C., Harris, B. T., Mantani, A., Ward, N. M., Paolella, B. R., Cuzon, V. C., et al. (2008). Id2 is required for specification of dopaminergic neurons during adult olfactory neurogenesis. *J. Neurosci.* 28, 14074–14087. doi: 10.1523/JNEUROSCI.3188-08.2008

Heng, X., Breer, H., Zhang, X., Tang, Y., Li, J., Zhang, S., et al. (2012). Sall3 correlates with the expression of TH in mouse olfactory bulb. *J. Mol. Neurosci.* 46, 293–302. doi: 10.1007/s12031-011-9563-x

Höglinger, G. U., Alvarez-Fischer, D., Arias-Carrión, O., Djufri, M., Windolph, A., Keber, U., et al. (2015). A new dopaminergic nigro-olfactory projection. *Acta Neuropathol.* 130, 333–348. doi: 10.1007/s00401-015-1451-y

Jin, B. K., Franzen, L., and Baker, H. (1996). Regulation of c-Fos mRNA and fos protein expression in olfactory bulbs from unilaterally odor-deprived adult mice. *Int. J. Devl. Neurosci.* 14, 971–982. doi: 10.1016/S0736-5748(96)00044-5

Kawano, T., and Margolis, F. L. (1982). Transsynaptic regulation of olfactory bulb catecholamines in mice and rats. *J. Neurochem.* 39, 342–348. doi: 10.1111/j.1471-4159.1982.tb03953.x

Kiyokage, E., Pan, Y.-Z., Shao, Z., Kobayashi, K., Szabo, G., Yanagawa, Y., et al. (2010). Molecular identity of periglomerular and short axon cells. *J. Neurosci.* 30, 1185–1196. doi: 10.1523/JNEUROSCI.3497-09.2010

Kohwi, M., Osumi, N., Rubenstein, J. L. R., and Alvarez-Buylla, A. (2005). Pax6 is required for making specific subpopulations of granule and periglomerular neurons in the olfactory bulb. *J. Neurosci.* 25, 6997–7003. doi: 10.1523/JNEUROSCI.1435-05.2005

Kohwi, M., Petryniak, M. A., Long, J. E., Ekker, M., Obata, K., Yanagawa, Y., et al. (2007). A subpopulation of olfactory bulb GABAergic interneurons is derived from Emx1- and Dlx5/6-expressing progenitors. *J. Neurosci.* 27, 6878–6891. doi: 10.1523/JNEUROSCI.0254-07.2007

Kosaka, T., and Kosaka, K. (2008). Tyrosine hydroxylase-positive GABAergic juxtaglomerular neurons are the main source of the interglomerular connections in the mouse main olfactory bulb. *Neurosci. Res.* 60, 349–354. doi: 10.1016/j.neures.2007.11.012

Kosaka, T., and Kosaka, K. (2009). Two types of tyrosine hydroxylase positive GABAergic juxtaglomerular neurons in the mouse main olfactory bulb are different in their time of origin. *Neurosci. Res.* 64, 436–441. doi: 10.1016/j.neures.2009.04.018

Kosaka, T., and Kosaka, K. (2011). "Interneurons" in the olfactory bulb revisited. *Neurosci. Res.* 69, 93–99. doi: 10.1016/j.neures.2010.10.002

Kruzich, P. J., and Grandy, D. K. (2004). Dopamine D2 receptors mediate two-odor discrimination and reversal learning in C57BL/6 mice. *BMC Neurosci.* 5:12. doi: 10.1186/1471-2202-5-12

Lazarini, F., Gabellec, M.-M., Moigneu, C., de Chaumont, F., Olivo-Marin, J.-C., and Lledo, P.-M. (2014). Adult neurogenesis restores dopaminergic neuronal loss in the olfactory bulb. *J. Neurosci.* 34, 14430–14442. doi: 10.1523/JNEUROSCI.5366-13.2014

Liu, S., Plachez, C., Shao, Z., Puche, A., and Shipley, M. T. (2013). Olfactory bulb short axon cell release of GABA and dopamine produces a temporally biphasic inhibition-excitation response in external tufted cells. *J. Neurosci.* 33, 2916–2926. doi: 10.1523/JNEUROSCI.3607-12.2013

Mandairon, N., Sacquet, J., Jourdan, F., and Didier, A. (2006). Long-term fate and distribution of newborn cells in the adult mouse olfactory bulb: influences of olfactory deprivation. *Neuroscience* 141, 443–451. doi: 10.1016/j.neuroscience.2006.03.066

McLean, J. H., and Shipley, M. T. (1988). Postmigrational olfactory bulb dopaminergic expression neurons of tyrosine hydroxylase in olfactory bulb dopaminergic neurons. *Methods* 8, 3658–3669.

Merkle, F. T., Mirzadeh, Z., and Alvarez-buylla, A. (2007). Mosaic organization of neural stem cells in the adult brain. *Science* 317, 381–384. doi: 10.1126/science.1144914

Nadi, N. S., Head, R., Grillo, M., Hempstead, J., Grannot-Reisfeld, N., and Margolis, F. L. (1981). Chemical deafferentation of the olfactory bulb: plasticity of the levels of tyrosine hydroxylase, dopamine and norepinephrine. *Brain Res.* 213, 365–377. doi: 10.1016/0006-8993(81)90241-9

Ninkovic, J., Pinto, L., Petricca, S., Lepier, A., Sun, J., Rieger, M. A., et al. (2010). The transcription factor Pax6 regulates survival of dopaminergic olfactory bulb neurons via crystallin αA. *Neuron* 68, 682–694. doi: 10.1016/j.neuron.2010.09.030

Parrish-Aungst, S., Kiyokage, E., Szabo, G., Yanagawa, Y., Shipley, M. T., and Puche, A. C. (2011). Sensory experience selectively regulates transmitter synthesis enzymes in interglomerular circuits. *Brain Res.* 1382, 70–76. doi: 10.1016/j.brainres.2011.01.068

Parrish-Aungst, S., Shipley, M. T., Erdelyi, F., Szabo, G., and Puche, A. C. (2007). Quantitative analysis of neuronal diversity in the mouse olfactory bulb. *J. Comp. Neurol.* 501, 825–836. doi: 10.1002/cne.21205

Pavlis, M., Feretti, C., Levy, A., Gupta, N., and Linster, C. (2006). (L)-DOPA improves odor discrimination learning in rats. *Physiol. Behav.* 87, 109–113. doi: 10.1016/j.physbeh.2005.09.011

Pignatelli, A., Ackman, J. B., Vigetti, D., Beltrami, A. P., Zucchini, S., and Belluzzi, O. (2009). A potential reservoir of immature dopaminergic replacement neurons in the adult mammalian olfactory bulb. *Pflugers Arch. Eur. J. Physiol.* 457, 899–915. doi: 10.1007/s00424-008-0535-0

Pignatelli, A., Borin, M., Fogli Iseppe, A., Gambardella, C., and Belluzzi, O. (2013). The h-current in periglomerular dopaminergic neurons of the mouse olfactory bulb. *PLoS ONE* 8:e56571. doi: 10.1371/journal.pone.0056571

Pignatelli, A., Kobayashi, K., Okano, H., and Belluzzi, O. (2005). Functional properties of dopaminergic neurones in the mouse olfactory bulb. *J. Physiol.* 564, 501–514. doi: 10.1113/jphysiol.2005.084632

Pinching, A. J., and Powell, T. P. (1971). The neuron types of the glomerular layer of the olfactory bulb. *J. Cell Sci.* 9, 305–345.

Rochefort, C., Gheusi, G., Vincent, J.-D., and Lledo, P.-M. (2002). Enriched odor exposure increases the number of newborn neurons in the adult olfactory bulb and improves odor memory. *J. Neurosci.* 22, 2679–2689.

Saino-Saito, S., Cave, J. W., Akiba, Y., Sasaki, H., Goto, K., Kobayashi, K., et al. (2007). ER81 and CaMKIV identify anatomically and phenotypically defined subsets of mouse olfactory bulb interneurons. *J. Comp. Neurol.* 502, 485–496. doi: 10.1002/cne.21293

Saino-Saito, S., Sasaki, H., Volpe, B. T., Kobayashi, K., Berlin, R., and Baker, H. (2004). Differentiation of the dopaminergic phenotype in the olfactory system of neonatal and adult mice. *J. Comp. Neurol.* 479, 389–398. doi: 10.1002/cne.20320

Sawada, M., Kaneko, N., Inada, H., Wake, H., Kato, Y., Yanagawa, Y., et al. (2011). Sensory input regulates spatial and subtype-specific patterns of neuronal turnover in the adult olfactory bulb. *J. Neurosci.* 31, 11587–11596. doi: 10.1523/JNEUROSCI.0614-11.2011

Sawamoto, K., Nakao, N., Kobayashi, K., Matsushita, N., Takahashi, H., Kakishita, K., et al. (2001). Visualization, direct isolation, and transplantation of midbrain dopaminergic neurons. *Proc. Natl. Acad. Sci. U.S.A.* 98, 6423–6428. doi: 10.1073/pnas.111152398

Serguera, C., Triaca, V., Kelly-Barrett, J., Banchaabouchi, M. A., and Minichiello, L. (2008). Increased dopamine after mating impairs olfaction and prevents odor interference with pregnancy. *Nat. Neurosci.* 11, 949–956. doi: 10.1038/nn.2154

Sternson, S. M., and Roth, B. L. (2014). Chemogenetic tools to interrogate brain functions. *Annu. Rev. Neurosci.* 37, 387–407. doi: 10.1146/annurev-neuro-071013-014048

Tillerson, J. L., Caudle, W. M., Parent, J. M., Gong, C., Schallert, T., and Miller, G. W. (2006). Olfactory discrimination deficits in mice lacking the dopamine transporter or the D2 dopamine receptor. *Behav. Brain Res.* 172, 97–105. doi: 10.1016/j.bbr.2006.04.025

Vergaño-Vera, E., Díaz-Guerra, E., Rodríguez-Traver, E., Méndez-Gómez, H. R., Solís, Ó., Pignatelli, J., et al. (2015). Nurr1 blocks the mitogenic effect of FGF-2 and EGF, inducing olfactory bulb neural stem cells to adopt dopaminergic and dopaminergic-GABAergic neuronal phenotypes. *Dev. Neurobiol.* 75, 823–841. doi: 10.1002/dneu.22251

Vergaño-Vera, E., Yusta-boyo, M. J., De Castro, F., Bernad, A., De Pablo, F., Vicario-abejón, C., et al. (2006). Generation of GABAergic and dopaminergic interneurons from endogenous embryonic olfactory bulb precursor cells. *Development* 133, 4367–4379. doi: 10.1242/dev.02601

Wei, C. J., Linster, C., and Cleland, T. A. (2006). Dopamine D(2) receptor activation modulates perceived odor intensity. *Behav. Neurosci.* 120, 393–400. doi: 10.1037/0735-7044.120.2.393

Zhou, X., Liu, F., Tian, M., Xu, Z., Liang, Q., Wang, C., et al. (2015). Transcription factors COUP-TFI and COUP-TFII are required for the production of granule cells in the mouse olfactory bulb. *Development* 142, 1593–1605. doi: 10.1242/dev.115279

15

Mosaic Subventricular Origins of Forebrain Oligodendrogenesis

Kasum Azim [1], Benedikt Berninger [1] and Olivier Raineteau [2]**

[1] Focus Translational Neuroscience, Institute of Physiological Chemistry, University of Mainz, Mainz, Germany, [2] Inserm U1208, Stem Cell and Brain Research Institute, Université Lyon 1, Bron, France

Edited by:
Laura López-Mascaraque, Instituto Cajal-CSIC, Spain

Reviewed by:
Fernando De Castro, Instituto Cajal-CSIC & Hospital Nacional de Parapléjicos, Spain
Eduardo Weruaga, Universidad de Salamanca, Spain

***Correspondence:**
Kasum Azim
kasumazim@gmail.com;
Olivier Raineteau
olivier.raineteau@inserm.fr

In the perinatal as well as the adult CNS, the subventricular zone (SVZ) of the forebrain is the largest and most active source of neural stem cells (NSCs) that generates neurons and oligodendrocytes (OLs), the myelin forming cells of the CNS. Recent advances in the field are beginning to shed light regarding SVZ heterogeneity, with the existence of spatially segregated microdomains that are intrinsically biased to generate phenotypically distinct neuronal populations. Although most research has focused on this regionalization in the context of neurogenesis, newer findings underline that this also applies for the genesis of OLs under the control of specific patterning molecules. In this mini review, we discuss the origins as well as the mechanisms that induce and maintain SVZ regionalization. These come in the flavor of specific signaling ligands and subsequent initiation of transcriptional networks that provide a basis for subdividing the SVZ into distinct lineage-specific microdomains. We further emphasize canonical Wnts and FGF2 as essential signaling pathways for the regional genesis of OL progenitors from NSCs of the dorsal SVZ. This aspect of NSC biology, which has so far received little attention, may unveil new avenues for appropriately recruiting NSCs in demyelinating diseases.

Keywords: subventricular, neural stem cell, oligodendrocyte precursor, oligodendrocyte, oligodendrogenesis, transcription factors, Wnt signaling, dorsal subventricular zone

INTRODUCTION

Adult CNS white matter consists largely of axons, astrocytes, NG2 glia, and OLs, that are all generated in sequential steps during late development. In the rodent forebrain, 3–4 weeks after birth oligodendrocytes (OLs) develop myelin sheaths (Hartman et al., 1982; Rowitch and Kriegstein, 2010) that will wrap around axons enabling insulation and saltatory conductance of action potentials traveling down axons (reviewed in Pfeiffer et al., 1993). Major advances in the field underline that neurogenesis but also gliogenesis persists lifelong in specific germinal niches (Capilla-Gonzalez et al., 2015). The major reservoir containing neural stem cells (NSCs) in the postnatal forebrain is the subventricular zone (SVZ also referred as ventricular SVZ or subependymal zone, SEZ) of the lateral ventricle (Quinones-Hinojosa et al., 2006; Fiorelli et al., 2015). Within this germinal niche, NSCs throughout life generate new neuronal and glial cells to replenish or expand onto preexisting cell

Abbreviations: NSC, neural stem cells; OLs, oligodendrocytes; OPs, oligodendrocyte progenitors; SVZ, subventricular; dSVZ, dorsal subventricular zone; dNSCs, dorsal neural stem cells; vNSCs, ventral neural stem cells; RGCs, radial glial cells; vSVZ, ventral subventricular zone.

populations (Imayoshi et al., 2008; Young et al., 2013). Several recent reviews have detailed adult neurogenesis thoroughly, but much is still to be learned regarding region specific properties of NSCs in generating various subtypes of glial cells. Here, novel findings obtained are discussed to raise awareness of the importance in studying the origin of OLs in the postnatal forebrain in order to shed light onto the mechanisms that regulate their specification from spatially segregated NSCs subpopulations.

ORIGINS OF POSTNATAL SVZ REGIONALIZATION

Immediately after birth, the SVZ undergoes major structural changes with radial glial cells [(RGCs), an embryonic form of NSCs] transforming into NSCs (Merkle et al., 2004; Tong and Alvarez-Buylla, 2014). Another subcategory of glia, ependymal glia, are generated by RGCs earlier during development (mostly between embryonic day 14 and 16, Spassky et al., 2005) and gradually mature following a caudo-rostral gradient around the lateral ventricle. NSCs, located in the SVZ during postnatal development and into adulthood are also termed as Type B1 cells (Doetsch et al., 1997) and give rise to transiently amplifying progenitors (TAPs). This latter progenitor type is identifiable by expression of Ascl1, an essential TF for the genesis of OPs from NSCs, and by short-term BrdU or EdU labeling regimes (Parras et al., 2004; Nakatani et al., 2013). Noticeable cytoarchitectural and transcriptional differences are observed between the different microdomains of the SVZ that are believe to dictate the timing and genesis of neuronal lineages (reviewed in Weinandy et al., 2011; Fiorelli et al., 2015) as well as astrocyte lineages (reviewed in Tabata, 2015). It is now evident that the diversity of neural subtypes generated after birth is larger than first believed (Merkle et al., 2007, 2014; Fiorelli et al., 2015), and emerging evidences suggest that this is now also apparent for the subtypes of glial cells.

Recent lineage tracing studies have revealed that embryonic day 10.5 NSCs (i.e., RGCs) generate all 3 major lineages, i.e., neuronal, astrocytic and oligodendroglial populations (Eckler et al., 2015). Thus, although the existence of lineage restricted RGCs clones has previously been suggested (Franco et al., 2012), it appears that multipotent NSCs prevail during early embryonic forebrain development. It is currently unknown if NSCs clones capable of giving rise to all 3 lineages are evident later in adulthood. Indeed, recent transcriptional and *in vitro* evidences suggest that segregated clones of lineage specific NSCs are observed in adulthood (Ortega et al., 2013; Llorens-Bobadilla et al., 2015), implying that adult NSCs may behave as restricted progenitors. Throughout postnatal life, the diversity in the genesis of different neural cell types is further complexed by their spatiotemporal origin within the SVZ, contrasting with previous beliefs of the SVZ as a reservoir containing a homogeneous NSC population. The events that drive genesis of OLs in a region-dependent manner within the SVZ is the focus of the present review.

Several studies have stressed regional differences in the embryonic origin and neural subtype generation from postnatal and adult SVZ-NSCs. Fate mapping approaches using Cre recombinase under the control of pallial and subpallial transcription factor (TF) promoters have collectively identified that SVZ microdomains are derived from their embryonic counterparts. For example, the medial ganglionic eminence, the lateral ganglionic eminence, and the embryonic cortex generate NSCs that populate the medial (i.e., septal), lateral (i.e., striatal), and dorsal (i.e., cortical) aspects of the adult SVZ, respectively (Ventura and Goldman, 2007; Young et al., 2007). These initial studies identified panels of key embryonic pallial regulators (Emx1, Pax6, Tbr2, Tbr1, Neurog2) whose expression is restricted to the dorsal most regions of the postnatal and adult SVZ. Subpallial markers (Dlx1/2/5, Gsh1/2, Ascl1, Nkx2.1, Nkx6.2) and septal markers (Zic1/3) are expressed more ventrally in the lateral and medial regions of the SVZ, respectively (Kohwi et al., 2007; Young et al., 2007; Batista-Brito et al., 2008; Winpenny et al., 2011; Azim et al., 2012a; Merkle et al., 2014; Sequerra, 2014). This implies that regionally segregated NSCs are primed and regulated in a timely manner for the generation of neural cells subtypes and suggests that intrinsic mechanisms coupled to environmental cues (see below) are major rate determinants of NSC fates in generating both neuronal and glial cells. In addition, recent retroviral barcode labeling of embryonic NSCs (or RGCs) have demonstrated the absence of direct linear relationship of adult or postnatal NSCs from their embryonic counterparts. Thus, the roots of postnatal and adult NSCs are apparently derived from subset of quiescent, segregated and clonally distinct embryonic progenitors from around E11.5 (Fuentealba et al., 2015). These specialized NSCs form by segregation into quiescent NSCs during embryonic development and retain their positional information onto different subregions of the postnatal SVZ through to adulthood, likely in the form of TFs.

Recently, the whole transcriptome of isolated region specific postnatal NSCs has been resolved and offers new avenues to pursue in-depth analyses of SVZ regionalization (Azim et al., 2015). This study identified transcriptional differences between region specific NSCs by means of TF expression (Azim et al., 2015), that could be dependent on environmental cues, some of which are discussed below (reviewed further in Tong and Alvarez-Buylla, 2014; Fiorelli et al., 2015). Additional network interaction analysis was performed on our recently published datasets, confirming many of the above described TFs, whose expression is enriched within specific postnatal SVZ microdomains (Supplementary Tables 8, 9, Azim et al., 2015). The numbers of generic and regionally enriched TFs in postnatal NSCs compared to embryonic or adult NSCs are illustrated in **Figure 1**. It is noticeable that transcriptional cues regulating the switch in glial subtype specification and TFs essential for oligodendrogenesis (e.g., Olig1/2) are abundantly expressed in isolated postnatal dorsal NSCs (dNSCs) (Fuentealba et al., 2015) (see **Figure 1** below) and are associated with the expression of more generic TFs, such as Ascl1 also known to be essential for oligodendrogenesis (Nakatani et al., 2013). These analyses underline the vast extent of TF complexity, which is prevalent in dNSCs compared to their ventral NSC (vNSC) counterparts, and which is likely to be causative for the greater diversities of neural lineages generated from the dorsal SVZ. Furthermore, these findings imply that the action or "networks" of multiple TFs are prerequisites in generating the large diversity of neural lineages observed during postnatal life. Future studies will identify such TF networks and foster further analyses in their relation to the timely genesis of defined neural lineages.

REGIONALIZED GERMINAL ORIGIN OF OLIGODENDROCYTES

Original studies of oligodendrogenesis had assumed that all SVZ-NSCs (RGCs) during embryonic development contribute and specify oligodendrocytes progenitors (OPs), based on cells of the oligodendroglial lineage being detected in all regions of the forebrain (reviewed in Richardson et al., 2006, see also Rubenstein and Rakic, 2013 for a comprehensive overview of OP migration in the forebrain). Most oligodendrogenesis studies to date assume the SVZ after birth to be a single homogeneous germinal zone. As a consequence, researchers in this field generally do not subdivide the SVZ into distinct microdomains for assessing their contribution to OL generation. Because of clear regional differences, this might result in underestimations or inconsistencies in reported findings. For example, Menn et al. (2006). described convincingly that approximately 1/20 of all newly generated cells from adult SVZ-NSCs generate OLs, but also present evidences that this ratio varies considerably depending of rostro-caudal coordinates. Other cre-lox transgenic approaches provide additional information on the origin of OL that are retained into adulthood by demonstrating that they are derived from Emx1+ dNSCs during early postnatal life (Kessaris et al., 2006). This dorsal origin of OLs at postnatal and adult stages contrast with embryonic development, when cohorts of OPs are generated from ventral or lateral forebrain sources, at E12.5 and E15.5 respectively. These OPs are eventually eliminated, presumably due to lack of appropriate survival factors (Richardson et al., 2006). Thus, the final surge of highly migratory dNSC-derived OPs ultimately fulfills its purpose in mediating forebrain myelination (Kessaris et al., 2006). It remains to be determined if postnatal dNSCs of the Emx1 lineage are intrinsically primed in generating new OL lineage cells as well as the role of dorsally enriched environmental cues in triggering OLs migration and maturation after birth. The identity of these signals may be similar to those acting earlier during development, as suggested by the dorsal enrichment of some TGFβ family members (e.g., BMP4) in the postnatal SVZ that have been described to drive OP migration into the cortex during embryonic development (Choe et al., 2014). Understanding the mechanisms that regulate oligodendrogenesis from a default origin and/or lineage restricted NSCs clones (Ortega et al., 2013; Llorens-Bobadilla et al., 2015) represents an essential first step for translational strategies aimed at stimulating endogenous forebrain NSCs.

EXTRINSIC REGULATION OF OLIGODENDROCYTE SPECIFICATION

During postnatal life, signaling ligands are expressed by multiple sources and regulate NSC behaviors in both autocrine and paracrine manners. Expression of these ligands is observed in the various cell types forming the niche, which they also reach by the vasculature (Tavazoie et al., 2008), or more distance sources such as the choroid plexus through the cerebral spinal fluid (Falcao et al., 2012). During postnatal development and to some extent into adulthood, several generic ligands, i.e., Notch ligands, FGFs, EGF, chemokines, members of the BMP family are detected (Johe et al., 1996; Tanigaki et al., 2001; Fiorelli et al., 2015; Grinspan, 2015), and influence NSCs maintenance (see **Figure 2**, reviewed elsewhere in broader SVZ-oligodendrogenesis contexts, El Waly et al., 2014; Capilla-Gonzalez et al., 2015). Other ligands show regional enrichment and participate in the regionalization of the postnatal SVZ. For example, ventrally secreted Shh, which act in concert with Fgf8 during embryonic development, initiates expression of TFs of the Gsh and Nkx families as inducers of the early medial (MGE (Nkx2.1+) and lateral ventricular zones [LGE (Gsh2+) (Cocas et al., 2009]. Noticeably, Shh expression persists into adulthood to maintain SVZ regionalization (Palma et al., 2005; Ihrie et al., 2011). Those enriched in cells of the postnatal dSVZ comprise IGF1, Bmp4, Bmp7, and potent canonical Wnt-ligands such as Rspo1,2, that have long been described to dorsalize the forebrain during development (Takahashi and Liu, 2006; Bond et al., 2012; Harrison-Uy and Pleasure, 2012; Choe et al., 2014; Azim et al., 2015; see **Figure 2**). Importantly, receptors of some distantly secreted patterning ligands are also showing preferential regional expression. For example, this is the case for FGFR1 and FGFR2 which show dorsal enrichment in the postnatal SVZ (Azim et al., 2012) and may therefore regionally integrate FGF2 signaling in promoting NP/OP specification, proliferation and migration (Garcia-Gonzalez et al., 2010; Murcia-Belmonte et al., 2014). Thus, local expression of morphogens combined with regional expression of receptors or downstream effectors of distantly secreted ones are likely to act together in initiating TF expression that stimulates and maintains microdomain heterogeneity during postnatal life. In the case of dorsalizing ligands that promote oligodendrogenesis, Wnt-signaling appears to be a central candidate onto which other signaling pathways converge (see below). Refer to Guo et al (Guo et al., 2015) for a recent comprehensive review of Wnt signaling in the distinct stages of OL differentiation and CNS regions.

The initial dorsalizing trigger of the forebrain and subsequent inducer of oligodendrogenesis at birth, are derived from the choroid plexus which releases several canonical Wnt-ligands (Harrison-Uy and Pleasure, 2012; Azim et al., 2014a). In turn, newly generated OL lineage cells provide further added autocrine support by secreting Wnt3 and possibly other canonical Wnt ligands (Harrison-Uy and Pleasure, 2012; Ortega et al., 2013; Azim et al., 2014a). In the postnatal SVZ, active Wnt-signaling as per the Wnt-reporter Bat-gal transgenic exhibits intense signal that is detected in dorsal NSCs and TAPs as well as within OL lineage cells in the overlying corpus callosum, which are still

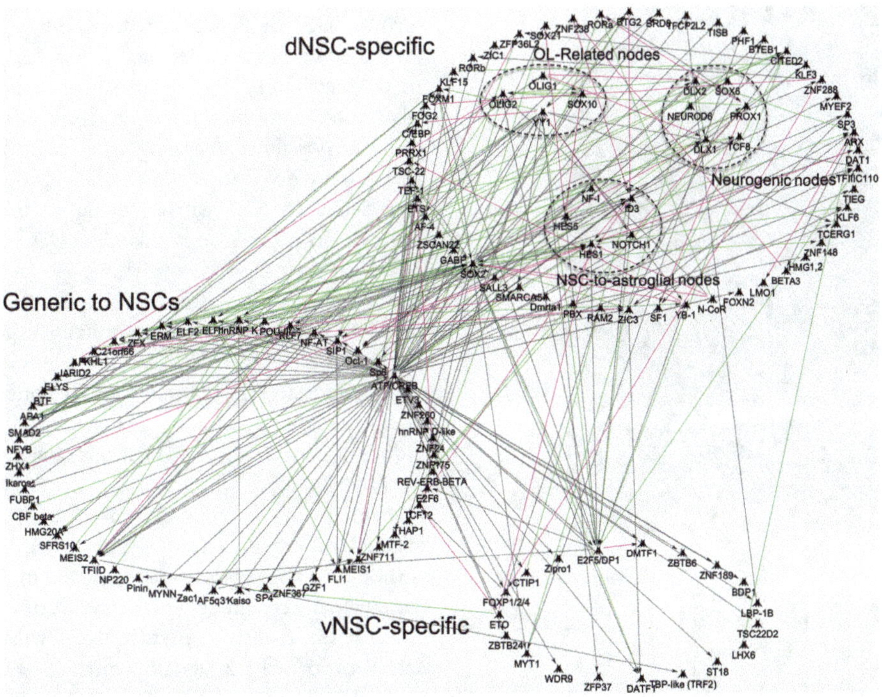

FIGURE 1 | Transcriptional network interactions in regionalized postnatal NSCs of the postnatal subventricular zone. Previously published datasets of genes enriched in postnatal: (1) dNSCs compared to E14 dorsal RGCs and Adult NSCs; (2) vNSCs compared to E14 ventral RGCs and Adult NSCs, were re-analyzed and processed onto Genego Metacore "Direct Interactions" algorithm coupled to Dijkstra's shortest path interface to connect genes based on literature evidences. TFs were focused for analysis and grouped into categories that show dNSC, vNSC or generic enrichment (i.e., common to both). Some nodes were grouped together for illustrative purposes, for example, TFs specific to oligodendrogenesis. Green, magenta and gray lines mark activation, inhibition or unspecified interaction respectively, in TF function or direct gene regulation.

maturing at this stage (**Figure 2**; Azim et al., 2014a). Canonical Wnt activation by either genetic or pharmacological means promotes the generation of OPs by dNSCs (Azim et al., 2014a,b). Wnt-signaling however appears to be an additive mechanism in enhancing the genesis of OL lineage cells. Indeed, ablation in the transcriptional activity of β-catenin does not alter the numbers of newly specified dNSC-derived OPs (Azim et al., 2014a). This is likely to be due to the presence of other Wnt effectors that positively regulates oligodendrocyte differentiation in a manner independent of Wnt/β-catenin signaling, i.e., Tcf7l2 (Hammond et al., 2015), (highly enriched in expression in dNSCs compared to vNSCs, Azim et al., 2015), as well as in the activity of other signaling pathways such as FGF2 (Azim et al., 2014b). Further studies are needed to address the mechanisms by which Tcf7l2 drives NSC-to-OP fates in this context, as well as the involvement of other signaling ligands in regulating this process. Interestingly, enforcing genetically downstream transcription of Wnt-signaling in vNSCs immediately after birth does not alter the numbers of newly generated OPs from adjacent NSC sources (Azim et al., 2014a), while pharmacological activation of Wnt-signaling and infusion of FGF2 only partly induces vNSC-to-OP specification (Azim et al., 2012, 2014b). Notably, even at embryonic stages when the developing forebrain is relatively more plastic, ectopic activation of downstream Wnt-signaling in vSVZ regions only partially promotes dorsalization, although few ventral markers, Nkx2.1, Gsh2, and Ascl1 are down-regulated (Backman et al., 2005). Altogether, these observations suggest the early appearance of epigenetic barriers, multiple inhibitory factors and lack of intrinsic TF networks permitting oligodendrogenesis in more ventral SVZ microdomains. Thus, signaling molecules such as Wnts together with FGF2 act in concert as major inducers of dorsally derived oligodendrogenesis during postnatal development and adulthood.

CROSS-TALK OF SIGNALING LIGANDS IN REGULATING DOWNSTREAM WNT-SIGNALING

In the postnatal forebrain, immediately following birth, relatively few specific lineage directive cues that boost the genesis of OPs from dNSCs have been identified. These, appear to ultimately converge onto activation of common TFs that are considered acting downstream of the Wnt-signaling machinery. As active Wnt canonical signaling is profusely detected in the dSVZ and absent in other SVZ microdomains (**Figure 2A**), few ligands have been identified that have the capacity to directly regulate dorsalization through β-catenin nuclear accumulation. These include, FGF2 as well as BMP4 or EGF that respectfully positively or negatively regulate β-catenin nuclear function, implying multiple modes of regulation by signaling ligands known to be present in the dorsal SVZ (Azim et al., 2014b). In this respect,

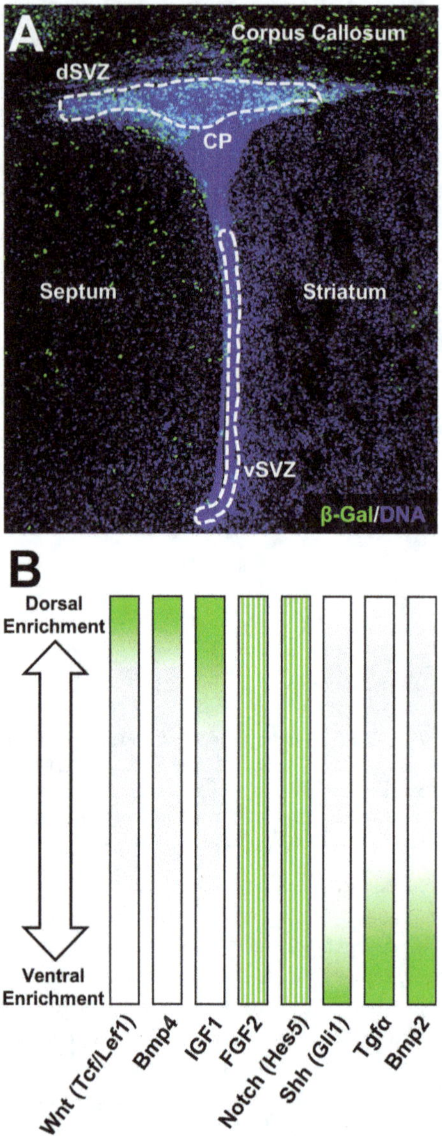

FIGURE 2 | Canonical Wnt-signaling demarcates dorsal forebrain germinal microdomains. (A) Overview of the β-Gal (β-galactosidase) intensity in canonical Wnt-report mouse line highlighting exclusive expression in the dSVZ and in the adjacent corpus callosum at postnatal day 4. For staining procedures (see Azim et al., 2014a). **(B)** Examples of pathway-specific target genes and signaling ligand expression gradients according to previous published studies (Azim et al., 2012, 2014a, 2015). FGF2 and Notch (Hes5) are homogeneously distributed in the P4 SVZ and gradients illustrate relative expression intensities based on previous qPCR validation.

high concentrations of FGF2 is one of few triggers able to induce some aspects of dorsal identity and oligodendrogenesis in the postnatal SVZ (Naruse et al., 2006). This is likely to occur, at least in part, by inhibition of GSK3β (Azim et al., 2014b), presumably via activation of FGFR1 and FGFR2 that are enriched in the dSVZ (Azim et al., 2012). The precise signaling machineries acting downstream of FGFRs and involved in this cross-talk are unknown since multiple developmentally relevant kinases are able to phosphorylate and therefore inhibit GSK3β (Grimes and Jope, 2001). At later differentiation stages *in vitro*, other ligands such as IGF1 or PDGF upregulate major myelin-related genes via β-catenin activity, dependent of GSK3β signaling (Ye et al., 2010; Chew et al., 2011). This suggests the existence of a cross-talk between multiple signaling pathways and the canonical Wnt pathway, possibly converging onto the inhibition of GSK3β. This kinase is involved in several cellular processes and is generally considered as a negative regulator in neurodevelopmental contexts. Its expression in postnatal NSCs is considerably higher compared to others cells in the SVZ (Azim et al., 2015), and developmentally it is often associated with regulation of the Wnt-signaling pathway, with lesser weight on other developmentally important pathways such as Notch, Shh, etc. (reviewed in Kim and Snider, 2011). This was recently confirmed within the SVZ microdomains, in which pharmacological inhibition of GSK3β induces the expression of Wnt target genes by multiple folds in parallel to oligodendrogenesis, whereas target genes specific to other pathways (i.e., Notch, Shh, Bmps) are either very subtly affected or are unaltered (Azim et al., 2014b). Additionally, GSK3β further regulates later stages of OL differentiation in parallel to other signaling pathways (Azim and Butt, 2011; Meffre et al., 2015). In this respect, it is noteworthy mentioning FGF2 activation of Erk1/2 signaling through FGFR1/2, and its cross talk with Akt/mTor signaling in regulating OL migration (Ishii et al., 2014; Murcia-Belmonte et al., 2015), differentiation and survival (Guardiola-Diaz et al., 2012; Dai et al., 2014). Further studies in the field are required to address the concerted role of "generic" (i.e., EGF, VEGFs, HGFs, etc.) and regionaly acting (i.e., FGF2, Wnt) signaling ligands in mediating these effects via the induction of specific TF networks (see **Figure 1**).

SUMMARY AND FUTURE OUTLOOK

In this review, the known mechanisms essential for inducing oligodendrogenesis have been discussed that altogether underline a strict spatial coding within segregated NSC populations of the postnatal dSVZ. Evidences for the existence of lineage specific microdomains in primates (Azim et al., 2013), coupled to the demonstrated origin of OLs from dorsal RGCs in developing human brain (Rakic and Zecevic, 2003), and activation of the SVZ in human Multiple Sclerosis lesions (Nait-Oumesmar et al., 2007), emphasizes that the SVZ should be sampled in 3D for recruitment of region-specific NSCs. Ultimately, identifying mechanisms that regulate oligodendrogenesis from specific subsets of NSCs, will serve as a starting basis for future translational studies.

AUTHOR CONTRIBUTIONS

KA: Main contributing author and wrote the article; BB and OR: Financial support, manuscript editing.

ACKNOWLEDGMENTS

We thank the Swiss National Science Foundation (SNF) for the SNF project grant NRP63; 406340_128291 to OR, SNF Advanced

Post-doc mobility fellowship P300P3_154614 to KA, research grant. Further funding for OR was obtained from the program "Investissements d'Avenir" (ANR-11-IDEX-0007) via the French National Research Agency (ANR). We gratefully thank also Misako Watanabe at Thomson Reuters for technical support for the Bioinformatic analysis performed. Finally we thank Dr Sophie Perron and Nicolas Marcolis for critical evaluation of this manuscript.

REFERENCES

Azim, K., and Butt, A. M. (2011). GSK3beta negatively regulates oligodendrocyte differentiation and myelination *in vivo*. *Glia* 59, 540–553. doi: 10.1002/glia.21122

Azim, K., Fiorelli, R., Zweifel, S., Hurtado-Chong, A., Yoshikawa, K., Slomianka, L., et al. (2012a). 3-dimensional examination of the adult mouse subventricular zone reveals lineage-specific microdomains. *PLoS ONE* 7:e49087. doi: 10.1371/journal.pone.0049087

Azim, K., Fischer, B., Hurtado-Chong, A., Draganova, K., Cantu, C., Zemke, M., et al. (2014a). Persistent Wnt/beta-catenin signaling determines dorsalization of the postnatal subventricular zone and neural stem cell specification into oligodendrocytes and glutamatergic neurons. *Stem Cells* 32, 1301–1312. doi: 10.1002/stem.1639

Azim, K., Hurtado-Chong, A., Fischer, B., Kumar, N., Zweifel, S., Taylor, V., et al. (2015). Transcriptional hallmarks of heterogeneous neural stem cell niches of the subventricular zone. *Stem Cells* 33, 2232–2242. doi: 10.1002/stem.2017

Azim, K., Raineteau, O., and Butt, A. M. (2012). bIntraventricular injection of FGF-2 promotes generation of oligodendrocyte-lineage cells in the postnatal and adult forebrain. *Glia* 60, 1977–1990. doi: 10.1002/glia.22413

Azim, K., Rivera, A., Raineteau, O., and Butt, A. M. (2014b). GSK3beta regulates oligodendrogenesis in the dorsal microdomain of the subventricular zone via Wnt-beta-catenin signaling. *Glia* 62, 778–779. doi: 10.1002/glia.22641

Azim, K., Zweifel, S., Klaus, F., Yoshikawa, K., Amrein, I., and Raineteau, O. (2013). Early decline in progenitor diversity in the marmoset lateral ventricle. *Cereb. Cortex* 23, 922–931. doi: 10.1093/cercor/bhs085

Backman, M., Machon, O., Mygland, L., van den Bout, C. J., Zhong, W., Taketo, M. M., et al. (2005). Effects of canonical Wnt signaling on dorso-ventral specification of the mouse telencephalon. *Dev. Biol.* 279, 155–168. doi: 10.1016/j.ydbio.2004.12.010

Batista-Brito, R., Close, J., Machold, R., and Fishell, G. (2008). The distinct temporal origins of olfactory bulb interneuron subtypes. *J. Neurosci.* 28, 3966–3975. doi: 10.1523/JNEUROSCI.5625-07.2008

Bond, A. M., Bhalala, O. G., and Kessler, J. A. (2012). The dynamic role of bone morphogenetic proteins in neural stem cell fate and maturation. *Dev. Neurobiol.* 72, 1068–1084. doi: 10.1002/dneu.22022

Capilla-Gonzalez, V., Herranz-Perez, V., and Garcia-Verdugo, J. M. (2015). The aged brain: genesis and fate of residual progenitor cells in the subventricular zone. *Front. Cell. Neurosci.* 9:365. doi: 10.3389/fncel.2015.00365

Chew, L. J., Shen, W., Ming, X., Senatorov, V. V. Jr., Chen, H. L., Cheng, Y., et al. (2011). SRY-box containing gene 17 regulates the Wnt/beta-catenin signaling pathway in oligodendrocyte progenitor cells. *J. Neurosci.* 31, 13921–13935. doi: 10.1523/JNEUROSCI.3343-11.2011

Choe, Y., Huynh, T., and Pleasure, S. J. (2014). Migration of oligodendrocyte progenitor cells is controlled by transforming growth factor beta family proteins during corticogenesis. *J. Neurosci.* 34, 14973–14983. doi: 10.1523/JNEUROSCI.1156-14.2014

Cocas, L. A., Miyoshi, G., Carney, R. S., Sousa, V. H., Hirata, T., Jones, K. R., et al. (2009). Emx1-lineage progenitors differentially contribute to neural diversity in the striatum and amygdala. *J. Neurosci.* 29, 15933–15946. doi: 10.1523/JNEUROSCI.2525-09.2009

Dai, J., Bercury, K. K., and Macklin, W. B. (2014). Interaction of mTOR and Erk1/2 signaling to regulate oligodendrocyte differentiation. *Glia* 62, 2096–2109. doi: 10.1002/glia.22729

Doetsch, F., Garcia-Verdugo, J. M., and Alvarez-Buylla, A. (1997). Cellular composition and three-dimensional organization of the subventricular germinal zone in the adult mammalian brain. *J. Neurosci.* 17, 5046–5061.

Eckler, M. J., Nguyen, T. D., McKenna, W. L., Fastow, B. L., Guo, C., Rubenstein, J. L., et al. (2015). Cux2-positive radial glial cells generate diverse subtypes of neocortical projection neurons and macroglia. *Neuron* 86, 1100–1108. doi: 10.1016/j.neuron.2015.04.020

El Waly, B., Macchi, M., Cayre, M., and Durbec, P. (2014). Oligodendrogenesis in the normal and pathological central nervous system. *Front. Neurosci.* 8:145. doi: 10.3389/fnins.2014.00145

Falcao, A. M., Marques, F., Novais, A., Sousa, N., Palha, J. A., and Sousa, J. C. (2012). The path from the choroid plexus to the subventricular zone: go with the flow! *Front. Cell. Neurosci.* 6:34. doi: 10.3389/fncel.2012.00034

Fiorelli, R., Azim, K., Fischer, B., and Raineteau, O. (2015). Adding a spatial dimension to postnatal ventricular-subventricular zone neurogenesis. *Development* 142, 2109–2120. doi: 10.1242/dev.119966

Franco, S. J., Gil-Sanz, C., Martinez-Garay, I., Espinosa, A., Harkins-Perry, S. R., Ramos, C., et al. (2012). Fate-restricted neural progenitors in the mammalian cerebral cortex. *Science* 337, 746–749. doi: 10.1126/science.1223616

Fuentealba, L. C., Rompani, S. B., Parraguez, J. I., Obernier, K., Romero, R., Cepko, C. L., et al. (2015). Embryonic origin of postnatal neural stem cells. *Cell* 161, 1644–1655. doi: 10.1016/j.cell.2015.05.041

Garcia-Gonzalez, D., Clemente, D., Coelho, M., Esteban, P. F., Soussi-Yanicostas, N., and de Castro, F. (2010). Dynamic roles of FGF-2 and Anosmin-1 in the migration of neuronal precursors from the subventricular zone during pre- and postnatal development. *Exp. Neurol.* 222, 285–295. doi: 10.1016/j.expneurol.2010.01.006

Grimes, C. A., and Jope, R. S. (2001). The multifaceted roles of glycogen synthase kinase 3beta in cellular signaling. *Prog. Neurobiol.* 65, 391–426. doi: 10.1016/S0301-0082(01)00011-9

Grinspan, J. B. (2015). Bone morphogenetic proteins: inhibitors of myelination in development and disease. *Vitam. Horm.* 99, 195–222. doi: 10.1016/bs.vh.2015.05.005

Guardiola-Diaz, H. M., Ishii, A., and Bansal, R. (2012). Erk1/2 MAPK and mTOR signaling sequentially regulates progression through distinct stages of oligodendrocyte differentiation. *Glia* 60, 476–486. doi: 10.1002/glia.22281

Guo, F., Lang, J., Sohn, J., Hammond, E., Chang, M., and Pleasure, D. (2015). Canonical Wnt signaling in the oligodendroglial lineage–puzzles remain. *Glia* 63, 1671–1693. doi: 10.1002/glia.22813

Hammond, E., Lang, J., Maeda, Y., Pleasure, D., Angus-Hill, M., Xu, J., et al. (2015). The Wnt effector transcription factor 7-like 2 positively regulates oligodendrocyte differentiation in a manner independent of Wnt/beta-catenin signaling. *J. Neurosci.* 35, 5007–5022. doi: 10.1523/JNEUROSCI.4787-14.2015

Harrison-Uy, S. J., and Pleasure, S. J. (2012). Wnt signaling and forebrain development. *Cold Spring Harb. Perspect. Biol.* 4:a008094. doi: 10.1101/cshperspect.a008094

Hartman, B. K., Agrawal, H. C., Agrawal, D., and Kalmbach, S. (1982). Development and maturation of central nervous system myelin: comparison of immunohistochemical localization of proteolipid protein and basic protein in myelin and oligodendrocytes. *Proc. Natl. Acad. Sci. U.S.A.* 79, 4217–4220. doi: 10.1073/pnas.79.13.4217

Ihrie, R. A., Shah, J. K., Harwell, C. C., Levine, J. H., Guinto, C. D., Lezameta, M., et al. (2011). Persistent sonic hedgehog signaling in adult brain determines neural stem cell positional identity. *Neuron* 71, 250–262. doi: 10.1016/j.neuron.2011.05.018

Imayoshi, I., Sakamoto, M., Ohtsuka, T., Takao, K., Miyakawa, T., Yamaguchi, M., et al. (2008). Roles of continuous neurogenesis in the structural and functional integrity of the adult forebrain. *Nat. Neurosci.* 11, 1153–1161. doi: 10.1038/nn.2185

Ishii, A., Furusho, M., Dupree, J. L., and Bansal, R. (2014). Role of ERK1/2 MAPK signaling in the maintenance of myelin and axonal integrity in the adult CNS. *J. Neurosci.* 34, 16031–16045. doi: 10.1523/JNEUROSCI.3360-14.2014

Johe, K. K., Hazel, T. G., Muller, T., Dugich-Djordjevic, M. M., and McKay, R. D. (1996). Single factors direct the differentiation of stem cells from the fetal and adult central nervous system. *Genes Dev.* 10, 3129–3140. doi: 10.1101/gad.10.24.3129

Kessaris, N., Fogarty, M., Iannarelli, P., Grist, M., Wegner, M., and Richardson, W. D. (2006). Competing waves of oligodendrocytes in the forebrain and postnatal elimination of an embryonic lineage. *Nat. Neurosci.* 9, 173–179. doi: 10.1038/nn1620

Kim, W. Y., and Snider, W. D. (2011). Functions of GSK-3 signaling in development of the nervous system. *Front. Mol. Neurosci.* 4:44. doi: 10.3389/fnmol.2011.00044

Kohwi, M., Petryniak, M. A., Long, J. E., Ekker, M., Obata, K., Yanagawa, Y., et al. (2007). A subpopulation of olfactory bulb GABAergic interneurons is derived from Emx1- and Dlx5/6-expressing progenitors. *J. Neurosci.* 27, 6878–6891. doi: 10.1523/JNEUROSCI.0254-07.2007

Llorens-Bobadilla, E., Zhao, S., Baser, A., Saiz-Castro, G., Zwadlo, K., and Martin-Villalba, A. (2015). Single-cell transcriptomics reveals a population of dormant neural stem cells that become activated upon brain injury. *Cell Stem Cell* 17, 329–340. doi: 10.1016/j.stem.2015.07.002

Meffre, D., Massaad, C., and Grenier, J. (2015). Lithium chloride stimulates PLP and MBP expression in oligodendrocytes via Wnt/beta-catenin and Akt/CREB pathways. *Neuroscience* 284, 962–971. doi: 10.1016/j.neuroscience.2014.10.064

Menn, B., Garcia-Verdugo, J. M., Yaschine, C., Gonzalez-Perez, O., Rowitch, D., and Alvarez-Buylla, A. (2006). Origin of oligodendrocytes in the subventricular zone of the adult brain. *J. Neurosci.* 26, 7907–7918. doi: 10.1523/JNEUROSCI.1299-06.2006

Merkle, F. T., Fuentealba, L. C., Sanders, T. A., Magno, L., Kessaris, N., and Alvarez-Buylla, A. (2014). Adult neural stem cells in distinct microdomains generate previously unknown interneuron types. *Nat. Neurosci.* 17, 207–214. doi: 10.1038/nn.3610

Merkle, F. T., Mirzadeh, Z., and Alvarez-Buylla, A. (2007). Mosaic organization of neural stem cells in the adult brain. *Science* 317, 381–384. doi: 10.1126/science.1144914

Merkle, F. T., Tramontin, A. D., Garcia-Verdugo, J. M., and Alvarez-Buylla, A. (2004). Radial glia give rise to adult neural stem cells in the subventricular zone. *Proc. Natl. Acad. Sci. U.S.A.* 101, 17528–17532. doi: 10.1073/pnas.0407893101

Murcia-Belmonte, V., Esteban, P. F., Martinez-Hernández, J., Gruart, A., Luján, R., Delgado-García, J. M., et al. (2015). Anosmin-1 over-expression regulates oligodendrocyte precursor cell proliferation, migration and myelin sheath thickness. *Brain Struct. Funct.* doi: 10.1007/s00429-014-0977-4. [Epub ahead of print].

Murcia-Belmonte, V., Medina-Rodriguez, E. M., Bribian, A., de Castro, F., and Esteban, P. F. (2014). ERK1/2 signaling is essential for the chemoattraction exerted by human FGF2 and human anosmin-1 on newborn rat and mouse OPCs via FGFR1. *Glia* 62, 374–386. doi: 10.1002/glia.22609

Nait-Oumesmar, B., Picard-Riera, N., Kerninon, C., Decker, L., Seilhean, D., Hoglinger, G. U., et al. (2007). Activation of the subventricular zone in multiple sclerosis: evidence for early glial progenitors. *Proc. Natl. Acad. Sci. U.S.A.* 104, 4694–4699. doi: 10.1073/pnas.0606835104

Nakatani, H., Martin, E., Hassani, H., Clavairoly, A., Maire, C. L., Viadieu, A., et al. (2013). Ascl1/Mash1 promotes brain oligodendrogenesis during myelination and remyelination. *J. Neurosci.* 33, 9752–9768. doi: 10.1523/JNEUROSCI.0805-13.2013

Naruse, M., Nakahira, E., Miyata, T., Hitoshi, S., Ikenaka, K., and Bansal, R. (2006). Induction of oligodendrocyte progenitors in dorsal forebrain by intraventricular microinjection of FGF-2. *Dev. Biol.* 297, 262–273. doi: 10.1016/j.ydbio.2006.05.017

Ortega, F., Gascon, S., Masserdotti, G., Deshpande, A., Simon, C., Fischer, J., et al. (2013). Oligodendrogliogenic and neurogenic adult subependymal zone neural stem cells constitute distinct lineages and exhibit differential responsiveness to Wnt signalling. *Nat. Cell Biol.* 15, 602–613. doi: 10.1038/ncb2736

Palma, V., Lim, D. A., Dahmane, N., Sanchez, P., Brionne, T. C., Herzberg, C. D., et al. (2005). Sonic hedgehog controls stem cell behavior in the postnatal and adult brain. *Development* 132, 335–344. doi: 10.1242/dev.01567

Parras, C. M., Galli, R., Britz, O., Soares, S., Galichet, C., Battiste, J., et al. (2004). Mash1 specifies neurons and oligodendrocytes in the postnatal brain. *EMBO J.* 23, 4495–4505. doi: 10.1038/sj.emboj.7600447

Pfeiffer, S. E., Warrington, A. E., and Bansal, R. (1993). The oligodendrocyte and its many cellular processes. *Trends Cell Biol.* 3, 191–197. doi: 10.1016/0962-8924(93)90213-K

Quinones-Hinojosa, A., Sanai, N., Soriano-Navarro, M., Gonzalez-Perez, O., Mirzadeh, Z., Gil-Perotin, S., et al. (2006). Cellular composition and cytoarchitecture of the adult human subventricular zone: a niche of neural stem cells. *J. Comp. Neurol.* 494, 415–434. doi: 10.1002/cne.20798

Rakic, S., and Zecevic, N. (2003). Early oligodendrocyte progenitor cells in the human fetal telencephalon. *Glia* 41, 117–127. doi: 10.1002/glia.10140

Richardson, W. D., Kessaris, N., and Pringle, N. (2006). Oligodendrocyte wars. *Nat. Rev. Neurosci.* 7, 11–18. doi: 10.1038/nrn1826

Rowitch, D. H., and Kriegstein, A. R. (2010). Developmental genetics of vertebrate glial-cell specification. *Nature* 468, 214–222. doi: 10.1038/nature09611

Rubenstein, J. L. R., and Rakic, P. (2013). *Comprehensive Developmental Neuroscience: Patterning and Cell Type Specification in the Developing CNS and PNS*. Oxford: Academic Press.

Sequerra, E. B. (2014). Subventricular zone progenitors in time and space: generating neuronal diversity. *Front. Cell. Neurosci.* 8:434. doi: 10.3389/fncel.2014.00434

Spassky, N., Merkle, F. T., Flames, N., Tramontin, A. D., Garcia-Verdugo, J. M., and Alvarez-Buylla, A. (2005). Adult ependymal cells are postmitotic and are derived from radial glial cells during embryogenesis. *J. Neurosci.* 25, 10–18. doi: 10.1523/JNEUROSCI.1108-04.2005

Tabata, H. (2015). Diverse subtypes of astrocytes and their development during corticogenesis. *Front. Neurosci.* 9:114. doi: 10.3389/fnins.2015.00114

Takahashi, H., and Liu, F. C. (2006). Genetic patterning of the mammalian telencephalon by morphogenetic molecules and transcription factors. *Birth Defects Res. C Embryo Today* 78, 256–266. doi: 10.1002/bdrc.20077

Tanigaki, K., Nogaki, F., Takahashi, J., Tashiro, K., Kurooka, H., and Honjo, T. (2001). Notch1 and Notch3 instructively restrict bFGF-responsive multipotent neural progenitor cells to an astroglial fate. *Neuron* 29, 45–55. doi: 10.1016/S0896-6273(01)00179-9

Tavazoie, M., Van der Veken, L., Silva-Vargas, V., Louissaint, M., Colonna, L., Zaidi, B., et al. (2008). A specialized vascular niche for adult neural stem cells. *Cell Stem Cell* 3, 279–288. doi: 10.1016/j.stem.2008.07.025

Tong, C. K., and Alvarez-Buylla, A. (2014). SnapShot: adult neurogenesis in the V-SVZ. *Neuron* 81, 220-220.e1. doi: 10.1016/j.neuron.2013.12.004

Ventura, R. E., and Goldman, J. E. (2007). Dorsal radial glia generate olfactory bulb interneurons in the postnatal murine brain. *J. Neurosci.* 27, 4297–4302. doi: 10.1523/JNEUROSCI.0399-07.2007

Weinandy, F., Ninkovic, J., and Gotz, M. (2011). Restrictions in time and space–new insights into generation of specific neuronal subtypes in the adult mammalian brain. *Eur. J. Neurosci.* 33, 1045–1054. doi: 10.1111/j.1460-9568.2011.07602.x

Winpenny, E., Lebel-Potter, M., Fernandez, M. E., Brill, M. S., Gotz, M., Guillemot, F., et al. (2011). Sequential generation of olfactory bulb glutamatergic neurons by Neurog2-expressing precursor cells. *Neural Dev.* 6:12. doi: 10.1186/1749-8104-6-12

Ye, P., Hu, Q., Liu, H., Yan, Y., and D'Ercole, A. J. (2010). beta-catenin mediates insulin-like growth factor-I actions to promote cyclin D1 mRNA expression, cell proliferation and survival in oligodendroglial cultures. *Glia* 58, 1031–1041. doi: 10.1002/glia.20984

Young, K. M., Fogarty, M., Kessaris, N., and Richardson, W. D. (2007). Subventricular zone stem cells are heterogeneous with respect to their embryonic origins and neurogenic fates in the adult olfactory bulb. *J. Neurosci.* 27, 8286–8296. doi: 10.1523/JNEUROSCI.0476-07.2007

Young, K. M., Psachoulia, K., Tripathi, R. B., Dunn, S. J., Cossell, L., Attwell, D., et al. (2013). Oligodendrocyte dynamics in the healthy adult CNS: evidence for myelin remodeling. *Neuron* 77, 873–885. doi: 10.1016/j.neuron.2013.01.006

Adult Neurogenesis 50 Years Later: Limits and Opportunities in Mammals

Luca Bonfanti [1,2]*

[1] *Neuroscience Institute Cavalieri Ottolenghi, Orbassano, Italy,* [2] *Department of Veterinary Sciences, University of Turin, Torino, Italy*

Keywords: neural stem cells, brain repair, parenchymal progenitors, astrocytes, comparative neurogenesis, mammalian brain

Edited by:
Alino Martinez-Marcos, Universidad de Castilla, Spain

Reviewed by:
Juan Manuel Encinas, Ikerbasque - the Basque Foundation for Science, Spain
David Díaz, Universidad de Salamanca, Spain

Correspondence:
Luca Bonfanti
luca.bonfanti@unito.it

After five decades of research in adult neurogenesis (AN) it is far from easy to make a balance. If this field was a movie genre, brain repair goals would be a dreary mystery (with cell replacement therapies approaching fantasy), opportunities would be high quality science fiction, and limits could well belong to a hopeless thriller. Though apparently depicting a pessimistic screenplay, these aspects actually represent very exciting plots in which the only pitfall had been the attitude of those main characters (the scientists) who, starting with the re-discovery of AN (Paton and Nottebohm, 1984; Lois and Alvarez-Buylla, 1994), looked for neuronal cell replacement. The chimera of regenerative outcomes led to an exponential burst of studies: more than 7500 articles on PubMed with the keyword "adult neurogenesis." Why such an interest many years after the first demonstration of AN (Altman and Das, 1965)? Maybe because the first isolation of neural stem cells (NSCs) took place in the same period (Reynolds and Weiss, 1992), thus making it possible to figure out continuous replenishment of new neurons throughout a brain's life (Gage, 2000; Alvarez-Buylla et al., 2001). At the same time, the possibility to play *in vitro* with the NSC plasticity (Galli et al., 2003) might explain why the AN articles in PubMed become 23,000 when the keyword "neural stem cell" is employed.

REVISITING THE HISTORY OF AN

Most AN review articles start with Altman's pioneering studies, disregarded at the time by most neurobiologists and then upgraded to the death of a dogma (Gross, 2000). What is more difficult to find is a critical evaluation of what happened after the nineties. Briefly, an intense phase of AN characterization contributed to persuade the scientific community that stem cells actually persist in the adult mammalian brain (Palmer et al., 1997; Doetsch et al., 1999), making the integration of new neurons a real phenomenon producing anatomical and functional changes (Gage, 2000; Alvarez-Buylla et al., 2001; Lledo et al., 2006). The stem cell niches of two main neurogenic sites (subventricular zone and hippocampal dentate gyrus) were identified and progressively defined in their structure and regulation (**Figure 1**). On these solid bases, a sort of gold rush-like fever aiming at demonstrating new sites of AN grew exponentially (Gould et al., 1999, 2001; Zhao et al., 2003; Dayer et al., 2005; Shapiro et al., 2007). Yet, some of the "alternative" neurogenic regions were subsequently denied by independent studies (references in Bonfanti and Peretto, 2011; Nacher and Bonfanti, 2015). In parallel, it was shown that neurogenesis can be induced by different types of injury or disease (lesion-induced, reactive neurogenesis), either by mobilization of cells from the neurogenic sites (Arvidsson et al., 2002) or by local activation of parenchymal progenitors (Magnusson et al., 2014; Nato et al., 2015; **Figure 1**). Nevertheless, though large numbers of neuroblasts can be produced in response to stroke or inflammation (Arvidsson et al., 2002; Ohira et al., 2010; Magnusson et al., 2014; Nato et al., 2015), the mechanisms of such responses as well as the ultimate fate of the newborn cells remain largely unknown, as acknowledged by leading experts in the field (Lindvall and Kokaia, 2015). In addition, only limited spontaneous recovery occurs (Sohur et al., 2006; Bonfanti, 2011) and some promising results published on megahit journals have not been reproduced (Magavi et al., 2000; Nakatomi et al., 2002). Finally, the huge effort for obtaining regenerative outcomes by using exogenous sources of stem/progenitor cells has also led, until now, to scarce results in terms of reliability and effectiveness (Li et al., 2010), although some therapeutic perspectives might come from the use of stem cell-derived dopaminergic cells in Parkinson disease (Barker et al., 2015).

How can we find an explanation for recurrent failures in obtaining cell replacement from AN? Maybe the answer resides in a psychological attitude: the initial burst of optimism affecting scientists with the biased vision that "new neurons equals brain repair" persisted too long under translational pressures, in forgetfulness of a basic fact: the mammalian central nervous system (CNS) evolved to be substantially nonrenewable, relatively hardwired, non-self repairing (Weil et al., 2008). Further proof come from examples of spontaneous "parenchymal" (non-canonical) neurogenesis detectable in other mammals: the outcome of these newly-produced neurons is quite different from that performed in canonical NSC niches (Feliciano et al., 2015) since "transient" neural cells are mostly produced (Gould et al., 2001; Luzzati et al., 2014). More recently, some neurogenic activity has been shown in the hypothalamus, starting from tanycytes harbored within a germinal layer-derived zone, linked with feeding regulation and energy balance, and responding to external stimuli (Migaud et al., 2010). Yet, low levels of neurons are generated in basal conditions, and their final outcome is far from clear.

Hence, if regarding AN as a "full biological process" (from NSC activation to neuronal integration), all neurogenic phenomena occurring out of the hippocampus and olfactory bulb should be classified as "incomplete" (Bonfanti and Peretto, 2011), both spontaneously-occurring and reactive neurogenic events appearing as "unwanted hosts" in the mature brain tissue (**Figure 1K**).

THE BIG QUESTIONS IN AN

By putting together data learned over 50 years of AN research with CNS evolutionary history, it appears clear that: (i) AN has lost most of its capacity for brain repair in mammals with respect to other vertebrates (Grandel and Brand, 2013), its role being largely restricted to physiological plasticity of specific systems (Peretto and Bonfanti, 2014); (ii) this feature might not primarily depend on the availability of stem cells (AN does exist in mammals!) rather on CNS structural, cellular, molecular organization, as a result of its postnatal development and immunological responses (Bonfanti, 2011). Hence, one big question concerns the intermix of biological events leading to such a loss of regenerative capacity.

Many scientists working in the field focus on the question: how NSCs divide and regulate their quiescent/active state *in vivo*? (in the perspective of modulating—usually intended as "increasing"—their mitotic activity and neuronal fate). These actually are crucial points in NSC basic biology. Yet, beside the common viewpoint considering the neurogenic potential of NSCs to be beneficial, the fact is emerging that having more new neurons or synapses is not always better (Tang et al., 2014; e.g., hippocampal AN can be implicated in memory erasure, Akers et al., 2014; Kitamura and Inokuchi, 2014). By contrast, I consider as essential questions: whether, how, when different types of progenitor cells can produce a progeny which can actually survive and functionally integrate in the brain regions in which they are needed, out of the two canonical niches. Even within the niches, specific subsets of progenitors occupying precise topographical subregions produce only selected neuronal types for selected tissue domains (Obernier et al., 2014), thus confirming that mature brain neurogenic plasticity occurs only within restricted bounds. Also in gliogenesis, the amount of oligodendrocyte precursor cells (OPCs) generated daily in the adult CNS (Young et al., 2013; Boda and Buffo, 2014) clashes with the slow rate of myelin turnover, suggesting that only a small fraction of them actually integrate. Moreover, they appear able to sustain remyelination after acute lesion or disease but not in chronic phases (Franklin, 2002).

A fundamental issue regards the molecular and cellular features which make the mature mammalian brain environment refractory to substantial reshaping or repair, both in physiological and pathological states, with respect to the permissive conditions existing in non-mammalian vertebrates (Kyritsis et al., 2014; **Figures 1J,K**). Unfortunately, the tools at present available to address such aspect are scarce. One possible way could reside in neurodevelopmental studies aimed at unraveling how the embryonic, permissive tissue environment shifts to mature, more restrictive conditions (Peretto et al., 2005), taking into account that a regulated balance of stability and plasticity is required for optimal functioning of neuronal circuits (Abraham and Robins, 2005; Akers et al., 2014). This approach could open new landscapes from the re-expression of developmental programs (Sohur et al., 2012) to the cutting edge frontier of homeosis (Arlotta and Hobert, 2015).

Another fundamental question remains substantially unanswered (and often skipped by scientists hurrying in search for reparative roles of AN): concerns the function of AN (**Figure 1M**). It seems clear that AN can play a physiological role in memory and learning, yet rapid adaptation of hippocampal neurogenesis to experimental challenges appears to be a characteristic of laboratory rodents, whereas low or missing AN in bats and dolphins argues against a critical role in spatial learning (Amrein and Lipp, 2009). Wild mammals show species-specific, rather stable hippocampal neurogenesis, which appears related to demands that characterize the niche exploited by a species rather than to acute events in the life of its members (Amrein, 2015). It is worthwhile to remember that AN itself should not be considered as a "function," rather a tool the brain can use to perform different functions (see also Hersman et al., 2016). As stated by Anderson and Finlay (2014), "Mounting evidence from allometric, developmental, comparative, systems-physiological, neuroimaging, and neurological studies suggests that brain elements are used and reused in multiple functional systems." They suggest that "this variable allocation can be seen in neuroplasticity over the life span," and that "the same processes

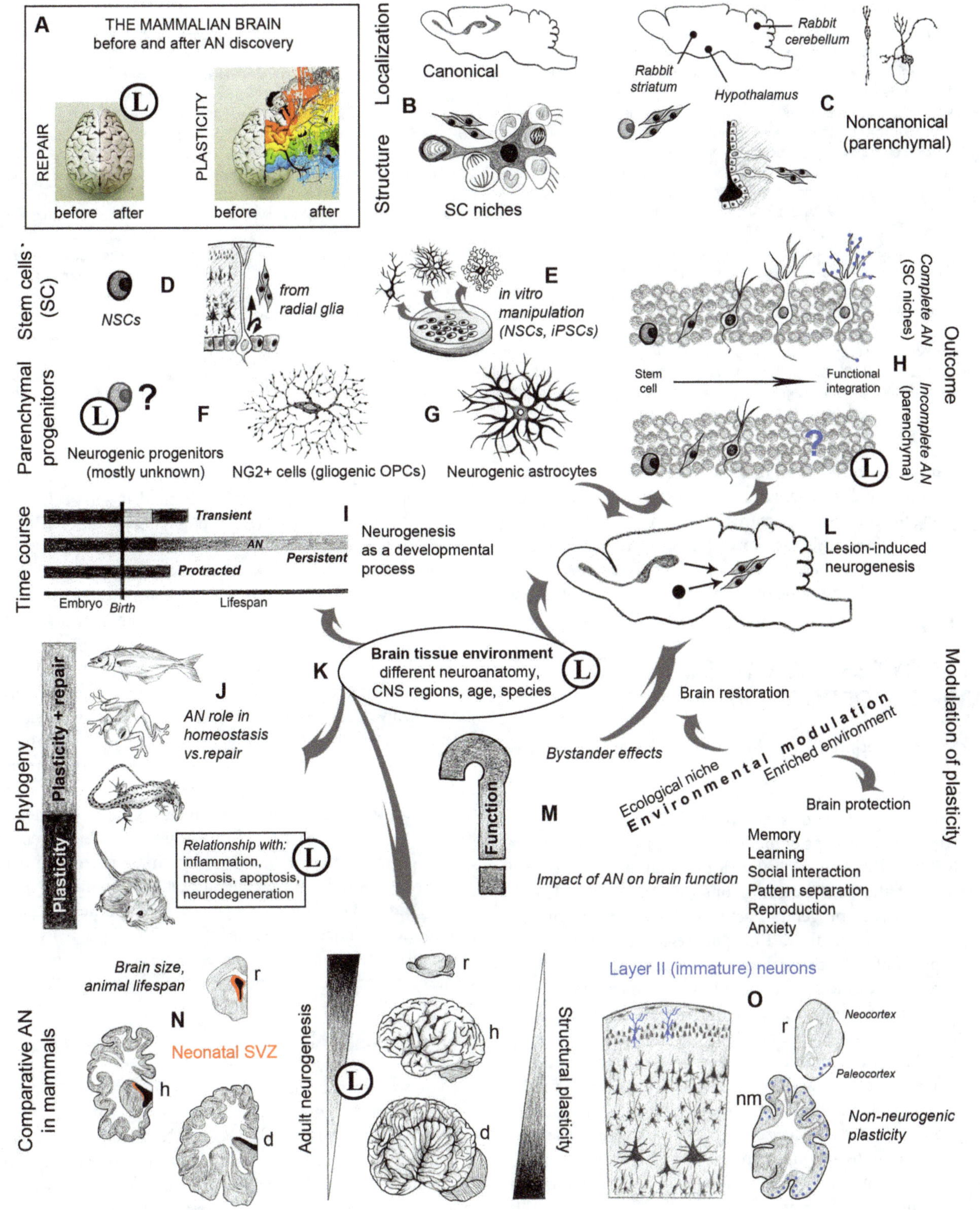

FIGURE 1 | Graphic representation of multifaceted aspects and new opportunities arisen in neurobiology by the study of adult neurogenesis (AN). Circled L indicate when substantial limits are also present. **(A)** An image originally referring to brain hemisphere asymmetry (http://thebiointernet.org/training-of-right-brain-hemisphere-and-intuitive-information-sight-in-bratislava/) is used here to represent the new vision of brain plasticity after AN discoveries; beside remarkable limits still existing in brain repair (pale pink), most opportunities involve new forms of structural plasticity with respect to the old dogma of a static brain (rainbow

(Continued)

FIGURE 1 | Continued
colors). **(B)** Canonical sites of AN, harboring well characterized stem cell niches (Tong and Alvarez-Buylla, 2014; Vadodaria and Gage, 2014). **(C)** Different types and locations of non-canonical neurogenesis do occur in various brain regions, depending on the species (Luzzati et al., 2006; Ponti et al., 2008; Feliciano et al., 2015). **(D)** NSCs are astrocytes originating from bipotent radial glia cells (Kriegstein and Alvarez-Buylla, 2009); **(E)** the occurrence of stem cells in the brain gives rise to (theoretically endless) in vitro manipulations. **(F)** Parenchymal progenitors are less known; most of them are gliogenic, yet some are responsible for species-specific/region-specific, non-canonical neurogenesis, and some others can be activated after lesion **(G)** (Nishiyama et al., 2009; Feliciano et al., 2015; Nato et al., 2015). **(H)** The outcome of canonical and non-canonical neurogenesis is different, only the former leading to functional integration of the newborn neurons (Bonfanti and Peretto, 2011); blue dots: synaptic contacts between the new neurons and the pre-existing neural circuits. **(I)** Strictly speaking, AN should be restricted to the continuous, "persistent" genesis of new neurons, which is different from "protracted" neurogenesis (delayed developmental processes, e.g., postnatal genesis of cerebellar granule cells, postnatal streams of neuroblasts directed to the cortex; Luzzati et al., 2003; Ponti et al., 2006, 2008), and "transient" genesis of neuronal populations within restricted temporal windows (e.g., striatal neurogenesis in guinea pig; Luzzati et al., 2014). **(L)** Reactive neurogenesis can be observed in different injury/disease states both as a cell mobilization from neurogenic sites and as a local activation of parenchymal progenitors (Arvidsson et al., 2002; Magnusson et al., 2014; Nato et al., 2015). **(J)** Evolutionary constraints have dramatically reduced the reparative role of AN, involving tissue reactions far more deleterious than in non-mammalian vertebrates (Weil et al., 2008; Bonfanti, 2011). **(K)** Failure in mammalian CNS repair/regeneration is likely linked to mature tissue environment, clearly refractory to new neuron integration outside the two canonical NSC niches and relative neural systems; this fact confines AN to physiological/homeostatic roles, which remain undefined in terms of "function." **(M)** The role of AN strictly depends on the animal species, evolutionary history and ecological niche; its rate and outcome is affected by different internal and external cues; although not being strictly a function, AN can impact several brain functions (Voss et al., 2013; Aimone et al., 2014; Amrein, 2015). **(N)** Different anatomy, physiology, and lifespan in mammals do affect AN rate and outcome; periventricular AN is highly reduced in large-brained mammals (Sanai et al., 2011; Paredes et al., 2015; Parolisi et al., 2015). **(O)** Studies on AN carried out by using markers of immaturity (e.g., DCX and PSA-NCAM) have revealed other forms of plasticity (non-neurogenic), being well represented in large-brained mammals (Gomez-Climent et al., 2008; Bonfanti and Nacher, 2012). r, rodents; h, humans; d, dolphins; nm, non-rodent mammals. Drawings by the Author.

are evident in brain evolution (interaction between evolutionary and developmental mechanisms to produce distributed and overlapping functional architectures in the brain)." That is to say: brain evolution is an ultimate expression of neuroplasticity, and more systematic information about evolutionary perspectives is needed to set out the question of the normal functionality of new neurons.

ASTROCYTES AND OTHER, WIDELY RAMIFIED, OPPORTUNITIES

The most counterintuitive discovery in half a century of AN research concerned the central role of astrocytes as primary progenitors for neuron production (Alvarez-Buylla et al., 2001). Across the years, new roles for these glial cells progressively emerged in different steps of the AN process, from maintenance of the NSC niche, through substrate for migration and functional integration of the newlyborn neurons (Sultan et al., 2015), to that of parenchymal progenitors activated by lesion (Magnusson et al., 2014; Nato et al., 2015). The regional and temporal heterogeneity of astrocytes should be among the big issues for future investigation of brain plasticity (Bayraktar et al., 2015), but this is only one example indicating how deeply different is our vision of brain structure and function before and after AN discovery. More recent breakthroughs concern the modulatory effects of lifestyle on AN (e.g., how exercise protects and restores the brain; Voss et al., 2013), and many emerging roles of the new neurons in impacting brain functions such as social interaction, reproduction, memory, learning, pattern separation, overgeneralization of sensory stimuli, and anxiety disorders (Leuner and Gould, 2010; Sahay et al., 2011; Feierstein, 2012; Kheirbek et al., 2012; **Figure 1M**). Furthermore, a vast range of "bystander effects" acting through paracrine or immunemodulatory mechanisms can exert beneficial effects by modifying the microenvironment at the injury site through the release of chemokines/cytokines (Martino et al., 2011; Kokaia et al., 2012; Pluchino and Cossetti, 2013). Other ramifications involve the big chapter of widespread gliogenesis (Nishiyama et al., 2009), whose effects are not limited to glial cell renewal, since bystander functions are also emerging for OPCs (Boda and Buffo, 2014; Birey et al., 2015). Yet, in the complex intermix of interactions involved in AN, most processes remain ill-defined as "ghost outcomes" of the stem cell activity (including the transient existence of the progeny), thus being worthwhile of further investigation.

Finally, unexpected trends are emerging from comparative studies showing how the spatial and temporal extent of AN dramatically decreases in large-brained, long-living species (e.g., humans and dolphins; Sanai et al., 2011; Parolisi et al., 2015; Patzke et al., 2015) with respect to small-brained, short-living rodents (Paredes et al., 2015; **Figure 1N**). The use of markers usually expressed in newly born neurons (e.g., doublecortin) led to reveal the existence of immature, non-newly generated cells (Gomez-Climent et al., 2008) which are more abundant in large-brained species (Luzzati et al., 2009; Bonfanti and Nacher, 2012; **Figure 1O**). This fact opens new hypothesis about the evolutionary choices in terms of structural plasticity among mammals, again underlining the importance of comparative studies (Lindsey and Tropepe, 2006; Bonfanti et al., 2011).

CONCLUSION

Even if we are still far from healing most brain lesions and neurodegenerative diseases, we have gained a fully new vision of brain plasticity (**Figure 1A**). In AN history, it seems that scientists have made serious sins in their approach. Yet, there are many reasons for forgiveness linked to the extremely innovative character of their work aimed at unraveling the dynamic nature of a brain tissue constrained within limits of invariability imposed by evolution. Five decades after the first demonstration of AN we still need to place it in the domain of basic research aimed at unraveling cellular, molecular, and evolutionary aspects of an extremely complex biological process. Maintaining a substantial independence from translational pressures (what implies hard work of teaching the values of fundamental research to grantmakers) could lead to higher achievements: the understanding of brain function and plasticity.

Looking back to its origin and forward to its future, the AN research field is maybe one of the best movies ever shot in the neurosciences, with passion and love for the unknown prevailing at the beginning of the story, then gradually shifting to magical realism toward the end.

AUTHOR CONTRIBUTIONS

The author confirms being the sole contributor of this work and approved it for publication.

ACKNOWLEDGMENTS

The author wishes to thank Barbara Finlay and Enrica Boda for helpful discussion, and Christopher Pullen for English revision.

REFERENCES

Abraham, W. C., and Robins, A. (2005). Memory retention - the synaptic stability versus plasticity dilemma. *Trends Neurosci.* 28, 73–78. doi: 10.1016/j.tins.2004.12.003

Aimone, J. B., Li, Y., Lee, S. W., Clemenson, G. D., Deng, W., and Gage, F. H. (2014). Regulation and function of adult neurogenesis: from genes to cognition. *Physiol. Rev.* 94, 1991–1026. doi: 10.1152/physrev.00004.2014

Akers, K. G., Martinez-Canabal, A., Restivo, L., Yiu, A. P., De Cristofaro, A., Hsiang, H. L., et al. (2014). Hippocampal neurogenesis regulates forgetting during adulthood and infancy. *Science* 344, 598–602. doi: 10.1126/science.1248903

Altman, J., and Das, G. D. (1965). Post-natal origin of microneurones in the rat brain. *Nature* 207, 953–956. doi: 10.1038/207953a0

Alvarez-Buylla, A., Garcia-Verdugo, J. M., and Tramontin, A. D. (2001). A unified hypothesis on the lineage of neural stem cells. *Nat. Rev. Neurosci.* 2, 287–293. doi: 10.1038/35067582

Amrein, I. (2015). Adult hippocampal neurogenesis in natural populations of mammals. *Cold Spring Harb. Perspect. Biol.* 7:a021295. doi: 10.1101/cshperspect.a021295

Amrein, I., and Lipp, H. P. (2009). Adult hippocampal neurogenesis of mammals: evolution and life history. *Biol. Lett.* 5, 141–144. doi: 10.1098/rsbl.2008.0511

Anderson, M. L., and Finlay, B. L. (2014). Allocating structure to function: the strong links between neuroplasticity and natural selection. *Front. Hum. Neurosci.* 7:918. doi: 10.3389/fnhum.2013.00918

Arlotta, P., and Hobert, O. (2015). Homeotic transformations of neuronal cell identities. *Trends Neurosci.* 38, 751–762. doi: 10.1016/j.tins.2015.10.005

Arvidsson, A., Collin, T., Kirik, D., Kokaia, Z., and Lindvall, O. (2002). Neuronal replacement from endogenous precursors in the adult brain after stroke. *Nat. Med.* 8, 963–970. doi: 10.1038/nm747

Barker, R. A., Drouin-Ouellet, J., and Parmar, M. (2015). Cell-based therapies for Parkinson disease-past insights and future perspectives. *Nat. Rev. Neurol.* 11, 492–503. doi: 10.1038/nrneurol.2015.123

Bayraktar, O. A., Fuentealba, L. C., Alvarez-Buylla, A., and Rowitch, D. H. (2015). Astrocyte development and heterogeneity. *Cold Spring Harb. Perspect. Biol.* 7:a020362. doi: 10.1101/cshperspect.a020362

Birey, F., Kloc, M., Chavali, M., Hussein, I., Wilson, M., Christoffel, D. J., et al. (2015). Genetic and stress-induced loss of NG2 glia triggers emergence of depressive-like behaviors through reduced secretion of FGF2. *Neuron* 88, 941–956. doi: 10.1016/j.neuron.2015.10.046

Boda, E., and Buffo, A. (2014). Beyond cell replacement: unresolved roles of NG2-expressing progenitors. *Front. Neurosci.* 8:122. doi: 10.3389/fnins.2014.00122

Bonfanti, L. (2011). From hydra regeneration to human brain structuralplasticity: a long trip through narrowing roads. *ScientificWorldJournal* 11, 1270–1299. doi: 10.1100/tsw.2011.113

Bonfanti, L., and Nacher, J. (2012). New scenarios for neuronal structural plasticity in non-neurogenic brain parenchyma: The case of cortical layer II immature neurons. *Prog. Neurobiol.* 98, 1–15. doi: 10.1016/j.pneurobio.2012.05.002

Bonfanti, L., and Peretto, P. (2011). Adult neurogenesis in mammals–a theme with many variations. *Eur. J. Neurosci.* 34, 930–950. doi: 10.1111/j.1460-9568.2011.07832.x

Bonfanti, L., Rossi, F., and Zupanc, G. K. (2011). Towards a comparative understanding of adult neurogenesis. *Eur. J. Neurosci.* 34, 845–846. doi: 10.1111/j.1460-9568.2011.07816.x

Dayer, A. G., Cleaver, K. M., Abouantoun, T., and Cameron, H. A. (2005). New GABAergic interneurons in the adult neocortex and striatum are generated from different precursors. *J. Cell Biol.* 168, 415–427. doi: 10.1083/jcb.200407053

Doetsch, F., Caille, I., Lim, D. A., Garcia-Verdugo, J. M., and Alvarez-Buylla, A. (1999). Subventricular zone astrocytes are neural stem cells in the adult mammalian brain. *Cell* 97, 703–716. doi: 10.1016/S0092-8674(00)80783-7

Feierstein, C. E. (2012). Linking adult olfactory neurogenesis to social behavior. *Front. Neurosci.* 6:173. doi: 10.3389/fnins.2012.00173

Feliciano, D. M., Bordey, A., and Bonfanti, L. (2015). Noncanonical sites of adult neurogenesis in the mammalian brain. *Cold Spring Harb. Perspect. Biol.* 7:a018846 doi: 10.1101/cshperspect.a018846

Franklin, R. J. (2002). Why does remyelination fail in multiple sclerosis? *Nat. Rev. Neurosci.* 3, 705–714. doi: 10.1038/nrn917

Gage, F. H. (2000). Mammalian neural stem cells. *Science* 287, 1433–1438. doi: 10.1126/science.287.5457.1433

Galli, R., Gritti, A., Bonfanti, L., and Vescovi, A. L. (2003). Neural stem cells: an overview. *Circ. Res.* 92, 598–608. doi: 10.1161/01.RES.0000065580.02404.F4

Gomez-Climent, M. A., Castillo-Gomez, E., Varea, E., Guirado, R., Blasco-Ibanez, J. M., Crespo, C., et al. (2008). A population of prenatallygenerated cells in the rat paleocortex maintains an immature neuronal phenotypeinto adulthood. *Cereb. Cortex* 18, 2229–2240. doi: 10.1093/cercor/bhm255

Gould, E., Reeves, A. J., Graziano, M. S., and Gross, C. G. (1999). Neurogenesis in the neocortex of adult primates. *Science* 286, 548–552. doi: 10.1126/science.286.5439.548

Gould, E., Vail, N., Wagers, M., and Gross, C. G. (2001). Adult-generated hippocampal and neocortical neurons in macaques have a transient existence. *Proc. Natl. Acad. Sci. U.S.A.* 98, 10910–10917. doi: 10.1073/pnas.181354698

Grandel, H., and Brand, M. (2013). Comparative aspects of adult neural stem cell activity in vertebrates. *Dev. Genes Evol.* 223, 131–147. doi: 10.1007/s00427-012-0425-5

Gross, C. G. (2000). Neurogenesis in the adult brain: death of a dogma. *Nat. Rev. Neurosci.* 1, 67–73. doi: 10.1038/35036235

Hersman, S., Rodriguez Barrera, V., and Fanselow, M. (2016). Assigning functions to adult-born neurons: a theoretical framework for characterizing neural manipulation of learning. *Front. Syst. Neurosci.* 9:182. doi: 10.3389/fnsys.2015.00182

Kheirbek, M. A., Klemenhagen, K. C., Sahay, A., and Hen, R. (2012). Neurogenesis and generalization: a new approach to stratify and treat anxiety disorders. *Nat. Neurosci.* 15, 1613–1620. doi: 10.1038/nn.3262

Kitamura, T., and Inokuchi, K. (2014). Role of adult neurogenesis in hippocampal-cortical memory consolidation. *Mol. Brain* 7:13. doi: 10.1186/1756-6606-7-13

Kokaia, Z., Martino, G., Schwartz, M., and Lindvall, O. (2012). Cross-talk between neural stem cells and immune cells: the key to better brain repair? *Nat. Neurosci.* 15, 1078–1087. doi: 10.1038/nn.3163

Kriegstein, A., and Alvarez-Buylla, A. (2009). The glial nature of embryonic and adult neural stem cells. *Annu. Rev. Neurosci.* 32, 149–184. doi: 10.1146/annurev.neuro.051508.135600

Kyritsis, N., Kizil, C., and Brand, M. (2014). Neuroinflammation and central nervous system regeneration in vertebrates. *Trends Cell Biol.* 24, 128–135. doi: 10.1016/j.tcb.2013.08.004

Leuner, B., and Gould, E. (2010). Structural plasticity and hippocampal function. *Annu. Rev. Psychol.* 61, 111–140. doi: 10.1146/annurev.psych.093008.100359

Li, L., Jiang, Q., Ding, G., Zhang, L., Zhang, Z. G., Li, Q., et al. (2010). Effects of administration route on migration and distribution of neural progenitor cells transplanted into rats with focal cerebral ischemia, an MRI study. *J. Cereb. Blood Flow Metab.* 30, 653–662. doi: 10.1038/jcbfm.2009.238

Lindsey, B. W., and Tropepe, V. (2006). A comparative framework for understanding the biological principles of adult neurogenesis. *Prog. Neurobiol.* 80, 281–307. doi: 10.1016/j.pneurobio.2006.11.007

Lindvall, O., and Kokaia, Z. (2015). Neurogenesis following stroke affecting the adult brain. *Cold Spring Harb. Perspect. Biol.* 7:a019034. doi: 10.1101/cshperspect.a019034

Lledo, P. M., Alonso, M., and Grubb, M. S. (2006). Adult neurogenesis and functional plasticity in neuronal circuits. *Nat. Rev. Neurosci.* 7, 179–193. doi: 10.1038/nrn1867

Lois, C., and Alvarez-Buylla, A. (1994). Long-distance neuronal migration in the adult mammalian brain. *Science* 264, 1145–1148. doi: 10.1126/science.81 78174

Luzzati, F., Bonfanti, L., Fasolo, A., and Peretto, P. (2009). DCX and PSA-NCAM expression identifies a population of neurons preferentially distributed in associative areas of different pallial derivatives and vertebrate species. *Cereb. Cortex* 19, 1028–1041. doi: 10.1093/cercor/bhn145

Luzzati, F., De Marchis, S., Fasolo, A., and Peretto, P. (2006). Neurogenesis in the caudate nucleus of the adult rabbit. *J. Neurosci.* 26, 609–621. doi: 10.1523/JNEUROSCI.4371-05.2006

Luzzati, F., Nato, G., Oboti, L., Vigna, E., Rolando, C., Armentano, M., et al. (2014). Quiescent neuronal progenitors are activated in the juvenile guinea pig lateral striatum and give rise to transient neurons. *Development* 141, 4065–4075. doi: 10.1242/dev.107987

Luzzati, F., Peretto, P., Aimar, P., Ponti, G., Fasolo, A., and Bonfanti, L. (2003). Glia-independent chains of neuroblasts through the subcortical parenchyma of the adult rabbit brain. *Proc. Natl. Acad. Sci. U.S.A.* 100, 13036–13041. doi: 10.1073/pnas.1735482100

Magavi, S. S., Leavitt, B. R., and Macklis, J. D. (2000). Induction of neurogenesis in the neocortex of adult mice. *Nature* 405, 951–955. doi: 10.1038/350 16083

Magnusson, J. P., Göritz, C., Tatarishvili, J., Dias, D. O., Smith, E. M. K., Lindvall, O. et al. (2014). A latent neurogenic program in astrocytes regulated by Notch signaling in the mouse. *Science* 346, 237–241. doi: 10.1126/science.346.62 06.237

Martino, G. V., Pluchino, S., Bonfanti, L., and Schwartz, M. (2011). Brain regeneration in physiology and pathology: the immune signature driving therapeutic plasticity of neural stem cells. *Phys. Rev.* 91, 1281–1304. doi: 10.1152/physrev.00032.2010

Migaud, M., Batailler, M., Segura, S., Duittoz, A., Franceschini, I., and Pillon, D. (2010). Emerging new sites for adult neurogenesis in the mammalian brain: a comparative study between the hypothalamus and the classical neurogenic zones. *Eur. J. Neurosci.* 32, 2042–2052. doi: 10.1111/j.1460-9568.2010.07521.x

Nacher, J., and Bonfanti, L. (2015). New neurons from old beliefs in the adult piriform cortex? *Front. Neuroanat.* 9:62. doi: 10.3389/fnana.2015.00062

Nakatomi, H., Kuriu, T., Okabe, S., Yamamoto, S., Hatano, O., Kawahara, N., et al. (2002). Regeneration of hippocampal pyramidal neurons after ischemic brain injury by recruitment of endogenous neural progenitors. *Cell* 110, 429–441. doi: 10.1016/S0092-8674(02)00862-0

Nato, G., Caramello, A., Trova, S., Avataneo, V., Rolando, C., Taylor, V., et al. (2015). Striatal astrocytes produce neuroblasts in an excitotoxic model of Huntington disease. *Development* 142, 840–845. doi: 10.1242/dev.116657

Nishiyama, A., Komitova, M., Suzuki, R., and Zhu, X. (2009). Polydendrocytes (NG2 cells): multifunctional cells with lineage plasticity. *Nat. Rev. Neurosci.* 10, 9–22. doi: 10.1038/nrn2495

Obernier, K., Tong, C. K., and Alvarez-Buylla, A. (2014). Restricted nature of adult neural stem cells: re-evaluation of their potential for brain repair. *Front. Neurosci.* 8:162. doi: 10.3389/fnins.2014.00162

Ohira, K., Furuta, T., Hioki, H., Nakamura, K. C., Kuramoto, E., Tanaka, Y., et al. (2010). Ischemia-induced neurogenesis of neocortical layer 1 progenitor cells. *Nat. Neurosci.* 13, 173–179. doi: 10.1038/nn.2473

Palmer, T. D., Takahashi, J., and Gage, F. H. (1997). The adult rat hippocampus contains primordial neural stem cells. *Mol. Cell. Neurosci.* 8, 389–404. doi: 10.1006/mcne.1996.0595

Paredes, M. F., Sorrells, S. F., Garcia-Verdugo, J. M., and Alvarez-Buylla, A. (2015). Brain sixe and limits to adult neurogenesis. *J. Comp. Neurol.* 524, 646–664. doi: 10.1002/cne.23896

Parolisi, R., Peruffo, A., Messina, S., Panin, M., Montelli, S., Giurisato, M., et al. (2015). Forebrain neuroanatomy of the neonatal and juvenile dolphin (*T. truncatus* & *S. coeruloalba*). *Front. Neuroanat.* 9:140. doi: 10.3389/fnana.2015.00140

Paton, J. A., and Nottebohm, F. (1984). Neurons generated in adult brain are recruited into functional circuits. *Science* 225, 1046–1048. doi: 10.1126/science.6474166

Patzke, N., Spocter, M. A., Karlsson, K. Æ., Bertelsen, M. F., Haagensen, M., Chawana, R., et al. (2015). In contrast to many other mammals, cetaceans have relatively small hippocampi that appear to lack adult neurogenesis. *Brain Struct. Funct.* 220, 361–383. doi: 10.1007/s00429-013-0660-1

Peretto, P., and Bonfanti, L. (2014). Major unsolved points in adult neurogenesis: doors open on a translational future? *Front. Neurosci.* 8:154. doi: 10.3389/fnins.2014.00154

Peretto, P., Giachino, C., Aimar, P., Fasolo, A., and Bonfanti, L. (2005). Chain formation and glial tube assembly in the shift from neonatal to adult subventricular zone of the rodent forebrain. *J. Comp. Neurol.* 487, 407–427.

Pluchino, S., and Cossetti, C. (2013). How stem cells speak with host immune cells in inflammatory brain diseases. *Glia* 61, 1379–1401. doi: 10.1002/glia.22500

Ponti, G., Aimar, P., and Bonfanti, L. (2006). Cellular composition and cytoarchitecture of the rabbit subventricular zone (SVZ) and its extensions in the forebrain. *J. Comp. Neurol.* 498, 491–507. doi: 10.1002/cne.21043

Ponti, G., Peretto, P., and Bonfanti, L. (2008). Genesis of neuronal and glial progenitors in the cerebellar cortex of peripuberal and adult rabbits. *PLoS ONE* 3:e2366. doi: 10.1371/journal.pone.0002366

Reynolds, B. A., and Weiss, S. (1992). Generation of neurons and astrocytes from isolated cells of the adult mammalian central nervous system. *Science* 255, 1707–1710. doi: 10.1126/science.1553558

Sahay, A., Wilson, D. A., and Hen, R. (2011). Pattern separation: a common function for new neurons in hippocampus and olfactory bulb. *Neuron* 70, 582–588. doi: 10.1016/j.neuron.2011.05.012

Sanai, N., Nguyen, T., Ihrie, R. A., Mirzadeh, Z., Tsai, H. H., Wong, M., et al. (2011). Corridors of migrating neurons in the human brain and their decline during infancy. *Nature* 478, 382–386. doi: 10.1038/nature10487

Shapiro, L. A., Ng, K. L., Kinyamu, R., Whitaker-Azmitia, P., Geisert, E. E., Blurton-Jones, M., et al. (2007). Origin, migration and fate of newly generated neurons in the adult rodent piriform cortex. *Brain Struct. Funct.* 212, 133–148. doi: 10.1007/s00429-007-0151-3

Sohur, U. S., Arlotta, P., and MacKlis, J. D. (2012). Developmental controls are re-expressed during induction of neurogenesis in the neocortex of young adult mice. *Front. Neurosci.* 6:12. doi: 10.3389/fnins.2012.00012

Sohur, U. S., Emsley, J. G., Mitchell, B. D., and MacKlis, J. D. (2006). Adult neurogenesis and repair of the adult CNS with neural progenitors, precursors, and stem cells. *Philos. Trans. R. Soc. Lond. B Biol. Sci.* 361, 1477–1497. doi: 10.1098/rstb.2006.1887

Sultan, S., Li, L., Moss, J., Petrelli, F., Casse, F., Gebara, E., et al. (2015). Synaptic integration of adult-born hippocampal neurons is locally controlled by astrocytes. *Neuron* 88, 1–16. doi: 10.1016/j.neuron.2015.10.037

Tang, G., Gudsnuk, K., Kuo, S.-H., Cotrina, M. L., Rosoklija, G., Sosunov, A., et al. (2014). Loss of mTOR-dependent macroautophagy causes autistic-like synaptic pruning deficits. *Neuron* 83, 1131–1143. doi: 10.1016/j.neuron.2014.07.040

Tong, C. K., and Alvarez-Buylla, A. (2014). SnapShot: adult neurogenesis in the V-SVZ. *Neuron* 81, 220–220. doi: 10.1016/j.neuron.2013.12.004

Vadodaria, K. C., and Gage, F. H. (2014). SnapShot: adult hippocampal neurogenesis. *Cell* 156, 1114–1114. doi: 10.1016/j.cell.2014.02.029

Voss, M. W., Vivar, C., Kramer, A. F., and van Praag, H. (2013). Bridging animal and human models of exercise-induced brain plasticity. *Trends Cogn. Sci.* 17, 525–544. doi: 10.1016/j.tics.2013.08.001

Weil, Z. M., Norman, G. J., DeVries, A. C., and Nelson, R. J. (2008). The injured nervous system: A Darwinian perspective. *Prog. Neurobiol.* 86, 48–59. doi: 10.1016/j.pneurobio.2008.06.001

Young, K. M., Psachoulia, K., Tripathi, R. B., Dunn, S.-J., Cossell, L., Attwell, D., et al. (2013). Oligodendrocyte dynamics in the healthy adult CNS: evidence for myelin remodeling. *Neuron* 77, 873–885. doi: 10.1016/j.neuron.2013.01.006

Zhao, M., Momma, S., Delfani, K., Carlen, M., Cassidy, R. M., Johansson, C. B., et al. (2003). Evidence for neurogenesis in the adult mammalian substantia nigra. *Proc. Natl. Acad. Sci. U.S.A.* 100, 7925–7930. doi: 10.1073/pnas.1131955100

17

Distinct Effects of Chronic Dopaminergic Stimulation on Hippocampal Neurogenesis and Striatal Doublecortin Expression in Adult Mice

Rachele Salvi[1†], *Tobias Steigleder*[2,3†], *Johannes C. M. Schlachetzki*[1,4], *Elisabeth Waldmann*[5], *Stefan Schwab*[2], *Beate Winner*[6], *Jürgen Winkler*[1*] and *Zacharias Kohl*[1*]

[1] Department of Molecular Neurology, Friedrich-Alexander University Erlangen-Nürnberg, Erlangen, Germany, [2] Department of Neurology, Friedrich-Alexander University Erlangen-Nürnberg, Erlangen, Germany, [3] Department of Palliative Medicine, Friedrich-Alexander University Erlangen-Nürnberg, Erlangen, Germany, [4] Department of Cellular and Molecular Medicine, University of California, San Diego, CA, USA, [5] Department of Medical Informatics, Biometry and Epidemiology, Friedrich-Alexander University Erlangen-Nürnberg, Erlangen, Germany, [6] IZKF Junior Research Group III and BMBF Research Group Neuroscience, Friedrich-Alexander University Erlangen-Nürnberg, Erlangen, Germany

Edited by:
José Luis Trejo,
Institute Cajal - CSIC, Spain

Reviewed by:
J. Martin Wojtowicz,
University of Toronto, Canada
Eric D. Laywell,
Florida State University, USA

***Correspondence:**
Jürgen Winkler
juergen.winkler@uk-erlangen.de;
Zacharias Kohl
zacharias.kohl@uk-erlangen.de

† These authors have contributed equally to this work.

While adult neurogenesis is considered to be restricted to the hippocampal dentate gyrus (DG) and the subventricular zone (SVZ), recent studies in humans and rodents provide evidence for newly generated neurons in regions generally considered as non-neurogenic, e.g., the striatum. Stimulating dopaminergic neurotransmission has the potential to enhance adult neurogenesis in the SVZ and the DG most likely via D_2/D_3 dopamine (DA) receptors. Here, we investigated the effect of two distinct preferential D_2/D_3 DA agonists, Pramipexole (PPX), and Ropinirole (ROP), on adult neurogenesis in the hippocampus and striatum of adult naïve mice. To determine newly generated cells in the DG incorporating 5-bromo-2′-deoxyuridine (BrdU) a proliferation paradigm was performed in which two BrdU injections (100 mg/kg) were applied intraperitoneally within 12 h after a 14-days-DA agonist treatment. Interestingly, PPX, but not ROP significantly enhanced the proliferation in the DG by 42% compared to phosphate buffered saline (PBS)-injected control mice. To analyze the proportion of newly generated cells differentiating into mature neurons, we quantified cells co-expressing BrdU and Neuronal Nuclei (NeuN) 32 days after the last of five BrdU injections (50 mg/kg) applied at the beginning of 14-days DA agonist or PBS administration. Again, PPX only enhanced neurogenesis in the DG significantly compared to ROP- and PBS-injected mice. Moreover, we explored the pro-neurogenic effect of both DA agonists in the striatum by quantifying neuroblasts expressing doublecortin (DCX) in the entire striatum, as well as in the dorsal and ventral sub-regions separately. We observed a significantly higher number of DCX^+ neuroblasts in the dorsal compared to the ventral sub-region of the striatum in PPX-injected mice. These results suggest that the stimulation of hippocampal and dorsal striatal neurogenesis may be up-regulated by PPX. The increased generation of neural cells, both in constitutively active and quiescent neurogenic niches, might be related to the proportional higher D_3 receptor affinity of PPX, non-dopaminergic effects of PPX, or altered motor behavior.

Keywords: adult neurogenesis, dentate gyrus, striatum, dopamine agonist, dopamine receptor, neuroblast, doublecortin, Parkinson's disease

INTRODUCTION

The generation of new neurons in the adult forebrain persists in the subgranular zone (SGZ) of the dentate gyrus (DG) and the subventricular zone (SVZ) of the lateral ventricles throughout the mammalian lifespan (Sanai et al., 2004; Ming and Song, 2005; Spalding et al., 2013), including non-human primates and humans (Eriksson et al., 1998; Ngwenya et al., 2006; Jabes et al., 2010; Spalding et al., 2013). Several extrinsic factors regulate proliferation and survival of neural precursor cells (NPCs) such as growth factors, hormones, and neurotransmitters in the "classical" constitutively active neurogenic niches (Brezun and Daszuta, 1999; Kulkarni et al., 2002). In this regard, the neurotransmitter dopamine (DA) plays a pivotal role (Winner et al., 2006; Berg et al., 2011) since dopaminergic fibers directly target hippocampal and SVZ NPCs (Hoglinger et al., 2004). Dopaminergic neurons in the midbrain, particularly from the substantia nigra pars compacta (SNc) and the ventral tegmental area (VTA) innervate the hippocampal formation, as well as the striatum (Bjorklund and Dunnett, 2007; Hoglinger et al., 2014). The SGZ is mainly targeted by dopaminergic projections of the caudal SNc (Hoglinger et al., 2004). In rodents, neurons of the SNc project toward the dorsal and lateral striatum in a topographically ordered medial-to-lateral arrangement forming the ascending nigrostriatal pathway (Perrone-Capano and Di Porzio, 2000). The previously defined non-neurogenic region, the striatum, possesses the ability to generate neuroblasts in response to cerebral ischemic stroke or traumatic injury and in corresponding animals models (Luzzati et al., 2011; Nato et al., 2015). Furthermore, striatal neurogenesis has also been observed in adult non-human primates, such as the squirrel monkey (Bedard et al., 2002). An indication for the generation of new neurons in the striatum also derives from a study in humans using a birth dating approach based on the incorporation of nuclear-bomb-test-derived ^{14}C in the DNA of proliferating cells. Strikingly, a postnatal turnover of cells was observed in the human striatum post-mortem (Ernst et al., 2014).

Adult hippocampal neurogenesis is severely impaired in neurodegenerative diseases, in particular Parkinson's disease (PD), the second most common neurodegenerative disorder (Maj et al., 1997). One of the well-known hallmarks in PD is the loss of dopaminergic neurons in the SNc with the consecutive reduction of dopaminergic projections to the DG and the striatum (Bernheimer et al., 1973; Hoglinger et al., 2004). Although, the current treatment in PD is mainly constituted by levodopa and/or DA agonists to alleviate the diminished dopaminergic tone within the striatum, a better understanding of the micro-environmental signals regulating the generation of NPCs will provide the possibility to regionally increase the neural pool in the hippocampal formation and possibly in quiescent neurogenic areas like the striatum. DA agonists act by binding to different subsets of postsynaptic DA receptors classified into two groups based on their intracellular signaling properties, the D_1- and the D_2-like family. D_1 and D_5 receptors, belonging to the D_1-like family, are coupled to G-proteins and thereby enhancing cyclic adenosine monophosphate (cAMP) levels, whereas D_2, D_3, and D_4 classified as D_2-like receptor, exert an opposite effect on cAMP resulting in decreased protein kinase A (PKA) activity (Missale et al., 1998). Pramipexole (PPX) is a D_2-like selective, non-ergolinic DA agonist with 5- to 7-fold higher affinity selectivity for the D_3 receptor compared to the D_2 receptor and minimal activity on the D_4 receptor (Mierau et al., 1995; Dooley and Markham, 1998). Ropinirole (ROP), another non-ergolinic DA agonist, has also a selectivity for D_2-like family receptors, but exhibit less specificity for the D_3 receptor in comparison to PPX (Tanaka et al., 2001). In rodents D_2-like family receptors are anatomically distributed in telencephalic regions receiving dopaminergic afferents from the VTA (A10), such as the hippocampus and the whole striatum as observed by *in situ* hybridization and by qPCR analysis of RNA extracted from hippocampal and striatal regions (Sokoloff et al., 1990; Bouthenet et al., 1991; Mu et al., 2011).

Several *in vivo* studies focused on dopaminergic stimulation of adult neurogenesis within the SVZ or the SGZ in rodents with dopaminergic lesions (Winner et al., 2006; Chiu et al., 2015). Initially, there was evidence that levodopa restores proliferation of NPCs within the SVZ after 6-hydroxydopamine (6-OHDA) lesioning (Hoglinger et al., 2004). Furthermore, the proliferation of NPCs was reduced in the SVZ of 6-OHDA-lesioned rats (Winner et al., 2006), and consequently, PPX administration induced the proliferation of NPCs in the SVZ of 6-OHDA lesioned rats (Winner et al., 2009). Recently, treatment of levodopa and PPX restored decreased neurogenesis in the DG and periglomerular layer of the olfactory bulb in mice with bilateral intra-nigral 6-OHDA lesions (Chiu et al., 2015). Since these studies were performed in lesioned animals only, we explored the effects of the DA agonists, PPX and ROP, frequently used for the treatment in PD patients, on adult neurogenesis in the hippocampal SGZ and striatum of adult naïve mice.

Abbreviations: 6-OHDA, 6-hydroxydopamine; BDNF, brain derived growth factor; BrdU, 5-bromo-2′-deoxyuridine; cAMP, cyclic adenosine monophosphate; d, days; DA, dopamine; DAB, 3,3′-diaminobenzidine; DCX, doublecortin; DG, dentate gyrus; D.Str., dorsal striatum; GCL, granule cell layer; GDNF, glial cell derived neurotrophic factor; HD, Huntington's disease; i.p., intraperitoneal; LED, levodopa equivalent dose; NA, not applicable; NeuN, neuronal nuclei; NPCs, neural precursor cells; PB, phosphate buffer; PBS, phosphate buffered saline; PD, Parkinson's disease; PFA, paraformaldehyde; PKA, protein kinase A; PPX, pramipexole; ROP, ropinirole; SEM, standard error of the mean; SGZ, subgranular zone; SNc, substantia nigra pars compacta; SVZ, subventricular zone; TBS, Tris-buffered saline; V.Str., ventral striatum; VTA, ventral tegmental area; wks, weeks.

MATERIALS AND METHODS

Animals

Naïve female C57BL/6 mice aged 3 months (obtained from Charles River Laboratories International, Inc.) were housed in a 12 h light/12 h dark cycle and had free access to food and water. All experiments were carried out in accordance with the European Communities Council Directive of November, 24th 1986 (86/609/ EEC) and were approved by the local governmental commission for animal health.

Experimental Design

Proliferation of NPCs and the survival of newly generated neurons in the DG were analyzed using three weight- and age-matched groups of animals [proliferation group: phosphate buffered saline (PBS), $n = 5$; PPX and ROP, $n = 6$; survival group: PBS, $n = 5$; PPX and ROP, $n = 7$]. For both designs, PPX, ROP, or PBS was administered by intraperitoneal injections (i.p., dissolved in 100 μl PBS) once per day for 14 consecutive days: animals received either PPX 0.3 mg/kg or ROP 3.0 mg/kg; the control animals were injected with 0.5% PBS only. The dose selection for PPX and ROP was based on previous studies where PPX treatment in a dose range between 0.1 and 1 mg/kg for up to 2 weeks was able to restore lesion-induced dopaminergic deficits in mice on a functional, biochemical, and structural level (Anderson et al., 2001; Jabes et al., 2010). Furthermore, ROP treatment for up to 1 week with doses between 0.5 and 3 mg/kg attenuated lesion-induced dopaminergic deficits in mice (Iida et al., 1999; Park et al., 2013). In addition, we referred to the levodopa equivalent dose (LED) representing an estimation of the DA agonist dose able to produce a similar antiparkinsonian effect as 100 mg of levodopa in humans. The standardized LED for PPX and ROP are 1 and 5 mg, respectively (Yamada et al., 1990). The 2-week treatment period with DA agonists was also based on previous studies reporting chronic DA agonist administration being more effective in enhancing adult neurogenesis than acute administration (Winner et al., 2009; Onoue et al., 2014; Takamura et al., 2014).

To label proliferating cells in the forebrain, 5-bromo-2′-deoxyuridine (BrdU) was injected i.p. twice on day 15 (100 mg/kg body weight; **Figure 2A**, proliferation paradigm). At day 15, animals were deeply anesthetized and transcardially perfused with 4% paraformaldehyde (PFA; Sigma) in 100 mM phosphate buffer (PB), pH 7.4. In order to detect the survival of newly generated cells in the DG, BrdU was administered once daily for the first 5 days (50 mg/kg, given in a volume of 100 μl) of the 14-days DA agonist treatment in a second cohort of mice, and after 2 weeks animals were perfused at day 37 (**Figure 3A**, survival paradigm).

Tissue Processing

Dissected brains were post-fixed in 4% PFA/PBS for 24 h, placed in a solution of 30% sucrose in PBS and cut into 40-μm coronal and sagittal sections using a sliding microtome (Leica, Germany) on dry ice. The sections were stored in cryoprotectant (ethylene glycol, glycerol, 0.1 M PB pH 7.4, 1:1:2 by volume) at −20°C until further processing for immunohistochemistry or -fluorescence.

Immunohistochemistry and -Fluorescence

Immunostainings were performed as previously described (Kohl et al., 2012). In order to detect BrdU, tissues were pre-treated with formamide and HCl in order to denature DNA. Free-floating sections in Tris-buffered saline (TBS; 0.15 M NaCl, 0.1 M Tris-HCl, pH 7.5) were treated with 0.6% H_2O_2 for 30 min. Following several washes in TBS, sections were blocked in 3% donkey serum and 0.1% Triton-X100 (Sigma) diluted in TBS for 1 h and incubated with primary antibodies in blocking solution overnight at 4°C. The primary antibodies used were monoclonal rat anti-BrdU (1:500, AbD Serotec, Oxford, UK), monoclonal mouse anti-Neuronal Nuclei (NeuN; 1:500, Millipore, Billerica, MA, USA), and polyclonal goat anti-DCX (1:250, Santa Cruz Biotechnology, CA, USA). For immunohistochemistry, tissues were treated with biotin-conjugated species-specific secondary antibodies followed by incubation with avidin-biotin-peroxidase complex (1:100) and 3, 3′-diaminobenzidine (DAB) substrate (both Vector Laboratories, Burlingame, CA, USA). For immunofluorescence, donkey-derived anti-mouse and anti-rat secondary antibodies were used conjugated with Alexa-568 and Alexa-488 or biotin (1:500, Dianova, Hamburg, Germany), respectively (all 1:1000, Invitrogen, Carlsbad, CA, USA). For all antibodies, control stainings without primary antibody showed no signal.

Counting Procedures

Slides were blind-coded and all counting procedures were performed on 40-μm sagittal sections. Every 6th section (240-μm interval) was selected and processed for immunohistochemistry. To analyze the number of $BrdU^+$ cells in the granule cell layer (GCL) of the DG, BrdU-labeled cells were exhaustively counted on each section excluding the uppermost focal plane (exclusion plane) and the obtained values multiplied by 6, as an estimation of the total number of $BrdU^+$ cells, both for the proliferation and survival paradigm (Williams and Rakic, 1988). All counting procedures and measurements of reference DG volumes (measured in mm^3) were conducted on a light/fluorescence microscope (Zeiss AxioImager M2, Göttingen, Germany) equipped with a semi-automatic stereology system (Stereoinvestigator, MicroBrightField, Colchester, VT, USA) as previously described (Kohl et al., 2012). The subsequent densities of $BrdU^+$ cells were calculated by dividing the number by the DG volume for each animal. To quantify the number of DCX^+ neuroblasts in the entire striatum and consequently in the dorsal and ventral sub-regions, we used sections at the following coordinates: interaural lateral 1.44 and 1.08 mm. By using this approach, the boundaries between the dorsal and ventral striatum are anatomically well-defined by the anterior commissure (see **Figure 1**, adopted from Franklin and Paxinos, 2013). The identical procedures as above described were applied for the assessment of DCX^+ cell numbers and striatal volumes. All bright-field images were obtained using the same microscope, as previously described.

To estimate the differentiation into a neuronal phenotype, every 12th section was stained for BrdU and NeuN by immunofluorescence and examined using a confocal laser microscope (ZEISS LSM780, Göttingen, Germany) equipped with a 40x PL APO oil objective and a pinhole setting that corresponds to a focal plane of 2 μm or less. In the DG, 40 to 50 $BrdU^+$ cells from each animal were analyzed, randomly selected, and examined by moving through the z-axis of each cell in order to exclude false double labeling. $BrdU^+$ cells were counted (newborn cells) and cells positive for both BrdU and NeuN ($BrdU^+/NeuN^+$ double-positive cells, newborn neurons) were assessed. The ratio of $BrdU^+/NeuN^+$ double positive cells by $BrdU^+$ cells was determined. Applying the ratio of

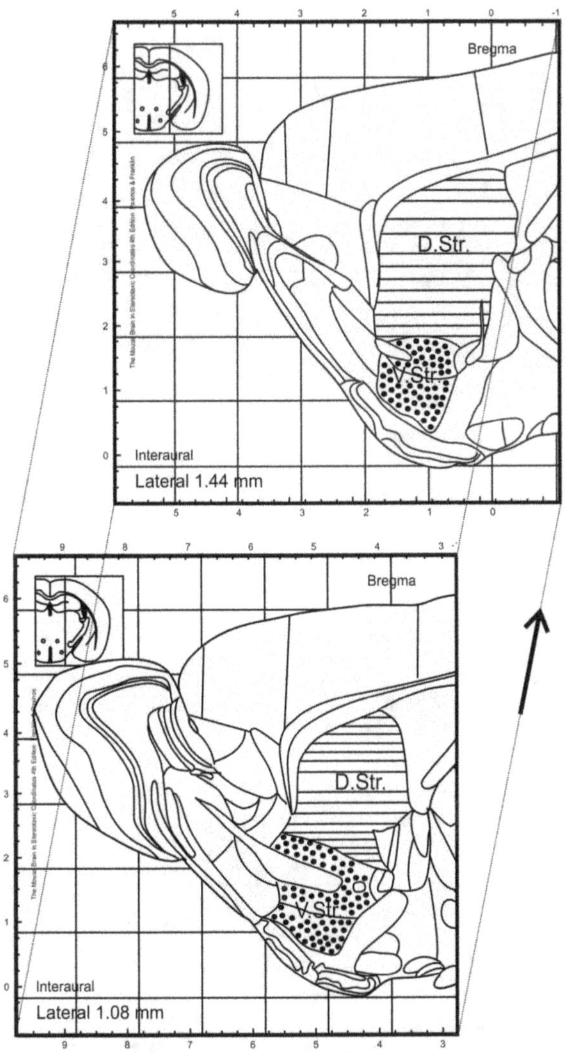

FIGURE 1 | Topographical map of sagittal sections of adult mice adopted from Franklin and Paxinos (2013). Regions analyzed within this study are marked and include the dorsal and ventral striatum. Sections analyzed between interaural lateral 1.44 and 1.08 mm. D.Str., dorsal striatum; V.Str., ventral striatum.

BrdU$^+$/NeuN$^+$ cells to the density of BrdU$^+$ cells the number of newborn neurons was calculated. Fluorescent images were obtained using the identical confocal laser microscope (40x APO objective).

Statistical Analysis

All values are expressed as mean ± standard error of the mean (SEM). Statistical analysis was performed using one-way ANOVA comparisons between treatment groups followed by Tukey's *post-hoc* analysis (Prism 5; GraphPad, San Diego, CA, USA). For the analysis of DCX$^+$ neuroblasts in the sub-regions of the striatum, we used a classical linear regression with a square root transformation of the dependent variable. Significance threshold was assumed at $p < 0.05$.

RESULTS

PPX, but Not ROP Administration Results in Increased Proliferation of NPCs in the Hippocampal DG

In order to investigate the effect of two different DA agonists on NPC proliferation in the adult DG, we compared the density of newborn cells between PPX-, ROP-, and PBS-injected animals. The groups were daily injected with PPX, ROP, or PBS for 14 days followed by two BrdU administrations at the same day prior to perfusion (**Figure 2A**). We quantified the number of BrdU$^+$ cells in the DG and calculated their density. PPX significantly increased the number of BrdU$^+$ cells compared to PBS-injected mice by 42% [PPX: 15421.3 ± 544.2, ROP: 12722.9 ± 129.4, PBS: 10864.2 ± 827.1, $F_{(2, 14)} = 17.65$, $p < 0.001$; **Figures 2B–D**; **Table 1**]. In contrast, there was no significant effect on the number of BrdU$^+$ cells after administration of ROP ($p > 0.05$; **Figures 2B,E**; **Table 1**). In addition, there was no effect of both DA agonists on the DG volume [PPX: 0.183 ± 0.01, ROP: 0.174 ± 0.01, PBS: 0.198 ± 0.02, $F_{(2, 14)} = 0.569, p > 0.05$].

PPX Doubles Adult Neurogenesis in the Murine DG

Next, we analyzed whether 14 days of administration with PPX or ROP has a pro-neurogenic effect by determining the survival of newborn neurons in the DG 32 days after the last BrdU injection (**Figures 3A,C–E**). Therefore, we quantified the density of surviving new DG cells and determined the number of cells colabelling BrdU$^+$ and the mature neuronal marker NeuN$^+$ in the DG. Interestingly, we observed that the percentage of NeuN/BrdU double-labeled cells was significantly increased in PPX-injected mice compared to ROP and PBS [PPX: 88% ± 0.99, ROP: 73% ± 1.25, PBS: 70% ± 0.93, $F_{(2, 16)} = 76.41$, $p < 0.05$]. However, there was no effect of ROP compared to PBS-injected mice. Calculating the density of newborn neurons (BrdU$^+$/NeuN$^+$), PPX significantly enhanced hippocampal neurogenesis by 91% in comparison with PBS-injected mice [PPX: 11468.0 ± 1254.0, ROP: 7369.0 ± 797.8, PBS: 6014.0 ± 928.2, $F_{(2, 16)} = 7.305$, PPX vs. PBS $p < 0.01$, PPX vs. ROP $p < 0.05$; **Figures 3B,F–H**; **Table 1**]. In contrast, the administration of ROP did not result in an increased number of new neurons compared to PBS-injected mice ($p > 0.05$; **Figure 3B**). Again, DG volumes were not different between groups [PPX: 0.152 ± 0.01, ROP: 0.151 ± 0.01, PBS: 0.150 ± 0.008, $F_{(2, 16)} = 0.008, p > 0.05$].

PPX Predominantly Promotes the Generation of DCX$^+$ Neuroblasts in the Dorsal Striatum

We further investigated whether chronic DA agonist treatment influences the number of neuroblasts within the striatum. We quantified the number of DCX$^+$ cells in the striatum of animals from the survival paradigm. We observed that PPX and ROP had no significant effect on the total number of neuroblasts in the entire striatum compared with PBS-treated mice [PPX: 257.1 ± 63.1, ROP: 157.7 ± 23.3, PBS: 134.4 ±

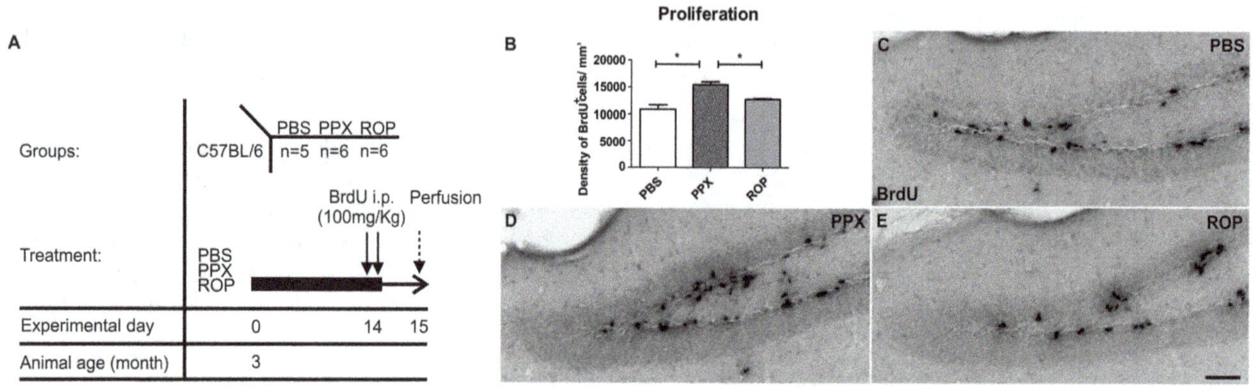

FIGURE 2 | Increased cell proliferation in the murine DG after chronic administration with PPX, but not after ROP treatment. (A) Proliferation paradigm. 3-month-old C57BL/6 received either i.p. PPX, ROP or PBS for 14 days. At day 14, animals were i.p. injected with BrdU (100 mg/kg) twice to label proliferating cells. Mice were perfused at day 15. **(B)** Quantification of BrdU$^+$ cells in the DG revealed an increased density of proliferating cells after PPX compared to ROP and PBS. Representative stainings of BrdU$^+$ cells in the DG of PBS- **(C)**, PPX- **(D)**, and ROP-injected animals **(E)**. Error bars represent mean ± SEM. One-way ANOVA followed by Tukey's *post-hoc* test, $^*p < 0.05$. Scale bar: 50 μm **(C–E)**.

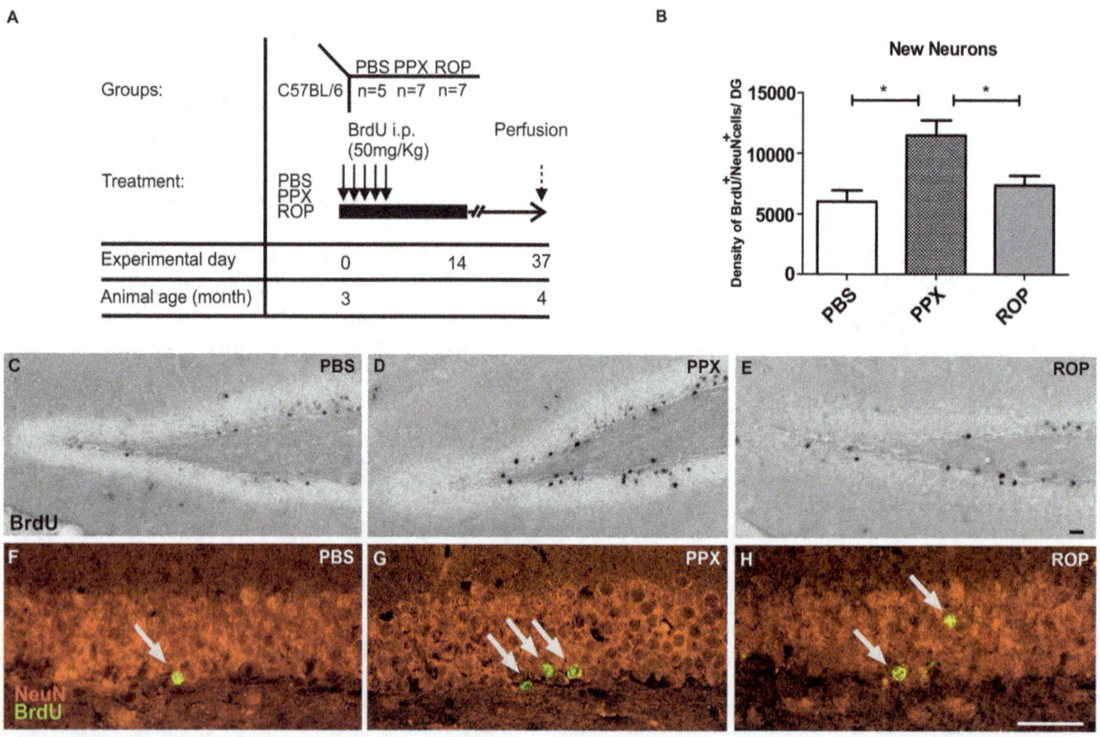

FIGURE 3 | PPX only increases the generation of new neurons in the murine DG. (A) Survival paradigm. At the beginning, 3-month-old animals received PPX, ROP or PBS i.p. for 14 days. During the first 5 days, all mice were i.p. injected with BrdU (50 mg/kg). Animals were perfused 32 days after the last BrdU injection. **(B)** Hippocampal neurogenesis (calculated density of BrdU$^+$/NeuN$^+$ neurons) was increased after PPX compared to PBS. No change in DG neurogenesis was observed after ROP treatment. Representative stainings of BrdU$^+$ in the DG of the hippocampus of PBS **(C)**, PPX **(D)**, and ROP **(E)** treated mice show a significant increase in PPX-injected animals compared to ROP- and PBS-injected controls. Confocal microscopy depicts double-labeled BrdU$^+$ (green)/NeuN$^+$ (red) neurons in the hippocampal DG of PBS **(F)**, PPX **(G)**, and ROP-injected mice **(H)**. Error bars represent mean ± SEM. One-way ANOVA followed by Tukey's *post-hoc* test, $^*p < 0.05$. Scale bars: 20 μm **(C–H)**.

13.9, $F_{(2, 16)} = 2.237$, $p > 0.05$; **Figures 4A–D**; **Table 1**]. To detect whether the dorsal striatum, being highly innervated by dopaminergic projections of the SNc, was affected by PPX or ROP administration to a greater extent in comparison to the ventral striatum, we analyzed the number of DCX$^+$ cells in both sub-regions separately (**Figure 1**). To analyse the impact of PPX and ROP simultaneously on the subregions (dorsal striatum, PPX: 185.1 ± 41.6, ROP: 104.6 ± 16.5, PBS: 103.2 ± 6.1; ventral

TABLE 1 | Summary of PPX and ROP treatment on hippocampal and striatal neurogenesis.

	PBS	PPX	ROP
Hippocampal neurogenesis			
Proliferation DG: density of BrdU$^+$ cells	10864.2 ± 827.1	15421.3 ± 544.2$^{\#\#\#,++}$	12722.9 ± 129.4
Newly generated neurons DG: density of BrdU$^+$/NeuN$^+$ cells	6014.0 ± 928.2	11468.0 ± 1254.0$^{\#\#,+}$	7369.0 ± 797.8
Striatal Neuroblasts			
DCX$^+$ cells overall	134.4 ± 13.9	257.1 ± 63.1	157.7 ± 23.3
DCX$^+$ dorsal striatum	103.2 ± 6.1	185.1 ± 41.6$^{\#}$	104.6 ± 16.5
DCX$^+$ ventral striatum	31.2 ± 10.5	72.0 ± 23.6	53.1 ± 24.1

PPX induced an increased number of dividing cells compared to ROP (by 21%) and PBS (by 42%) in the DG. A significant increased survival of newly generated neurons, identified by BrdU/NeuN co-labeling, was observed in the DG of PPX-injected mice in comparison to ROP (56%) and PBS (91%). PPX-injected mice showed a non-significant increase of DCX$^+$ neuroblasts in the entire striatum compared to PBS- or ROP-injected mice. Data is shown as mean ± SEM. Comparison between groups in the DG and the entire striatum was performed by one-way ANOVA followed by Tukey's post-hoc test and in the dorsal and ventral striatum by using a classical linear regression. BrdU, 5-bromo-2'-deoxyuridine; NeuN, neuronal nuclei, DCX: doublecortin.

$^{\#\#\#}$Significance level $p < 0.001$ compared to PBS; $^{\#\#}$Significance level $p < 0.01$ compared to PBS; $^{\#}$Significance level $p < 0.05$ compared to PBS; $^{++}$Significance level $p < 0.01$ compared to ROP; $^{+}$Significance level $p < 0.05$ compared to ROP.

striatum, PPX: 72.0 ± 23.6, ROP: 53.1 ± 24. 1, PBS: 31.2 ± 10.5; **Figure 4E**), we fit a linear regression model on the number of DCX$^+$ cells. To gain normality in the dependent variable a square root transformation was used. The effect of *region* was significant with a coefficient of −4.73 ($sd = 1.00$, $p < 0.001$, reference category: *dorsal*). In the categorical variable *treatment* (reference category: *PBS*) the effect of PPX was significant with a coefficient of 3.01 ($sd = 1.28$, $p = 0.0246$), while the effect of ROP was not significant with a coefficient of 0.606 ($sd = 1.28$, $p = 0.639$). The intercept of the model was 9.88. The volumes of the entire striatum did not differ significantly between groups [PPX: 3.065 ± 0.233, ROP: 2.788 ± 0.313, PBS: 2.962 ± 0.471, $F_{(2, 16)} = 0.201, p > 0.05$].

DISCUSSION

The chronic administration of the non-ergoline D_2/D_3-receptor agonist PPX is able to strongly stimulate cell proliferation as well as adult neurogenesis in the hippocampal DG of naive mice. In contrast, the D_2/D_3-receptor agonist ROP shows no pro-neurogenic effects, neither on cell proliferation nor on the survival of newly generated DG neurons. Moreover, PPX only resulted in an increased number of DCX$^+$ neuroblasts in the dorsal striatum suggesting a specific PPX mediated effect in the mouse forebrain, both for constitutively active and quiescent neurogenic niches.

While increasing experimental evidence supports the pro-neurogenic effect of dopaminergic compounds such as levodopa or DA agonists for enhancing adult neurogenesis in the SVZ (Van Kampen et al., 2004; Borta and Hoglinger, 2007; Winner et al., 2009) their role in stimulating adult hippocampal neurogenesis is rather limited. In the present study we observed that mice injected with PPX (0.3 mg/kg) over 14 days showed an increase of proliferating cells by 42% in the hippocampal DG compared to PBS-injected controls. In contrast, chronic ROP administration (3 mg/kg) failed to stimulate hippocampal cell proliferation. So far, two studies examined the effect of DA agonists on cell proliferation in the hippocampus in naïve rats: Onoue and colleagues described a reduction of proliferating BrdU$^+$ cells in the SGZ by 34% after administration of PPX for 14 days in Wistar rats using a higher dosage of PPX (1 mg/kg; Onoue et al., 2014; **Table 2**). Another study observed no changes in SGZ proliferation of Sprague Dawley rats following PPX administration for 21 days at two different dosages (0.3 or 1 mg/kg; Takamura et al., 2014). These apparent discrepancies between the present and previous studies in enhancing adult hippocampal neurogenesis after chronic PPX administration may be very likely explained by species differences related to distinct characteristics of the hippocampal neurogenic niche of mice and rats. Interestingly, there is a species difference in relation to the duration necessary for the maturation of new DG neurons (Snyder et al., 2009).

Besides analyzing the effect of PPX on the proliferation of hippocampal NPCs, the aim of this study was to determine whether these newly generated cells were able to differentiate toward a neuronal lineage. Here, we observed that PPX administration significantly enhanced the proportion of neuronal differentiation resulting in an increased density of newly generated neurons by 91% in the DG of adult naïve mice compared to PBS-injected controls. Again, ROP administration failed to enhance hippocampal neurogenesis. The present effect of PPX on the survival and differentiation of newly generated neurons in the DG is in contrast to the previous study by Takamura et al. in rats where PPX at two different dosages (0.3 and 1 mg/kg) failed to enhance the survival of newly generated cells (Takamura et al., 2014). However, the D3-receptor DA agonist SKF38393 increased the survival of newly generated cells by 53%, however without determining the cellular phenotype (Takamura et al., 2014). While the majority of previous findings are in contrast to the present study (see **Table 2**), it is very likely that in particular species differences may account for the divergent response to chronic DA agonist administration. This notion is supported by our previous study in 6-OHDA lesioned Sprague-Dawley rats, where chronic PPX administration was

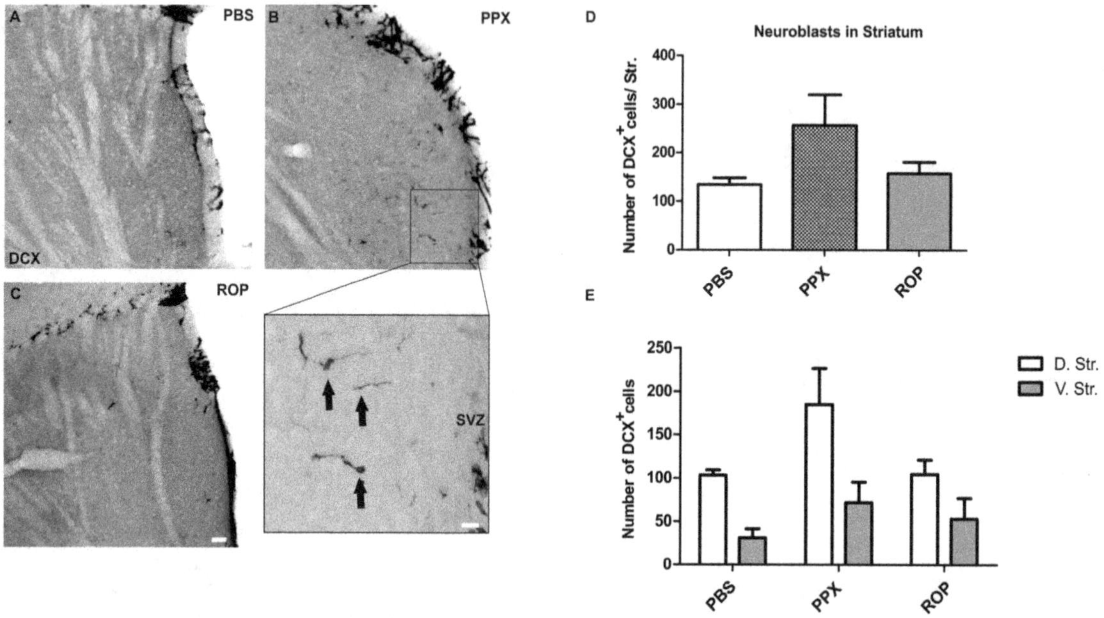

FIGURE 4 | PPX induces the generation of neuroblasts in the dorsal compared to the ventral striatum. Representative stainings of DCX^+ cells in the striatum showing a low number of neuroblasts in the PBS **(A)** and in the ROP group **(C)**, and a higher number in the PPX group **(B)**. Insert displays the region of interest with DCX^+ cells at higher magnification. **(D–E)** Quantification of DCX^+ neuroblasts in the entire striatum, and separately in the dorsal vs. ventral striatal sub-regions. No significant difference in the number of DCX^+ cells was observed in the entire striatum for all groups (One-way ANOVA followed by Tukey's *post-hoc* test). In contrast, the analysis of striatal sub-regions by using a linear regression model revealed a significant effect of PPX, but not with ROP treatment. Please note that the regression model was calculated based on the square root transformed numbers of DCX neuroblasts, whereas the untransformed numbers are displayed in **E**. Error bars represent mean ± SEM. Scale bars: 50 μm **(A–C)**, 10 μm (insert). D.Str, dorsal striatum; V.Str, ventral striatum.

TABLE 2 | Overview of studies addressing the effects of DA agonists on hippocampal neurogenesis in naïve rodents.

Study	Species/background, age, gender	BrdU dosage/paradigm	Treatment		Proliferation	Survival
Present study	C57BL/6 mice; 12 wks, female	2 × 100 mg/kg 24 h before perfusion or 5 × 50 mg/kg 32 d before perfusion	0.3 mg/kg PPX	14 d	1 d: 42% ⇑ (BrdU)	32 d: 91% ⇑ (BrdU/NeuN)
			3 mg/kg ROP	14 d	1 d: ⇔ (BrdU)	32 d: ⇔ (BrdU/NeuN)
Onoue et al., 2014	Wistar rat; male	4 × 75 mg/kg 6 h before perfusion	1 mg/kg PPX	14 d	1 d: ⇓ 34.2% (BrdU)	NA
Takamura et al., 2014	Sprague–Dawley rat; 7 wks, male	1 × 75 mg/kg 24 h before perfusion or 21 d before perfusion	0.3 or 1 mg/kg PPX	21 d	1 d: ⇔ (BrdU)	23 d: ⇔ (BrdU)
			10 or 30 mg/kg SKF38393	21 d	1d: ⇔ (BrdU)	23 d: 53% ⇑ (BrdU)

Values indicate the percentage increase or decrease of $BrdU^+$ and $BrdU^+/NeuN^+$ cells in the DG compared to the control groups of the respective studies. The age of the animals at the beginning of the experiments is given. ⇔; no effect vs. control, ⇑: increased effect vs. control; ⇓:: reduced effect vs. control. NA, not applicable, d, days, wks: weeks, BrdU, 5-bromo-2′-deoxyuridine; NeuN, neuronal nuclei.

not able to enhance adult neurogenesis in the hippocampal DG (Winner et al., 2009). In support of this striking species difference in regard to the response to dopaminergic stimuli, a very recent study showed that PPX administration rescued an impaired DG neurogenesis in 6-OHDA lesioned mice (Chiu et al., 2015).

PPX, but not ROP had a strong pro-neurogenic effect on adult hippocampal neurogenesis in mice although both compounds are D_2-like selective DA agonists. One possible explanation for the different efficacy between both DA agonists may be related to the distinct receptor binding profile of PPX with its proportional higher affinity to the D_3 receptor. In addition, the chosen dosage for ROP may be too low, although recovery of dopaminergic parameters after lesioning has been observed in the range of 0.5–2.0 mg/kg in mice (Iida et al., 1999; Park et al., 2013). Furthermore, Li and colleagues demonstrated that PPX administered both at a low (0.1 mg/kg) or high dosage (0.5 mg/kg) showed neuroprotective effects in a murine PD model with an impaired ubiquitin-proteasome system (Li et al., 2010). Interestingly, pretreatment with the D_3 receptor antagonist U99194 blocked the PPX-mediated neuroprotection implying a selectivity of PPX for the D_3 subtype (Li et al., 2010). However, there is also evidence for the selectivity of ROP for the D_3 subtype over human D_2 and D_4 receptors based on radio-ligand binding studies (Eden et al., 1991). Alternatively, the effect of DA agonists on proliferation and differentiation of hippocampal NPCs may be mediated by non-dopaminergic, pro-neurogenic mechanisms, e.g., the stimulation of distinct growth factors such as brain derived growth factor (BDNF) and glial cell derived neurotrophic factor (GDNF; Du et al., 2005), or altered physical activity (Yamada et al., 1990; Maj et al., 1997).

The recent discovery of adult neurogenesis in the human striatum and previously in the rodent striatum showed that the generation of new neurons takes place in regions generally considered as non-neurogenic (Bedard et al., 2002; Dayer et al., 2005; Ernst et al., 2014; Inta et al., 2015). In the present study, we addressed the question whether the DA agonists, PPX or ROP, promote the generation of DCX^+ neuroblasts in the striatum of naïve adult C57BL/6 mice. Indeed, we observed DCX^+ neuroblasts throughout the striatum possibly constituting an endogenous cellular pool with the potential to further differentiate into neurons under physiological conditions, in the context of a compromised striatal microenvironment or upon specific exogenous stimuli. Interestingly, the number of DCX^+ neuroblasts was significantly higher in the dorsal compared to the ventral sub-region of the striatum in the PPX group only. This dorsal-ventral gradient may reflect the fact that the dorsal striatum receives the majority of dopaminergic projections from the SNc (Haber, 2014).

Previously, a 10-fold increase in the number of $BrdU^+$ cells was observed in the dorsal striatum of adult Sprague-Dawley rats following the intraventricular administration of the D_3-receptor agonist 7-hydroxy-N,N-di-n-propyl-2-aminotetralin (Van Kampen et al., 2004). However, systemic treatment with PPX both in 6-OHDA and PBS medial forebrain bundle injected rats did not increase the number of DCX^+ neuroblasts in the dorsal striatum (Winner et al., 2009). At present, it is still an open question whether DCX^+ neuroblasts or newly generated neurons within the striatum evade from the adjacent SVZ or are locally generated from an endogenous progenitor pool within the striatal parenchyma. Interestingly and similar to the post-mortem analysis in humans, we observed an increased number of DCX^+ neuroblasts in the striatum adjacent to the SVZ in transgenic mouse and rat models of Huntington's disease (HD) suggesting that the damaged striatum may attract to some extent immature neuroblasts from the adjacent SVZ (Kohl et al., 2010; Kandasamy et al., 2015). However, it is important to note that the lesioned striatum in PD models even after stimulation with growth factors such as the epidermal growth factor or the fibroblast growth factor-2 failed to provide a sufficient stimulus for immature DCX^+ neuroblasts to obtain a mature neuronal phenotype (Winner et al., 2008). More recently, a long-lasting inflammatory response within the striatum after lesioning was observed and may explain the failure to differentiate into mature neurons (Schlachetzki et al., 2014). Taken together, this study provides evidence that species and the specific strain largely matter when investigating effects of the generation of new neurons in neurogenic and non-neurogenic regions following compound treatment.

AUTHOR CONTRIBUTIONS

RS and TS performed experiments, collected and analyzed data, interpreted results, and partially wrote the manuscript. EW performed statistical analyses and interpreted the data. JS and SS discussed and interpreted the data. BW conceived the study and planned experiments. JW and ZK conceived the study, planned experiments, interpreted the data and edited the entire manuscript.

ACKNOWLEDGMENTS

This study was supported by the Bavarian State Ministry of Education, Science and the Arts (ForIPS grant), the University Hospital Erlangen (IZKF grants E12 and N3), and the Deutsche Forschungsgemeinschaft (DFG grant INST 410/45-1 FUGG). The authors would like to thank Robert Aigner for excellent technical assistance and Dr. Kathrin Utz for helpful comments on the statistical analysis.

REFERENCES

Anderson, D. W., Neavin, T., Smith, J. A., and Schneider, J. S. (2001). Neuroprotective effects of pramipexole in young and aged MPTP-treated mice. *Brain Res.* 905, 44–53. doi: 10.1016/S0006-8993(01)02466-0

Bedard, A., Cossette, M., Levesque, M., and Parent, A. (2002). Proliferating cells can differentiate into neurons in the striatum of normal adult monkey. *Neurosci. Lett.* 328, 213–216. doi: 10.1016/S0304-3940(02)00530-X

Berg, D. A., Kirkham, M., Wang, H., Frisen, J., and Simon, A. (2011). Dopamine controls neurogenesis in the adult salamander midbrain in homeostasis and during regeneration of dopamine neurons. *Cell Stem Cell* 8, 426–433. doi: 10.1016/j.stem.2011.02.001

Bernheimer, H., Birkmayer, W., Hornykiewicz, O., Jellinger, K., and Seitelberger, F. (1973). Brain dopamine and the syndromes of Parkinson and Huntington. *Clinical, morphological and neurochemical correlations. J. Neurol. Sci.* 20, 415–455. doi: 10.1016/0022-510X(73)90175-5

Bjorklund, A., and Dunnett, S. B. (2007). Dopamine neuron systems in the brain: an update. *Trends Neurosci.* 30, 194–202. doi: 10.1016/j.tins.2007.03.006

Borta, A., and Hoglinger, G. U. (2007). Dopamine and adult neurogenesis. *J. Neurochem.* 100, 587–595. doi: 10.1111/j.1471-4159.2006.04241.x

Bouthenet, M. L., Souil, E., Martres, M. P., Sokoloff, P., Giros, B., and Schwartz, J. C. (1991). Localization of dopamine D3 receptor mRNA in the rat brain using *in situ* hybridization histochemistry: comparison with dopamine D2 receptor mRNA. *Brain Res.* 564, 203–219. doi: 10.1016/0006-8993(91)91456-B

Brezun, J. M., and Daszuta, A. (1999). Depletion in serotonin decreases neurogenesis in the dentate gyrus and the subventricular zone of adult rats. *Neuroscience* 89, 999–1002. doi: 10.1016/S0306-4522(98)00693-9

Chiu, W. H., Depboylu, C., Hermanns, G., Maurer, L., Windolph, A., Oertel, W. H., et al. (2015). Long-term treatment with L-DOPA or pramipexole affects adult neurogenesis and corresponding non-motor behavior in a mouse model of Parkinson's disease. *Neuropharmacology* 95, 367–376. doi: 10.1016/j.neuropharm.2015.03.020

Dayer, A. G., Cleaver, K. M., Abouantoun, T., and Cameron, H. A. (2005). New GABAergic interneurons in the adult neocortex and striatum are generated from different precursors. *J. Cell Biol.* 168, 415–427. doi: 10.1083/jcb.200407053

Dooley, M., and Markham, A. (1998). Pramipexole. a review of its use in the management of early and advanced Parkinson's disease. *Drugs Aging* 12, 495–514. doi: 10.2165/00002512-199812060-00007

Du, F., Li, R., Huang, Y., Li, X., and Le, W. (2005). Dopamine D3 receptor-preferring agonists induce neurotrophic effects on mesencephalic dopamine neurons. *Eur. J. Neurosci.* 22, 2422–2430. doi: 10.1111/j.1460-9568.2005.04438.x

Eden, R. J., Costall, B., Domeney, A. M., Gerrard, P. A., Harvey, C. A., Kelly, M. E., et al. (1991). Preclinical pharmacology of ropinirole (SK&F 101468-A) a novel dopamine D2 agonist. *Pharmacol. Biochem. Behav.* 38, 147–154. doi: 10.1016/0091-3057(91)90603-Y

Eriksson, P. S., Perfilieva, E., Bjork-Eriksson, T., Alborn, A. M., Nordborg, C., Peterson, D. A., et al. (1998). Neurogenesis in the adult human hippocampus. *Nat. Med.* 4, 1313–1317. doi: 10.1038/3305

Ernst, A., Alkass, K., Bernard, S., Salehpour, M., Perl, S., Tisdale, J., et al. (2014). Neurogenesis in the striatum of the adult human brain. *Cell* 156, 1072–1083. doi: 10.1016/j.cell.2014.01.044

Franklin, K. B., and Paxinos, G. (2013). *The Mouse Brain in Stereotaxic Coordinates, 4th Edn.* San Diego, CA: Elsevier.

Haber, S. N. (2014). The place of dopamine in the cortico-basal ganglia circuit. *Neuroscience* 282C, 248–257. doi: 10.1016/j.neuroscience.2014.10.008

Hoglinger, G. U., Arias-Carrion, O., Ipach, B., and Oertel, W. H. (2014). Origin of the dopaminergic innervation of adult neurogenic areas. *J. Comp. Neurol.* 522, 2336–2348. doi: 10.1002/cne.23537

Hoglinger, G. U., Rizk, P., Muriel, M. P., Duyckaerts, C., Oertel, W. H., Caille, I., et al. (2004). Dopamine depletion impairs precursor cell proliferation in Parkinson disease. *Nat. Neurosci.* 7, 726–735. doi: 10.1038/nn1265

Iida, M., Miyazaki, I., Tanaka, K., Kabuto, H., Iwata-Ichikawa, E., and Ogawa, N. (1999). Dopamine D2 receptor-mediated antioxidant and neuroprotective effects of ropinirole, a dopamine agonist. *Brain Res.* 838, 51–59. doi: 10.1016/S0006-8993(99)01688-1

Inta, D., Cameron, H. A., and Gass, P. (2015). New neurons in the adult striatum: from rodents to humans. *Trends Neurosci.* 38, 517–523. doi: 10.1016/j.tins.2015.07.005

Jabes, A., Lavenex, P. B., Amaral, D. G., and Lavenex, P. (2010). Quantitative analysis of postnatal neurogenesis and neuron number in the macaque monkey dentate gyrus. *Eur. J. Neurosci.* 31, 273–285. doi: 10.1111/j.1460-9568.2009.07061.x

Kandasamy, M., Rosskopf, M., Wagner, K., Klein, B., Couillard-Despres, S., Reitsamer, H. A., et al. (2015). Reduction in subventricular zone-derived olfactory bulb neurogenesis in a rat model of Huntington's disease is accompanied by striatal invasion of neuroblasts. *PLoS ONE* 10:e0116069. doi: 10.1371/journal.pone.0116069

Kohl, Z., Regensburger, M., Aigner, R., Kandasamy, M., Winner, B., Aigner, L., et al. (2010). Impaired adult olfactory bulb neurogenesis in the R6/2 mouse model of Huntington's disease. *BMC Neurosci.* 11:114. doi: 10.1186/1471-2202-11-114

Kohl, Z., Winner, B., Ubhi, K., Rockenstein, E., Mante, M., Munch, M., et al. (2012). Fluoxetine rescues impaired hippocampal neurogenesis in a transgenic A53T synuclein mouse model. *Eur. J. Neurosci.* 35, 10–19. doi: 10.1111/j.1460-9568.2011.07933.x

Kulkarni, V. A., Jha, S., and Vaidya, V. A. (2002). Depletion of norepinephrine decreases the proliferation, but does not influence the survival and differentiation, of granule cell progenitors in the adult rat hippocampus. *Eur. J. Neurosci.* 16, 2008–2012. doi: 10.1046/j.1460-9568.2002.02268.x

Li, C., Guo, Y., Xie, W., Li, X., Janokovic, J., and Le, W. (2010). Neuroprotection of pramipexole in UPS impairment induced animal model of Parkinson's disease. *Neurochem. Res.* 35, 1546–1556. doi: 10.1007/s11064-010-0214-3

Luzzati, F., De Marchis, S., Parlato, R., Gribaudo, S., Schutz, G., Fasolo, A., et al. (2011). New striatal neurons in a mouse model of progressive striatal degeneration are generated in both the subventricular zone and the striatal parenchyma. *PLoS ONE* 6:e25088. doi: 10.1371/journal.pone.0025088

Maj, J., Rogoz, Z., Skuza, G., and Kolodziejczyk, K. (1997). The behavioural effects of pramipexole, a novel dopamine receptor agonist. *Eur. J. Pharmacol.* 324, 31–37. doi: 10.1016/S0014-2999(97)00066-6

Mierau, J., Schneider, F. J., Ensinger, H. A., Chio, C. L., Lajiness, M. E., and Huff, R. M. (1995). Pramipexole binding and activation of cloned and expressed dopamine D2, D3 and D4 receptors. *Eur. J. Pharmacol.* 290, 29–36. doi: 10.1016/0922-4106(95)90013-6

Ming, G. L., and Song, H. (2005). Adult neurogenesis in the mammalian central nervous system. *Annu. Rev. Neurosci.* 28, 223–250. doi: 10.1146/annurev.neuro.28.051804.101459

Missale, C., Nash, S. R., Robinson, S. W., Jaber, M., and Caron, M. G. (1998). Dopamine receptors: from structure to function. *Physiol. Rev.* 78, 189–225.

Mu, Y., Zhao, C., and Gage, F. H. (2011). Dopaminergic modulation of cortical inputs during maturation of adult-born dentate granule cells. *J. Neurosci.* 31, 4113–4123. doi: 10.1523/JNEUROSCI.4913-10.2011

Nato, G., Caramello, A., Trova, S., Avataneo, V., Rolando, C., Taylor, V., et al. (2015). Striatal astrocytes produce neuroblasts in an excitotoxic model of Huntington's disease. *Development* 142, 840–845. doi: 10.1242/dev.116657

Ngwenya, L. B., Peters, A., and Rosene, D. L. (2006). Maturational sequence of newly generated neurons in the dentate gyrus of the young adult rhesus monkey. *J. Comp. Neurol.* 498, 204–216. doi: 10.1002/cne.21045

Onoue, Y., Kuwatsuka, K., Miyazaki, I., Asanuma, M., Kitamura, Y., and Sendo, T. (2014). Effects of bupropion and pramipexole on cell proliferation in the hippocampus of adrenocorticotropic hormone-treated rats. *Biol. Pharm. Bull.* 37, 327–330. doi: 10.1248/bpb.b13-00749

Park, G., Park, Y. J., Yang, H. O., and Oh, M. S. (2013). Ropinirole protects against 1-methyl-4-phenyl-1, 2, 3, 6-tetrahydropyridine (MPTP)-induced neurotoxicity in mice via anti-apoptotic mechanism. *Pharmacol. Biochem. Behav.* 104, 163–168. doi: 10.1016/j.pbb.2013.01.017

Perrone-Capano, C., and Di Porzio, U. (2000). Genetic and epigenetic control of midbrain dopaminergic neuron development. *Int. J. Dev. Biol.* 44, 679–687.

Sanai, N., Tramontin, A. D., Quinones-Hinojosa, A., Barbaro, N. M., Gupta, N., Kunwar, S., et al. (2004). Unique astrocyte ribbon in adult human brain contains neural stem cells but lacks chain migration. *Nature* 427, 740–744. doi: 10.1038/nature02301

Schlachetzki, J. C., Marxreiter, F., Regensburger, M., Kulinich, A., Winner, B., and Winkler, J. (2014). Increased tyrosine hydroxylase expression accompanied by glial changes within the non-lesioned hemisphere in the 6-hydroxydopamine model of Parkinson's disease. *Restor. Neurol. Neurosci.* 32, 447–462. doi: 10.3233/RNN-130371

Snyder, J. S., Choe, J. S., Clifford, M. A., Jeurling, S. I., Hurley, P., Brown, A., et al. (2009). Adult-born hippocampal neurons are more numerous, faster maturing, and more involved in behavior in rats than in mice. *J. Neurosci.* 29, 14484–14495. doi: 10.1523/JNEUROSCI.1768-09.2009

Sokoloff, P., Giros, B., Martres, M. P., Bouthenet, M. L., and Schwartz, J. C. (1990). Molecular cloning and characterization of a novel dopamine receptor (D3) as a target for neuroleptics. *Nature* 347, 146–151. doi: 10.1038/347146a0

Spalding, K. L., Bergmann, O., Alkass, K., Bernard, S., Salehpour, M., Huttner, H. B., et al. (2013). Dynamics of hippocampal neurogenesis in adult humans. *Cell* 153, 1219–1227. doi: 10.1016/j.cell.2013.05.002

Takamura, N., Nakagawa, S., Masuda, T., Boku, S., Kato, A., Song, N., et al. (2014). The effect of dopamine on adult hippocampal neurogenesis. *Prog. Neuropsychopharmacol. Biol. Psychiatry* 50, 116–124. doi: 10.1016/j.pnpbp.2013.12.011

Tanaka, K., Miyazaki, I., Fujita, N., Haque, M. E., Asanuma, M., and Ogawa, N. (2001). Molecular mechanism in activation of glutathione system by ropinirole, a selective dopamine D2 agonist. *Neurochem. Res.* 26, 31–36. doi: 10.1023/A:1007672414239

Van Kampen, J. M., Hagg, T., and Robertson, H. A. (2004). Induction of neurogenesis in the adult rat subventricular zone and neostriatum following dopamine D3 receptor stimulation. *Eur. J. Neurosci.* 19, 2377–2387. doi: 10.1111/j.0953-816X.2004.03342.x

Williams, R. W., and Rakic, P. (1988). Three-dimensional counting: an accurate and direct method to estimate numbers of cells in sectioned material. *J. Comp. Neurol.* 278, 344–352. doi: 10.1002/cne.902780305

Winner, B., Couillard-Despres, S., Geyer, M., Aigner, R., Bogdahn, U., Aigner, L., et al. (2008). Dopaminergic lesion enhances growth factor-induced striatal neuroblast migration. *J. Neuropathol. Exp. Neurol.* 67, 105–116. doi: 10.1097/nen.0b013e3181630cff

Winner, B., Desplats, P., Hagl, C., Klucken, J., Aigner, R., Ploetz, S., et al. (2009). Dopamine receptor activation promotes adult neurogenesis in an acute Parkinson model. *Exp. Neurol.* 219, 543–552. doi: 10.1016/j.expneurol.2009.07.013

Winner, B., Geyer, M., Couillard-Despres, S., Aigner, R., Bogdahn, U., Aigner, L., et al. (2006). Striatal deafferentation increases dopaminergic neurogenesis in the adult olfactory bulb. *Exp. Neurol.* 197, 113–121. doi: 10.1016/j.expneurol.2005.08.028

Yamada, K., Nagashima, M., Kimura, H., Matsumoto, S., and Furukawa, T. (1990). Possible involvement of differing classes of dopamine D-2 receptors in yawning and stereotypy in rats. *Psychopharmacology* 100, 141–144. doi: 10.1007/BF02244396

18

Sexual Behavior Increases Cell Proliferation in the Rostral Migratory Stream and Promotes the Differentiation of the New Cells into Neurons in the Accessory Olfactory Bulb of Female Rats

*Rebeca Corona [1], Socorro Retana-Márquez [2], Wendy Portillo [1] and Raúl G. Paredes [1]**

[1] Instituto de Neurobiología, Universidad Nacional Autónoma de México, Mexico, Mexico, [2] Departamento de Biología de la Reproducción, Universidad Autónoma Metropolitana-Iztapalapa, Mexico, Mexico

Edited by:
Laura López-Mascaraque, Instituto Cajal-Consejo Superior de Investigaciones Científicas, Spain

Reviewed by:
Luis Miguel Garcia-Segura, Consejo Superior de Investigaciones Científicas, Spain
Carmen Agustín-Pavón, Universitat Jaume I, Spain

***Correspondence:**
Raúl G. Paredes
rparedes@unam.mx

We have previously demonstrated, that 15 days after female rats pace the sexual interaction, there is an increase in the number of new cells that reach the granular cell layer (GrL) of the accessory olfactory bulb (AOB). The aim of the present study was to evaluate, if the first sexual experience in the female rat increases cell proliferation in the subventricular zone (SVZ) and the rostral migratory stream (RMS). We also tested if this behavior promotes the survival of the new cells that integrate into the main olfactory bulb (MOB) and AOB 45 days after the behavioral test. Sexually, naive female rats were injected with the DNA synthesis marker 5′-bromo-2′-deoxyuridine (BrdU) on the day of the behavioral test. They were randomly divided into the following groups: Female rats placed alone in the mating cage (1); Females exposed to amyl acetate odor [banana scent, (2)]; Females that could see, hear, and smell the male but physical contact was not possible [exposed to male, (3)]; Female rats that could pace the sexual interaction (4); and females that mated without the possibility of pacing the sexual interaction (5). Animals were sacrificed 2 days after the behavioral test (proliferation) or 45 days later (survival). Our results show that 2 days after females were exposed to banana scent or to the male, they had a higher number of cells in the SVZ. Females, that mated in pace and no-paced conditions had more new cells in the RMS. At 45 days, no significant differences were found in the number of new cells that survived in the MOB or in the AOB. However, mating increased the percentage of new cells, that differentiated into neurons in the GrL of the AOB. These new cells expressed c-Fos after a second sexual encounter just before the females were sacrificed. No significant differences in plasma levels of estradiol and progesterone were observed between groups. Our results indicate that the first sexual experience increases cell proliferation in the RMS and mating 45 days later enhances the number of new cells that differentiate into neurons in the AOB. These new neurons are activated by sexual stimulation.

Keywords: neurogenesis and sexual behavior, cell proliferation, cell survival, paced mating, olfactory bulbs

INTRODUCTION

Paced mating increases the probability of reproductive success and augments, the rewarding properties of mating. In pacing behavior, the female controls the sexual interaction by regulating the frequency and the temporal pattern of the stimuli received from the male, favoring long periods between each intromission, making the sexual interaction less intense and more efficient (Erskine, 1995; Paredes and Vazquez, 1999; Sugai et al., 2006; Corona and Paredes, 2012). Pacing promotes the acute secretion of luteinizing hormone (LH), prolactin (PRL), and extracellular dopamine in the nucleus accumbens and striatum (Erskine and Hanrahan, 1997). The vaginocervical stimulation received in paced mating increases PRL secretion raising the percentage of pregnant females in comparison to females that did not pace the sexual interaction (McClintock and Adler, 1978; McClintock and Anisko, 1982; Sugai et al., 2006). In female rats, olfactory cues are involved in mate selection as well as in the display and maintenance of the sexual interaction. There are two anatomically separated areas within the OB that process these sexually relevant cues: the main (MOB) and the accessory olfactory bulb (AOB) (Portillo and Paredes, 2004; Bagley et al., 2007). Both the MOB and the AOB continuously add new cells (interneurons) throughout life. Addition of the new interneurons (periglomerular and granular cells) is important for the normal function of the OB since they regulate the activity of projection neurons (mitral cells). Mitral cells process and send the olfactory signal to the rest of the olfactory circuit to control social and reproductive behaviors (Brennan, 2004). The new OB cells proliferate mainly in the lateral walls of the ventricles, the subventricular zone (SVZ), but also in the rostral migratory stream (RMS) (Alvarez-Buylla et al., 2002; Gritti et al., 2002). After the new cells are born, they migrate tangentially for about 2 weeks until reaching the OB and incorporating into their final location in the MOB and AOB. Regulation of the neurogenesis process is highly sensitive to internal and external changes, and since the OB is involved in controlling reproductive behaviors in most mammals, the relevance of the neurogenesis process in OB mediated behaviors is well documented (see Oboti et al., 2009; Nunez-Parra et al., 2011; Peretto et al., 2014). For example, in male hamsters the majority of new cells that incorporate into the MOB and AOB are activated in response to mating and a low percentage of them respond to estrous female odors or to the female presence without physical contact (Huang and Bittman, 2002), suggesting a possible role of the new cells in the processing of sexual related odors and sexual behavior. In female mice, where recognition of the sexual partner is essential for the display of sexual behavior and maintenance of pregnancy, the simple exposure to male pheromones increases proliferation in the SVZ and the number of new cells in the MOB (Mak et al., 2007), and in the AOB (Takahashi et al., 2009). It is well documented that in mice a recently mated female exposed to chemosignals from an unfamiliar male will undergo pregnancy block and will return to estrous, a phenomenon known as the Bruce effect (Bruce, 1959). In contrast, if the female is exposed to the same male she mated with, pregnancy will continue. Females treated with cytosine arabinose (Ara-C), an antimitotic drug that inhibits cell proliferation, show a high rate of pregnancy failure as if the treatment switched the effect from familiar odor to an unfamiliar one (Oboti et al., 2011), further suggesting that the new cells that reach the OB have an important role in reproductive behaviors. The changes during the reproductive cycle seem to be related to OB neurogenesis, since the induction of estrous promotes an increase in proliferation in the SVZ in the female prairie vole (Smith et al., 2001) and in the RMS of female rats (Díaz et al., 2009).

Results from our research group have shown that sexual behavior *per se* could also regulate OB neurogenesis. Sexually experienced male rats injected with the DNA synthesis marker 5′-Bromo-2′-deoxyuridine (BrdU) and allowed to copulate the same day, showed 15 days later an increase in the number of new cells in the granular cell layer (GrL) of the AOB only when males regulate the pattern of copulation and ejaculated one or 3 times (Portillo et al., 2012). In female rats, one paced sexual encounter significantly increased the incorporation of new cells into the GrL of the AOB 15 days after mating (Corona et al., 2011). If the stimulus is repeated, that is, if the females experienced additional paced mating once weekly for 3 consecutive weeks the number of new cells incorporated into the GrL of the AOB is further increased. Moreover, these females also showed a higher incorporation of new cells into the MOB (Arzate et al., 2013). Together, these findings suggest, that paced mating promotes clear changes in OB neurogenesis in a short time interval (15 days). However, it is not known if the presence of these new cells in the AOB could result from increased cell proliferation in the SVZ and RMS. We also need to determine if the increase in the new cells is maintained after 15 days and if the new cells actually survive and integrate into the OB circuits. In order to address these possibilities we evaluated cell proliferation in the SVZ and RMS (two days after mating) and cell survival in the OB 45 days after the first sexual encounter in female rats. We also tested the participation of the new cells in sexual behavior by evaluating the immediate early gene expression (c-Fos) after a sexual interaction. We hypothesized that cell proliferation and survival would be increased in those female rats that paced the sexual interaction, and that the new cells that survived would be activated by sexual behavior.

MATERIALS AND METHODS

To examine the effects of sexual behavior on cell proliferation in the SVZ and RMS and on cell survival in the MOB and AOB we compared females that were allowed to pace (paced) and females that could not pace (non-paced) the sexual interaction. We also included two olfactory stimuli: females that were exposed to a sexually experienced male (without physical contact) and females exposed to amyl acetate (banana scent). An additional group of females was placed alone in the mating cage.

Animals

Seventy female rats (Wistar), bred in a local colony at the Instituto de Neurobiologia, Universidad Nacional Autónoma de México were used. They weighed between 230–270 g and were bilaterally ovariectomized (ovx) under deep anesthesia (30% xylazine—70% ketamine; Procin, PiSA A099884, and Cheminova KTCHH11L05, respectively). They were allowed to recover from surgery for 1 week before the experiments began. Forty sexually experienced male rats (300–350 g) of the same strain were used for the behavioral tests. Females were housed in a room without males, with controlled temperature (25 ± 1°C) and humidity and under a reverse light-dark cycle (12 h:12 h). They received tap water and food *ad libitum* (Lab Diet Feed PMI, USA). All behavioral tests were performed during the dark phase of the light-dark cycle, under red dim illumination. Experiments were carried out in accordance with the "Reglamento de la Ley General de Salud en Materia de Investigación para la Salud" of the Mexican Health Ministry that follows NIH guidelines for the use and care of animals and approved by the Instituto de Neurobiologia animal care committee.

Hormonal Treatment

To induce sexual receptivity in the experimental females, they were subcutaneously injected (sc) with estradiol benzoate (EB, 25 μg/rat; Sigma Aldrich, E-8515) 48 h and with progesterone (P, 1 mg/rat; Sigma Aldrich, P0130-25G) 4 h before the behavioral test (**Figure 1A**).

Hormonal Levels Measurement

In experiment 2, 45 days after BrdU administration ovx females were treated with EB and P and tested according to their corresponding group. At the end of testing, they were anesthetized whit pentoparbital and the blood samples were obtained by cardiac puncture. Plasma levels of estrogen (E2) and progesterone (P) were determined using ELISA (enzyme-linked immunosorbent assay; Diagnostica Internacional Foster City, California, USA). We followed the procedure previously reported (Arzate et al., 2013). Briefly, 25 μl samples of standards or plasma from control and experimental animals were placed in a 96-well microtiter plates; hormone-horseradish per-oxidase conjugated to E2 or P and either rabbit anti-E2 or anti-P, respectively were added and incubated. The microwells were rinsed and incubated with 3,3′,5,5′-tetramethylbenzidine reagent and finally with 1N HCl to stop the reaction. The absorbance was read at 450 nm in an automatic ELISA Microplate Reader (Bio-Rad Hercules, CA, USA). The inter-assay and intra-assay coefficients of variation were: for E2 18.82 and 9.35%, and for P 16.02 and 7.91%, respectively (Tietz, 1995; Pettit et al., 2012).

Experimental Procedure

In order to evaluate the effect of female sexual behavior on OB neurogenesis, we designed two experiments. In experiment 1 (cell

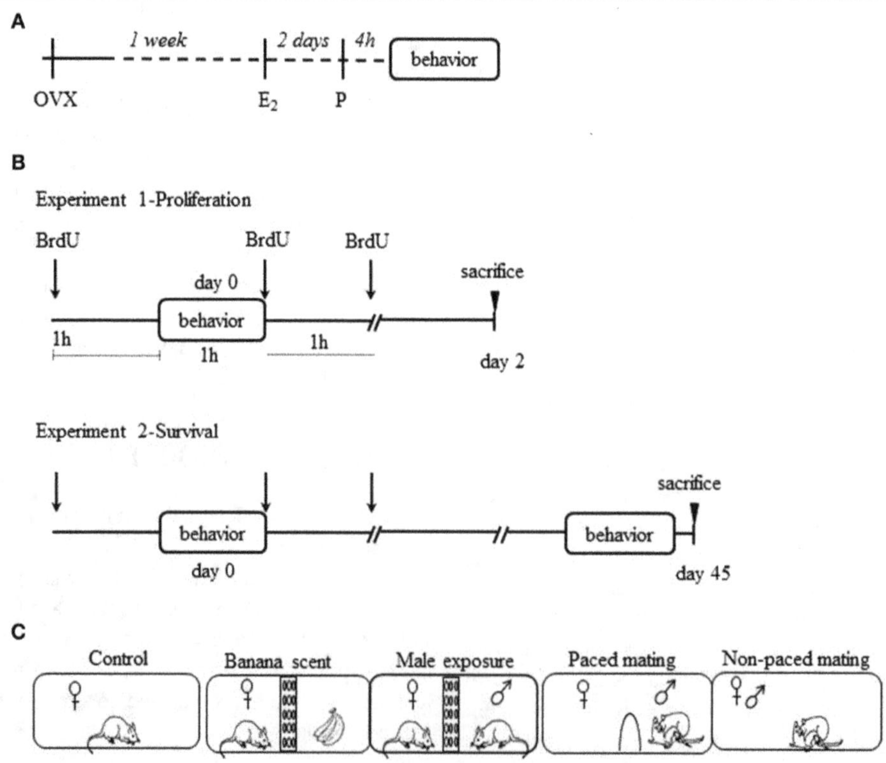

FIGURE 1 | Experimental Procedure. (A) ovariectomized (ovx) females were treated with estradiol benzoate (E_2) and progesterone (P) to induce sexual receptivity. **(B)** Ovx females were injected with 5′-bromo-2′-deoxyuridine (BrdU) three times: 1 h before the behavioral test, immediately after the test and 1 h after the test. They were sacrificed 2 days later for the proliferation experiment and the other groups were sacrificed 45 days later for the survival experiment. **(C)** Schematic representation of the experimental groups.

proliferation) 35 females of the different groups were sacrificed 2 days after the behavioral tests and cellular proliferation was evaluated in the SVZ and the RMS (**Figure 1B**). In experiment 2 (cell survival) 35 females of the different groups were sacrificed 45 days after the behavioral tests (**Figure 1B**). Cell survival, percentage of new cells that differentiated into neurons, and new cells activated after mating (as evaluated by Fos expression) were quantified in the AOB and MOB. The groups and behavioral tests were identical in both experiments. The behavioral tests lasted 1 h and were performed in odorless acrylic cages (62 × 29 × 42 cm) with fresh sawdust covering the floor. Sexually naive females were randomly distributed in the following groups (n = 7 per group): (1) Control, females were gently placed in the mating cages, without sexual or olfactory stimulation; (2) Females exposed to amyl acetate (banana scent), subjects were placed in a cage divided in two equal compartments by an acrylic screen with small holes (1 cm diameter). A container fixed to the wall of the screen contained a filter paper moistened with 10 μl of a 10% solution of amyl acetate (Sigma Aldrich, W50400-9); (3) Exposed to male, females were placed in a cage as for group 2, but instead of the container with the banana scent a sexually experienced male was placed in the opposite compartment. In this way females were able to hear, see and smell the active male, but no physical contact was possible; (4) Paced mating, females in this group were allowed to mate pacing the sexual interaction. The tests were performed in the mating cage divided in two equal compartments by an acrylic screen. In the bottom of the screen there was a hole (7 × 4 cm), that allowed the female, but not the male, to go back and forth from the compartment where the male was placed. The hole was too small for the male to go through and in this way the female controlled the rate of the sexual stimulation; (5) Non-paced mating, females in this group mated with a sexually active male without the barrier; in this condition females were not able to pace the sexual interaction (**Figure 1C**). For experiment 1, females were left in their home cage for the next 2 days. For experiment 2 females were housed with other females of the same group (3 or 4 females per cage) for 45 days. On day 45 they were tested 1 h for sexual behavior with the same male they had mated before and 30 min later they were sacrificed in order to evaluate the activation of the new cells after mating. Females were placed in a separate room with reduce noise, they were gently anesthetized to minimize unspecific c-fos activation.

Behavioral Measures

The lordosis quotient (LQ) was used as a measure of sexual receptivity, and was calculated as the total number of lordosis responses divided by the number of mounts multiplied by 100. Lordosis responses were scored from 0 to 2 as follows: 0 no lordosis displayed; 1 Slight flexion of the back, 2 flexion of the back, head and tail. Lordosis intensity (LI) was calculated as the sum of lordosis score divided by the number of mounts received from the male (Hardy and DeBold, 1972). The number and latencies of mounts, intromissions and ejaculations, and the inter-intromission interval (III) were also recorded. In the paced mating group, the percentage of exits after a mount, intromission, and ejaculation and the return latencies after a mount, intromission, and ejaculation were also recorded.

Cell Proliferation and Survival Detection by Brdu (5′-Bromo-2′Deoxyuridine)

BrdU is broadly used to label new born cells, and is an indicator of DNA synthesis (Shingo et al., 2003; Ming and Song, 2005, 2011). BrdU (Sigma Aldrich, B5002-5G) was administrated three times (each 100 mg/kg in 0.9% NaCl for a total dose of 300 mg/kg): 1 h before the test, immediately after the behavioral test and 1 h after the test (**Figure 1B**).

Brain-Tissue Preparation

At the end of each experiment, proliferation (2 days) and survival (45 days) the brain tissue was obtained. All the females received a lethal dose of sodium pentobarbital (100 mg/kg, Cheminova). They were intracardially perfused with 0.1 M phosphate-buffered solution (PBS, pH 7.4) followed by 4% paraformaldehyde (Sigma Aldrich, P-6148) in 0.1 M PBS. The brains were removed and post-fixed in 4% paraformaldehyde for 1 h before they were placed in 30% sucrose for cryoprotection. The right hemisphere of all the subjects was sliced in the sagittal plane at 30 μm intervals using a microtome (Leica, SM2000R) obtaining serial sections. Only this hemisphere was used because there are no significant differences in cell proliferation in the SVZ, RMS and RMS-OB, between the two brain hemispheres (Díaz et al., 2009). Five sections containing the SVZ and RMS were selected for the proliferation experiment and five slices with the AOB and MOB for the survival experiment and processed for immunohistochemical labeling. To analyse cell proliferation we used BrdU-labeling, and BrdU/DCX labeling to identify the cells committed to the neuronal phenotype. BrdU/NeuN labeling was used to identify the mature neuronal phenotype of the new cells, and BrdU/cFos to evaluate the activation of the new cells.

Immunohistochemistry

Protocol for BrdU Labeling with Peroxidase

Brain slices were processed for floating immunohistochemistry as previously reported (Corona et al., 2011; Portillo et al., 2012; Arzate et al., 2013). Briefly, tissue samples were repeatedly washed in buffer phosphates (Tris hydrochloride, Tris base, and Sodium chloride; J.T Baker) and incubated in 0.5% sodium borohydride (Sigma Aldrich, 452882). Later, the slices were incubated in 1% Triton X-100 (J. T Baker, X198-07), 1% H_2O2 (J. T Baker, 2189-01), and 1% DMSO (Dimethyl sulfoxide, J. T Baker, 9224-01) solution. Then, cells were incubated with 2N HCl at 36°C for 1 h (J. T Baker, 5616-02). Non-specific epitopes were blocked with 0.1% bovine albumin (Sigma Aldrich A-91418) and 0.3% Triton X-100. Tissues were incubated with primary antibody against BrdU for 48 h at 4°C then washed and incubated for 2 h at room temperature with the secondary antibody diluted in 0.32% Triton X-100 and 0.1% bovine albumin. Brain sections were then rinsed and incubated in Avidin Biotin Complex (AB elite kit; Vector Laboratories, PK-6100) for 90 min at room temperature. Brain sections were rinsed and revealed with the chromogen solution nickel chloride-3,3'-diaminobenzidine

(DAB; Vector Laboratories, D5637) and H_2O_2. Finally, the reaction was stopped by washing the slices in buffer solution. The brain slices were mounted onto gelatin-coated slides and cover slipped using permount (Fisher, SP 15-500; see list of antibodies, **Table 1**).

Protocol for Double Labeling with Fluorescence

Bran slices were incubated with one of the primary antibodies (BrdU, DCX, NeuN, cFos) for 48 h at 4°C in albumin (0.1%) and Triton X-100 (0.32%). The tissues were washed in TBS containing 0.02% Triton X-100 and 1 % albumin to remove primary antibodies and then were incubated with both secondary fluorescent antibodies for 2 h (**Table 1**). After the incubation, the samples were rinsed with Triton X-100 (0.02%) in TBS followed by TBS, the brain slices were then mounted onto slides and covered with aqua poly/mount (Polysciences, Inc, 18606).

Quantification of the Cells

Images of the five sections of each subject were taken at 10X magnification with a light microscope (Olympus BX60F-3) connected to a motorized slide (Prior ProScan) and the number of BrdU positive cells was counted using the Image Pro software 6.1. During this process, the researcher was blind to the group being analyzed. Reconstructions of these images were used to quantify the BrdU-labeled cells localized in the SVZ, the RMS, the MOB and the AOB (**Figure 2**).

For experiment 1 (proliferation), the quantification was performed throughout the SVZ and the RMS. Evidence shows that the new OB cells are born in different regions of the SVZ and the RMS (Lois and Alvarez-Buylla, 1993, 1994; Carani et al., 1999; Alonso et al., 2008), therefore we divided the SVZ into dorsal, anterior-medial, ventral, and anterior regions, and the RMS into posterior, medial and anterior regions (**Figure 2**). Each zone was defined as an area of interest (AOI) with a known area surface and BrdU-labeled cells within its limits were counted. Data are expressed as the number of cells per mm^2.

For experiment 2, quantification was performed in the glomerular (GlL) and GrL of the MOB and AOB. For the MOB, three circular AOI's (400 μm diameter) were placed in the apical zone of the GlL and GrL. The AOB, was subdivided into the anterior and posterior regions based on the different functions suggested for them (Martínez-Marcos and Halpern, 1999). Three circular AOI's (200 μm diameter) were placed on the anterior or posterior portion of the GlL and GrL. Five brain sections containing both the MOB and the AOB were counted per subject and seven subjects per group were analyzed. Representative photomicrographs of the BrdU positive cells in the RMS, SVZ and OB are shown in **Figures 3D, 5C**.

Double-labeled cells for BrdU/DCX, BrdU/NeuN, and Brdu/cFos were counted using a confocal microscope (Zeiss Inverted LSM 510 and LSM 780) and the image examiner software Aim Image Examiner (Carl Zeiss Microscopy, Jena, Germany). For both experiments, three images were obtained with a 25X objective in each ROI: SVZ (dorsal, anterior-medial, ventral, and anterior), RMS (posterior, medial, and anterior), MOB and AOB (GlL and GrL). For each ROI a z-stack of 12 slices (2 μm per slice) was obtained. Co-localization was verified with the orthogonal tool in the Image Examiner software. Each image was divided into four sections for counting. All the BrdU-labeled cells in each section were counted. We then quantified all the BrdU-labeled cells that colocalized (**Figure 6**). An average of the four sections was obtained for the three images, and from this data, the percentage of colocalization was calculated as the number of colocalized cells multiplied by 100 and divided by the number of BrdU-labeled cells.

Statistical Analysis

The statistical analysis was performed with SigmaPlot 11.0 software. Since none of the data had a normal distribution, as determined by the Shapiro-Wilk test, non-parametric tests were used. To compare the behavior of paced mating vs. non-paced mating, a Mann-Whitney test was used. The number of cells was analyzed by a Kruskal Wallis test followed by a Mann-Whitney test in case of significant effects. Differences with $p < 0.05$ were considered significant.

TABLE 1 | List of antibodies used in both experiments.

Antibody	Species	Dilution	Suuplier
PRIMARY ANTIBODIES			
BrdU	Mice	1:2000	BD bioscience
BrdU	Rat	1:800	AbD serotec
DCX	Guinea pig	1:500	Millipore
NeuN	Mice	1:250	Millipore
cFos	Rabbit	1:250	Santa Cruz Biotech
SECONDARY ANTIBODIES			
IgG biotinylated	Mice	1:500	Vector
Alexa 488	Rat	1:1250	Invitrogen
CY2	Guinea pig	1:1000	Jackson immuno
CY3	Mice	1:1000	Jackson immuno
Alexa 488	Rabbit	1:1250	Invitrogen

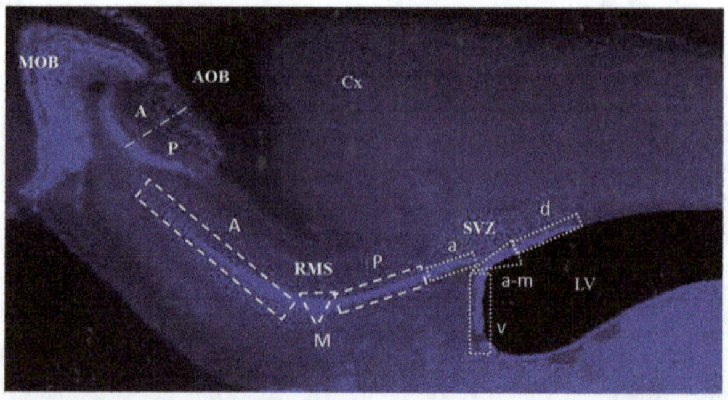

FIGURE 2 | Photomicrograph showing the different regions where cells were quantified in the subventricular zone (SVZ), the rostral migratory stream (RMS), the main olfactory bulb (MOB), and the accessory olfactory bulb (AOB) in the anterior (A) and posterior (P) region. The SVZ anterior (A), M (medial) and P (posterior), and in the RMS a (anterior), v (ventral), a-m (anterior-medial), and d (dorsal). The Cortex (Cx) and lateral ventricles (LV) are also indicated.

RESULTS

Experiment 1-Proliferation

Behavioral Measures

Paced vs. non-paced mating

All the females were equally receptive at the time of the behavioral test (**Table 2**). No significant differences were found in the LQ or the LI between paced and non-paced mating (LQ: $U = 32$, $p = 0.409$; LS: $U = 34$, $p = 0.883$). No significant differences were found in the number of mounts ($U = 22$, $p = 0.536$), intromissions ($U = 16.5$, $p = 0.067$), and ejaculations ($U = 22$, $p = 0.313$) or in mount ($U = 10$, $p = 0.081$), intromission ($U = 23$, $p = 0.229$) and ejaculation latencies ($U = 35$, $p = 0.962$). As expected, and as described in previous studies comparing paced and non-paced mating, the inter intromission interval was higher in the pacing group ($U = 10$, $p = 0.014$). As well the percent of exits and return latencies was higher after ejaculation than after intromissions, which in turn was higher than after mounts.

Cell proliferation in the SVZ

Females exposed to banana scent ($U = 17$, $p = 0.032$) and those exposed to the male ($U = 16$, $p = 0.009$) showed a significant increase in the total number of new cells in the SVZ in comparison to the control group (**Figure 3A**). When we analyzed cell proliferation in the different regions of the SVZ (anterior, anterior-medial, dorsal, and ventral), the highest density of new cells was localized in the ventral part ($H = 13.109$, $p = 0.011$), in the groups exposed to the banana scent ($U = 0$, $p = 0.008$), and the male ($U = 2$, $p = 0.017$) in comparison to the control group. No differences were found in the other regions of the SVZ (**Figure 3B**).

TABLE 2 | Sexual behavior parameters in the proliferation experiment in females that did or did not pace the sexual interaction.

Behavioral measures	Groups	
	Paced mating	Non-paced mating
LQ (%)	99.6 ± 0.44	100
LI	1.86 ± 0.04	1.86 ± 0.05
NUMBER		
Mounts	11.1 ± 3	15.7 ± 4.3
Intromissions	30.1 ± 30.7	40 ± 2.8
Ejaculations	2.4 ± 0.24	3 ± 0.4
LATENCIES (SEC)		
Mounts	69.4 ± 25.9	276.8 ± 120.1
Intromissions	371.2 ± 211.9	479.9 ± 168.3
Ejaculations	1418.9 ± 330.3	1297.5 ± 164.6
III (sec)	105.1 ± 10.6*	64.4 ± 7.7
PERCENTAGE OF EXITS AFTER		
Mounts	20.44 ± 6.9	
Intromissions	61.9 ± 4.2	
Ejaculations	100	
RETURN LATENCIES (SEC) AFTER		
Mounts	46.6 ± 27.8	
Intromissions	51.7 ± 14.4	
Ejaculations	366.7 ± 79.7	

LQ, lordosis coefficient; LI, lordosis intensity, III, inter intromission interval.
**Different from the non-paced mating group, Mann-Whitney U test ($U = 10$, $p = 0.014$).*

Cell proliferation in the RMS

Cell proliferation in the RMS was significantly different between groups ($H = 11.140$, $p = 0.025$). We found, that the group, that paced the sexual interaction showed a higher density of BrdU-immunoreactive (BrdU-IR) cells compared to control females ($U = 1$, $p = 0.017$). Females, that did not pace the sexual interaction showed an increase in the number of BrdU-IR cells that was not statistically significant ($U = 4$, $p = 0.052$; **Figure 3A**). When the cell density was analyzed in the different regions of the RMS, the differences were located in the anterior region ($H = 16.634$, $p = 0.002$). Subjects from both paced ($U = 3$, $p = 0.015$) and non-paced mating ($U = 2$, $p = 0.009$) groups had a higher density of new cells than control animals. The number of BrdU-IR cells found in the medial and posterior regions was similar for all groups (**Figure 3C**).

Migrating neuroblasts in the SVZ and RMS

The percentage of new cells (BrdU-IR), that were already committed to the neuronal phenotype and were migrating (DCX-IR) was evaluated in the SVZ and RMS (**Figure 4**). We found no differences in the total number of the migrating neuroblasts (BrdU-IR/DCX-IR cells) in the SVZ and RMS. When the different regions were analyzed we found, that the groups exposed to banana scent ($U = 0$, $p = 0.029$) and to the male ($H = 9.947$, $p = 0.041$) both had a higher percentage of migrating neuroblasts than the control group in the anterior region of the SVZ (**Table 3**). No differences were found in the other regions of the SVZ. In the posterior, RMS the group exposed to banana scent had a higher percentage of neuroblasts ($H = 11.679$, $p = 0.020$) than the control group. No differences were found in other areas of the RMS.

Experiment 2-Survival

Behavioral Measures

Paced vs. non-paced mating

To evaluate the effect of sexual behavior on the survival of the new cells in the OB, and the activation of these new cells after sexual behavior, females mated twice with the same male. The first mating test was done on day 0, when BrdU was administered and the second test was 45 days later. No significant differences were found in the LQ and the LI between the paced and non-paced mating groups in either test (**Table 4**). There was a significant reduction in the number of mounts in test 2 in the females that paced the sexual interaction ($U = 9.5$, $p = 0.029$) in comparison to the females that didn't pace the sexual interaction in the same test. The III was higher in the groups that paced the sexual interaction than in those that didn't. Although these differences were not significant (test 1 $U = 24$, $p = 0.442$; test 2 $U = 14.5$, $p = 0.065$) the change is on the same direction as seen in previous studies (Corona et al., 2011). As observed in experiment 1 the percent of exits and return latencies were higher after ejaculation than after intromissions, which in turn were higher than after mounts.

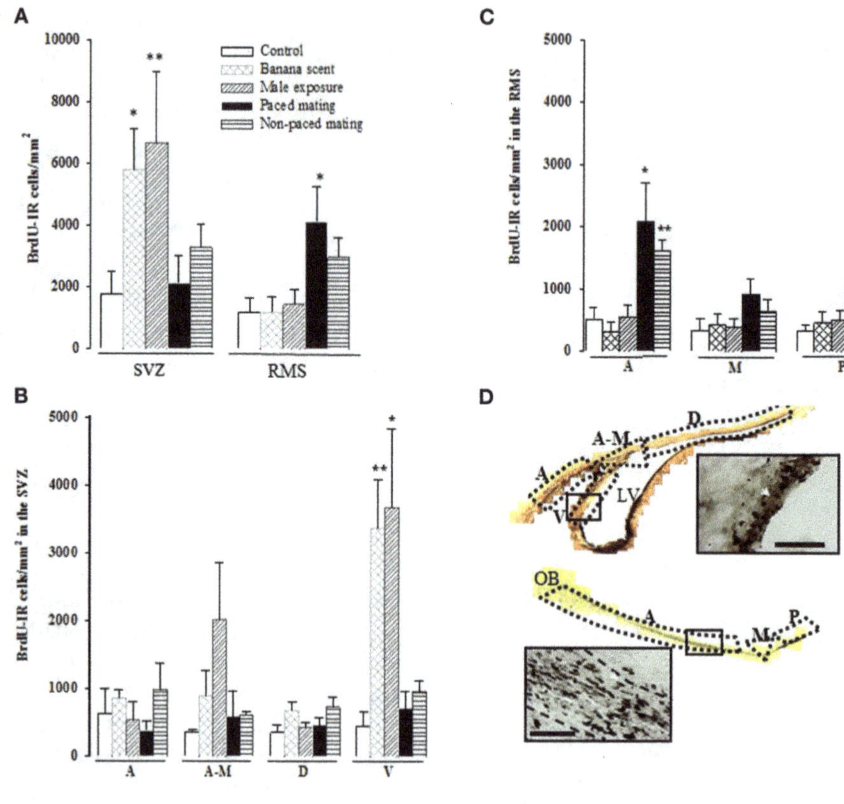

FIGURE 3 | Cell proliferation in the Subventricular Zone (SVZ) and the Rostral Migratory Stream (RMS) two days after BrdU injection. (A) BrdU immunoreactive (BrdU-IR) cells in the whole SVZ and RMS; **(B)** BrdU-IR cells in the anterior (A), anterior-medial (A-M), dorsal (D), and ventral (V) sub-regions of the SVZ; **(C)** BrdU positive cells in the anterior (A), medial (M), and posterior (P) sub-regions of the RMS and **(D)** representative photomicrographs of BrdU positive cells in the SVZ and RMS. Arrow heads point to BrdU positive cells. Scale bar = 50 μm. The lateral ventricles (LV) and the olfactory bulb (OB) are also indicated. *Different from control $P < 0.05$, $^{**}P < 0.01$.

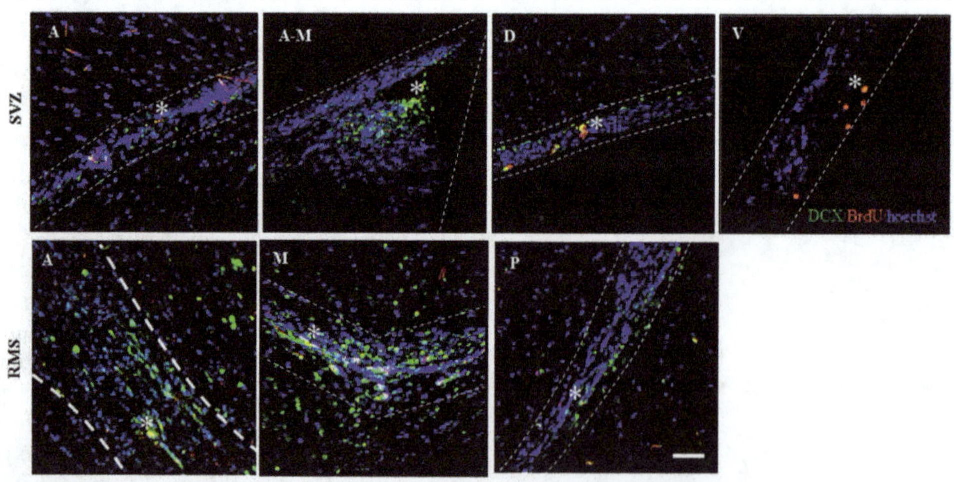

FIGURE 4 | Representative photomicrographs of the migrating neuroblasts localized in the regions of the Subventricular Zone (SVZ) in the anterior (A), anterior-medial (A-M), dorsal (D), and ventral (V) sub-regions and in the Rostral Migratory Stream (RMS), anterior (A), medial (M), and posterior (P). Doublecortin (DCX) positive cells are labeled in green, BrdU positive cells in red, and the cell nuclei in blue (Hoechst). Scale bar = 50 μm. *BrdU/DCX positive cells.

TABLE 3 | Percentage of migrating neuroblasts in the Subventricular Zone (SVZ) and in the Rostral Migratory Stream (RMS).

Regions		Control	Banana scent	Male exposure	Paced mating	Non-paced mating
		Percentage of BrdU-IR/DCX-IR cells				
		Groups				
	SVZ (complete)	35.9 ± 3.8	67.7 ± 3.4	67.5 ± 4.1	53.5 ± 8.1	58.3 ± 14.3
SVZ	Anterior	35.9 ± 6.8	78.8 ± 7.3*	73.7 ± 5.1*	52.1 ± 5.2	60.8 ± 15.4
	Anterior-Medial	50.5 ± 9.4	65.8 ± 5.5	70.8 ± 10.5	80.6 ± 10	52.8 ± 13.7
	Dorsal	25 ± 16	69.2 ± 7.1	64.3 ± 14.5	58.3 ± 14.4	66.7 ± 15.6
	Ventral	32.4 ± 6.1	57.2 ± 13.6	61.3 ± 5.2	43.1 ± 6.4	70.5 ± 5.8
	RMS (complete)	44.9 ± 7.3	62.4 ± 2.3	50.9 ± 5.7	47.5 ± 4.6	60.6 ± 3.4
RMS	Anterior	36.6 ± 15.5	59.7 ± 7.5	63.8 ± 21.9	68 ± 12.0	71 ± 4.2
	Medial	43.7 ± 8.0	54.6 ± 6.7	56.8 ± 2.4	35.5 ± 3.5	54.8 ± 8.1
	Posterior	54.4 ± 8.5	72.9 ± 7.1*	32.1 ± 6.6	39.6 ± 6.3	56.2 ± 5.4

**p < 0.05 different from Control, Mann-Whitney U test.*

TABLE 4 | Sexual behavior parameters in the survival experiment in females that paced and in those not allowed to pace the sexual interaction in test 1, when BrdU was administered, and 45 days latter.

Behavioral measures	Groups			
	Paced mating		Non-paced mating	
	Test 1 day 0	Test 2 day 45	Test 1 day 0	Test 2 day 45
LQ (%)	99.02 ± 0.65	100	100	100
LI	1.84 ± 0.04	1.85 ± 0.07	1.84 ± 0.04	1.85 ± 0.05
NUMBER				
Mounts	9.1 ± 2.5	7.6 ± 1.9*	21.9 ± 6.5	27.5 ± 6.5
Intromissions	26 ± 5.1	24.6 ± 6.3	34 ± 3.9	32.5 ± 6.4
Ejaculations	3 ± 0.3	3.3 ± 0.6	3.4 ± 0.5	4 ± 0.4
LATENCIES (SEC)				
Mounts	88.5 ± 40.6	556.2 ± 372.8	21.8 ± 6.5	27.5 ± 6.0
Intromissions	459.8 ± 208.2	369.1 ± 196.1	34 ± 3.8	32.5 ± 6.4
Ejaculations	1092.9 ± 210.4	1182.6 ± 189.5	1382.2 ± 292.1	901.4 ± 203.2
III (sec)	127.7 ± 24	161.9 ± 28	94.1 ± 5.4	92.5 ± 8.7
PERCENTAGE OF EXITS AFTER				
Mounts	42.75 ± 9.9	39.5 ± 11.2		
Intromissions	57.38 ± 7.5	78.25 ± 7.8		
Ejaculations	98.88 ± 3.12	100		
RETURN LATENCIES (SEC) AFTER				
Mounts	50.8 ± 25.4	56.2 ± 39.4		
Intromissions	72.6 ± 21.2	57 ± 11.6		
Ejaculations	164.9 ± 50.4	200.1 ± 61.6		

LQ, lordosis coefficient; LI, lordosis intensity, III, inter intromission interval.
**Different from non-paced mating group on test 2, p < 0.05.*

Hormonal levels

The plasma levels of E2 and P were quantified in order to exclude the possibility, that the effects on new cell survival were due to hormonal differences. The plasma levels of E2 and P were similar in all the groups (E2: $F = 1.033$, $p = 0.419$; P: $F = 0.930$, $p = 0.467$). The plasma levels (expressed as pg/ml mean ± sem) for E2 were: control 38.8 ± 12, odor exposure 25.1 ± 7.5, exposed to male 33.4 ± 2.5, paced mating 40 ± 3.5, non-paced mating 35.9 ± 4.7. For P: control 15.4 ± 6.4, odor exposure 25.2 ± 2.7, exposed to male 15 ± 4.4, paced mating 17.1 ± 4.1, non-paced mating 21.6 ± 5.2.

Cell survival in the OB

No significant differences were found in the number of BrdU-IR cells that survived 45 days after mating in the different layers of the MOB and the AOB (**Figure 5A**). Similarly, no differences were found between the anterior and posterior regions of the AOB (**Figure 5B**).

New neurons in the MOB and AOB

In order to characterize the mature neuronal phenotype of the new cells, the colocalization of BrdU and NeuN markers was counted and the results expressed as the percentage of newborn cells that are neurons in the MOB and AOB (see **Table 5A**). No differences were found in the different layers of the MOB. In the GrL of the AOB the group that paced the sexual interaction had a higher percentage of new neurons ($U = 0$, $p = 0.029$) than the control group. In the anterior and posterior layers of the AOB no differences were observed in the GlL but in the GrL significant differences were found. Both mating groups had a significantly higher percentages of BrdU-NeuN IR cells (Paced $U = 0$, $p = 0.029$; non-paced $U = 0$, $p = 0.029$) than the control group. The group exposed to the male had significantly lower percentage of new neurons ($U = 0$, $p = 0.029$) in comparison to the control group. No changes were observed in the percentage of new neurons in the AOB or the MOB in the animals expose to banana scent.

New cell activation in the MOB and AOB

The new cells (BrdU-IR) that were also activated, as evaluated by cFos-IR, were quantified and the results are reported as percentage of BrdU-IR/cFos-IR (**Table 5B**). No differences were found in the percentage of new cells activated in the MOB.

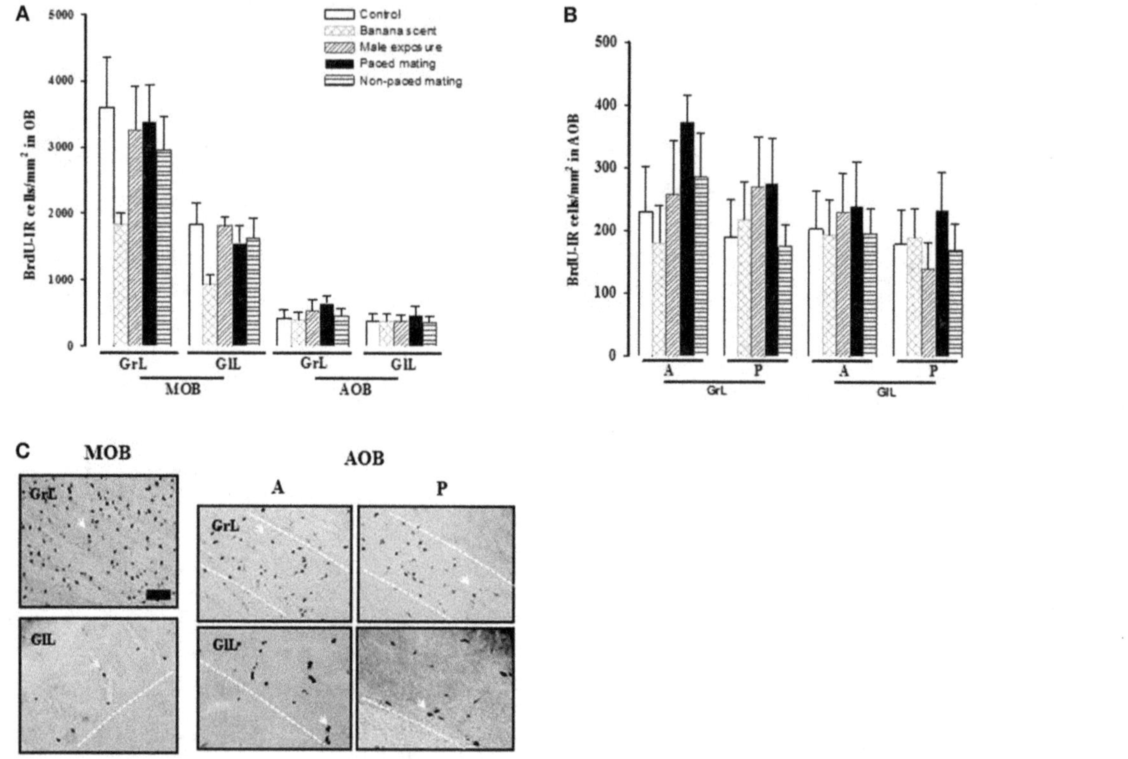

FIGURE 5 | Number of new cells that survive (A) in the granular (GrL) and glomerular cell layer (GlL) of the Main Olfactory Bulb (MOB) and Accesory Olfactory Bulb (AOB) 45 days after BrdU injection. (B) Number of BrdU positive cells in the anterior (A) and posterior (P) region in the GrL and GlL of the AOB). **(C)** Representative photomicrographs of the BrdU positive cells in the GrL and GlL of the MOB and in the A and P regions of the AOB. Arrow heads point to BrdU positive cells. Scale bar = 50 μm.

Significant differences were found in the AOB. In the GrL, the paced mating group had a significantly higher percentage of activated new neurons than the control group ($U = 0$, $p = 0.029$). In the GlL, the non-paced mating group had the highest percentage of new neurons that were activated ($U = 0$, $p = 0.029$). When the anterior and posterior regions of the AOB were analyzed, the paced mating group had a significantly higher number of activated new neurons in the anterior region of the GrL ($U = 0$, $p = 0.029$) and GlL ($U = 0$, $p = 0.029$) than the control group. In the anterior GlL the non-paced group also showed a higher number of activated neurons than the control group ($U = 0$, $p = 0.029$). In the banana scent group, no changes were observed in the percentage of BrdU-/cFos- IR cells in the AOB and MOB.

DISCUSSION

Cell Proliferation

In the present study, we hypothesized that paced sexual behavior would increase cell proliferation in the SVZ and RMS of female rats. However, in the SVZ a significant increase in cell proliferation was observed only in the groups exposed to amyl acetate (a non-sexual odor) and in the group exposed to the male (without physical contact), suggesting that olfactory stimulation favors the proliferation of new cells in the SVZ. This cell proliferation was higher specifically in the ventral part of the SVZ. In the RMS females displaying sexual behavior either paced or not, showed a higher density of new cells. This suggests that sexual behavior is important for cell proliferation in females independently of the possibility of pacing the sexual interaction. Sexual behavior enhances the number of cells in the anterior region of the RMS. In this region, the number of BrdU-labeled cells was about three times higher than, that found in the other groups. Together, the results of the proliferation study indicate that odors induce cell proliferation in the SVZ and sexual behavior increases cell proliferation in the anterior RMS, independently of whether the female can or cannot pace the sexual interaction.

Cell proliferation in the SVZ and RMS appears to be differentially regulated. It has been shown that pregnancy and mating with vasectomized males increases the production of neural progenitors in the SVZ (Shingo et al., 2003). In sheep, estrous females in contact with an experienced male did not change the rate of proliferation in the SVZ, but parturient females in contact with their lamb showed decreased proliferation in the SVZ (Brus et al., 2010). It has also been shown that the induction of maternal behavior and exposure of nulliparous female rats to pups, increased the number of new cells in the SVZ, independently of pregnancy or lactation (Furuta and Bridges, 2009). When female mice were exposed to odors from male

TABLE 5 | Percentage of new neurons (A) and percentage of new cells activated (B) after the second mating test in the different groups in the MOB and AOB.

A. Percentage of BrdU-IR/NeuN-IR cells

Regions			Groups			
		Control	Banana scent	Male exposure	Paced mating	Non-paced mating
MOB	*GrL*	78.71 ± 4.8	81.7 ± 8.5	69.3 ± 7.5	85.2 ± 2.3	79.2 ± 4.5
	GlL	33.3 ± 11.8	25 ± 14.4	58.9 ± 22.3	35.4 ± 14.6	37.5 ± 23.9
AOB	*GrL*	19.6 ± 1.5	16.3 ± 2.6	11.6 ± 1.2	46.1 ± 11.1*	26.5 ± 5
	GlL	25 ± 14.4	76.3 ± 10.3	37.1 ± 10.3	27.1 ± 10.4	18.8 ± 12
	GrL					
	A	19.8 ± 1.3	14.8 ± 2.3	12.5 ± 1.2*	37.8 ± 8.2*	35.5 ± 9.5*
	P	19.5 ± 2.7	17.8 ± 4.2	10.8 ± 3.5	55 ± 19.3	18 ± 3
	GlL					
	A	13 ± 12.5	90 ± 10	28 ± 11.1	59.5 ± 21.2	37.5 ± 23.9
	P	50 ± 28.8	53 ± 21	54.3 ± 20.6	54.2 ± 20.8	37.5 ± 23.9

B. Percentage of BrdU-IR/cFos-IR cells

Regions		Control	Banana scent	Male exposure	Paced mating	Non-paced mating
MOB	*GrL*	32.2 ± 12.3	51.4 ± 3.3	28 ± 10	47.1 ± 5	32.2 ± 9
	GlL	25.3 ± 11.8	40 ± 17	32.6 ± 6.3	60 ± 16.3	60.4 ± 7.5
AOB	*GrL*	35.1 ± 5.4	3.1 ± 8.5	36.2 ± 3.7	65.1 ± 8*	49.4 ± 7.5
	GlL	18.1 ± 7.2	36.5 ± 2.1	27 ± 7	49.2 ± 13	59.1 ± 5.6*
	GrL					
	A	26.8 ± 7.5	28 ± 10	47.1 ± 5	64.3 ± 4.2*	59 ± 15
	P	43.3 ± 3.6	32.2 ± 9	25.3 ± 11.8	66 ± 12	40.1 ± 10
	GlL					
	A	12 ± 8	27.4 ± 7.1	23 ± 11.1	68 ± 15*	54 ± 5*
	P	24.4 ± 12	46 ± 8.0	31.5 ± 7.7	31 ± 12.2	65 ± 8.6

**Different from the control group in the same layer, $p < 0.05$.*

mice for 7 days a significant increase in BrdU labeled cells was observed in the SVZ and dentate gyrus (Mak et al., 2007). This effect appears to be mediated by the MOB because females treated with $ZnSO_4$, which eliminates the function of the main olfactory epithelium, didn't show the increase in proliferation (Mak et al., 2007). These observations suggest that cellular proliferation in the SVZ is highly sensitive to sexually and socially relevant olfactory cues. This is consistent with the results of the present study where a significant increase in cell proliferation in the SVZ was observed only in the groups exposed to amyl acetate (a non-sexual odor) or to the male (without physical contact). It is possible that the cellular proliferation in the SVZ could be due to novelty of an olfactory stimulus and/or to the acquisition of a new olfactory memory generated from sexually relevant olfactory cues.

The RMS is primarily recognized as a migratory pathway and its proliferative role is less known (Alonso et al., 2008). In the female prairie vole, cell proliferation in the RMS is promoted by sexually relevant male olfactory cues that induce sexual receptivity (Smith et al., 2001). In addition, the RMS shows differences in cellular proliferation depending on the day of the estrous cycle. When female rats are in estrous, the proliferation rate is increased in the RMS, but not in the SVZ, (Díaz et al., 2009). These changes are not associated with cell death in the RMS but rather they appear to be associated with an increase in the number of new cells (Díaz et al., 2009). Our data indicate that females displaying sexual behavior either paced or not, showed a higher density of new cells in the RMS.

In the present experiment, we characterized the neural phenotype of the new cells using doublecortin (DCX, widely used to identify immature neurons and migrating neuroblast) labeling. In the anterior-SVZ the groups exposed to banana scent and to male odors showed more than 70% of the new cells label as DCX-IR compared to 30% of the control females. In the posterior RMS, a significant increase in the percentage of DCX-IR cells was observed in the group exposed to banana scent compared to the control females. These results suggest, that the olfactory stimuli promote or facilitate neuronal phenotype determination in the new cells in the anterior SVZ and in the posterior RMS. It has been described that each proliferative region of

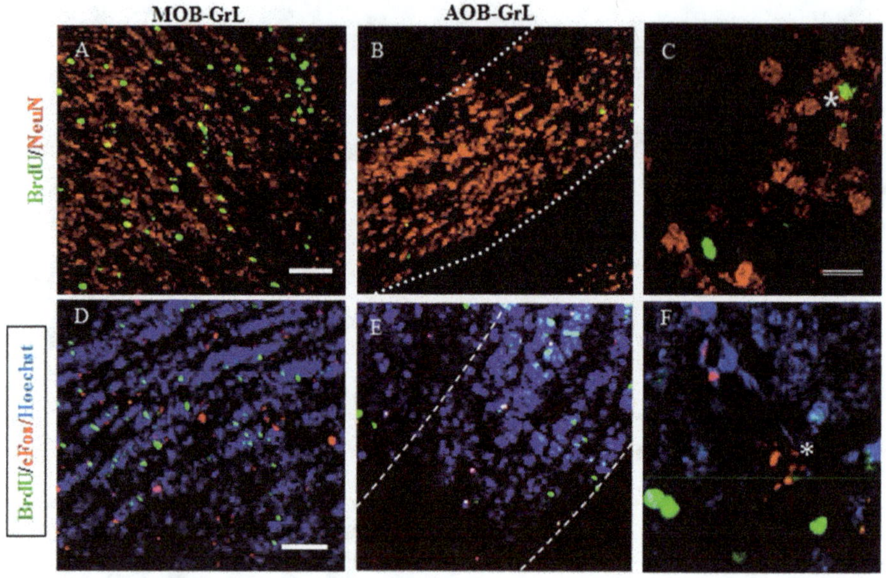

FIGURE 6 | Representative photomicrographs of new neurons (A–C) in: (A) the granular layer (GrL) of the Main Olfactory Bulb (MOB) and (B) the Accesory Olfactory Bulb (AOB). (C) High magnification of the BrdU/NeuN positive cells. **(D–F)** new cells that are activated after the second sexual behavior test (BrdU/cFos) in the GrL of the MOB **(D)** and the GrL of the AOB **(E)**. High magnification of a BrdU/cFos positive cell. Scale bar = 50 μm. *Double positive cells for BrdU and NeuN.

the SVZ and RMS could be regulated by particular information from their microenvironment. The dorsal regions produce periglomerular interneurons that express tyrosine hydroxylase (TH), and the superficial granule cells. The ventral regions generate the periglomerual interneurons that express calbindin-IR, and the deep granular cells; and the anterior region in general produce calretinin expressing periglomerual interneurons, and most of the granular cells (Carani et al., 1999; Merkle et al., 2007). Future studies will need to evaluate the type of cells induced by olfactory stimulus and mating.

Cell Survival

To evaluate the effect of sexual behavior on cell survival in the MOB and AOB, females were injected with BrdU the same day, that they had the first behavioral test and were sacrificed 45 days later. The survival rate observed in the MOB and AOB was the same for all groups of females, suggesting that one stimulation, either olfactory or mating, was not enough to modify the survival rate of the new cells that reach the OB. We also quantified, cell survival in the anterior and posterior divisions of the AOB, since there is an anatomical, functional, and chemical distinction between them (Bonfanti et al., 1997; Halpern et al., 1998; Martínez-Marcos et al., 2001; Larriva-Sahd, 2008). The anterior division of the AOB has been extensively related to processing of sexually relevant information, and thus an increase in neurogenesis and the activation of the new cells may contribute to process this specific information. The sensory olfactory neurons located in the apical region of the VNO are connected to the anterior division of the AOB, and are activated by male pheromones present in male urine (Inamura et al., 1999a). As well, exposure to male urine induces cFos expression in the anterior division of the AOB (Inamura et al., 1999a,b). When male mice are exposed to urine of female in estrous, increased activation in the anterior division of the GrL and GlL of the BOA is observed (Honda et al., 2008). All of this evidence suggests, that sexually relevant odors activate preferentially cells in the anterior division of the AOB. However, in the present study we did not find differences in the number of new cells between the anterior and posterior divisions of the AOB. We have previously shown that in female rats that paced the sexual interaction once, there is a significant increase in the number of cells that reach the GrL of the AOB 15 days after mating (Corona et al., 2011). If the stimulus is repeated; that is if the females paced the sexual interaction in 3 more sessions a higher number of cells reach the GrL of the AOB. Moreover, a significantly higher number of cells reach the GlL of the AOB and the mitral and GrL of the MOB (Arzate et al., 2013). When the number of neurons was analyzed, a significant increase was observed in the GrL in both, the AOB and MOB suggesting that repeated paced mating promotes the arrival of more new born neurons to the OB (Arzate et al., 2013). Preliminary observations from our group indicate that repeated paced mating also induces a higher number of neurons 45 days after the first mating session. It has been shown that in the process of OB neurogenesis, the new cells have to go through critical steps that will allow them to reach their final destination (Petreanu and Alvarez-Buylla, 2002; Lledo et al., 2006; Ming and Song, 2011). The time that the new cells require to arrive to the OB and incorporate into their respective layers and preexistent circuits is around 45 days in rodents (Petreanu and Alvarez-Buylla, 2002; Ming and Song, 2011). New neurons between 15 and 22 days old show a mature morphology and it has been suggested that the activity of the OB, specifically the mitral and tufted cells, regulates the incorporation of the new cells into the pre-existent circuits, thereby enhancing their survival (Petreanu and Alvarez-Buylla, 2002). During this critical period, 15 days after generation of the new cells, if they don't receive information or are not stimulated the cells will not survive. For example, it has been demonstrated that in anosmic mice with a mutation in a channel of the olfactory sensory neurons of the main olfactory epithelium where odor information does not arrive to the OB a high proportion of the new cells died between days 15 and 45 days after being born, suggesting that constant information from the OB during this critical period is necessary for the survival of the new cells (Petreanu and Alvarez-Buylla, 2002).

Neuronal Phenotype of the New Cells

We evaluated the neuronal phenotype of the new cells, that reached the AOB 45 days after mating and found that the percentage of new neurons (BrdU/NeuN-IR cells) in the GrL was higher in the females that paced the sexual interactions (46%) compared with the control females (20%). This increase was specifically observed in the anterior division of the AOB, in which females, that paced and non-paced the sexual interaction showed the highest level of new neurons (38 and 36%, respectively) compared with the control females (20%), and females exposed to males showed the lowest percentage of new neurons (13%). These results suggest, that sexual behavior could influence the neuronal fate of the new OB cells. The percentage of new neurons found in the MOB GlL and GrL was the same for all groups (80 and 30%, respectively). The effect of sexual behavior on the determination of the new AOB cells is exclusively neuronal, since no differences were observed in the percentage of new glial cells (BrdU/GFAP-IR cells; data not shown). We don't have a clear explanation as to why the group exposed to the male showed a significantly lower percentage of new cells in the anterior region of the GrL of the AOB. Since we haven't seen this effect in our previous studies where groups of females have been exposed to male it could be a spurious effect.

Activation of the New Cells in the OB after Mating

Once the new OB cells have survived and arrived at their final destination, they become fully integrated into the pre-existent circuits and present synaptic activity and electric responses after stimulation of OB circuits (Carani et al., 1999; Saghatelyan et al., 2003). The new OB cells, in particular the granular cells have unique properties compared to the preexistent granular cells, including an enhanced synaptic plasticity with a higher response to odors, and greater sensitivity to new odors than the preexistent OB granular cells (Magavi et al., 2005; Sinchak et al., 2007; Nissant et al., 2009). In the present study in order to evaluate if the new cells, that reach the OB are activated, females were tested again for sexual behavior before being sacrificed. No differences in the percentage of BrdU/Fos-IR cells were found in the MOB. In the AOB clear differences were observed in the activation of the new cells. Non-paced mating significantly increased the activation of new cells in the GlL, specifically in the anterior region, of the AOB. Paced mating also increased the percentage of BrdU/Fos-IR cells in the GrL, and in the anterior region of the GrL and GlL of the AOB. These results suggest that the new cells that reach the AOB label 45 day before, after a sexual behavior test are preferentially activated by sexual behavior and not by olfactory cues (banana scent) or by sexually relevant olfactory cues. The new cells incorporated into the OB are more sensitive to stimuli between days 28 and 56 after being born because in this period the density of dendritic spines is increased resulting in an intensified production of synaptic contacts; as a result the new cells are more readily activated (Sinchak et al., 2007).

The activation of the new cells in the AOB found in the present study is consistent with the role of the AOB in sexual behavior. Female sexual behavior is initially regulated by the detection of male pheromones by the AOB. Lesions of the vomeronasal organ (VNO), which projects to the AOB, eliminates receptive behavior in hamsters (Mackay-Sim and Rose, 1986), prairie voles (Wysocki et al., 1991), rats (Guarraci and Clark, 2006), and mice (Keller et al., 2006). The AOB receives information directly from several central brain regions like the bed nucleus of the stria terminalis (BNST), rostral and medial portion of the medial amygdala (MeA) and the posteromedial amygdala (Keller et al., 2009). The posteromedial amygdala and the BNST are two of the regions that are activated (measured by Fos expression) after females receive natural or artificial vaginocervical stimulation (VCS; Erskine, 1993; Hosokawa and Chiba, 2005; Sugai et al., 2006). This implies the possibility, that when females receive stimulation from the male during sexual behavior these structures are activated. This activation together with the information that arrives to the AOB could promote the activation of the new neurons. The new neurons in the GrL receive and are activated by centrifugal inputs from the central regions. The periglomerular interneurons, which are also activated after sexual behavior, could be associated with mate discrimination.

Sexual behavior induces a reward state that could enhance the effects observed on OB neurogenesis. Our group has demonstrated that females and males that paced the sexual interaction develop a positive affective, reward, state as evaluated by conditioned place preference (CPP). If the subjects do not pace the sexual interaction they don't develop CPP (Paredes and Alonso, 1997; Martínez and Paredes, 2001; Arzate et al., 2011). The reward state in females can be induced by 10 paced intromissions (Paredes and Alonso, 1997) or by 1 h of paced mating (Arzate et al., 2011). The reward state generated by paced mating is mediated by opioids since the administration of naloxone, an opioid antagonist, blocks the CPP induced by paced mating in males (Agmo and Berenfeld, 1990) and females (Paredes and Martínez, 2001; García-Horsman et al., 2008). Since, opioids are involved in the process of cell death and survival (Tegeder and Geisslinger, 2004) and inhibit neurogenesis in the adult rat hippocampus (Eisch et al., 2000), future studies will need to address if neurogenesis induced by paced mating can be block by opioid antagonists.

The results observed in the present experiment are not due to differences in E2 or P plasma levels. All groups had the same hormonal levels when sacrificed. Similar results were obtained when females were mated repeatedly under pacing conditions. We found a higher number of cells and neurons (see above) but no differences were found in E2 and P levels 15 days after mating (Arzate et al., 2013).

To summarize, one sexual encounter promotes changes in the OB neurogenesis process. Mating increases the proliferation of new cells in the RMS particularly in the anterior region, favors the incorporation of new cells in the GrL of the AOB and promotes commitment to the neuronal lineage of the new cells, increasing the percentage of new neurons in the GrL of the AOB, especially in the anterior division. The new cells, that reach the GrL of the AOB anterior division are preferentially activated by mating. Together, these results strongly suggest, that mating behavior influences the process of OB neurogenesis and that the new cells that incorporate into the AOB have a relevant function in female sexual behavior.

AUTHOR CONTRIBUTIONS

RC help in the design of the study, performed the experiments and help writing the paper. SR performed the hormonal assay of the study and help writing the paper. WP supervised the behavioral tests, analyzed the data and help writing the paper. RP designed the study, help in data analysis, help writing the paper, and obtained funding.

ACKNOWLEDGMENTS

This work was supported by CONACyT grants 167101, 252756, and fronteras 374; and by DGAPA grants IN210215, IN203615. We thank Francisco J. Camacho, Leonor Casanova, Omar González, Ma. De Lourdes Lara, Martín García, Alejandra Castilla, Francisco Javier Valles, Deisy Gasca, and Elsa Nydia Hernández for their excellent technical assistance.

REFERENCES

Agmo, A., and Berenfeld, R. (1990). Reinforcing properties of ejaculation in the male rat: role of opioids and dopamine. *Behav. Neurosci.* 104, 177–182. doi: 10.1037/0735-7044.104.1.177

Alonso, M., Ortega-Pérez, I., Grubb, M. S., Bourgeois, J. P., Charneau, P., and Lledo, P. M. (2008). Turning astrocytes from the rostral migratory stream into neurons: a role for the olfactory sensory organ. *J. Neurosci.* 28, 11089–11102. doi: 10.1523/JNEUROSCI.3713-08.2008

Alvarez-Buylla, A., Seri, B., and Doetsch, F. (2002). Identification of neural stem cells in the adult vertebrate brain. *Brain Res. Bull.* 57, 751–758. doi: 10.1016/S0361-9230(01)00770-5

Arzate, D. M., Portillo, W., Corona, R., and Paredes, R. G. (2013). Repeated paced mating promotes the arrival of more newborn neurons in the main and accessory olfactory bulbs of adult female rats. *Neuroscience* 232, 151–160. doi: 10.1016/j.neuroscience.2012.12.014

Arzate, D. M., Portillo, W., Rodríguez, C., Corona, R., and Paredes, R. G. (2011). Extended paced mating tests induces conditioned place preference without affecting sexual arousal. *Horm. Behav.* 59, 674–680. doi: 10.1016/j.yhbeh.2010.08.016

Bagley, J., LaRocca, G., Jimenez, D. A., and Urban, N. N. (2007). Adult neurogenesis and specific replacement of interneuron subtypes in the mouse main olfactory bulb. *BMC Neurosci.* 8:92. doi: 10.1186/1471-2202-8-92

Bonfanti, L., Peretto, P., Merighi, A., and Fasolo, A. (1997). Newly-generated cells from the rostral migratory stream in the accessory olfactory bulb of the adult rat. *Neuroscience* 81, 489–502. doi: 10.1016/S0306-4522(97)00090-0

Brennan, P. A. (2004). The nose knows who's who: chemosensory individuality and mate recognition in mice. *Horm. Behav.* 46, 231–240. doi: 10.1016/j.yhbeh.2004.01.010

Bruce, H. M. (1959). An exteroceptive block to pregnancy in the mouse. *Nature* 184, 105. doi: 10.1038/184105a0

Brus, M., Meurisse, M., Franceschini, I., Keller, M., and Lévy, F. (2010). Evidence for cell proliferation in the sheep brain and its down-regulation by parturition and interactions with the young. *Horm. Behav.* 58, 737–746. doi: 10.1016/j.yhbeh.2010.07.006

Carani, C., Rochira, V., Faustini-Fustini, M., Balestrieri, A., and Granata, A. R. (1999). Role of oestrogen in male sexual behaviour: insights from the natural model of aromatase deficiency. *Clin. Endocrinol.* 51, 517–524. doi: 10.1046/j.1365-2265.1999.00849.x

Corona, R., Larriva-Sahd, J., and Paredes, R. G. (2011). Paced-mating increases the number of adult new born cells in the internal cellular (granular) layer of the accessory olfactory bulb. *PLoS ONE* 6:e19380. doi: 10.1371/journal.pone.0019380

Corona, R. P. W., and Paredes, R. (2012). *Neuronas y Sexo*. Mexico, MX: Publicaciones cbs y Universidad Autónoma Metropolitana.

Díaz, D., Valero, J., Airado, C., Baltanás, F. C., Weruaga, E., and Alonso, J. R. (2009). Sexual dimorphic stages affect both proliferation and serotonergic innervation in the adult rostral migratory stream. *Exp. Neurol.* 216, 357–364. doi: 10.1016/j.expneurol.2008.12.013

Eisch, A. J., Barrot, M., Schad, C. A., Self, D. W., and Nestler, E. J. (2000). Opiates inhibit neurogenesis in the adult rat hippocampus. *Proc. Natl. Acad. Sci. U.S.A.* 97, 7579–7584. doi: 10.1073/pnas.120552597

Erskine, M. S. (1993). Mating-induced increases in FOS protein in preoptic area and medial amygdala of cycling female rats. *Brain Res. Bull.* 32, 447–451. doi: 10.1016/0361-9230(93)90289-N

Erskine, M. S. (1995). Prolactin release after mating and genitosensory stimulation in females. *Endocr. Rev.* 16, 508–528.

Erskine, M. S., and Hanrahan, S. B. (1997). Effects of paced mating on c-fos gene expression in the female rat brain. *J. Neuroendocrinol.* 9, 903–912. doi: 10.1046/j.1365-2826.1997.00660.x

Furuta, M., and Bridges, R. S. (2009). Effects of maternal behavior induction and pup exposure on neurogenesis in adult, virgin female rats. *Brain Res. Bull.* 80, 408–413. doi: 10.1016/j.brainresbull.2009.08.011

Garcia-Horsman, S. P., Agmo, A., and Paredes, R. G. (2008). Infusions of naloxone into the medial preoptic area, ventromedial nucleus of the hypothalamus, and amygdala block conditioned place preference induced by paced mating behavior. *Horm. Behav.* 54, 709–716. doi: 10.1016/j.yhbeh.2008.07.011

Gritti, A., Bonfanti, L., Doetsch, F., Caille, I., Alvarez-Buylla, A., Lim, D. A., et al. (2002). Multipotent neural stem cells reside into the rostral extension and olfactory bulb of adult rodents. *J. Neurosci.* 22, 437–445.

Guarraci, F. A., and Clark, A. S. (2006). Ibotenic acid lesions of the medial preoptic area disrupt the expression of partner preference in sexually receptive female rats. *Brain Res.* 1076, 163–170. doi: 10.1016/j.brainres.2005.12.120

Halpern, M., Shapiro, L. S., and Jia, C. (1998). Heterogeneity in the accessory olfactory system. *Chem. Senses* 23, 477–481. doi: 10.1093/chemse/23.4.477

Hardy, D. F., and DeBold, J. F. (1972). Effects of coital stimulation upon behavior of the female rat. *J. Comp. Physiol. Psychol.* 78, 400–408. doi: 10.1037/h0032536

Honda, N., Sakamoto, H., Inamura, K., and Kashiwayanagi, M. (2008). Changes in Fos expression in the accessory olfactory bulb of sexually experienced male rats after exposure to female urinary pheromones. *Eur. J. Neurosci.* 27, 1980–1988. doi: 10.1111/j.1460-9568.2008.06169.x

Hosokawa, N., and Chiba, A. (2005). Effects of sexual experience on conspecific odor preference and estrous odor-induced activation of the vomeronasal projection pathway and the nucleus accumbens in male rats. *Brain Res.* 1066, 101–108. doi: 10.1016/j.brainres.2005.10.036

Huang, L., and Bittman, E. L. (2002). Olfactory bulb cells generated in adult male golden hamsters are specifically activated by exposure to estrous females. *Horm. Behav.* 41, 343–350. doi: 10.1006/hbeh.2002.1767

Inamura, K., Kashiwayanagi, M., and Kurihara, K. (1999a). Regionalization of Fos immunostaining in rat accessory olfactory bulb when the vomeronasal organ was exposed to urine. *Eur. J. Neurosci.* 11, 2254–2260. doi: 10.1046/j.1460-9568.1999.00646.x

Inamura, K., Matsumoto, Y., Kashiwayanagi, M., and Kurihara, K. (1999b). Laminar distribution of pheromone-receptive neurons in rat vomeronasal epithelium. *J. Physiol.* 517(Pt 3), 731–739. doi: 10.1111/j.1469-7793.1999.0731s.x

Keller, M., Baum, M. J., Brock, O., Brennan, P. A., and Bakker, J. (2009). The main and the accessory olfactory systems interact in the control of mate recognition and sexual behavior. *Behav. Brain Res.* 200, 268–276. doi: 10.1016/j.bbr.2009.01.020

Keller, M., Pierman, S., Douhard, Q., Baum, M. J., and Bakker, J. (2006). The vomeronasal organ is required for the expression of lordosis behaviour, but not sex discrimination in female mice. *Eur. J. Neurosci.* 23, 521–530. doi: 10.1111/j.1460-9568.2005.04589.x

Larriva-Sahd, J. (2008). The accessory olfactory bulb in the adult rat: a cytological study of its cell types, neuropil, neuronal modules, and interactions with the main olfactory system. *J. Comp. Neurol.* 510, 309–350. doi: 10.1002/cne.21790

Lledo, P. M., Alonso, M., and Grubb, M. S. (2006). Adult neurogenesis and functional plasticity in neuronal circuits. *Nat. Rev. Neurosci.* 7, 179–193. doi: 10.1038/nrn1867

Lois, C., and Alvarez-Buylla, A. (1993). Proliferating subventricular zone cells in the adult mammalian forebrain can differentiate into neurons and glia. *Proc. Natl. Acad. Sci. U.S.A.* 90, 2074–2077. doi: 10.1073/pnas.90.5.2074

Lois, C., and Alvarez-Buylla, A. (1994). Long-distance neuronal migration in the adult mammalian brain. *Science* 264, 1145–1148. doi: 10.1126/science.8178174

Mackay-Sim, A., and Rose, J. D. (1986). Removal of the vomeronasal organ impairs lordosis in female hamsters: effect is reversed by luteinising hormone-releasing hormone. *Neuroendocrinology* 42, 489–493. doi: 10.1159/000124492

Magavi, S. S., Mitchell, B. D., Szentirmai, O., Carter, B. S., and Macklis, J. D. (2005). Adult-born and preexisting olfactory granule neurons undergo distinct experience-dependent modifications of their olfactory responses *in vivo*. *J. Neurosci.* 25, 10729–10739. doi: 10.1523/JNEUROSCI.2250-05.2005

Mak, G. K., Enwere, E. K., Gregg, C., Pakarainen, T., Poutanen, M., Huhtaniemi, I., et al. (2007). Male pheromone-stimulated neurogenesis in the adult female brain: possible role in mating behavior. *Nat. Neurosci.* 10, 1003–1011. doi: 10.1038/nn1928

Martínez, I., and Paredes, R. G. (2001). Only self-paced mating is rewarding in rats of both sexes. *Horm. Behav.* 40, 510–517. doi: 10.1006/hbeh.2001.1712

Martínez-Marcos, A., and Halpern, M. (1999). Differential projections from the anterior and posterior divisions of the accessory olfactory bulb to the medial amygdala in the opossum, Monodelphis domestica. *Eur. J. Neurosci.* 11, 3789–3799. doi: 10.1046/j.1460-9568.1999.00797.x

Martínez-Marcos, A., Ubeda-Bañón, I., and Halpern, M. (2001). Cell migration to the anterior and posterior divisions of the granule cell layer of the accessory olfactory bulb of adult opossums. *Brain Res. Dev. Brain Res.* 127, 95–98. doi: 10.1016/S0165-3806(01)00106-7

McClintock, M. K., and Adler, N. T. (1978). The role of the female during copulation in wild domestic Norway rats (*Rattus norvegicus*). *Behaviour* 67, 67–96. doi: 10.1163/156853978X00260

McClintock, M. K., and Anisko, J. J. (1982). Group mating among Norway rats I. Sex differences in the pattern and neuroendocrine consequences of copulation. *Animal Behav.* 30, 12. doi: 10.1016/S0003-3472(82)80051-1

Merkle, F. T., Mirzadeh, Z., and Alvarez-Buylla, A. (2007). Mosaic organization of neural stem cells in the adult brain. *Science* 317, 381–384. doi: 10.1126/science.1144914

Ming, G. L., and Song, H. (2005). Adult neurogenesis in the mammalian central nervous system. *Annu. Rev. Neurosci.* 28, 223–250. doi: 10.1146/annurev.neuro.28.051804.101459

Ming, G. L., and Song, H. (2011). Adult neurogenesis in the mammalian brain: significant answers and significant questions. *Neuron* 70, 687–702. doi: 10.1016/j.neuron.2011.05.001

Nissant, A., Bardy, C., Katagiri, H., Murray, K., and Lledo, P. M. (2009). Adult neurogenesis promotes synaptic plasticity in the olfactory bulb. *Nat. Neurosci.* 12, 728–730. doi: 10.1038/nn.2298

Nunez-Parra, A., Pugh, V., and Araneda, R. C. (2011). Regulation of adult neurogenesis by behavior and age in the accessory olfactory bulb. *Mol. Cell. Neurosci.* 47, 274–285. doi: 10.1016/j.mcn.2011.05.003

Oboti, L., Savalli, G., Giachino, C., De Marchis, S., Panzica, G. C., Fasolo, A., et al. (2009). Integration and sensory experience-dependent survival of newly-generated neurons in the accessory olfactory bulb of female mice. *Eur. J. Neurosci.* 29, 679–692. doi: 10.1111/j.1460-9568.2009.06614.x

Oboti, L., Schellino, R., Giachino, C., Chamero, P., Pyrski, M., Leinders-Zufall, T., et al. (2011). Newborn interneurons in the accessory olfactory bulb promote mate recognition in female mice. *Front. Neurosci.* 5:113. doi: 10.3389/fnins.2011.00113

Paredes, R. G., and Alonso, A. (1997). Sexual behavior regulated (paced) by the female induces conditioned place preference. *Behav. Neurosci.* 111, 123–128. doi: 10.1037/0735-7044.111.1.123

Paredes, R. G., and Martínez, I. (2001). Naloxone blocks place preference conditioning after paced mating in female rats. *Behav. Neurosci.* 115, 1363–1367. doi: 10.1037/0735-7044.115.6.1363

Paredes, R. G., and Vazquez, B. (1999). What do female rats like about sex? Paced mating. *Behav. Brain Res.* 105, 117–127. doi: 10.1016/S0166-4328(99)00087-X

Peretto, P., Schellino, R., De Marchis, S., and Fasolo, A. (2014). The interplay between reproductive social stimuli and adult olfactory bulb neurogenesis. *Neural Plast.* 2014:497657. doi: 10.1155/2014/497657

Petreanu, L., and Alvarez-Buylla, A. (2002). Maturation and death of adult-born olfactory bulb granule neurons: role of olfaction. *J. Neurosci.* 22, 6106–6113.

Pettit, A. S., Desroches, R., and Bennett, S. A. (2012). The opiate analgesic buprenorphine decreases proliferation of adult hippocampal neuroblasts and increases survival of their progeny. *Neuroscience* 200, 211–222. doi: 10.1016/j.neuroscience.2011.10.039

Portillo, W., and Paredes, R. G. (2004). Sexual incentive motivation, olfactory preference, and activation of the vomeronasal projection pathway by sexually relevant cues in non-copulating and naive male rats. *Horm. Behav.* 46, 330–340. doi: 10.1016/j.yhbeh.2004.03.001

Portillo, W., Unda, N., Camacho, F. J., Sánchez, M., Corona, R., Arzate, D. M., et al. (2012). Sexual activity increases the number of newborn cells in the accessory olfactory bulb of male rats. *Front. Neuroanat.* 6:25. doi: 10.3389/fnana.2012.00025

Saghatelyan, A., Carleton, A., Lagier, S., de Chevigny, A., and Lledo, P. M. (2003). Local neurons play key roles in the mammalian olfactory bulb. *J. Physiol. Paris* 97, 517–528. doi: 10.1016/j.jphysparis.2004.01.009

Shingo, T., Gregg, C., Enwere, E., Fujikawa, H., Hassam, R., Geary, C., et al. (2003). Pregnancy-stimulated neurogenesis in the adult female forebrain mediated by prolactin. *Science* 299, 117–120. doi: 10.1126/science.1076647

Sinchak, K., Dewing, P., Cook, M., and Micevych, P. (2007). Release of orphanin FQ/nociceptin in the medial preoptic nucleus and ventromedial nucleus of the hypothalamus facilitates lordosis. *Horm. Behav.* 51, 406–412. doi: 10.1016/j.yhbeh.2006.12.008

Smith, M. T., Pencea, V., Wang, Z., Luskin, M. B., and Insel, T. R. (2001). Increased number of BrdU-labeled neurons in the rostral migratory stream of the estrous prairie vole. *Horm. Behav.* 39, 11–21. doi: 10.1006/hbeh.2000.1630

Sugai, T., Yoshimura, H., Kato, N., and Onoda, N. (2006). Component-dependent urine responses in the rat accessory olfactory bulb. *Neuroreport* 17, 1663–1667. doi: 10.1097/01.wnr.0000239950.14954.59

Takahashi, T., Zhu, Y., Hata, T., Shimizu-Okabe, C., Suzuki, K., and Nakahara, D. (2009). Intracranial self-stimulation enhances neurogenesis in hippocampus of adult mice and rats. *Neuroscience* 158, 402–411. doi: 10.1016/j.neuroscience.2008.10.048

Tegeder, I., and Geisslinger, G. (2004). Opioids as modulators of cell death and survival–unraveling mechanisms and revealing new indications. *Pharmacol. Rev.* 56, 351–369. doi: 10.1124/pr.56.3.2

Tietz, N. W. (ed.) (1995). *Clinical/Guide to Laboratory Tests, 3rd Edn.* Philadelphia, PA: W.B. Saunders, CO.

Wysocki, C. J., Kruczek, M., Wysocki, L. M., and Lepri, J. J. (1991). Activation of reproduction in nulliparous and primiparous voles is blocked by vomeronasal organ removal. *Biol. Reprod.* 45, 611–616. doi: 10.1095/biolreprod45.4.611

19

The Ever-Changing Morphology of Hippocampal Granule Neurons in Physiology and Pathology

María Llorens-Martín[1,2*], *Alberto Rábano*[2,3] *and Jesús Ávila*[1,2*]

[1] *Molecular Neurobiology, Function of Microtubular Proteins, Centro de Biología Molecular Severo Ochoa (Consejo Superior de Investigaciones Científicas-Universidad Autónoma de Madrid), Madrid, Spain,* [2] *Centro de Investigación Biomédica en Red sobre Enfermedades Neurodegenerativas (Instituto de Salud Carlos III), Madrid, Spain,* [3] *Neuropathology Department, CIEN Foundation, Madrid, Spain*

Edited by:
José Luis Trejo, Instituto Cajal, Spain

Reviewed by:
Janice R. Naegele, Wesleyan University, USA
Francesca Ciccolini, Heidelberg University, Germany
Juan Manuel Encinas, Ikerbasque and University of the Basque Country, Spain

***Correspondence:**
María Llorens-Martín
m.llorens@csic.es;
Jesús Ávila
javila@cbm.csic.es

Newborn neurons are continuously added to the hippocampal dentate gyrus throughout adulthood. In this review, we analyze the maturational stages that newborn granule neurons go through, with a focus on their unique morphological features during each stage under both physiological and pathological circumstances. In addition, the influence of deleterious (such as schizophrenia, stress, Alzheimer's disease, seizures, stroke, inflammation, dietary deficiencies, or the consumption of drugs of abuse or toxic substances) and neuroprotective (physical exercise and environmental enrichment) stimuli on the maturation of these cells will be examined. Finally, the regulation of this process by proteins involved in neurodegenerative and neurological disorders such as Glycogen synthase kinase 3β, Disrupted in Schizophrenia 1 (DISC-1), Glucocorticoid receptor, pro-inflammatory mediators, Presenilin-1, Amyloid precursor protein, Cyclin-dependent kinase 5 (CDK5), among others, will be evaluated. Given the recently acquired relevance of the dendritic branch as a functional synaptic unit required for memory storage, a full understanding of the morphological alterations observed in newborn neurons may have important consequences for the prevention and treatment of the cognitive and affective alterations that evolve in conjunction with impaired adult hippocampal neurogenesis.

Keywords: neurogenesis, hippocampus, morphology, neurodegeneration, neuroprotection, retrovirus, golgi, newborn granule neuron

Despite increasing knowledge regarding the developmental steps that control the proliferation, differentiation, and integration of adult-born granule neurons in the hippocampal circuit, the regulatory genes required for morphological maturation and neurite growth of newborn granule cells remain largely unknown. Given that alterations in adult hippocampal neurogenesis (AHN) may be key components in hippocampus-associated neurological diseases, such as major depression (Malberg et al., 2000; Santarelli et al., 2003), schizophrenia (Suh et al., 2013), Alzheimer's disease (AD) (Perry et al., 2012), and epilepsy (Lothman et al., 1992), understanding the molecular mechanisms underlying neuronal migration, neurite extension, and dendrite pathfinding of newborn neurons will be crucial if headway is to be made in the prevention and treatment of neurological and neurodegenerative diseases.

In this review, the fundamental aspects regulating the establishment of the classical morphology of the hippocampal granule neuron will be evaluated under physiological conditions. Pathological aspects will be also discussed. Given the recently acquired relevance of the dendritic branch as a functional synaptic unit needed for memory storage (Govindarajan et al., 2011), alterations in the appropriate branching, structure, and pathfinding of neurites might have far-reaching effects on the synaptic integration and activity of these newborn neurons, phenomena demonstrated to be dysregulated in the aforementioned disorders.

VARIATIONS IN THE MORPHOLOGY OF NEWBORN GRANULE NEURONS UNDER PHYSIOLOGICAL CONDITIONS

Morphological Maturation of Newborn Granule Neurons

Under physiological conditions, the generation of newborn neurons in the adult brain of vertebrates occurs mainly in two regions, namely the subventricular zone of the lateral ventricles and the subgranular zone (SGZ) of the hippocampal dentate gyrus (DG) (Kempermann et al., 1998). Adult hippocampal neurogenesis (AHN) occurs in several vertebrate species, including humans (Eriksson et al., 1998; Spalding et al., 2013). In the latter, AHN is quantitatively much more important than adult neurogenesis in the subventricular zone. In addition, while a net age-related reduction of AHN occurs in rodents, in humans only a modest decline in turnover rate has been reported (Spalding et al., 2013), thus supporting the predominant role played by the hippocampus in cognitive processing in our species (Spalding et al., 2013). The maturational stages that newborn neurons go through before becoming fully mature can be identified on the basis not only of the expression of specific molecular markers but also of unique morphological features, as shown in **Figure 1A**. In the DG, Type-1 cells have a triangular soma and a single apical prolongation that enters the granule cell layer (GL), branching sparsely in the inner molecular layer (IML), where it disperses into many small processes (Kempermann et al., 2004). After dividing asymmetrically, radial-glia-like progenitor (or Type 1) cells give rise to a transiently amplifying population of intermediate neuronal precursors (Type 2 cells). From an electrophysiological and morphological perspective, the transiently amplifying progenitor stage comprises a heterogeneous population of cells. During their initial stages of differentiation (Type-2 cells), they have flabby short processes oriented tangentially and an irregularly shaped dense nucleus. However, during more advanced stages of differentiation, such as the neuroblast stage (Type-3 cells), the greatest morphological and electrophysiological changes occur, and the expression of neuronal markers progressively increases. At the end of this stage, cells are oriented vertically and they present a rounded or slightly triangular nucleus and a clearly visible apical dendrite (Kempermann et al., 2004). By means of retroviral labeling of newborn neurons, Zhao et al. demonstrated that the apical dendrite of these cells reaches the IML and the edge of the molecular layer (ML) at 10 and 21 days post-injection, respectively (Zhao et al., 2006). The complexity of the dendritic tree of immature newborn neurons increases sequentially during subsequent maturational stages. Dendritic spines can be observed for the first time around 16 days after retroviral injection (Zhao et al., 2006). Excitatory synapses appear around the third week of cell life (Kelsch et al., 2008). Once dendritic spines have formed, their number, volume and complexity progressively increase until reaching a plateau at 8–10 weeks of cell age (van Praag et al., 2002). At the end of this maturational process, newborn neurons are fully integrated into tri-synaptic circuits and are electrophysiologically and morphologically indistinguishable from surrounding mature granule neurons (Zhao et al., 2006; Llorens-Martin et al., 2015). Mature granule neurons generally have only one primary apical dendrite emerging from the soma and which is vertically oriented toward the ML. This dendrite remains poorly bifurcated until it reaches the ML, where it branches extensively in order to receive its main afferents, namely the perforant pathway from the Entorhinal cortex (EC). We refer to this characteristic morphology of granule neurons as "Y-shape," which contrasts with the other shapes present in several pathological conditions, as will be further commented. In this regard, it is noteworthy that, under physiological conditions, the length of the primary apical dendrite is generally inversely correlated to the position that the cell occupies in the GL. Thus, cells whose nuclei are placed in the outer third of the GL have much shorter primary apical dendrites than cells located in the inner section of this layer. While this empirical observation has been systematically reported in the literature, it has received little attention. However, whether migration to the outer sections of the GL is accompanied by and related to the retraction of the primary apical dendrite merits further study. The shortening of the primary apical dendrite should be considered a physiological difference between newborn granule neurons and those generated during development (which are generally located in the outer third of the GL) and should not be confused with the pathological shortening of that occurs in some pathologies. As pointed out by Redila et al., cells with more than one primary apical dendrite appear almost exclusively in the outer third of the GL under physiological conditions and do not seem to correspond to adult-generated neurons but rather to old granule neurons generated during development (Redila and Christie, 2006).

Figure 1 shows the characteristic morphology of the stages of granule cell development previously mentioned (**Figure 1A**), as well as the representative Sholl's analysis of the dendritic tree of these retrovirally labeled cells at various ages (**Figure 1B**). As can be observed, the most outstanding outgrowth of the dendritic tree occurs between 2 and 4 weeks after retroviral injections.

During differentiation, newborn neurons progressively lengthen their axons [the mossy fibers (MFs)] and send them toward the CA3 (Zhao et al., 2006) and CA2 (Llorens-Martin et al., 2015) hippocampal regions. Kohara et al. (2014) have recently demonstrated that mature granule neurons establish functional synapses not only with CA3 but also with CA2 pyramidal neurons. We have further confirmed these results and also shown that newborn neurons also establish synapses with the pyramidal neurons in CA2. The time-course of this latter connection follows a similar one to that observed for CA3 (Zhao et al., 2006; Llorens-Martin et al., 2015). The first axonal processes appear in the hilus 10 days after retroviral injection and subsequently reach CA3 and CA2 at 12–13 days (Zhao et al.,

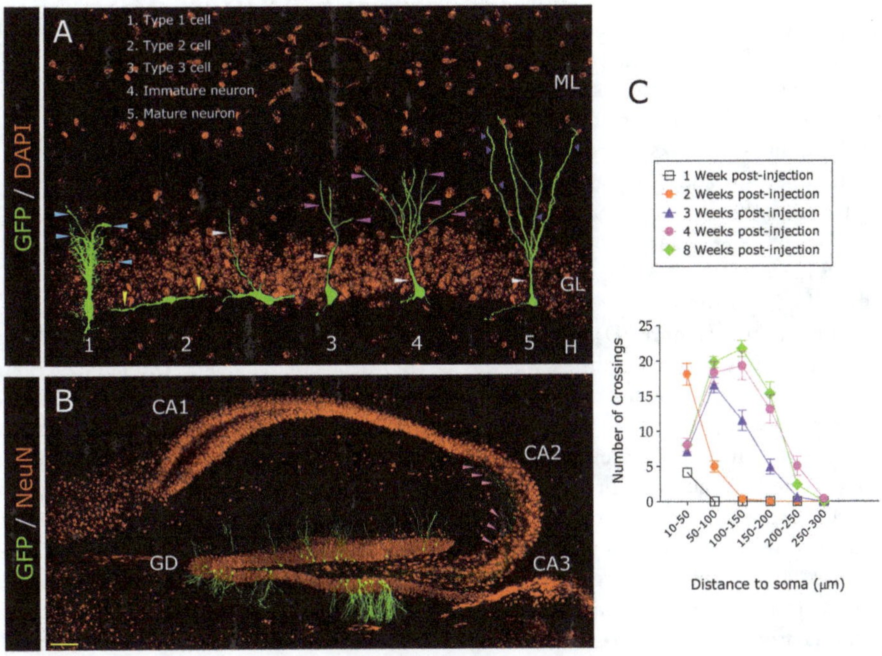

FIGURE 1 | Morphological maturation of newborn granule neurons under physiological conditions. In **(A)** the different morphological stages newborn neurons go through before becoming mature are shown. Type-1 cells have a triangular soma and a single apical prolongation that enters the granule cell layer, branching sparsely in the inner molecular layer, where it disperses into many small processes (pale blue triangles). Type-1 cells divide asymmetrically and give rise to transient amplifying progenitors. During their initial stages of differentiation, Type-2 cells have short processes oriented tangentially (yellow triangles) and an irregularly shaped dense nucleus. However, during more advanced stages of differentiation such as the neuroblast stage (Type-3 cells), the greatest morphological changes occur. At the end of this stage, cells are oriented vertically and present a rounded or slightly triangular nucleus and a clearly visible apical dendrite (white triangle). Immature newborn neurons sequentially increase the complexity of their dendritic trees (purple triangles) during subsequent maturational stages until they are indistinguishable from surrounding mature granule neurons. **(B)** Newborn neurons progressively enlarge their axons and send them toward the CA3 and the CA2 regions (pink triangles). In **(C)** the Sholl's analysis of 1-, 2-, 3-, 4-, and 8-, week-old newborn granule neurons is shown. Dendritic branching progressively increases with age. The greatest morphological changes occur between 2 and 4 weeks post-injection. H, Hilus; GL, Granule cell layer; ML, Molecular layer. Yellow scale bar: 100 μm. Dark blue triangles, Dendritic spines.

2006; Llorens-Martin et al., 2015). **Figure 1C** shows how the axons of mature granule neurons labeled with GFP-expressing retroviruses reach the CA3 and CA2 regions.

Differences among Mammalian Species

As previously commented, the dendritic tree of rodent granule neurons has a "Y-shape." The lack of basal dendrites in mature granule neurons is a hallmark of these cells in rodents under physiological conditions (Seress and Pokorny, 1981; Shapiro et al., 2005). In fact, granule cells with basal dendrites appear to be a recent formation in phylogeny. In this regard, their morphological variability is greater in humans (Seress and Mrzljak, 1987) than in rats and primates (Seress and Frotscher, 1990; Frotscher et al., 1991; Senitz and Beckmann, 2003). In rats, only up to 2% of granule cells show basal dendrites (Seress and Pokorny, 1981; Spigelman et al., 1998). In primates, 10% of these cells present these structures (Seress, 1992; Seress and Ribak, 1992), while 30% of granule cells from human control subjects show basal dendrites (Seress and Mrzljak, 1987; Senitz and Beckmann, 2003). As an exception, the presence of basal dendrites in rodent granule neurons has been described only in very immature neurons (Ribak et al., 2004) and in organotypic hippocampal cultures. In the latter case, it has been proposed that these structures are due to deafferentation caused by hippocampus sectioning (Heimrich and Frotscher, 1991).

Regarding the morphology of granule neurons in the human brain, in 1987, two simultaneous studies by de Ruiters et al. and Flood et al. were published, in which the morphology of these cells in non-demented aged subjects was described (de Ruiter and Uylings, 1987; Flood et al., 1987). Using Golgi staining, these authors indicated that, as in rodents, inverted-cone morphology is typical of human granule neurons. They showed that the highest branching of the dendritic tree occurs in the inner third of the ML. Although the presence of basal dendrites did not take place in all the subjects studied, the presence of thick basal dendrites full of spines was found to be a common feature of granule neurons. In a later study, Einstein et al. (1994) labeled granule neurons intracellularly with Lucifer Yellow and further confirmed the previous results obtained with Golgi staining, corroborating the presence of numerous spines of distinct shapes in the apical dendrites of these cells. In addition, Senitz et al. described four types of granule neuron in humans on the basis of the positioning and branching of the dendrites (Lauer et al., 2003; Senitz and Beckmann, 2003). In addition, Flood et al. reported age-related dendritic shortening in very elderly humans (Flood et al., 1985, 1987).

In non-human primates, the morphology of granule neurons has received little attention. Kohler et al. reported significant differences in the timing of the maturation of newborn neurons in Macaque monkeys compared to rodents (Kohler et al., 2011). Whereas newborn granule neurons in rodents complete their morphological maturation within 8–10 weeks (Zhao et al., 2006), these authors demonstrated that 4th and 5th branching order dendrites occur only after 11 or 23 weeks of maturation in the newborn granule neurons of the Macaque monkey (Kohler et al., 2011). **Figure 2** shows the appearance of the Golgi-stained DGs of the mouse (**Figure 2A**), Capuchine monkey (**Figure 2B**), Chimpanzee (**Figure 2C**), and human (**Figure 2D**). It should be noted that murine granule neurons lack basal dendrites, whereas chimpanzee and human ones present numerous ramified basal dendrites with abundant spines.

Only a few other species of mammals have received attention regarding the morphology of granule neurons. For example, the granule neurons of megachiropteran bats (flying fox) have been reported to be more similar to those of primates than to those of rodents (Buhl and Dann, 1990). The main difference observed between these bats and rodents is that the latter have functional basal dendrites in granule neurons, while these structures are largely absent in the former under physiological conditions.

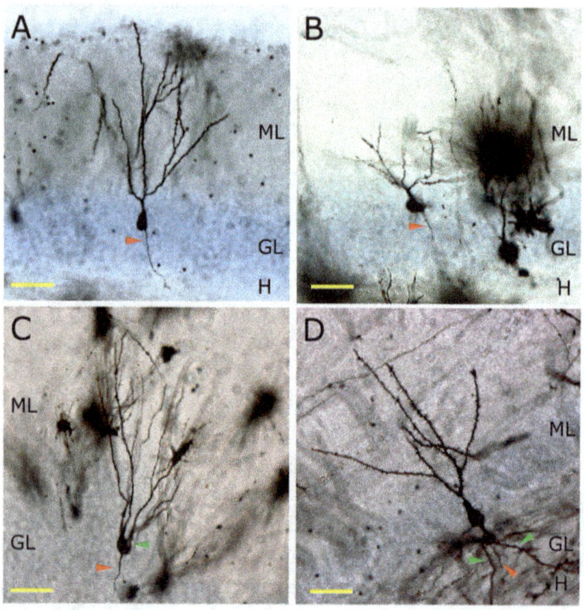

FIGURE 2 | The morphology of granule neurons among different mammalian species. In **(A)** the morphology of a Golgi-impregnated murine granule neuron is shown. The total lack of basal dendrites, as well as the presence of one single primary apical dendrite and one axonal process (red triangle) can be observed. In the Capuchine monkey, a great variability of morphologies is observed. A representative neuron lacking basal dendrites and having one apical dendrite and one axonal process is shown **(B)**. Conversely, one of the most remarkable morphological features of the granule neurons of the Chimpanzee **(C)** is the presence of basal dendrites (green triangle). The same feature can be observed in human granule neurons **(D)**, in which a profusely branched basal dendrite emerges from the bottom of the cell soma and ramifies in the hilus. H, Hilus; GL, Granule cell layer; ML, Molecular layer. Yellow scale bar: 50 μm.

REGULATION OF THE MORPHOLOGICAL MATURATION OF NEWBORN NEURONS BY NEUROPROTECTIVE STIMULI

In general terms, neuroprotective stimuli such as physical exercise or environmental enrichment promote morphological maturation of newborn granule neurons, as will be further discussed in this section.

Physical Exercise

Physical activity is one of the most potent stimulators of AHN (van Praag et al., 1999a,b). It exerts anti-depressant (Bjornebekk et al., 2005; Duman, 2005) and anxiolytic (Duman et al., 2008; Trejo et al., 2008; Salam et al., 2009) actions and stimulates hippocampal-dependent memory (Cotman and Berchtold, 2002; Parle et al., 2005; van Praag et al., 2005; Creer et al., 2010). These beneficial effects have been observed not only in young (van Praag et al., 1999b; Llorens-Martin et al., 2006) but also in aged (Kronenberg et al., 2006; Hollmann et al., 2007; Fabel and Kempermann, 2008) individuals, and physical exercise has been proposed as a co-adjuvant for the treatment of several neurodegenerative and mood disorders (Cotman and Engesser-Cesar, 2002), since it delays the progression of the disease in several animal models (Adlard et al., 2005) and human patients (Cotman and Berchtold, 2002; Hoffmann et al., 2013). Among the hypotheses aiming to explain the beneficial effects exerted by physical activity on the brain, the "neurotrophic hypothesis of physical exercise" postulates that these favorable actions critically depend on the increase in the levels of growth factors that it induces (reviewed in Llorens-Martin et al., 2008). Physical activity increases the levels of brain-derived neurotrophic factor (BDNF) (Neeper et al., 1995, 1996; Oliff et al., 1998), insulin-like growth factor I (Trejo et al., 2001), vascular-endothelial growth factor (VEGF) (Fabel et al., 2003), and nerve growth factor (NGF) (Chae et al., 2012), among others. In the adult hippocampus, running stimulates neuron precursor proliferation (van Praag et al., 1999b; Olson et al., 2006), a process that is mediated by an increase in the circulating levels of IGF-I (Trejo et al., 2001), VEGF (Fabel et al., 2003; During and Cao, 2006), and BDNF (Vaynman et al., 2004). The downstream molecular pathways triggered by these factors converge in the stimulation of the AKT pro-survival pathway and, interestingly, in the inhibition of GSK-3β (Chen and Russo-Neustadt, 2005; Bruel-Jungerman et al., 2009), a pivotal kinase involved in several neurodegenerative disorders (Llorens-Martin et al., 2014b) and that dramatically impairs AHN (Fuster-Matanzo et al., 2013; Llorens-Martin et al., 2013).

Regarding the enhancement of newborn neuron development by physical activity, several studies involving Golgi staining have shown that it increases the percentage of cells with a single primary apical dendrite and also the total dendritic length of granule cells (Redila and Christie, 2006; Stranahan et al., 2007). The use of the same technique revealed that physical activity increases the number of dendritic spines in these cells (Stranahan et al., 2009; Glasper et al., 2010). Using 3R-Tau, a novel marker for newborn neuron axons, we have demonstrated that physical exercise accelerates the appearance of these nerve fibers in newborn neurons (Llorens-Martin et al., 2012) and enhances the innervation of the CA2 region by these cells (Llorens-Martin et al., 2015). Importantly, using a retroviral labeling approach, Zhao et al. demonstrated that physical exercise accelerates the morphological maturation of newborn neurons. In addition to these morphological changes, physical exercise increases the number of mushroom spines in newborn neurons (Zhao et al., 2006).

Of all the neurotrophic factors increased by physical exercise, BDNF seems to play a crucial role in the dendritic alterations caused by running. In fact, BDNF has been demonstrated to exert autocrine actions on the morphological development of newborn neurons, and hence, BDNF knockdown in newborn neurons dramatically reduces the total length and branching of dendrites and prevents the stimulatory effects of exercise on these parameters (Wang et al., 2015). Accordingly, the central knockdown of BDNF causes the same effect on newborn neurons: both the total dendritic length and the number of branches are reduced in mutant mice (Chan et al., 2008). In addition, the overexpression of BDNF leads to an increased dendritic complexity in granule neurons (Tolwani et al., 2002). These observations thus support the pivotal role played by this growth factor in the maturation and integration of newborn granule neurons and emphasize its essential role as mediator of the stimulatory effects of physical exercise.

Environmental Enrichment

Environmental enrichment (EE), an experimental manipulation that consists of a combination of physical activity, social interaction, and cognitive stimulation, is neuroprotective under both physiological and pathological circumstances (van Praag et al., 2000). EE increases AHN both in combination and in the absence of physical activity. In addition to the pro-proliferative actions of physical activity, EE is also a pro-survival stimulus and it triggers the maturation of newborn neurons (Llorens-Martin et al., 2011).

The first studies on the effects of EE on the brain showed that a period of enhanced environmental complexity increases dendritic branching in hippocampal neurons during development (Fiala et al., 1978). In the adult, these studies revealed that EE increased neurite branching and synapse formation in the cortex (Holloway, 1966; Greenough and Volkmar, 1973; Greenough et al., 1973; Diamond et al., 1976). Subsequent research demonstrated that EE triggers similar morphological changes in granule neurons. In particular, this stimulatory procedure increases the number of dendrites per neuron and the complexity of the dendritic tree (Juraska et al., 1985). Using Golgi staining, Faherty et al. showed that EE also increases the total dendritic length of granule neurons (Faherty et al., 2003). By analyzing dendritic complexity in DCX-expressing cells, Choi et al., demonstrated that EE increases the total length and complexity of dendrites in immature neuroblasts (Choi et al., 2008). In addition, these authors further confirmed the notion that BDNF is required for normal dendritic development under standard housing conditions; however, BDNF-independent effects of EE were suggested, since the stimulatory effects of this exposure also occur in BDNF knockout mice (Choi et al., 2008). Using a retroviral labeling approach, we demonstrated that EE increases the maturation and connectivity of newborn granule neurons in control animals and also in a model of AD (Llorens-Martin et al., 2013). These data, together with numerous reports in the literature demonstrating the positive effects of EE on various neurodegenerative and neurological diseases, points to the promise of this approach as a suitable adjuvant treatment for these disorders.

CREB Signaling Pathway

One potential mechanism underlying the effects of physical exercise and EE on the dendritic plasticity of newborn granule neurons involves the cAMP response element-binding protein (CREB). Several studies have shown that blocking CREB signaling leads to a dramatic decrease in hippocampal neurogenesis and dendritic arborization in newborn neurons (Jagasia et al., 2009), although the opposite results have also been reported (Gur et al., 2007). Among the many factors activated by CREB cascade, of particular importance are the microRNAs miR-212 and miR-132. The overexpression of miR-132 in cortical neurons increases dendritic branches *in vitro* (Vo et al., 2005). Using a Cre-recombinase-based system, Magill et al. demonstrated that the knockdown of miR-212/132 in newborn granule neurons dramatically decreases dendritic length and branching, and the number of dendritic spines. These authors also reported a drastic distal shrinkage and that most of the neurons lack secondary or tertiary dendrites (Magill et al., 2010).

Melatonin

Melatonin promotes microtubule polymerization, neuritogenesis, and the formation of dendritic spines *in vitro* (Bellon et al., 2007). In addition, it promotes the survival of newborn neurons in the hippocampus thus contributing to a net increase in the rate of AHN (Ramirez-Rodriguez et al., 2009). A marked decrease in the levels of melatonin has been described both during aging and during the course of neuropsychiatric disorders (Liu et al., 1999; Brusco et al., 2000). Using immunohistochemistry against DCX to label immature newborn neurons, Ramirez-Rodriguez et al. found that chronic melatonin treatment increases the complexity of the dendritic tree of immature neurons. Although melatonin increases dendritic branching in all the domains of the dendritic tree, the changes are more accentuated in the distal parts of the tree, as revealed Sholl's analysis (Ramirez-Rodriguez et al., 2011).

REGULATION OF THE MORPHOLOGY OF NEWBORN GRANULE NEURONS BY DETRIMENTAL STIMULI

Several detrimental stimuli have been demonstrated to be negative regulators of AHN. The particular effects exerted by several of them on the morphology of newborn neurons will be discussed in the following section.

Epilepsy-Induced Changes in the Morphology of Newborn Granule Neurons

In the nineties, Timm staining was used to show that the MFs of granule neurons of patients with temporal lobe epilepsy (TLE) present a marked sprouting toward the IML (Franck et al., 1995). In addition, von Campe et al. described an increased and aberrant branching of apical dendrites in the IML of TLE patients, as revealed by the injection of Lucifer Yellow into individual granule neurons. It was then proposed that the abnormal morphology of granule neurons contributes to the hyper-excitability of the DG (von Campe et al., 1997). However, whether the morphological features of the individual dysplastic cells give rise to increased susceptibility to seizures or whether these dysplastic cells contribute to seizure activity by establishing abnormal circuits is still a matter of debate. Abnormal basal dendrites, MF sprouting, and recurrent axonal collaterals contacting the dendritic spines of granule neurons have been described in various animal models of epilepsy (Sutula et al., 1988; Holmes et al., 1998, 1999; Dashtipour et al., 2002; Ribak and Dashtipour, 2002; Patel et al., 2004) and in human tissue (Houser, 1992; Lurton et al., 1998; El Bahh et al., 1999). Interestingly, it has been recently described that intrahippocampal kainic acid injection results also in MF sprouting in the CA2 region (Haussler et al., 2015).

These aberrant features are thought to contribute to the establishment of recurrent circuits, which affects the overall balance between excitation and inhibition in the DG (Patel et al., 2004). The abnormal basal dendrites form additional recurrent synapses with the aberrant axonal collaterals of the MF, thus aggravating the recurrent nature of the circuit (Patel et al., 2004). Although not all the experimental data support the idea of individual cell hyper-excitability in epilepsy (Patel et al., 2004), computational (Tejada et al., 2012, 2014) and *in vitro* (Beck et al., 1996; Bausch and McNamara, 2000) models do strongly reinforce this notion. In addition, the electrophysiological properties of granule cells aberrantly located in the hilar region were studied in a rat model of TLE and in epileptic patients by Althaus et al. The authors found an increased excitability in rat neurons whereas neurons obtained from patients displayed a clear reduction in excitability. They affirmed that the discrepancies may reflect differences between the late-stage disease tissue available from human patients and the earlier disease stage examined in the rat TLE model (Althaus et al., 2015). In line with this, Hester et al., found a correlation between severity and duration of seizure and the degree of aberrant integration of newborn granule neurons (namely, their aberrant location, hilar sprouting, and MF loss), thus suggesting that the aberrant synaptic integration of newborn granule neurons directly correlates with epileptogenesis (Hester and Danzer, 2013).

Regarding the specific participation of adult-born neurons to the epileptogenesis of the DG, it has been proposed that only newborn neurons present MF sprouting (Jessberger et al., 2007; Kron et al., 2010) and contribute to the hyper-excitability of the DG. In this regard, it is known that during the development of epilepsy in adult animals, newly generated granule cells integrate abnormally into the hippocampus. These newly generated cells migrate to ectopic locations in the hilus, develop aberrant basal dendrites, contribute to mossy fiber sprouting, and exhibit changes in apical dendrite structure and dendritic spine number (Santos et al., 2011). Using retroviral labeling to visualize newborn neurons, Jessberger et al. described, in a seminal work, a significant number of these cells with aberrant morphology comprising additional basal dendrites directed into the hilus and an ectopic positioning of the cells after seizures (Jessberger et al., 2007). In addition, Cho et al. demonstrated that ablation of neurogenesis is sufficient to alleviate the cognitive decline produced by seizure activity and to prevent the development of subsequent seizures for at least 1 year. This observation thus supports the prevalent role of these cells in the epileptogenesis of the DG (Cho et al., 2015). Moreover, Hester et al., suggested that the accumulation of aberrantly generated newborn neurons directly and specifically contributes to the development of epilepsy (Hester and Danzer, 2013). Interestingly, Santos et al., demonstrated that the apical dendrites of mature newborn neurons generated 2 months before the induction of the status epilepticus, do not undergo morphological changes when they were exposed to *status epilepticus*, although synaptic rearrangement was observed (Santos et al., 2011).

Regarding the morphological changes affecting the apical dendrites of newborn neurons, doublecortin (DCX)-expressing neuroblasts undergo changes in the pilocarpine model of epilepsy (Parent et al., 1997; Arisi and Garcia-Cairasco, 2007). An increased branching of apical dendrites has been shown to occur in the regions in which MF sprouting is most evident, namely the GL and the IML (Arisi and Garcia-Cairasco, 2007). In addition, Overstreet et al. demonstrated that seizures accelerate the morphological maturation and functional integration of 2-week-old newborn neurons into the trisynaptic circuit (Overstreet-Wadiche et al., 2006). Nevertheless, Gao et al. have recently demonstrated that newborn neurons generated 5 days after pilocarpine injection were morphologically indistinguishable from control neurons, although an increase in the percentage of mushroom spines were found in pilocarpine-treated neurons (Gao et al., 2015). The normal integration of newborn neurons generated after status epilepticus into the trisynaptic circuit was further confirmed by the use of retroviral tracing in a work published by Hu et al. (2015).

An finally, in contrast to the data involving newborn neurons in the development of epilepsy, other data suggest that a reduction in neurogenesis increases brain susceptibility to the effects of kainic acid (Iyengar et al., 2015) and that neurogenesis plays a protective role in epileptogenesis (Kempermann, 2006).

Taken together, these data point to the tightly regulated role of newborn neurons in epilepsy. Further studies will be needed to elucidate the individual contribution of cells with varying degrees of maturation to this process. Although it is known that the abnormal networks in which newborn neurons are involved during epilepsy promote abnormal neuronal firing and hyperexcitability, it has yet to be established whether they directly contribute to seizure generation (Hester and Danzer, 2013). In addition, an inspiring idea has been suggested by Murphy et al. (2011). The authors proposed the existence of heterogeneous morphological and synaptic adaptations among the different newborn granule neurons to epilepsy. They observed that, while some newborn neurons underwent certain types of morphological and functional adaptations, other neurons showed the opposite changes, thus suggesting that newborn granule neurons may play diverse homeostatic and contradictory roles in epileptogenesis (Murphy et al., 2011).

Schizophrenia

Abnormal neuronal development and function of the DG have been proposed as risk factors for schizophrenia (Kobayashi, 2009). Neuropathological studies of patients with schizophrenia revealed cytoarchitectural disturbances in the DG and CA3 regions, including impaired dendritic arborizations (Christison et al., 1989; Arnold et al., 1995) and alterations in synaptic density and MF terminal structure (Kobayashi, 2009).

DISC-1 (Disrupted in Schizophrenia 1) protein, a molecule that determines susceptibility to schizophrenia, is crucial during embryogenesis due to its stimulatory actions on the non-canonical Wnt signaling pathway and its inhibition of glycogen synthase kinase 3-β (GSK-3β) (De Rienzo et al., 2011; Lipina et al., 2011). GSK-3β inhibition by DISC-1 is pivotal for the regulation of AHN (Mao et al., 2009; Ming and Song, 2009). DISC-1 regulates newborn neuron morphology, the synaptic integration of these cells into the trisynaptic circuit (Duan et al., 2007), and their migration within the GL (Meyer and Morris, 2009; Namba et al., 2011). In contrast to the widespread expression of this protein during development, in the adult brain it is greatly restricted, being particularly high in hippocampal granule neurons and the interneurons of the olfactory bulb (Austin and Buckmaster, 2004). DISC-1 knockdown in newborn neurons by means of a retroviral strategy leads to soma hypertrophy, accelerated aberrant dendritic outgrowth with the appearance of ectopic dendrites, overextended migration, enhanced intrinsic excitability, and accelerated synapse formation (Duan et al., 2007). DISC-1 knockout neurons exhibit multiple primary dendrites and show basal dendrites (Duan et al., 2007). In addition, the use of a mouse with a truncated lesion in endogenous DISC-1 revealed that newborn neurons present deficits in axonal targeting in CA3, altered excitability, and increased levels of cAMP (Kvajo et al., 2011). As further demonstrated, some of these morphological alterations are rescued by genetic inactivation of GSK-3 (Lee et al., 2011).

Stress-Exposed Granule Neurons Show Altered Morphology

The stress-induced increase in the levels of glucocorticoids (GCs) serves many beneficial homeostatic functions (Frank et al., 2013). However, dysregulation of the GC system is associated with cognitive impairments and depression (Snyder et al., 2011). At the cellular level, GCs regulate numerous central processes such as cell proliferation, survival, and death. Due to the involvement of this structure in stress-related neurological diseases, the hippocampal regulation of these processes by GCs has been studied both during development (Gould et al., 1991; Tanapat et al., 1998) and adulthood (Gould et al., 1992; Cameron and Gould, 1994; Gould and Tanapat, 1999).

Glucocorticoid receptor (GR) is highly expressed by hippocampal neurons, especially by CA1 and CA2 pyramidal and granule neurons (Nishi et al., 2007). In addition, the time-course of GR expression during AHN has been addressed by several groups (Gould et al., 1992; Garcia et al., 2004; Llorens-Martin and Trejo, 2011) and has been demonstrated to occur in immature neurons from 1 week after cell birth and onwards (Llorens-Martin and Trejo, 2011). Although a strong dependence of GC effects on the type, duration and strength of the stressor has been observed, in general terms, the stress-induced increase in GCs is thought to suppress AHN (Gould et al., 1997; Kim et al., 2005; Mitra et al., 2006; Llorens-Martin and Trejo, 2011; Ortega-Martinez and Trejo, 2015). Interestingly, AHN has been made responsible for buffering the effects of stress on various behaviors, and its abolishment impairs the restoration of normal levels of GCs after exposure to stress (Opendak and Gould, 2011; Snyder et al., 2011).

However, adrenalectomy (ADX) has been described to exert equivalent suppressive effects on AHN (Liposits et al., 1997; Trejo et al., 2000), thus suggesting that physiological levels of GCs are required for the proper development of hippocampal neurons. Gould, Woolley and McEwen (Gould et al., 1990; Woolley et al., 1990) were the first to report that ADX induces dendritic remodeling in the hippocampus. Golgi staining revealed a shrinkage of the dendritic tree and a reduction in the number of branches per cell 7 days after surgery (Gould et al., 1990). These results are further supported by other studies (Liposits et al., 1997).

In addition, data from other groups unveiled that prenatal stress causes a decrease in the total dendritic length and branching of granule neurons. These changes were observed during adulthood, thus supporting the permanent character of the effects of GCs on granule neurons. A net reduction in distal branching is the most outstanding feature of these alterations (Hosseini-Sharifabad and Hadinedoushan, 2007). Furthermore, the crucial role played by GCs in regulating the temporal dynamics of AHN was demonstrated by Fitzsimons et al. several years ago. They found that the knockdown of GR in hippocampal precursor cells accelerates the morphological maturation, migration into the GL, and functional integration of newborn neurons in the hippocampal circuit (Fitzsimons et al., 2013), thus confirming the specific functions played by GCs in the morphological and synaptic maturation of newborn neurons. Interestingly, the regulation of AHN exerted by GCs appears to have the same inverted "U-shape" characteristic of most of GC actions on the adult brain (Joels, 2006).

Inflammation

The inflammatory micro-environment strongly influences the survival, maturation, and recruitment of newborn neurons into behaviorally relevant circuits (Belarbi et al., 2012). In this regard, it has been hypothesized that the negative effects of inflammation on hippocampal-related memory are caused by alterations in AHN (Belarbi and Rosi, 2013; Enciu and Popescu, 2013; Kohman and Rhodes, 2013). Microglia, the population of resident macrophage cells within the brain, play continuous role of surveillance, phagocytosis and chemoattraction, among other functions, under both pathological and physiological conditions (Sierra et al., 2013). Although strongly dependent on the type and duration of the pro-inflammatory stimulus, neuroinflammation is considered to impair AHN (Monje et al., 2003; Biscaro et al., 2012). However, the interaction between microglia and newborn neurons is multi-faceted, as both neuroprotective and suppressive effects have been demonstrated (Sierra et al., 2013; Shigemoto-Mogami et al., 2014). In addition, neuroinflammation is a hallmark shared by numerous psychiatric and neurodegenerative diseases, such as schizophrenia (Khandaker and Dantzer, 2015), epileptic seizures (Johnson et al., 2011), depression (Dantzer et al., 2008), and AD (Meraz-Rios et al., 2013). It is thought that microglia orchestrate the transition between innate and adaptive immune responses in the brain (Town et al., 2005). In this respect, the phenotype expressed by microglial cells under either acute or chronic neuroinflammation differs (Boche et al., 2013). Microglia acquire a rapidly induced so-called "M1 classically activated" phenotype when acutely exposed to a pro-inflammatory stimulus (Varnum and Ikezu, 2012). When biased toward this phenotype, these cells secrete pro-inflammatory and chemoattractant mediators (Llorens-Martin et al., 2014a). In contrast, under chronic low-grade inflammation, microglia acquire a "M2 alternatively activated" phenotype (Varnum and Ikezu, 2012), which is characterized by the secretion of both pro- and anti-inflammatory cytokines. This phenotype is considered to be neuroprotective for newborn neurons. In most neurodegenerative diseases, microglial cells are skewed toward the M2 phenotype (Llorens-Martin et al., 2014a).

Using Golgi staining, Jurgens et al. demonstrated that influenza infection causes morphological alterations in hippocampal granule neurons (Jurgens et al., 2012). Influenza induces the retraction and reduces the number of branches in the outer portions of the dendritic tree, whereas it increases total branching near the cell soma. Although the technique used did not allow the determination of the age of the cells studied, the authors described more accentuated morphological and synaptic changes in granule cells located in the inner portion of the GL.

To the best of our knowledge, we were the first to describe that a pro-inflammatory stimulus alters the morphology of newborn granule neurons (Llorens-Martin et al., 2014a). We used the peripheral administration of LPS via subcutaneous osmotic pumps to induce chronic brain inflammation during a range of periods. Using this system in combination with the stereotaxic injection of a Postsynaptic density protein 95 (PSD95) fused to GFP (PSD95-GFP) expressing retrovirus, we subjected newborn neurons to inflammation at various stages of cell maturation and examined its effects. LPS induced striking and long-lasting morphological alterations, namely a marked reduction in distal branching and an increase in proximal branching of the dendritic tree in all the developmental stages studied (Llorens-Martin et al., 2014a). We named this inflammation-induced morphology "V-shape," due to the presence of several primary apical dendrites in many of the newborn neurons. In addition to these pronounced morphological changes, LPS impaired the connectivity of these cells, thus reducing both afferent (number and size of postsynaptic densities) and efferent (size of the MF terminals) connectivity. These changes in synaptic integration were also long-lasting and, unlike the morphological alterations, they were not fully reversed by an anti-inflammatory treatment with Ibuprofen. This observation suggests that inflammation causes permanent damage to newborn neurons when applied in critical periods of their development.

In the same year, Chugh et al. (2013) described that the intracerebroventricular injection of LPS to retrovirus-injected mice (1 or 4 weeks after retroviral injections) induces changes in the inhibitory synapses produced in newborn neurons. In this case, the authors did not report morphological alterations caused by LPS injection. However, the second stereotaxic injection itself is likely to produce a pro-inflammatory insult strong enough (even in the vehicle-injected animals) to mask some of the putative effects of LPS. It can be hypothesized that this may be the reason why these authors did not observe changes in morphology, although they did describe changes in the migration of newborn neurons (Belarbi and Rosi, 2013; Llorens-Martin et al., 2014a).

Drugs of Abuse

Although numerous studies have focused on the effects of various drugs of abuse on the rate of AHN (reviewed in Powrozek et al., 2004), only a few have examined the consequences of these substances on the morphology of newborn neurons. Ethanol exposure decreases neural stem cell proliferation in the DG (Svanidze et al., 2001; Miki et al., 2003; Powrozek et al., 2004; Redila et al., 2006). However, the effects of ethanol on granule neuron morphology have only recently been addressed. While ethanol exposure increases dendritic complexity in CA3 pyramidal neurons, it reduces the dendritic branching of granule neurons (Staples et al., 2015). In addition, exposure of adult rats to cocaine decreases progenitor cell proliferation in the DG but does not affect the survival or the morphology of newly generated neurons. No changes in dendritic arborization or in positioning in the GL were observed (Dominguez-Escriba et al., 2006; Hauser and Knapp, 2014).

Neurodegenerative Diseases

Alzheimer's Disease

The most relevant histopathological hallmarks of AD are the extracellular deposits of Amyloid-β (Aβ) and the intracellular tangles formed mainly by hyperphosphorylated Tau protein. The molecular pathways responsible for these two types of aberrant structures converge in a common step, namely the dysregulation of GSK-3β activity (Hernandez et al., 2010). This kinase is one of the most important molecules triggering the hyperphosphorylation of Tau and the subsequent destabilization of the cytoskeleton, Tau aggregation, and neuronal death. Interestingly, GSK-3β is required for the manifestation of the toxic effects of Aβ (Takashima et al., 1993), thus making it one of the most relevant molecules affecting the progression of AD.

It has been widely described that numerous animal models of AD, including GSK-3β-overexpressing mice under the control of the neuronal promoter CamKII, present alterations in the rate of AHN (Fuster-Matanzo et al., 2013). Although the general consensus in the field is that the generation of fully mature and functional neurons is impaired in AD (Li et al., 2008), both increases (Jin et al., 2004a,b), decreases (Crews et al., 2010; Demars et al., 2010; Faure et al., 2011), no changes (Boekhoorn et al., 2006), and changes dependent on the stage of the disease (Chen et al., 2008) have been described in AD patients and animal models. In addition, alterations varying in function of the stage of cell differentiation have been reported in AD patients (Perry et al., 2012; Gomez-Nicola et al., 2014). The in-depth study of the alterations in the AHN rate is not in the scope in this review, which rather focuses on the morphological alterations in granule neurons.

In 1987, de Ruiter et al., described that granule neurons undergo a profound morphological transformation in advanced stages of AD (de Ruiter and Uylings, 1987). By means of Golgi staining, these authors observed a significant reduction in the length of the distal segments of the dendritic trees of mature neurons. In addition, granule neurons from patients suffering senile dementia were described to present increased branching in the proximal domains of dendritic trees (Flood et al., 1987), in contrast to control newborn neurons which showed a single primary apical dendrite and a "Y-shape" (**Figure 3A**). It has been proposed that the decreased branching in the outer ML occurs as a result of denervation from the EC or alternatively of aberrant sprouting emerging from cell body (de Ruiter and Uylings, 1987). Given that no differences in the morphological or connectivity alterations were found between neurons located near or distant to the Aβ plaques in AD patients, an Aβ-independent mechanism was put forward to explain the aberrant morphology and reduced connectivity of granule neurons in AD (Einstein et al., 1994). We have proposed that one of these mechanisms might be GSK-3β. The rationale supporting this hypothesis is that the morphological alterations in newborn granule neurons of mice overexpressing GSK-3β are strikingly similar to those described in AD patients (Llorens-Martin et al., 2013; **Figure 3B**). In this regard, we observed an increased degree of branching in the proximal domain of the dendritic tree and a retraction of the distal domain in the ML. In contrast to the 30% of cells with more than one primary apical dendrite in control subjects, most cells (roughly 90%) in AD patients presented several. Hence, we adopted the terminology of "V-shape" for the granule cells predominant in AD brains. This aberrant morphology might have far-reaching functional consequences, especially taking into account that major afferent connections received by granule neurons arise from the EC and take place within the two outer thirds of the ML (Kharatishvili et al., 2006). Both in these mice and in AD patients, the increased number of proximal branches may favor recurrent connectivity from adjacent granule neurons, whereas the unbranched dendritic tree in the outer ML could account, to some extent, for the DG "disconnection" from the EC, a phenomenon that occurs in AD (Hyman et al., 1984). This disconnection might have important consequences for the function of the hippocampal circuit, since the innervation from the EC drives the dendritic maturation of newborn granule neurons (Frotscher et al., 2000). We have proposed that GSK-3β impairs the maturation of newborn neurons through at least three distinct mechanisms. First, it phosphorylates Tau protein, thereby destabilizing the developing cytoskeleton and its polarity, and hence impairing the establishment of a correct morphology; second, it impairs newborn neuron connectivity by internalizing AMPA receptor GluR1 and triggering the disappearance of synapses (Arendt, 2003; Peineau et al., 2007); and third, it promotes a series of indirect effects linked to neuroinflammation (Jope et al., 2007; Llorens-Martin et al., 2014a), thus aggravating maturational alterations through non-cell-autonomous mechanisms. It has been described, on the one hand, that GSK-3β leads neurons to secrete pro-inflammatory mediators (Martin et al., 2005). On the other, GSK-3β overexpression triggers the death of mature granule neurons (Sirerol-Piquer et al., 2011), a phenomenon that activates microglia and promotes the secretion of more pro-inflammatory cytokines (Pais et al., 2008), thus accentuating the pro-inflammatory nature of the whole process. As previously commented, this pro-inflammatory environment has negative effects on the development of newborn neurons (Belarbi

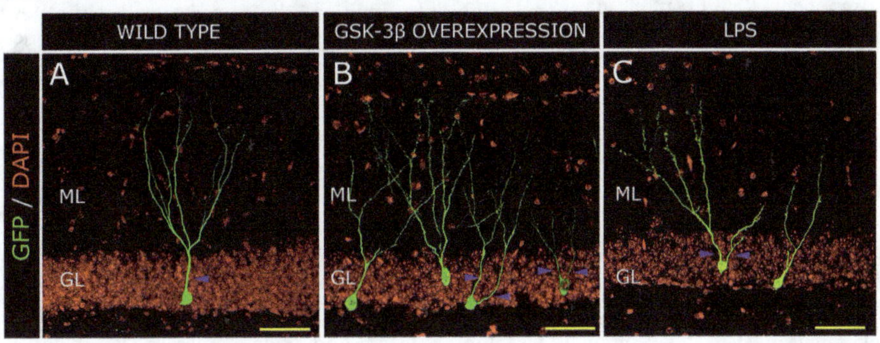

FIGURE 3 | Morphological alterations in a model of Alzheimer disease (AD) and inflammation. Retrovirus-labeled newborn neurons from control mice present one apical primary dendrite (blue triangles) and the dendritic tree resembles a "Y-shape" in the control mouse **(A)**. In contrast, in GSK-3β-overexpressing mice (a murine model of AD), cells acquire a "V-shape" morphology, characterized by the presence of several apical dendrites and atrophy of the distal branching of the dendritic tree **(B)**. In a model of brain inflammation induced by the peripheral infusion of LPS, newborn granule neurons also acquire a "V-shape" and show increased branching in the proximal domain of the dendritic tree, whereas distal domains appear to be atrophied **(C)**. H, Hilus; GL, Granule cell layer; ML, Molecular layer. Yellow scale bar: 50 μm.

and Rosi, 2013) and is responsible, to some extent, for the maturational alterations found in GSK-3β-overexpressing mice (Llorens-Martin et al., 2014a). In fact, the newborn granule neurons of mice injected peripherally with LPS show a marked "V-shape" (**Figure 3C**). Thus, whether through direct, cell-autonomous (namely Tau phosphorylation and synapsis removal) or indirect non-cell-autonomous, (neuroinflammation) mechanisms, GSK-3β—a pivotal kinase in AD—dramatically impairs newborn neuron maturation.

However, GSK-3β-overexpressing mice are not the only AD model in which the morphological maturation of newborn granule neurons has been addressed. Using a retroviral labeling technique, Biscaro et al. demonstrated that the expression of familial AD-causing mutations in the amyloid precursor protein and presenilin-1 genes in mice cause a profound impairment of mature granule neuron morphology and connectivity. In this regard, dendritic branching is reduced throughout the dendritic tree and a marked decrease in the number of dendritic spines also occurs in this model (Biscaro et al., 2009, 2012).

Interestingly, CDK5 has attracted great interest due to its involvement in Tau phosphorylation (Maccioni et al., 2001). Similar to the mechanisms proposed to explain the dysregulation of GSK-3β in AD, it has been demonstrated that Aβ also stimulates the activation of CDK5. Thus, inactivating CDK5 prevents the toxic effects of Aβ (Alvarez et al., 1999). GSK-3β and CDK5 are the main kinases phosphorylating Tau and triggering neuronal degeneration in AD (Wen et al., 2008).

CDK5 participates in the signaling pathway of Class 3 Semaphorins (SEM3) (Ng et al., 2013). These molecules play key roles in axonal guidance during development. By silencing the semaphorin receptors neuropilin (NRP) 1 or 2 in newborn neurons, Ng et al., demonstrated a reduction in the length and branching of these cells (Ng et al., 2013). In addition, overexpression of CDK5 in these cells rescues the dendritic phenotypes seen in NRP1- and NRP2-deficient neurons (Ng et al., 2013).

The CDK5 system is formed by the catalytic component (CDK5) and the regulatory proteins P35, P25, and P39 (Maccioni et al., 2001). CDK5 activation in neurons requires association with its regulatory component P35 (Tsai et al., 1994) and this system plays a crucial role both during development and adulthood. CDK5 participates in neuronal migration, neurite extension (Cheung et al., 2007; Ohshima et al., 2007), dendritic pathfinding, synaptic plasticity, and learning (Hawasli et al., 2007; Ohshima et al., 2007). Jessberger et al. used a retrovirus-based approach to overexpress and knockdown CDK5 in newly generated neurons (Jessberger et al., 2008) and to examine the effects of this manipulation on the morphological maturation of these cells. It was found that CDK5 overexpression does not alter the morphology of newborn granule neurons. On the contrary, knocked-down neurons for CDK5 activity lose the typical polarity of granule neurons and extend several dendrites along the GL or even toward the hilus (Jessberger et al., 2008). In addition, they showed a reduced total dendritic length and number of dendritic branches. These morphological alterations appeared from the seventh day after retroviral injections and were maintained thereafter. Interestingly, the knockdown of CDK5 also reduces the number of dendritic spines and the percentage of mushroom spines in these cells (Jessberger et al., 2008). These observations therefore support the prominent role played by this kinase in newborn neuron maturation, as has been further confirmed by other groups (Ng et al., 2013).

Synucleopathies: Parkinson Disease, and Lewy Body Dementia

Synucleinopathies are characterized by a marked cognitive decline, which has a severe impact on the patient's life quality (Possin et al., 2008). Clinical and imaging studies have linked cognitive decline in Parkinson's disease (PD) and Lewy body dementia (LBD) to the malfunction of hippocampal circuitries (Possin et al., 2008; Politis et al., 2010). The most relevant histopathological hallmark of these two conditions is the aggregation of α-synuclein to form Lewy bodies (Spillantini et al., 1997). Impaired AHN has been reported in the brains of PD patients and in murine models of synucleinopathies (Hoglinger et al., 2004). In addition, the expression of α-synuclein in neural progenitors has been observed in PD patients, but not in controls (Winner et al., 2012). Winner et al. demonstrated that the knockdown of α/β synuclein increases the rate of AHN (Winner et al., 2012). In contrast, the overexpression of human α-synuclein in mice dramatically impairs the morphological maturation of newborn granule neurons. In addition, the number of dendritic spines is severely reduced. However, the authors also revealed the cell-autonomous nature of these effects by constructing a retrovirus to overexpress α-synuclein in newborn cells. In this regard, they obtained the same results (Winner et al., 2012).

The morphological alterations in newborn granule neurons of other PD models have also been studied. Mutations in leucine-rich repeat kinase 2 (LRRK2) are considered a risk factor for the development of this disease (Zimprich et al., 2004). Mutation G2019S in Lrrk2 presents the highest genotype- and population-attributable risk (Hulihan et al., 2008). In transgenic mice, the expression of the Lrrk2 G2019S transgene occurs mainly in the neurogenic regions and leads to a drastic reduction in cellular proliferation and survival in the SGZ (Winner et al., 2011). In addition, the morphology of the newly generated neurons is dramatically altered by Lrrk2 G2019S expression. The total length, degree of branching, and branch length of are reduced in G2019S mice (Winner et al., 2011).

Lead Exposure

Epidemiological studies have established a link between ambient air pollutants and health (Verina et al., 2007). Lead is a ubiquitous, highly neurotoxic, environmental and industrial pollutant that particularly affects the developing central nervous system and leads to disease (Block and Calderon-Garciduenas, 2009). This metal has been related to a broad range of physiological, biochemical, and behavioral dysfunctions in humans and in animal models (Ahamed et al., 2009; Dabidi et al., 2013). Chronic exposure to lead impairs synaptic plasticity and cognitive function in animal models (Toscano and Guilarte, 2005; Toscano et al., 2005; Verina et al., 2007).

After subjecting adult rats to 2 months of lead exposure, Selvin-Testa et al. reported the appearance of irregular and dark-condensed cytoplasm in hippocampal granule cells. In addition, smooth dendrites, axons, and synaptic terminals were found to be condensed and darker than the surrounding elements (Selvin-Testa, 1991). These authors proposed that these ultrastructural modifications were a morphological substrate for the behavioral alterations caused by exposure to this neurotoxic substance during childhood.

The effects of lead exposure on the maturation of granule newborn neurons have been addressed by Verina et al. They demonstrated that such exposure causes a reduction in both the proliferation and survival of newborn neurons in the hippocampus (Verina et al., 2007). In addition, lead exposure causes a decrease in the length of the dendrites of immature DCX^+ cells. Specifically, newborn neurons extend dendrites along the GL, and branching in the ML is drastically reduced (Verina et al., 2007). In addition, they also observed a decrease in size of the MF bundle in lead-exposed rats (Verina et al., 2007).

Dietary Factors

It has been demonstrated that a certain prenatal period of malnutrition has adverse effects on spatial memory during adulthood, and the hippocampus has been pinpointed as one of the brain regions most sensitive to nutritional deficits during development. In particular, a reduction in the number of granule neurons and an alteration of the synapse/neuron ratio has been reported in pups of rats subjected to malnutrition during pregnancy (Ahmed et al., 1987). Similar effects have been reported after periods of malnutrition during adulthood (Andrade et al., 1995). In a subsequent study, despite not finding differences in neuron numbers, the same authors reported that food restriction causes a decrease in the total number of dendritic branches of granule neurons. In addition, under these conditions, they observed that the area of the postsynaptic densities in the outer regions of granule neuron dendritic trees tends to decrease (Andrade et al., 2002).

In particular, the effects caused by a deficiency in iodine uptake during development have been systematically studied, since such a deficiency is the most common cause of hypothyroidism and the single most important cause of preventable mental defects (Yu et al., 2014). Iodine deficiency during development downregulates the expression of DCX in the DG (Gong et al., 2010). In iodine-deficient rats, DCX^+ cells in the DG do not develop dendrites or are significantly shorter than those of control animals (Yu et al., 2014). Accordingly, hypothyroidism during developmental periods leads to a reduction in the number of granule neurons and volume of the DG (Madeira et al., 1991) and to alterations in the morphology of mature granule neurons (Rami et al., 1986), thus supporting the critical role played by the thyroid system in regulating hippocampal development.

On the other hand, it has been proposed that calorie restriction (CR) increases health and lifespan (Levenson and Rich, 2007). Intermittent fasting (IF) has been demonstrated to increase long-term potentiation (LTP) and the expression of the NMDA receptor subunit NR2B in the hippocampus, resulting in enhanced learning (Fontan-Lozano et al., 2007). The molecular mechanisms responsible for the neuroprotective role of CR and IF may be mediated by an increase in AHN in young animals (Lee et al., 2002) and a reduction in the age-related decline in AHN in older animals (Bondolfi et al., 2004). It is thought that both CR and IF increase the survival of neuronal stem cells by boosting the levels of neurotrophic factors (Lee et al., 2002; Bondolfi et al., 2004) and decreasing neuroinflammation (reviewed in Murphy et al., 2014). Despite a prominent increase in the number of dendritic spines in animal models subjected to CR, this regime has not demonstrated to alter the morphology of mature granule neurons (Stranahan et al., 2009), as revealed by means of Golgi staining method. However, specific effects on newborn neurons cannot be ruled out. Furthermore, given the relevant changes induced in both the neurotrophic and inflammatory milieu, it is reasonable to hypothesize that CR has a considerable effect on the morphological maturation of newborn granule neurons. Further studies are required to elucidate this issue.

Interestingly, a high-fat diet decreases the total length and branching of dendrites of newborn neurons, thus drastically impairing the morphological maturation of these cells (Tozuka et al., 2010).

X-ray Irradiation

Exposure of the hippocampus to focal X-ray irradiation during infancy causes a dramatic reduction in granule cell genesis in adulthood (Diaz-Granados et al., 1994; Barlind et al., 2010), thus preventing the MF connection in CA3 (Collet et al., 1999). Furthermore, such exposure impairs hippocampal-dependent learning (Wojtowicz et al., 2008; Hernandez-Rabaza et al., 2009). In addition, it destabilizes the cytoskeleton, leading to morphological alterations in hippocampal neurons (Zhang et al., 2012). Brain inflammation appears to play a key role in radiation-induced abolishment of AHN, since inflammatory blockade restores AHN in a model of cranial irradiation (CI) (Monje et al., 2003). In 2008, Naylor et al. demonstrated that CI alters the angle of orientation of the leading apical process in DCX^+ cells and that these alterations are reversed by physical exercise (Naylor et al., 2008). In addition, CI during adulthood alters the number and morphology of the dendritic spines in granule neurons. Using Golgi staining, Chakraborti et al. reported a marked reduction in the number and an increase in the proportion of immature, thin and stubby dendritic spines 1 week or 1 month after CI (Chakraborti et al., 2012).

Stroke

After brain ischemia, the proliferation and differentiation of neuronal progenitors in the DG is strongly stimulated, leading to a significant increase in neurogenesis (Liu et al., 1998; Arvidsson et al., 2001a,b; Kernie and Parent, 2010). Niv et al. used retroviral labeling to visualize newborn neuron morphology and found that stroke leads to a morphologically aberrant integration of adult newborn cells into the DG and that the extent of abnormalities increases with the extent of ischemic damage (Niv et al., 2012). They found that, although most of the neurons had a normally differentiated morphology, a small percentage of newborn granule neurons displayed a marked aberrant morphology, namely bipolar neurons with several basal dendrites, in addition to several long apical dendrites and ectopic neurons located near the hilus (Niv et al., 2012).

CONCLUDING REMARKS AND FURTHER DIRECTIONS

In summary, it can be concluded that the physiological process of morphological development comprises drastic modifications in the morphology of the dendritic tree of newborn neurons, namely, a vertical orientation of the apical dendrite and a profuse branching of the apical dendrite in the ML, thus conferring these cells a characteristic "Y-shape" (**Figure 4A**). The elongation and orientation of the apical dendrite seem to be a process particularly important, on one hand, and particularly vulnerable on the other. Most of the stimuli impairing AHN usually concur in similar morphological alterations of the dendritic tree of granule neurons. For instance, a significant shortening of the primary apical dendrite has been demonstrated to be triggered by inflammation, AD, stress and stroke (**Figure 4D**), whereas seizures and schizophrenia are known to induce an aberrant positioning and retention og basal dendrites by granule neurons (**Figure 4C**). In addition, the identity of the primary apical dendrite appears to be lost in most of these pathologies, and cells with more than one primary apical dendrite are commonly found in these conditions, in which granule cells acquire a "V-shape" (**Figure 4D**). It can be hypothesized that the several apical dendrites present in these "V-shape" neurons after their maturation derive from a defective elimination of the undifferentiated projections present at early maturative stages. Alternatively, a shortening of the primary apical dendrite can result in a "V-shape-like" morphology in these cells. Another crucial unanswered question is whether newborn neurons are equally vulnerable to the different insults during all their maturative stages or whether there are critical checkpoints at which the physiological maturation can be truncated. Intriguingly, an increased migration toward the GL accompanies the shortening of the primary apical dendrite, although these two processes (migration and primary apical dendrite formation) occur at different points of the maturational process. Whether these two processes are causally related or occur only in parallel still remains largely unknown. It can be hypothesized that once the cell migrates toward deeper zones of the GL, the apical dendrite must be shortened to maintain the previously established synaptic contacts. An alternative

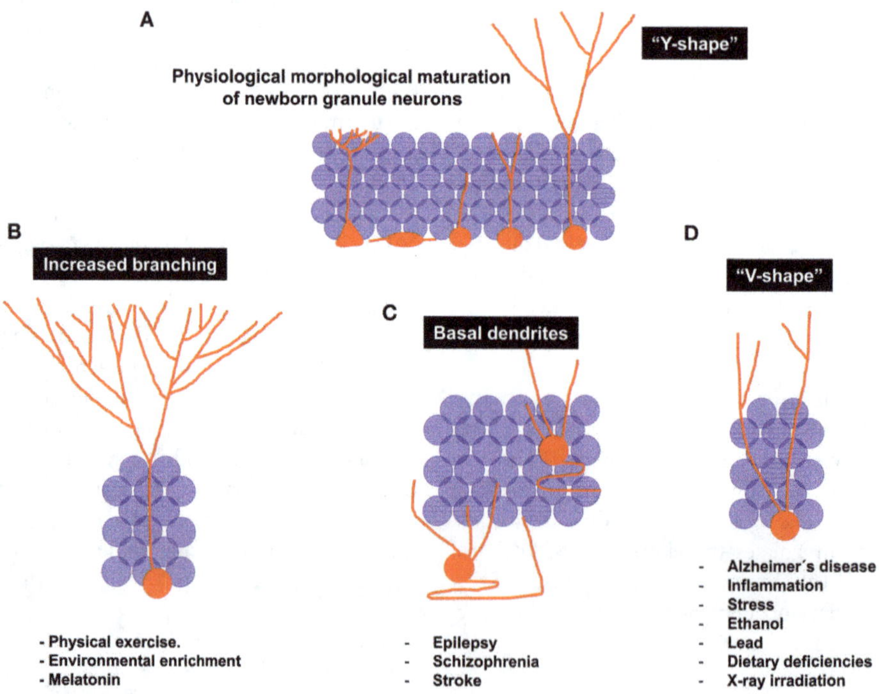

FIGURE 4 | Schematic diagram of the regulation of newborn granule neuron morphological maturation under physiological and pathological conditions. (A) Morphological maturation under physiological conditions. It should be noted that, at the end of the maturational process, newborn neurons generally acquire a "Y-shape," displaying one single primary apical dendrite emerging from the soma. The high dendritic branching observed in the molecular layer lead them to resemble to the aforementioned "Y" shape. **(B)** Neuroprotective stimuli are considered stimulators of newborn neuron maturation. For instance, physical exercise and Environmental enrichment increase dendritic branching of newborn granule neurons. **(C)** Pathological maturation of newborn neurons occurs in epilepsy, schizophrenia and stroke. Under these circumstances, newborn neurons are aberrantly located in the Hilus or in deeper layers of the Granule layer. In addition, recurrent basal dendrites are commonly observed. **(D)** Other pathological circumstances, including neurodegenerative disorders, inflammation, stress, alcohol consumption, dietary deficiencies, lead exposure, or X-ray irradiation result in impaired maturation of newborn neurons. Interestingly, a reduced branching in the molecular layer and the presence of several apical dendrites emerging from the cell soma are observed in these pathological circumstances. These morphological features lead granule neurons to acquire a "V-shape," in contrast to the "Y-shape" displayed by them under physiological conditions.

explanation of these complex phenomena is that the shortening of the apical dendrite is triggered by processes such as cellular aging and oxidative stress. As a consequence of these processes, cytoskeleton destabilization and apical dendrite shortening may trigger the retraction of the nucleus, which would acquire a deeper position in the GL.

Conversely, elements favoring AHN and newborn neuron maturation, such as physical exercise, EE, and melatonin coincide in causing a lengthening of the primary apical dendrite and an increase in branching in the distal domain of the dendritic tree of granule neurons (**Figure 4B**). Importantly, neuroprotective stimuli, also known to potentiate hippocampal-dependent learning, trigger morphological changes in newborn neurons that drive them toward the perforant pathway, thus giving them greater access to information from the EC. Conversely, insults impairing hippocampal function tend to increase the branching of proximal dendrites aberrantly located in the GL, thereby making newborn neurons more prone to be innervated by and also to contribute to recurrent connections, thus promoting the disconnection of the DC from the physiological hippocampal circuit, a phenomenon known to occur in several neurodegenerative and neurological disorders.

Understanding the molecular mechanisms that underlie the establishment of a correct morphology in newborn neurons is of crucial importance in order to advance in the design of therapeutic approaches to prevent and treat these diseases. In addition, investigating the mechanisms linking morphology and function will be crucial for understanding why this neuronal population undergoing adult regeneration throughout lifetime is so crucial for hippocampal functioning.

AUTHOR CONTRIBUTIONS

ML did the immunohistochemistry experiments and acquired the optical and confocal microscope images. ML and JÁ wrote the manuscript and obtained necessary funding. AR provided the human samples. ML, JÁ, and AR discussed available data and revised and approved the final version of the manuscript.

FUNDING

This study was funded by grants from the Spanish Ministry of Health (SAF-2014-5040-P), and the *Centro de Investigación Biomédica en Red sobre Enfermedades Neurodegenerativas* (CIBERNED, ISCIII; JÁ); and the *Alzheimer's Association* (2015-NIRG-340709; MLL-M).

ACKNOWLEDGMENTS

Human control samples were generously provided by the *Biobanco del Hospital Universitario Reina Sofia* (Córdoba, Spain). The authors thank Dr. R. Sánchez Sánchez for facilitating access to human control samples. AD samples were generously provided by the *Banco de Tejidos de la Fundación CIEN* (Madrid, Spain). The authors thank C. Lois for providing the plasmids used for the production of the PSD95-GFP virus.

REFERENCES

Adlard, P. A., Perreau, V. M., Pop, V., and Cotman, C. W. (2005). Voluntary exercise decreases amyloid load in a transgenic model of Alzheimer's disease. *J. Neurosci.* 25, 4217–4221. doi: 10.1523/JNEUROSCI.0496-05.2005

Ahamed, M., Mehrotra, P. K., Kumar, P., and Siddiqui, M. K. (2009). Placental lead-induced oxidative stress and preterm delivery. *Environ. Toxicol. Pharmacol.* 27, 70–74. doi: 10.1016/j.etap.2008.08.013

Ahmed, M. G., Bedi, K. S., Warren, M. A., and Kamel, M. M. (1987). Effects of a lengthy period of undernutrition from birth and subsequent nutritional rehabilitation on the synapse: granule cell neuron ratio in the rat dentate gyrus. *J. Comp. Neurol.* 263, 146–158. doi: 10.1002/cne.902630113

Althaus, A. L., Sagher, O., Parent, J. M., and Murphy, G. G. (2015). Intrinsic neurophysiological properties of hilar ectopic and normotopic dentate granule cells in human temporal lobe epilepsy and a rat model. *J. Neurophysiol.* 113, 1184–1194. doi: 10.1152/jn.00835.2014

Alvarez, A., Toro, R., Caceres, A., and Maccioni, R. B. (1999). Inhibition of tau phosphorylating protein kinase cdk5 prevents beta-amyloid-induced neuronal death. *FEBS Lett.* 459, 421–426. doi: 10.1016/S0014-5793(99)01279-X

Andrade, J. P., Lukoyanov, N. V., and Paula-Barbosa, M. M. (2002). Chronic food restriction is associated with subtle dendritic alterations in granule cells of the rat hippocampal formation. *Hippocampus* 12, 149–164. doi: 10.1002/hipo.1102

Andrade, J. P., Madeira, M. D., and Paula-Barbosa, M. M. (1995). Effects of long-term malnutrition and rehabilitation on the hippocampal formation of the adult rat. A morphometric study. *J. Anat.* 187 (Pt 2), 379–393.

Arendt, T. (2003). Synaptic plasticity and cell cycle activation in neurons are alternative effector pathways: the 'Dr. Jekyll and Mr. Hyde concept' of Alzheimer's disease or the yin and yang of neuroplasticity. *Progress Neurobiol.* 71, 83–248. doi: 10.1016/j.pneurobio.2003.09.007

Arisi, G. M., and Garcia-Cairasco, N. (2007). Doublecortin-positive newly born granule cells of hippocampus have abnormal apical dendritic morphology in the pilocarpine model of temporal lobe epilepsy. *Brain Res.* 1165, 126–134. doi: 10.1016/j.brainres.2007.06.037

Arnold, S. E., Franz, B. R., Gur, R. C., Gur, R. E., Shapiro, R. M., Moberg, P. J., et al. (1995). Smaller neuron size in schizophrenia in hippocampal subfields that mediate cortical-hippocampal interactions. *Am. J. Psychiatry* 152, 738–748. doi: 10.1176/ajp.152.5.738

Arvidsson, A., Kokaia, Z., Airaksinen, M. S., Saarma, M., and Lindvall, O. (2001a). Stroke induces widespread changes of gene expression for glial cell line-derived neurotrophic factor family receptors in the adult rat brain. *Neuroscience* 106, 27–41. doi: 10.1016/S0306-4522(01)00268-8

Arvidsson, A., Kokaia, Z., and Lindvall, O. (2001b). N-methyl-D-aspartate receptor-mediated increase of neurogenesis in adult rat dentate gyrus following stroke. *Eur. J. Neurosci.* 14, 10–18. doi: 10.1046/j.0953-816x.2001.01611.x

Austin, J. E., and Buckmaster, P. S. (2004). Recurrent excitation of granule cells with basal dendrites and low interneuron density and inhibitory postsynaptic current frequency in the dentate gyrus of macaque monkeys. *J. Comp. Neurol.* 476, 205–218. doi: 10.1002/cne.20182

Barlind, A., Karlsson, N., Bjork-Eriksson, T., Isgaard, J., and Blomgren, K. (2010). Decreased cytogenesis in the granule cell layer of the hippocampus and impaired place learning after irradiation of the young mouse brain evaluated using the IntelliCage platform. *Exp. Brain Res.* 201, 781–787. doi: 10.1007/s00221-009-2095-8

Bausch, S. B., and McNamara, J. O. (2000). Synaptic connections from multiple subfields contribute to granule cell hyperexcitability in hippocampal slice cultures. *J. Neurophysiol.* 84, 2918–2932.

Beck, H., Blumcke, I., Kral, T., Clusmann, H., Schramm, J., Wiestler, O. D., et al. (1996). Properties of a delayed rectifier potassium current in dentate granule cells isolated from the hippocampus of patients with chronic temporal lobe epilepsy. *Epilepsia* 37, 892–901. doi: 10.1111/j.1528-1157.1996.tb00043.x

Belarbi, K., Arellano, C., Ferguson, R., Jopson, T., and Rosi, S. (2012). Chronic neuroinflammation impacts the recruitment of adult-born neurons into behaviorally relevant hippocampal networks. *Brain Behav. Immun.* 26, 18–23. doi: 10.1016/j.bbi.2011.07.225

Belarbi, K., and Rosi, S. (2013). Modulation of adult-born neurons in the inflamed hippocampus. *Front. Cell. Neurosci.* 7:145. doi: 10.3389/fncel.2013.00145

Bellon, A., Ortiz-Lopez, L., Ramirez-Rodriguez, G., Anton-Tay, F., and Benitez-King, G. (2007). Melatonin induces neuritogenesis at early stages in N1E-115 cells through actin rearrangements via activation of protein kinase C and Rho-associated kinase. *J. Pineal Res.* 42, 214–221. doi: 10.1111/j.1600-079X.2006.00408.x

Biscaro, B., Lindvall, O., Hock, C., Ekdahl, C. T., and Nitsch, R. M. (2009). Abeta immunotherapy protects morphology and survival of adult-born neurons in doubly transgenic APP/PS1 mice. *J. Neurosci.* 29, 14108–14119. doi: 10.1523/JNEUROSCI.2055-09.2009

Biscaro, B., Lindvall, O., Tesco, G., Ekdahl, C. T., and Nitsch, R. M. (2012). Inhibition of microglial activation protects hippocampal neurogenesis and improves cognitive deficits in a transgenic mouse model for Alzheimer's disease. *Neurodegener. Dis.* 9, 187–198. doi: 10.1159/000330363

Bjornebekk, A., Mathe, A. A., and Brene, S. (2005). The antidepressant effect of running is associated with increased hippocampal cell proliferation. *Int. J. Neuropsychopharmacol.* 8, 357–368. doi: 10.1017/S1461145705005122

Block, M. L., and Calderon-Garciduenas, L. (2009). Air pollution: mechanisms of neuroinflammation and CNS disease. *Trends Neurosci.* 32, 506–516. doi: 10.1016/j.tins.2009.05.009

Boche, D., Perry, V. H., and Nicoll, J. A. (2013). Review: activation patterns of microglia and their identification in the human brain. *Neuropathol. Appl. Neurobiol.* 39, 3–18. doi: 10.1111/nan.12011

Boekhoorn, K., Joels, M., and Lucassen, P. J. (2006). Increased proliferation reflects glial and vascular-associated changes, but not neurogenesis in the presenile Alzheimer hippocampus. *Neurobiol. Dis.* 24, 1–14. doi: 10.1016/j.nbd.2006.04.017

Bondolfi, L., Ermini, F., Long, J. M., Ingram, D. K., and Jucker, M. (2004). Impact of age and caloric restriction on neurogenesis in the dentate gyrus of C57BL/6 mice. *Neurobiol. Aging* 25, 333–340. doi: 10.1016/S0197-4580(03)00083-6

Bruel-Jungerman, E., Veyrac, A., Dufour, F., Horwood, J., Laroche, S., and Davis, S. (2009). Inhibition of PI3K-Akt signaling blocks exercise-mediated enhancement of adult neurogenesis and synaptic plasticity in the dentate gyrus. *PLoS ONE* 4:e7901. doi: 10.1371/journal.pone.0007901

Brusco, L. I., Marquez, M., and Cardinali, D. P. (2000). Melatonin treatment stabilizes chronobiologic and cognitive symptoms in Alzheimer's disease. *Neuro Endocrinol. Lett.* 21, 39–42.

Buhl, E. H., and Dann, J. F. (1990). Basal dendrites are a regular feature of hippocampal granule cells in flying fox hippocampus. *Neurosci. Lett.* 116, 263–268. doi: 10.1016/0304-3940(90)90084-M

Cameron, H. A., and Gould, E. (1994). Adult neurogenesis is regulated by adrenal steroids in the dentate gyrus. *Neuroscience* 61, 203–209. doi: 10.1016/0306-4522(94)90224-0

Collet, J., Pollard, H., Moreau, J., Diabira, D., Ben, A. Y., and Khrestchatisky, M. (1999). Gene expression in developing rat hippocampal pyramidal neurons appears independent of mossy fiber innervation. *Neurochem. Int.* 34, 279–286. doi: 10.1016/S0197-0186(99)00011-X

Cotman, C. W., and Berchtold, N. C. (2002). Exercise: a behavioral intervention to enhance brain health and plasticity. *Trends Neurosci.* 25, 295–301. doi: 10.1016/S0166-2236(02)02143-4

Cotman, C. W., and Engesser-Cesar, C. (2002). Exercise enhances and protects brain function. *Exerc. Sport Sci. Rev.* 30, 75–79. doi: 10.1097/00003677-200204000-00006

Creer, D. J., Romberg, C., Saksida, L. M., Van Praag, H., and Bussey, T. J. (2010). Running enhances spatial pattern separation in mice. *Proc. Natl. Acad. Sci. U.S.A.* 107, 2367–2372. doi: 10.1073/pnas.0911725107

Crews, L., Adame, A., Patrick, C., Delaney, A., Pham, E., Rockenstein, E., et al. (2010). Increased BMP6 levels in the brains of Alzheimer's disease patients and APP transgenic mice are accompanied by impaired neurogenesis. *J. Neurosci.* 30, 12252–12262. doi: 10.1523/JNEUROSCI.1305-10.2010

Chae, C. H., Lee, H. C., Jung, S. L., Kim, T. W., Kim, J. H., Kim, N. J., et al. (2012). Swimming exercise increases the level of nerve growth factor and stimulates neurogenesis in adult rat hippocampus. *Neuroscience* 212, 30–37. doi: 10.1016/j.neuroscience.2012.03.030

Chakraborti, A., Allen, A., Allen, B., Rosi, S., and Fike, J. R. (2012). Cranial irradiation alters dendritic spine density and morphology in the hippocampus. *PLoS ONE* 7:e40844. doi: 10.1371/journal.pone.0040844

Chan, J. P., Cordeira, J., Calderon, G. A., Iyer, L. K., and Rios, M. (2008). Depletion of central BDNF in mice impedes terminal differentiation of new granule neurons in the adult hippocampus. *Mol. Cell. Neurosci.* 39, 372–383. doi: 10.1016/j.mcn.2008.07.017

Chen, M. J., and Russo-Neustadt, A. A. (2005). Exercise activates the phosphatidylinositol 3-kinase pathway. *Brain Res. Mol. Brain Res.* 135, 181–193. doi: 10.1016/j.molbrainres.2004.12.001

Chen, Q., Nakajima, A., Choi, S. H., Xiong, X., Sisodia, S. S., and Tang, Y. P. (2008). Adult neurogenesis is functionally associated with AD-like neurodegeneration. *Neurobiol. Dis.* 29, 316–326. doi: 10.1016/j.nbd.2007.09.005

Cheung, Z. H., Chin, W. H., Chen, Y., Ng, Y. P., and Ip, N. Y. (2007). Cdk5 is involved in BDNF-stimulated dendritic growth in hippocampal neurons. *PLoS Biol.* 5:e63. doi: 10.1371/journal.pbio.0050063

Cho, K. O., Lybrand, Z. R., Ito, N., Brulet, R., Tafacory, F., Zhang, L., et al. (2015). Aberrant hippocampal neurogenesis contributes to epilepsy and associated cognitive decline. *Nat. Commun.* 6, 6606. doi: 10.1038/ncomms7606

Choi, S. H., Veeraraghavalu, K., Lazarov, O., Marler, S., Ransohoff, R. M., Ramirez, J. M., et al. (2008). Non-cell-autonomous effects of presenilin 1 variants on enrichment-mediated hippocampal progenitor cell proliferation and differentiation. *Neuron* 59, 568–580. doi: 10.1016/j.neuron.2008.07.033

Christison, G. W., Casanova, M. F., Weinberger, D. R., Rawlings, R., and Kleinman, J. E. (1989). A quantitative investigation of hippocampal pyramidal cell size, shape, and variability of orientation in schizophrenia. *Arch. Gen. Psychiatry* 46, 1027–1032. doi: 10.1001/archpsyc.1989.01810110069010

Chugh, D., Nilsson, P., Afjei, S. A., Bakochi, A., and Ekdahl, C. T. (2013). Brain inflammation induces post-synaptic changes during early synapse formation in adult-born hippocampal neurons. *Exp. Neurol.* 250, 176–188. doi: 10.1016/j.expneurol.2013.09.005

Dabidi, R. V., Hosseinzadeh, S., Mahjoub, S., Hosseinzadeh, M., and Myers, J. (2013). Endurance exercise training and diferuloyl methane supplement: changes in neurotrophic factor and oxidative stress induced by lead in rat brain. *Biol. Sport* 30, 41–46. doi: 10.5604/20831862.1029820

Dantzer, R., O'connor, J. C., Freund, G. G., Johnson, R. W., and Kelley, K. W. (2008). From inflammation to sickness and depression: when the immune system subjugates the brain. *Nat. Rev. Neurosci.* 9, 46–56. doi: 10.1038/nrn2297

Dashtipour, K., Yan, X. X., Dinh, T. T., Okazaki, M. M., Nadler, J. V., and Ribak, C. E. (2002). Quantitative and morphological analysis of dentate granule cells with recurrent basal dendrites from normal and epileptic rats. *Hippocampus* 12, 235–244. doi: 10.1002/hipo.1114

De Rienzo, G., Bishop, J. A., Mao, Y., Pan, L., Ma, T. P., Moens, C. B., et al. (2011). Disc1 regulates both beta-catenin-mediated and noncanonical Wnt signaling during vertebrate embryogenesis. *FASEB J.* 25, 4184–4197. doi: 10.1096/fj.11-186239

de Ruiter, J. P., and Uylings, H. B. (1987). Morphometric and dendritic analysis of fascia dentata granule cells in human aging and senile dementia. *Brain Res.* 402, 217–229. doi: 10.1016/0006-8993(87)90028-X

Demars, M., Hu, Y. S., Gadadhar, A., and Lazarov, O. (2010). Impaired neurogenesis is an early event in the etiology of familial Alzheimer's disease in transgenic mice. *J. Neurosci. Res.* 88, 2103–2117. doi: 10.1002/jnr.22387

Diamond, M. C., Ingham, C. A., Johnson, R. E., Bennett, E. L., and Rosenzweig, M. R. (1976). Effects of environment on morphology of rat cerebral cortex and hippocampus. *J. Neurobiol.* 7, 75–85. doi: 10.1002/neu.480070108

Diaz-Granados, J. L., Greene, P. L., and Amsel, A. (1994). Selective activity enhancement and persistence in weanling rats after hippocampal X-irradiation in infancy: possible relevance for ADHD. *Behav. Neural Biol.* 61, 251–259. doi: 10.1016/S0163-1047(05)80008-1

Dominguez-Escriba, L., Hernandez-Rabaza, V., Soriano-Navarro, M., Barcia, J. A., Romero, F. J., Garcia-Verdugo, J. M., et al. (2006). Chronic cocaine exposure impairs progenitor proliferation but spares survival and maturation of neural precursors in adult rat dentate gyrus. *Eur. J. Neurosci.* 24, 586–594. doi: 10.1111/j.1460-9568.2006.04924.x

Duan, X., Chang, J. H., Ge, S., Faulkner, R. L., Kim, J. Y., Kitabatake, Y., et al. (2007). Disrupted-In-Schizophrenia 1 regulates integration of newly generated neurons in the adult brain. *Cell* 130, 1146–1158. doi: 10.1016/j.cell.2007.07.010

Duman, C. H., Schlesinger, L., Russell, D. S., and Duman, R. S. (2008). Voluntary exercise produces antidepressant and anxiolytic behavioral effects in mice. *Brain Res.* 1199, 148–158. doi: 10.1016/j.brainres.2007.12.047

Duman, R. S. (2005). Neurotrophic factors and regulation of mood: role of exercise, diet and metabolism. *Neurobiol. Aging* 26 (Suppl. 1), 88–93. doi: 10.1016/j.neurobiolaging.2005.08.018

During, M. J., and Cao, L. (2006). VEGF, a mediator of the effect of experience on hippocampal neurogenesis. *Curr. Alzheimer Res.* 3, 29–33. doi: 10.2174/156720506775697133

Einstein, G., Buranosky, R., and Crain, B. J. (1994). Dendritic pathology of granule cells in Alzheimer's disease is unrelated to neuritic plaques. *J. Neurosci.* 14, 5077–5088.

El Bahh, B., Lespinet, V., Lurton, D., Coussemacq, M., Le Gal La Salle, G., and Rougier, A. (1999). Correlations between granule cell dispersion, mossy fiber sprouting, and hippocampal cell loss in temporal lobe epilepsy. *Epilepsia* 40, 1393–1401. doi: 10.1111/j.1528-1157.1999.tb02011.x

Enciu, A. M., and Popescu, B. O. (2013). Is there a causal link between inflammation and dementia? *Biomed. Res. Int.* 2013:316495. doi: 10.1155/2013/316495

Eriksson, P. S., Perfilieva, E., Bjork-Eriksson, T., Alborn, A. M., Nordborg, C., Peterson, D. A., et al. (1998). Neurogenesis in the adult human hippocampus. *Nat. Med.* 4, 1313–1317. doi: 10.1038/3305

Fabel, K., Fabel, K., Tam, B., Kaufer, D., Baiker, A., Simmons, N., et al. (2003). VEGF is necessary for exercise-induced adult hippocampal neurogenesis. *Eur. J. Neurosci.* 18, 2803–2812. doi: 10.1111/j.1460-9568.2003.03041.x

Fabel, K., and Kempermann, G. (2008). Physical activity and the regulation of neurogenesis in the adult and aging brain. *Neuromol. Med.* 10, 59–66. doi: 10.1007/s12017-008-8031-4

Faherty, C. J., Kerley, D., and Smeyne, R. J. (2003). A Golgi-Cox morphological analysis of neuronal changes induced by environmental enrichment. *Dev. Brain Res.* 141, 55–61. doi: 10.1016/S0165-3806(02)00642-9

Faure, A., Verret, L., Bozon, B., El Tannir El Tayara, N., Ly, M., Kober, F., et al. (2011). Impaired neurogenesis, neuronal loss, and brain functional deficits in the APPxPS1-Ki mouse model of Alzheimer's disease. *Neurobiol. Aging* 32, 407–418. doi: 10.1016/j.neurobiolaging.2009.03.009

Fiala, B. A., Joyce, J. N., and Greenough, W. T. (1978). Environmental complexity modulates growth of granule cell dendrites in developing but not adult hippocampus of rats. *Exp. Neurol.* 59, 372–383. doi: 10.1016/0014-4886(78)90229-7

Fitzsimons, C. P., Van Hooijdonk, L. W., Schouten, M., Zalachoras, I., Brinks, V., Zheng, T., et al. (2013). Knockdown of the glucocorticoid receptor alters functional integration of newborn neurons in the adult hippocampus and impairs fear-motivated behavior. *Mol. Psychiatry* 18, 993–1005. doi: 10.1038/mp.2012.123

Flood, D. G., Buell, S. J., Defiore, C. H., Horwitz, G. J., and Coleman, P. D. (1985). Age-related dendritic growth in dentate gyrus of human brain is followed by regression in the 'oldest old'. *Brain Res.* 345, 366–368. doi: 10.1016/0006-8993(85)91018-2

Flood, D. G., Buell, S. J., Horwitz, G. J., and Coleman, P. D. (1987). Dendritic extent in human dentate gyrus granule cells in normal aging and senile dementia. *Brain Res.* 402, 205–216. doi: 10.1016/0006-8993(87)90027-8

Fontan-Lozano, A., Saez-Cassanelli, J. L., Inda, M. C., De Los Santos-Arteaga, M., Sierra-Dominguez, S. A., Lopez-Lluch, G., et al. (2007). Caloric restriction increases learning consolidation and facilitates synaptic plasticity through mechanisms dependent on NR2B subunits of the NMDA receptor. *J. Neurosci.* 27, 10185–10195. doi: 10.1523/JNEUROSCI.2757-07.2007

Franck, J. E., Pokorny, J., Kunkel, D. D., and Schwartzkroin, P. A. (1995). Physiologic and morphologic characteristics of granule cell circuitry in human epileptic hippocampus. *Epilepsia* 36, 543–558. doi: 10.1111/j.1528-1157.1995.tb02566.x

Frank, M. G., Watkins, L. R., and Maier, S. F. (2013). Stress-induced glucocorticoids as a neuroendocrine alarm signal of danger. *Brain Behav. Immun.* 33, 1–6. doi: 10.1016/j.bbi.2013.02.004

Frotscher, M., Drakew, A., and Heimrich, B. (2000). Role of afferent innervation and neuronal activity in dendritic development and spine maturation of fascia dentata granule cells. *Cereb. Cortex* 10, 946–951. doi: 10.1093/cercor/10.10.946

Frotscher, M., Seress, L., Schwerdtfeger, W. K., and Buhl, E. (1991). The mossy cells of the fascia dentata: a comparative study of their fine structure and synaptic connections in rodents and primates. *J. Comp. Neurol.* 312, 145–163. doi: 10.1002/cne.903120111

Fuster-Matanzo, A., Llorens-Martin, M., Sirerol-Piquer, M. S., Garcia-Verdugo, J. M., Avila, J., and Hernandez, F. (2013). Dual effects of increased glycogen synthase kinase-3beta activity on adult neurogenesis. *Hum. Mol. Genet.* 22, 1300–1315. doi: 10.1093/hmg/dds533

Gao, F., Song, X., Zhu, D., Wang, X., Hao, A., Nadler, J. V., et al. (2015). Dendritic morphology, synaptic transmission, and activity of mature granule cells born following pilocarpine-induced status epilepticus in the rat. *Front. Cell. Neurosci.* 9:384. doi: 10.3389/fncel.2015.00384

Garcia, A., Steiner, B., Kronenberg, G., Bick-Sander, A., and Kempermann, G. (2004). Age-dependent expression of glucocorticoid- and mineralocorticoid receptors on neural precursor cell populations in the adult murine hippocampus. *Aging Cell* 3, 363–371. doi: 10.1111/j.1474-9728.2004.00130.x

Glasper, E. R., Llorens-Martin, M. V., Leuner, B., Gould, E., and Trejo, J. L. (2010). Blockade of insulin-like growth factor-I has complex effects on structural plasticity in the hippocampus. *Hippocampus* 20, 706–712. doi: 10.1002/hipo.20672

Gomez-Nicola, D., Suzzi, S., Vargas-Caballero, M., Fransen, N. L., Al-Malki, H., Cebrian-Silla, A., et al. (2014). Temporal dynamics of hippocampal neurogenesis in chronic neurodegeneration. *Brain* 137, 2312–2328. doi: 10.1093/brain/awu155

Gong, J., Liu, W., Dong, J., Wang, Y., Xu, H., Wei, W., et al. (2010). Developmental iodine deficiency and hypothyroidism impair neural development in rat hippocampus: involvement of doublecortin and NCAM-180. *BMC Neurosci.* 11:50. doi: 10.1186/1471-2202-11-50

Gould, E., Daniels, D. C., Cameron, H. A., and Mcewen, B. S. (1992). Expression of adrenal steroid receptors by newly born cells and pyknotic cells in the dentate gyrus of the postnatal rat. *Mol. Cell. Neurosci.* 3, 44–48. doi: 10.1016/1044-7431(92)90007-O

Gould, E., Mcewen, B. S., Tanapat, P., Galea, L. A., and Fuchs, E. (1997). Neurogenesis in the dentate gyrus of the adult tree shrew is regulated by psychosocial stress and NMDA receptor activation. *J. Neurosci.* 17, 2492–2498.

Gould, E., and Tanapat, P. (1999). Stress and hippocampal neurogenesis. *Biol. Psychiatry* 46, 1472–1479. doi: 10.1016/S0006-3223(99)00247-4

Gould, E., Woolley, C. S., and Mcewen, B. S. (1990). Short-term glucocorticoid manipulations affect neuronal morphology and survival in the adult dentate gyrus. *Neuroscience* 37, 367–375. doi: 10.1016/0306-4522(90)90407-U

Gould, E., Woolley, C. S., and Mcewen, B. S. (1991). Adrenal steroids regulate postnatal development of the rat dentate gyrus: I. Effects of glucocorticoids on cell death. *J. Comp. Neurol.* 313, 479–485. doi: 10.1002/cne.903130308

Govindarajan, A., Israely, I., Huang, S. Y., and Tonegawa, S. (2011). The dendritic branch is the preferred integrative unit for protein synthesis-dependent LTP. *Neuron* 69, 132–146. doi: 10.1016/j.neuron.2010.12.008

Greenough, W. T., and Volkmar, F. R. (1973). Pattern of dendritic branching in occipital cortex of rats reared in complex environments. *Exp. Neurol.* 40, 491–504. doi: 10.1016/0014-4886(73)90090-3

Greenough, W. T., Volkmar, F. R., and Juraska, J. M. (1973). Effects of rearing complexity on dendritic branching in frontolateral and temporal cortex of the rat. *Exp. Neurol.* 41, 371–378. doi: 10.1016/0014-4886(73)90278-1

Gur, T. L., Conti, A. C., Holden, J., Bechtholt, A. J., Hill, T. E., Lucki, I., et al. (2007). cAMP response element-binding protein deficiency allows for increased neurogenesis and a rapid onset of antidepressant response. *J. Neurosci.* 27, 7860–7868. doi: 10.1523/JNEUROSCI.2051-07.2007

Hauser, K. F., and Knapp, P. E. (2014). Interactions of HIV and drugs of abuse: the importance of glia, neural progenitors, and host genetic factors. *Int. Rev. Neurobiol.* 118, 231–313. doi: 10.1016/B978-0-12-801284-0.00009-9

Haussler, U., Rinas, K., Kilias, A., Egert, U., and Haas, C. A. (2015). Mossy fiber sprouting and pyramidal cell dispersion in the hippocampal CA2 region in a mouse model of temporal lobe epilepsy. *Hippocampus.* doi: 10.1002/hipo.22543. [Epub ahead of print].

Hawasli, A. H., Benavides, D. R., Nguyen, C., Kansy, J. W., Hayashi, K., Chambon, P., et al. (2007). Cyclin-dependent kinase 5 governs learning and synaptic plasticity via control of NMDAR degradation. *Nat. Neurosci.* 10, 880–886. doi: 10.1038/nn1914

Heimrich, B., and Frotscher, M. (1991). Differentiation of dentate granule cells in slice cultures of rat hippocampus: a Golgi/electron microscopic study. *Brain Res.* 538, 263–268. doi: 10.1016/0006-8993(91)90438-2

Hernandez-Rabaza, V., Llorens-Martin, M., Velazquez-Sanchez, C., Ferragud, A., Arcusa, A., Gumus, H. G., et al. (2009). Inhibition of adult hippocampal neurogenesis disrupts contextual learning but spares spatial working memory, long-term conditional rule retention and spatial reversal. *Neuroscience* 159, 59–68. doi: 10.1016/j.neuroscience.2008.11.054

Hernandez, F., Gomez De Barreda, E., Fuster-Matanzo, A., Lucas, J. J., and Avila, J. (2010). GSK3: a possible link between beta amyloid peptide and tau protein. *Exp. Neurol.* 223, 322–325. doi: 10.1016/j.expneurol.2009.09.011

Hester, M. S., and Danzer, S. C. (2013). Accumulation of abnormal adult-generated hippocampal granule cells predicts seizure frequency and severity. *J. Neurosci.* 33, 8926–8936. doi: 10.1523/JNEUROSCI.5161-12.2013

Hoffmann, K., Frederiksen, K. S., Sobol, N. A., Beyer, N., Vogel, A., Simonsen, A. H., et al. (2013). Preserving cognition, quality of life, physical health and functional ability in Alzheimer's disease: the effect of physical exercise (ADEX trial): rationale and design. *Neuroepidemiology* 41, 198–207. doi: 10.1159/000354632

Hoglinger, G. U., Rizk, P., Muriel, M. P., Duyckaerts, C., Oertel, W. H., Caille, I., et al. (2004). Dopamine depletion impairs precursor cell proliferation in Parkinson disease. *Nat. Neurosci.* 7, 726–735. doi: 10.1038/nn1265

Holmes, G. L., Gairsa, J. L., Chevassus-Au-Louis, N., and Ben-Ari, Y. (1998). Consequences of neonatal seizures in the rat: morphological and behavioral effects. *Ann. Neurol.* 44, 845–857. doi: 10.1002/ana.410440602

Holmes, G. L., Sarkisian, M., Ben-Ari, Y., and Chevassus-Au-Louis, N. (1999). Mossy fiber sprouting after recurrent seizures during early development in rats. *J. Comp. Neurol.* 404, 537–553.

Hollmann, W., Struder, H. K., Tagarakis, C. V., and King, G. (2007). Physical activity and the elderly. *Eur. J. Cardiovasc. Prev. Rehabil.* 14, 730–739. doi: 10.1097/HJR.0b013e32828622f9

Holloway, R. L. Jr. (1966). Dendritic branching: some preliminary results of training and complexity in rat visual cortex. *Brain Res.* 2, 393–396. doi: 10.1016/0006-8993(66)90009-6

Hosseini-Sharifabad, M., and Hadinedoushan, H. (2007). Prenatal stress induces learning deficits and is associated with a decrease in granules and CA3 cell dendritic tree size in rat hippocampus. *Anat. Sci. Int.* 82, 211–217. doi: 10.1111/j.1447-073X.2007.00186.x

Houser, C. R. (1992). Morphological changes in the dentate gyrus in human temporal lobe epilepsy. *Epilepsy Res.* 7, 223–234.

Hu, M., Zhu, K., Chen, X. L., Zhang, Y. J., Zhang, J. S., Xiao, X. L., et al. (2015). Newly generated neurons at 2 months post-status epilepticus are functionally integrated into neuronal circuitry in mouse hippocampus. *Exp. Neurol.* 273, 273–287. doi: 10.1016/j.expneurol.2015.09.007

Hulihan, M. M., Ishihara-Paul, L., Kachergus, J., Warren, L., Amouri, R., Elango, R., et al. (2008). LRRK2 Gly2019Ser penetrance in Arab-Berber patients from Tunisia: a case-control genetic study. *Lancet Neurol.* 7, 591–594. doi: 10.1016/S1474-4422(08)70116-9

Hyman, B. T., Van Hoesen, G. W., Damasio, A. R., and Barnes, C. L. (1984). Alzheimer's disease: cell-specific pathology isolates the hippocampal formation. *Science* 225, 1168–1170. doi: 10.1126/science.6474172

Iyengar, S. S., Lafrancois, J. J., Friedman, D., Drew, L. J., Denny, C. A., Burghardt, N. S., et al. (2015). Suppression of adult neurogenesis increases the acute effects of kainic acid. *Exp. Neurol.* 264, 135–149. doi: 10.1016/j.expneurol.2014.11.009

Jagasia, R., Steib, K., Englberger, E., Herold, S., Faus-Kessler, T., Saxe, M., et al. (2009). GABA-cAMP response element-binding protein signaling regulates maturation and survival of newly generated neurons in the adult hippocampus. *J. Neurosci.* 29, 7966–7977. doi: 10.1523/JNEUROSCI.1054-09.2009

Jessberger, S., Aigner, S., Clemenson, G. D. Jr., Toni, N., Lie, D. C., Karalay, O., et al. (2008). Cdk5 regulates accurate maturation of newborn granule cells in the adult hippocampus. *PLoS Biol.* 6:e272. doi: 10.1371/journal.pbio.0060272

Jessberger, S., Zhao, C., Toni, N., Clemenson, G. D. Jr., Li, Y., and Gage, F. H. (2007). Seizure-associated, aberrant neurogenesis in adult rats characterized with retrovirus-mediated cell labeling. *J. Neurosci.* 27, 9400–9407. doi: 10.1523/JNEUROSCI.2002-07.2007

Jin, K., Galvan, V., Xie, L., Mao, X. O., Gorostiza, O. F., Bredesen, D. E., et al. (2004a). Enhanced neurogenesis in Alzheimer's disease transgenic (PDGF-APPSw, Ind) mice. *Proc. Natl. Acad. Sci. U.S.A.* 101, 13363–13367. doi: 10.1073/pnas.0403678101

Jin, K., Peel, A. L., Mao, X. O., Xie, L., Cottrell, B. A., Henshall, D. C., et al. (2004b). Increased hippocampal neurogenesis in Alzheimer's disease. *Proc. Natl. Acad. Sci. U.S.A.* 101, 343–347. doi: 10.1073/pnas.2634794100

Joels, M. (2006). Corticosteroid effects in the brain: U-shape it. *Trends Pharmacol. Sci.* 27, 244–250. doi: 10.1016/j.tips.2006.03.007

Johnson, E. A., Dao, T. L., Guignet, M. A., Geddes, C. E., Koemeter-Cox, A. I., and Kan, R. K. (2011). Increased expression of the chemokines CXCL1 and MIP-1alpha by resident brain cells precedes neutrophil infiltration in the brain following prolonged soman-induced status epilepticus in rats. *J. Neuroinflammation* 8:41. doi: 10.1186/1742-2094-8-41

Jope, R. S., Yuskaitis, C. J., and Beurel, E. (2007). Glycogen synthase kinase-3 (GSK3): inflammation, diseases, and therapeutics. *Neurochem. Res.* 32, 577–595. doi: 10.1007/s11064-006-9128-5

Juraska, J. M., Fitch, J. M., Henderson, C., and Rivers, N. (1985). Sex differences in the dendritic branching of dentate granule cells following differential experience. *Brain Res.* 333, 73–80. doi: 10.1016/0006-8993(85)90125-8

Jurgens, H. A., Amancherla, K., and Johnson, R. W. (2012). Influenza infection induces neuroinflammation, alters hippocampal neuron morphology, and impairs cognition in adult mice. *J. Neurosci.* 32, 3958–3968. doi: 10.1523/JNEUROSCI.6389-11.2012

Kelsch, W., Lin, C. W., and Lois, C. (2008). Sequential development of synapses in dendritic domains during adult neurogenesis. *Proc. Natl. Acad. Sci. U.S.A.* 105, 16803–16808. doi: 10.1073/pnas.0807970105

Kempermann, G. (2006). They are not too excited: the possible role of adult-born neurons in epilepsy. *Neuron* 52, 935–937. doi: 10.1016/j.neuron.2006.12.004

Kempermann, G., Jessberger, S., Steiner, B., and Kronenberg, G. (2004). Milestones of neuronal development in the adult hippocampus. *Trends Neurosci.* 27, 447–452. doi: 10.1016/j.tins.2004.05.013

Kempermann, G., Kuhn, H. G., and Gage, F. H. (1998). Experience-induced neurogenesis in the senescent dentate gyrus. *J. Neurosci.* 18, 3206–3212.

Kernie, S. G., and Parent, J. M. (2010). Forebrain neurogenesis after focal Ischemic and traumatic brain injury. *Neurobiol. Dis.* 37, 267–274. doi: 10.1016/j.nbd.2009.11.002

Khandaker, G. M., and Dantzer, R. (2015). Is there a role for immune-to-brain communication in schizophrenia? *Psychopharmacology (Berl).* [Epub ahead of print].

Kharatishvili, I., Nissinen, J. P., Mcintosh, T. K., and Pitkanen, A. (2006). A model of posttraumatic epilepsy induced by lateral fluid-percussion brain injury in rats. *Neuroscience* 140, 685–697. doi: 10.1016/j.neuroscience.2006.03.012

Kim, S. J., Lee, K. J., Shin, Y. C., Choi, S. H., Do, E., Kim, S., et al. (2005). Stress-induced decrease of granule cell proliferation in adult rat hippocampus: assessment of granule cell proliferation using high doses of bromodeoxyuridine before and after restraint stress. *Mol. Cells* 19, 74–80.

Kobayashi, K. (2009). Targeting the hippocampal mossy fiber synapse for the treatment of psychiatric disorders. *Mol. Neurobiol.* 39, 24–36. doi: 10.1007/s12035-008-8049-5

Kohara, K., Pignatelli, M., Rivest, A. J., Jung, H. Y., Kitamura, T., Suh, J., et al. (2014). Cell type-specific genetic and optogenetic tools reveal hippocampal CA2 circuits. *Nat. Neurosci.* 17, 269–279. doi: 10.1038/nn.3614

Kohler, S. J., Williams, N. I., Stanton, G. B., Cameron, J. L., and Greenough, W. T. (2011). Maturation time of new granule cells in the dentate gyrus of adult macaque monkeys exceeds six months. *Proc. Natl. Acad. Sci. U.S.A.* 108, 10326–10331. doi: 10.1073/pnas.1017099108

Kohman, R. A., and Rhodes, J. S. (2013). Neurogenesis, inflammation and behavior. *Brain Behav. Immun.* 27, 22–32. doi: 10.1016/j.bbi.2012.09.003

Kron, M. M., Zhang, H., and Parent, J. M. (2010). The developmental stage of dentate granule cells dictates their contribution to seizure-induced plasticity. *J. Neurosci.* 30, 2051–2059. doi: 10.1523/JNEUROSCI.5655-09.2010

Kronenberg, G., Bick-Sander, A., Bunk, E., Wolf, C., Ehninger, D., and Kempermann, G. (2006). Physical exercise prevents age-related decline in precursor cell activity in the mouse dentate gyrus. *Neurobiol. Aging* 27, 1505–1513. doi: 10.1016/j.neurobiolaging.2005.09.016

Kvajo, M., Mckellar, H., Drew, L. J., Lepagnol-Bestel, A. M., Xiao, L., Levy, R. J., et al. (2011). Altered axonal targeting and short-term plasticity in the hippocampus of Disc1 mutant mice. *Proc. Natl. Acad. Sci. U.S.A.* 108, E1349–E1358. doi: 10.1073/pnas.1114113108

Lauer, M., Beckmann, H., and Senitz, D. (2003). Increased frequency of dentate granule cells with basal dendrites in the hippocampal formation of schizophrenics. *Psychiatry Res.* 122, 89–97. doi: 10.1016/S0925-4927(02)00122-1

Lee, F. H., Kaidanovich-Beilin, O., Roder, J. C., Woodgett, J. R., and Wong, A. H. (2011). Genetic inactivation of GSK3alpha rescues spine deficits in Disc1-L100P mutant mice. *Schizophr. Res.* 129, 74–79. doi: 10.1016/j.schres.2011.03.032

Lee, J., Seroogy, K. B., and Mattson, M. P. (2002). Dietary restriction enhances neurotrophin expression and neurogenesis in the hippocampus of adult mice. *J. Neurochem.* 80, 539–547. doi: 10.1046/j.0022-3042.2001.00747.x

Levenson, C. W., and Rich, N. J. (2007). Eat less, live longer? New insights into the role of caloric restriction in the brain. *Nutr. Rev.* 65, 412–415. doi: 10.1111/j.1753-4887.2007.tb00319.x

Li, B., Yamamori, H., Tatebayashi, Y., Shafit-Zagardo, B., Tanimukai, H., Chen, S., et al. (2008). Failure of neuronal maturation in Alzheimer disease dentate gyrus. *J. Neuropathol. Exp. Neurol.* 67, 78–84. doi: 10.1097/nen.0b013e318160c5db

Lipina, T. V., Kaidanovich-Beilin, O., Patel, S., Wang, M., Clapcote, S. J., Liu, F., et al. (2011). Genetic and pharmacological evidence for schizophrenia-related Disc1 interaction with GSK-3. *Synapse* 65, 234–248. doi: 10.1002/syn.20839

Liposits, Z., Kallo, I., Hrabovszky, E., and Gallyas, F. (1997). Ultrastructural pathology of degenerating "dark" granule cells in the hippocampal dentate gyrus of adrenalectomized rats. *Acta Biol. Hung.* 48, 173–187.

Liu, J., Solway, K., Messing, R. O., and Sharp, F. R. (1998). Increased neurogenesis in the dentate gyrus after transient global ischemia in gerbils. *J. Neurosci.* 18, 7768–7778.

Liu, R. Y., Zhou, J. N., Van Heerikhuize, J., Hofman, M. A., and Swaab, D. F. (1999). Decreased melatonin levels in postmortem cerebrospinal fluid in relation to aging, Alzheimer's disease, and apolipoprotein E-epsilon4/4 genotype. *J. Clin. Endocrinol. Metab.* 84, 323–327.

Llorens-Martin, M., Fuster-Matanzo, A., Teixeira, C. M., Jurado-Arjona, J., Ulloa, F., Defelipe, J., et al. (2013). GSK-3beta overexpression causes reversible alterations on postsynaptic densities and dendritic morphology of hippocampal granule neurons *in vivo*. *Mol. Psychiatry* 18, 451–460. doi: 10.1038/mp.2013.4

Llorens-Martin, M., Jurado-Arjona, J., Avila, J., and Hernandez, F. (2015). Novel connection between newborn granule neurons and the hippocampal CA2 field. *Exp. Neurol.* 263, 285–292. doi: 10.1016/j.expneurol.2014.10.021

Llorens-Martin, M., Jurado-Arjona, J., Fuster-Matanzo, A., Hernandez, F., Rabano, A., and Avila, J. (2014a). Peripherally triggered and GSK-3beta-driven brain inflammation differentially skew adult hippocampal neurogenesis, behavioral pattern separation and microglial activation in response to ibuprofen. *Transl. Psychiatry* 4, e463. doi: 10.1038/tp.2014.92

Llorens-Martin, M., Jurado, J., Hernandez, F., and Avila, J. (2014b). GSK-3beta, a pivotal kinase in Alzheimer disease. *Front. Mol. Neurosci.* 7:46. doi: 10.3389/fnmol.2014.00046

Llorens-Martin, M., Teixeira, C. M., Fuster-Matanzo, A., Jurado-Arjona, J., Borrell, V., Soriano, E., et al. (2012). Tau isoform with three microtubule binding domains is a marker of new axons generated from the subgranular zone in the hippocampal dentate gyrus: implications for Alzheimer's disease. *J. Alzheimers. Dis.* 29, 921–930. doi: 10.3233/JAD-2012-112057

Llorens-Martin, M., Tejeda, G. S., and Trejo, J. L. (2011). Antidepressant and proneurogenic influence of environmental enrichment in mice: protective effects vs recovery. *Neuropsychopharmacology* 36, 2460–2468. doi: 10.1038/npp.2011.134

Llorens-Martin, M., Torres-Aleman, I., and Trejo, J. L. (2006). Pronounced individual variation in the response to the stimulatory action of exercise on immature hippocampal neurons. *Hippocampus* 16, 480–490. doi: 10.1002/hipo.20175

Llorens-Martin, M., Torres-Aleman, I., and Trejo, J. L. (2008). Growth factors as mediators of exercise actions on the brain. *Neuromolecular Med.* 10, 99–107. doi: 10.1007/s12017-008-8026-1

Llorens-Martin, M., and Trejo, J. L. (2011). Mifepristone prevents stress-induced apoptosis in newborn neurons and increases AMPA receptor expression in the dentate gyrus of C57/BL6 mice. *PLoS ONE* 6:e28376. doi: 10.1371/journal.pone.0028376

Lothman, E. W., Stringer, J. L., and Bertram, E. H. (1992). The dentate gyrus as a control point for seizures in the hippocampus and beyond. *Epilepsy Res.* 7, 301–313.

Lurton, D., El Bahh, B., Sundstrom, L., and Rougier, A. (1998). Granule cell dispersion is correlated with early epileptic events in human temporal lobe epilepsy. *J. Neurol. Sci.* 154, 133–136. doi: 10.1016/S0022-510X(97)00220-7

Maccioni, R. B., Otth, C., Concha, I.I, and Munoz, J. P. (2001). The protein kinase Cdk5. Structural aspects, roles in neurogenesis and involvement in A.lzheimer's pathology. *Eur. J. Biochem.* 268, 1518–1527. doi: 10.1046/j.1432-1327.2001.02024.x

Madeira, M. D., Cadete-Leite, A., Andrade, J. P., and Paula-Barbosa, M. M. (1991). Effects of hypothyroidism upon the granular layer of the dentate gyrus in male and female adult rats: a morphometric study. *J. Comp. Neurol.* 314, 171–186. doi: 10.1002/cne.903140116

Magill, S. T., Cambronne, X. A., Luikart, B. W., Lioy, D. T., Leighton, B. H., Westbrook, G. L., et al. (2010). microRNA-132 regulates dendritic growth and arborization of newborn neurons in the adult hippocampus. *Proc. Natl. Acad. Sci. U.S.A.* 107, 20382–20387. doi: 10.1073/pnas.1015691107

Malberg, J. E., Eisch, A. J., Nestler, E. J., and Duman, R. S. (2000). Chronic antidepressant treatment increases neurogenesis in adult rat hippocampus. *J. Neurosci.* 20, 9104–9110.

Mao, Y., Ge, X., Frank, C. L., Madison, J. M., Koehler, A. N., Doud, M. K., et al. (2009). Disrupted in schizophrenia 1 regulates neuronal progenitor proliferation via modulation of GSK3beta/beta-catenin signaling. *Cell* 136, 1017–1031. doi: 10.1016/j.cell.2008.12.044

Martin, M., Rehani, K., Jope, R. S., and Michalek, S. M. (2005). Toll-like receptor-mediated cytokine production is differentially regulated by glycogen synthase kinase 3. *Nat. Immunol.* 6, 777–784. doi: 10.1038/ni1221

Meraz-Rios, M. A., Toral-Rios, D., Franco-Bocanegra, D., Villeda-Hernandez, J., and Campos-Pena, V. (2013). Inflammatory process in Alzheimer's Disease. *Front. Integr. Neurosci.* 7:59. doi: 10.3389/fnint.2013.00059

Meyer, K. D., and Morris, J. A. (2009). Disc1 regulates granule cell migration in the developing hippocampus. *Hum. Mol. Genet.* 18, 3286–3297. doi: 10.1093/hmg/ddp266

Miki, T., Harris, S. J., Wilce, P. A., Takeuchi, Y., and Bedi, K. S. (2003). Effects of alcohol exposure during early life on neuron numbers in the rat hippocampus. I. Hilus neurons and granule cells. *Hippocampus* 13, 388–398. doi: 10.1002/hipo.10072

Ming, G. L., and Song, H. (2009). DISC1 partners with GSK3beta in neurogenesis. *Cell* 136, 990–992. doi: 10.1016/j.cell.2009.03.005

Mitra, R., Sundlass, K., Parker, K. J., Schatzberg, A. F., and Lyons, D. M. (2006). Social stress-related behavior affects hippocampal cell proliferation in mice. *Physiol. Behav.* 89, 123–127. doi: 10.1016/j.physbeh.2006.05.047

Monje, M. L., Toda, H., and Palmer, T. D. (2003). Inflammatory blockade restores adult hippocampal neurogenesis. *Science* 302, 1760–1765. doi: 10.1126/science.1088417

Murphy, B. L., Pun, R. Y., Yin, H., Faulkner, C. R., Loepke, A. W., and Danzer, S. C. (2011). Heterogeneous integration of adult-generated granule cells into the epileptic brain. *J. Neurosci.* 31, 105–117. doi: 10.1523/JNEUROSCI.2728-10.2011

Murphy, T., Dias, G. P., and Thuret, S. (2014). Effects of diet on brain plasticity in animal and human studies: mind the gap. *Neural Plast.* 2014:563160. doi: 10.1155/2014/563160

Namba, T., Ming, G. L., Song, H., Waga, C., Enomoto, A., Kaibuchi, K., et al. (2011). NMDA receptor regulates migration of newly generated neurons in the adult hippocampus via Disrupted-In-Schizophrenia 1 (DISC1). *J. Neurochem.* 118, 34–44. doi: 10.1111/j.1471-4159.2011.07282.x

Naylor, A. S., Bull, C., Nilsson, M. K., Zhu, C., Bjork-Eriksson, T., Eriksson, P. S., et al. (2008). Voluntary running rescues adult hippocampal neurogenesis after irradiation of the young mouse brain. *Proc. Natl. Acad. Sci. U.S.A.* 105, 14632–14637. doi: 10.1073/pnas.0711128105

Neeper, S. A., Gomez-Pinilla, F., Choi, J., and Cotman, C. (1995). Exercise and brain neurotrophins. *Nature* 373, 109. doi: 10.1038/373109a0

Neeper, S. A., Gomez-Pinilla, F., Choi, J., and Cotman, C. W. (1996). Physical activity increases mRNA for brain-derived neurotrophic factor and nerve growth factor in rat brain. *Brain Res.* 726, 49–56. doi: 10.1016/0006-8993(96)00273-9

Ng, T., Ryu, J. R., Sohn, J. H., Tan, T., Song, H., Ming, G. L., et al. (2013). Class 3 semaphorin mediates dendrite growth in adult newborn neurons through Cdk5/FAK pathway. *PLoS ONE* 8:e65572. doi: 10.1371/journal.pone.0065572

Nishi, M., Usuku, T., Itose, M., Fujikawa, K., Hosokawa, K., Matsuda, K. I., et al. (2007). Direct visualization of glucocorticoid receptor positive cells in the hippocampal regions using green fluorescent protein transgenic mice. *Neuroscience* 146, 1555–1560. doi: 10.1016/j.neuroscience.2007.03.020

Niv, F., Keiner, S., Krishna, W. O. W., Lie, D. C., and Redecker, C. (2012). Aberrant neurogenesis after stroke: a retroviral cell labeling study. *Stroke* 43, 2468–2475. doi: 10.1161/STROKEAHA.112.660977

Ohshima, T., Hirasawa, M., Tabata, H., Mutoh, T., Adachi, T., Suzuki, H., et al. (2007). Cdk5 is required for multipolar-to-bipolar transition during radial neuronal migration and proper dendrite development of pyramidal neurons in the cerebral cortex. *Development* 134, 2273–2282. doi: 10.1242/dev.02854

Oliff, H. S., Berchtold, N. C., Isackson, P., and Cotman, C. W. (1998). Exercise-induced regulation of brain-derived neurotrophic factor (BDNF) transcripts in the rat hippocampus. *Brain Res. Mol. Brain Res.* 61, 147–153. doi: 10.1016/S0169-328X(98)00222-8

Olson, A. K., Eadie, B. D., Ernst, C., and Christie, B. R. (2006). Environmental enrichment and voluntary exercise massively increase neurogenesis in the adult hippocampus via dissociable pathways. *Hippocampus* 16, 250–260. doi: 10.1002/hipo.20157

Opendak, M., and Gould, E. (2011). New neurons maintain efficient stress recovery. *Cell Stem Cell* 9, 287–288. doi: 10.1016/j.stem.2011.09.003

Ortega-Martinez, S., and Trejo, J. L. (2015). The postnatal origin of adult neural stem cells and the effects of glucocorticoids on their genesis. *Behav. Brain Res.* 279, 166–176. doi: 10.1016/j.bbr.2014.11.013

Overstreet-Wadiche, L. S., Bromberg, D. A., Bensen, A. L., and Westbrook, G. L. (2006). Seizures accelerate functional integration of adult-generated granule cells. *J. Neurosci.* 26, 4095–4103. doi: 10.1523/JNEUROSCI.5508-05.2006

Pais, T. F., Figueiredo, C., Peixoto, R., Braz, M. H., and Chatterjee, S. (2008). Necrotic neurons enhance microglial neurotoxicity through induction of glutaminase by a MyD88-dependent pathway. *J. Neuroinflammation* 5:43. doi: 10.1186/1742-2094-5-43

Parent, J. M., Yu, T. W., Leibowitz, R. T., Geschwind, D. H., Sloviter, R. S., and Lowenstein, D. H. (1997). Dentate granule cell neurogenesis is increased by seizures and contributes to aberrant network reorganization in the adult rat hippocampus. *J. Neurosci.* 17, 3727–3738.

Parle, M., Vasudevan, M., and Singh, N. (2005). Swim everyday to keep dementia away. *J. Sports Sci. Med.* 4, 37–46.

Patel, L. S., Wenzel, H. J., and Schwartzkroin, P. A. (2004). Physiological and morphological characterization of dentate granule cells in the p35 knock-out mouse hippocampus: evidence for an epileptic circuit. *J. Neurosci.* 24, 9005–9014. doi: 10.1523/JNEUROSCI.2943-04.2004

Peineau, S., Taghibiglou, C., Bradley, C., Wong, T. P., Liu, L., Lu, J., et al. (2007). LTP inhibits LTD in the hippocampus via regulation of GSK3beta. *Neuron* 53, 703–717. doi: 10.1016/j.neuron.2007.01.029

Perry, E. K., Johnson, M., Ekonomou, A., Perry, R. H., Ballard, C., and Attems, J. (2012). Neurogenic abnormalities in Alzheimer's disease differ between stages of neurogenesis and are partly related to cholinergic pathology. *Neurobiol. Dis.* 47, 155–162. doi: 10.1016/j.nbd.2012.03.033

Politis, M., Wu, K., Loane, C., Turkheimer, F. E., Molloy, S., Brooks, D. J., et al. (2010). Depressive symptoms in PD correlate with higher 5-HTT binding in raphe and limbic structures. *Neurology* 75, 1920–1927. doi: 10.1212/WNL.0b013e3181feb2ab

Possin, K. L., Filoteo, J. V., Song, D. D., and Salmon, D. P. (2008). Spatial and object working memory deficits in Parkinson's disease are due to impairment in different underlying processes. *Neuropsychology* 22, 585–595. doi: 10.1037/a0012613

Powrozek, T. A., Sari, Y., Singh, R. P., and Zhou, F. C. (2004). Neurotransmitters and substances of abuse: effects on adult neurogenesis. *Curr. Neurovasc. Res.* 1, 251–260. doi: 10.2174/1567202043362225

Rami, A., Patel, A. J., and Rabie, A. (1986). Thyroid hormone and development of the rat hippocampus: morphological alterations in granule and pyramidal cells. *Neuroscience* 19, 1217–1226. doi: 10.1016/0306-4522(86)90135-1

Ramirez-Rodriguez, G., Klempin, F., Babu, H., Benitez-King, G., and Kempermann, G. (2009). Melatonin modulates cell survival of new neurons in the hippocampus of adult mice. *Neuropsychopharmacology* 34, 2180–2191. doi: 10.1038/npp.2009.46

Ramirez-Rodriguez, G., Ortiz-Lopez, L., Dominguez-Alonso, A., Benitez-King, G. A., and Kempermann, G. (2011). Chronic treatment with melatonin stimulates dendrite maturation and complexity in adult hippocampal neurogenesis of mice. *J. Pineal Res.* 50, 29–37. doi: 10.1111/j.1600-079X.2010.00802.x

Redila, V. A., and Christie, B. R. (2006). Exercise-induced changes in dendritic structure and complexity in the adult hippocampal dentate gyrus. *Neuroscience* 137, 1299–1307. doi: 10.1016/j.neuroscience.2005.10.050

Redila, V. A., Olson, A. K., Swann, S. E., Mohades, G., Webber, A. J., Weinberg, J., et al. (2006). Hippocampal cell proliferation is reduced following prenatal ethanol exposure but can be rescued with voluntary exercise. *Hippocampus* 16, 305–311. doi: 10.1002/hipo.20164

Ribak, C. E., and Dashtipour, K. (2002). Neuroplasticity in the damaged dentate gyrus of the epileptic brain. *Prog. Brain Res.* 136, 319–328. doi: 10.1016/S0079-6123(02)36027-8

Ribak, C. E., Korn, M. J., Shan, Z., and Obenaus, A. (2004). Dendritic growth cones and recurrent basal dendrites are typical features of newly generated dentate granule cells in the adult hippocampus. *Brain Res.* 1000, 195–199. doi: 10.1016/j.brainres.2004.01.011

Salam, J. N., Fox, J. H., Detroy, E. M., Guignon, M. H., Wohl, D. F., and Falls, W. A. (2009). Voluntary exercise in C57 mice is anxiolytic across several measures of anxiety. *Behav. Brain Res.* 197, 31–40. doi: 10.1016/j.bbr.2008.07.036

Santarelli, L., Saxe, M., Gross, C., Surget, A., Battaglia, F., Dulawa, S., et al. (2003). Requirement of hippocampal neurogenesis for the behavioral effects of antidepressants. *Science* 301, 805–809. doi: 10.1126/science.1083328

Santos, V. R., De Castro, O. W., Pun, R. Y., Hester, M. S., Murphy, B. L., Loepke, A. W., et al. (2011). Contributions of mature granule cells to structural plasticity in temporal lobe epilepsy. *Neuroscience* 197, 348–357. doi: 10.1016/j.neuroscience.2011.09.034

Selvin-Testa, A. (1991). Chronic lead exposure induces alterations on local circuit neurons. *Microsc. Electron. Biol. Celular* 15, 25–39.

Senitz, D., and Beckmann, H. (2003). Granule cells of the dentate gyrus with basal and recurrent dendrites in schizophrenic patients and controls. *A comparative Golgi study. J Neural Transm* 110, 317–326. doi: 10.1007/s00702-002-0776-6

Seress, L. (1992). Morphological variability and developmental aspects of monkey and human granule cells: differences between the rodent and primate dentate gyrus. *Epilepsy Res.* 7, 3–28.

Seress, L., and Frotscher, M. (1990). Morphological variability is a characteristic feature of granule cells in the primate fascia dentata: a combined Golgi/electron microscope study. *J. Comp. Neurol.* 293, 253–267. doi: 10.1002/cne.902930208

Seress, L., and Mrzljak, L. (1987). Basal dendrites of granule cells are normal features of the fetal and adult dentate gyrus of both monkey and human hippocampal formations. *Brain Res.* 405, 169–174. doi: 10.1016/0006-8993(87)91003-1

Seress, L., and Pokorny, J. (1981). Structure of the granular layer of the rat dentate gyrus. A light microscopic and Golgi study. *J. Anat.* 133, 181–195.

Seress, L., and Ribak, C. E. (1992). Ultrastructural features of primate granule cell bodies show important differences from those of rats: axosomatic synapses, somatic spines and infolded nuclei. *Brain Res.* 569, 353–357. doi: 10.1016/0006-8993(92)90651-O

Shapiro, L. A., Korn, M. J., and Ribak, C. E. (2005). Newly generated dentate granule cells from epileptic rats exhibit elongated hilar basal dendrites that align along GFAP-immunolabeled processes. *Neuroscience* 136, 823–831. doi: 10.1016/j.neuroscience.2005.03.059

Shigemoto-Mogami, Y., Hoshikawa, K., Goldman, J. E., Sekino, Y., and Sato, K. (2014). Microglia enhance neurogenesis and oligodendrogenesis in the early postnatal subventricular zone. *J. Neurosci.* 34, 2231–2243. doi: 10.1523/JNEUROSCI.1619-13.2014

Sierra, A., Abiega, O., Shahraz, A., and Neumann, H. (2013). Janus-faced microglia: beneficial and detrimental consequences of microglial phagocytosis. *Front. Cell. Neurosci.* 7:6. doi: 10.3389/fncel.2013.00006

Sirerol-Piquer, M., Gomez-Ramos, P., Hernandez, F., Perez, M., Moran, M. A., Fuster-Matanzo, A., et al. (2011). GSK3beta overexpression induces neuronal death and a depletion of the neurogenic niches in the dentate gyrus. *Hippocampus* 21, 910–922. doi: 10.1002/hipo.20805

Snyder, J. S., Soumier, A., Brewer, M., Pickel, J., and Cameron, H. A. (2011). Adult hippocampal neurogenesis buffers stress responses and depressive behaviour. *Nature* 476, 458–461. doi: 10.1038/nature10287

Spalding, K. L., Bergmann, O., Alkass, K., Bernard, S., Salehpour, M., Huttner, H. B., et al. (2013). Dynamics of hippocampal neurogenesis in adult humans. *Cell* 153, 1219–1227. doi: 10.1016/j.cell.2013.05.002

Spigelman, I., Yan, X. X., Obenaus, A., Lee, E. Y., Wasterlain, C. G., and Ribak, C. E. (1998). Dentate granule cells form novel basal dendrites in a rat model of temporal lobe epilepsy. *Neuroscience* 86, 109–120. doi: 10.1016/S0306-4522(98)00028-1

Spillantini, M. G., Schmidt, M. L., Lee, V. M., Trojanowski, J. Q., Jakes, R., and Goedert, M. (1997). Alpha-synuclein in Lewy bodies. *Nature* 388, 839–840. doi: 10.1038/42166

Staples, M. C., Kim, A., and Mandyam, C. D. (2015). Dendritic remodeling of hippocampal neurons is associated with altered NMDA receptor expression in alcohol dependent rats. *Mol. Cell. Neurosci.* 65, 153–162. doi: 10.1016/j.mcn.2015.03.008

Stranahan, A. M., Khalil, D., and Gould, E. (2007). Running induces widespread structural alterations in the hippocampus and entorhinal cortex. *Hippocampus* 17, 1017–1022. doi: 10.1002/hipo.20348

Stranahan, A. M., Lee, K., Martin, B., Maudsley, S., Golden, E., Cutler, R. G., et al. (2009). Voluntary exercise and caloric restriction enhance hippocampal dendritic spine density and BDNF levels in diabetic mice. *Hippocampus* 19, 951–961. doi: 10.1002/hipo.20577

Suh, J., Foster, D. J., Davoudi, H., Wilson, M. A., and Tonegawa, S. (2013). Impaired hippocampal ripple-associated replay in a mouse model of schizophrenia. *Neuron* 80, 484–493. doi: 10.1016/j.neuron.2013.09.014

Sutula, T., He, X. X., Cavazos, J., and Scott, G. (1988). Synaptic reorganization in the hippocampus induced by abnormal functional activity. *Science* 239, 1147–1150. doi: 10.1126/science.2449733

Svanidze, I. K., Didimova, E. V., and Tsaishvili Ts, S. (2001). Proliferative activity of the matrix cells in lateral ventricles and granule cells in the dentate gyrus of the hippocampus in rats after pre- and postnatal alcoholic intoxication. *Izv. Akad. Nauk Ser. Biol.* 1, 117–120.

Takashima, A., Noguchi, K., Sato, K., Hoshino, T., and Imahori, K. (1993). Tau protein kinase I is essential for amyloid beta-protein-induced neurotoxicity. *Proc. Natl. Acad. Sci. U.S.A.* 90, 7789–7793. doi: 10.1073/pnas.90.16.7789

Tanapat, P., Galea, L. A., and Gould, E. (1998). Stress inhibits the proliferation of granule cell precursors in the developing dentate gyrus. *Int. J. Dev. Neurosci.* 16, 235–239. doi: 10.1016/S0736-5748(98)00029-X

Tejada, J., Arisi, G. M., Garcia-Cairasco, N., and Roque, A. C. (2012). Morphological alterations in newly born dentate gyrus granule cells that emerge after status epilepticus contribute to make them less excitable. *PLoS ONE* 7:e40726. doi: 10.1371/journal.pone.0040726

Tejada, J., Garcia-Cairasco, N., and Roque, A. C. (2014). Combined role of seizure-induced dendritic morphology alterations and spine loss in newborn granule cells with mossy fiber sprouting on the hyperexcitability of a computer model of the dentate gyrus. *PLoS Comput. Biol.* 10:e1003601. doi: 10.1371/journal.pcbi.1003601

Tolwani, R. J., Buckmaster, P. S., Varma, S., Cosgaya, J. M., Wu, Y., Suri, C., et al. (2002). BDNF overexpression increases dendrite complexity in hippocampal dentate gyrus. *Neuroscience* 114, 795–805. doi: 10.1016/S0306-4522(02)00301-9

Toscano, C. D., and Guilarte, T. R. (2005). Lead neurotoxicity: from exposure to molecular effects. *Brain Res. Brain Res. Rev.* 49, 529–554. doi: 10.1016/j.brainresrev.2005.02.004

Toscano, C. D., O'callaghan, J. P., and Guilarte, T. R. (2005). Calcium/calmodulin-dependent protein kinase II activity and expression are altered in the hippocampus of Pb2+-exposed rats. *Brain Res.* 1044, 51–58. doi: 10.1016/j.brainres.2005.02.076

Town, T., Nikolic, V., and Tan, J. (2005). The microglial "activation" continuum: from innate to adaptive responses. *J. Neuroinflammation* 2:24. doi: 10.1186/1742-2094-2-24

Tozuka, Y., Kumon, M., Wada, E., Onodera, M., Mochizuki, H., and Wada, K. (2010). Maternal obesity impairs hippocampal BDNF production and spatial learning performance in young mouse offspring. *Neurochem. Int.* 57, 235–247. doi: 10.1016/j.neuint.2010.05.015

Trejo, J. L., Carro, E., and Torres-Aleman, I. (2001). Circulating insulin-like growth factor I mediates exercise-induced increases in the number of new neurons in the adult hippocampus. *J. Neurosci.* 21, 1628–1634.

Trejo, J. L., Cuchillo, I., Machin, C., and Rua, C. (2000). Maternal adrenalectomy at the early onset of gestation impairs the postnatal development of the rat hippocampal formation: effects on cell numbers and differentiation, connectivity and calbindin-D28k immunoreactivity. *J. Neurosci. Res.* 62, 644–667. doi: 10.1002/1097-4547(20001201)62:5<644::AID-JNR4>3.0.CO;2-3

Trejo, J. L., Llorens-Martin, M. V., and Torres-Aleman, I. (2008). The effects of exercise on spatial learning and anxiety-like behavior are mediated by an IGF-I-dependent mechanism related to hippocampal neurogenesis. *Mol. Cell. Neurosci.* 37, 402–411. doi: 10.1016/j.mcn.2007.10.016

Tsai, L. H., Delalle, I., Caviness, V. S. Jr., Chae, T., and Harlow, E. (1994). p35 is a neural-specific regulatory subunit of cyclin-dependent kinase 5. *Nature* 371, 419–423. doi: 10.1038/371419a0

van Praag, H., Christie, B. R., Sejnowski, T. J., and Gage, F. H. (1999a). Running enhances neurogenesis, learning, and long-term potentiation in mice. *Proc. Natl. Acad. Sci. U.S.A.* 96, 13427–13431.

van Praag, H., Kempermann, G., and Gage, F. H. (1999b). Running increases cell proliferation and neurogenesis in the adult mouse dentate gyrus. *Nat. Neurosci.* 2, 266–270.

van Praag, H., Kempermann, G., and Gage, F. H. (2000). Neural consequences of environmental enrichment. *Nat. Rev. Neurosci.* 1, 191–198. doi: 10.1038/35044558

van Praag, H., Schinder, A. F., Christie, B. R., Toni, N., Palmer, T. D., and Gage, F. H. (2002). Functional neurogenesis in the adult hippocampus. *Nature* 415, 1030–1034. doi: 10.1038/4151030a

van Praag, H., Shubert, T., Zhao, C., and Gage, F. H. (2005). Exercise enhances learning and hippocampal neurogenesis in aged mice. *J. Neurosci.* 25, 8680–8685. doi: 10.1523/JNEUROSCI.1731-05.2005

Varnum, M. M., and Ikezu, T. (2012). The classification of microglial activation phenotypes on neurodegeneration and regeneration in Alzheimer's disease brain. *Arch. Immunol. Ther. Exp. (Warsz).* 60, 251–266. doi: 10.1007/s00005-012-0181-2

Vaynman, S., Ying, Z., and Gomez-Pinilla, F. (2004). Hippocampal BDNF mediates the efficacy of exercise on synaptic plasticity and cognition. *Eur. J. Neurosci.* 20, 2580–2590. doi: 10.1111/j.1460-9568.2004.03720.x

Verina, T., Rohde, C. A., and Guilarte, T. R. (2007). Environmental lead exposure during early life alters granule cell neurogenesis and morphology in the hippocampus of young adult rats. *Neuroscience* 145, 1037–1047. doi: 10.1016/j.neuroscience.2006.12.040

Vo, N., Klein, M. E., Varlamova, O., Keller, D. M., Yamamoto, T., Goodman, R. H., et al. (2005). A cAMP-response element binding protein-induced microRNA regulates neuronal morphogenesis. *Proc. Natl. Acad. Sci. U.S.A.* 102, 16426–16431. doi: 10.1073/pnas.0508448102

von Campe, G., Spencer, D. D., and De Lanerolle, N. C. (1997). Morphology of dentate granule cells in the human epileptogenic hippocampus. *Hippocampus* 7, 472–488.

Wang, L., Chang, X., She, L., Xu, D., Huang, W., and Poo, M. M. (2015). Autocrine action of BDNF on dendrite development of adult-born hippocampal neurons. *J. Neurosci.* 35, 8384–8393. doi: 10.1523/JNEUROSCI.4682-14.2015

Wen, Y., Planel, E., Herman, M., Figueroa, H. Y., Wang, L., Liu, L., et al. (2008). Interplay between cyclin-dependent kinase 5 and glycogen synthase kinase 3 beta mediated by neuregulin signaling leads to differential effects on tau phosphorylation and amyloid precursor protein processing. *J. Neurosci.* 28, 2624–2632. doi: 10.1523/JNEUROSCI.5245-07.2008

Winner, B., Melrose, H. L., Zhao, C., Hinkle, K. M., Yue, M., Kent, C., et al. (2011). Adult neurogenesis and neurite outgrowth are impaired in LRRK2 G2019S mice. *Neurobiol. Dis.* 41, 706–716. doi: 10.1016/j.nbd.2010.12.008

Winner, B., Regensburger, M., Schreglmann, S., Boyer, L., Prots, I., Rockenstein, E., et al. (2012). Role of alpha-synuclein in adult neurogenesis and neuronal maturation in the dentate gyrus. *J. Neurosci.* 32, 16906–16916. doi: 10.1523/JNEUROSCI.2723-12.2012

Wojtowicz, J. M., Askew, M. L., and Winocur, G. (2008). The effects of running and of inhibiting adult neurogenesis on learning and memory in rats. *Eur. J. Neurosci.* 27, 1494–1502. doi: 10.1111/j.1460-9568.2008.06128.x

Woolley, C. S., Gould, E., and Mcewen, B. S. (1990). Exposure to excess glucocorticoids alters dendritic morphology of adult hippocampal pyramidal neurons. *Brain Res.* 531, 225–231. doi: 10.1016/0006-8993(90)90778-A

Yu, F., Wang, Y., Xu, H., Dong, J., Wei, W., Wang, Y., et al. (2014). Developmental iodine deficiency delays the maturation of newborn granule neurons associated with downregulation of p35 in postnatal rat hippocampus. *Environ. Toxicol.* 29, 847–855. doi: 10.1002/tox.21811

Zhang, W., Wang, P. J., Li, P., Li, M. H., and Gao, X. L. (2012). Effects of low-dose X-ray on morphology of neuron and expression of microtubule associated protein-2 in hippocampus of young rats. *Zhonghua Yi Xue Za Zhi* 92, 336–340.

Zhao, C., Teng, E. M., Summers, R. G. Jr., Ming, G. L., and Gage, F. H. (2006). Distinct morphological stages of dentate granule neuron maturation in the adult mouse hippocampus. *J. Neurosci.* 26, 3–11. doi: 10.1523/JNEUROSCI.3648-05.2006

Zimprich, A., Biskup, S., Leitner, P., Lichtner, P., Farrer, M., Lincoln, S., et al. (2004). Mutations in LRRK2 cause autosomal-dominant parkinsonism with pleomorphic pathology. *Neuron* 44, 601–607. doi: 10.1016/j.neuron.2004.11.005

20

Hypocellularity in the Murine Model for Down Syndrome Ts65Dn is not Affected by Adult Neurogenesis

Rosa López-Hidalgo[1,2], *Raul Ballestín*[1,2], *Jessica Vega*[1,2], *José M. Blasco-Ibáñez*[1,2], *Carlos Crespo*[1,2], *Javier Gilabert-Juan*[1,2,3,4,5], *Juan Nácher*[1,2,3,4,5] *and Emilio Varea*[1,2]*

[1] Neurobiology Unit and Program in Basic and Applied Neurosciences, Cell Biology Department, Universitat de València, València, Spain, [2] Estructura de Recerca Interdisciplinar en Biotecnologia i Biomedicina (BIOTECMED), Universitat de València, València, Spain, [3] Fundación Investigación Hospital Clínico de Valencia, INCLIVA, València, Spain, [4] CIBERSAM, Spanish National Network for Research in Mental Health, València, Spain, [5] Genetics Department, CIBERSAM, Universitat de València, València, Spain

Edited by:
Alino Martinez-Marcos,
Universidad de Castilla, Spain

Reviewed by:
Armen Saghatelyan,
Université Laval, Canada
John W. Cave,
Weill Cornell Medical College Brain and Mind Research Institute, USA

***Correspondence:**
Emilio Varea
emilio.varea@uv.es

Down syndrome (DS) is caused by the presence of an extra copy of the chromosome 21 and it is the most common aneuploidy producing intellectual disability. Neural mechanisms underlying this alteration may include defects in the formation of neuronal networks, information processing and brain plasticity. The murine model for DS, Ts65Dn, presents reduced adult neurogenesis. This reduction has been suggested to underlie the hypocellularity of the hippocampus as well as the deficit in olfactory learning in the Ts65Dn mice. Similar alterations have also been observed in individuals with DS. To determine whether the impairment in adult neurogenesis is, in fact, responsible for the hypocellularity in the hippocampus and physiology of the olfactory bulb, we have analyzed cell proliferation and neuronal maturation in the two major adult neurogenic niches in the Ts656Dn mice: the subgranular zone (SGZ) of the hippocampus and the subventricular zone (SVZ). Additionally, we carried out a study to determine the survival rate and phenotypic fate of newly generated cells in both regions, injecting 5′BrdU and sacrificing the mice 21 days later, and analyzing the number and phenotype of the remaining 5′BrdU-positive cells. We observed a reduction in the number of proliferating (Ki67 positive) cells and immature (doublecortin positive) neurons in the subgranular and SVZ of Ts65Dn mice, but we did not observe changes in the number of surviving cells or in their phenotype. These data correlated with a lower number of apoptotic cells (cleaved caspase 3 positive) in Ts65Dn. We conclude that although adult Ts65Dn mice have a lower number of proliferating cells, it is compensated by a lower level of cell death. This higher survival rate in Ts65Dn produces a final number of mature cells similar to controls. Therefore, the reduction of adult neurogenesis cannot be held responsible for the neuronal hypocellularity in the hippocampus or for the olfactory learning deficit of Ts65Dn mice.

Keywords: adult neurogenesis, down syndrome, Ts65Dn mice, hippocampus, olfactory bulb, Ki67, doublecortin

INTRODUCTION

Down Syndrome (DS) is the most common chromosomal aneuploidy, with an incidence of one in 1000 live births (Roizen and Patterson, 2003). This chromosomal alteration induces a variable phenotype that may include immune deficiencies, heart defects, increased risk of leukemia, and early development of Alzheimer's disease (Ball and Nuttall, 1980; Hof et al., 1995; Holland et al., 2000; Folin et al., 2003; Nadel, 2003; Lott and Head, 2005). The common feature among all DS subjects is the presence of intellectual disability reflected by impairment in learning and memory. Neural mechanisms underlying this alteration may include defects in the formation of neuronal networks, information processing and brain structural plasticity.

Brain plasticity can be defined as the ability to perform adaptive changes related to the structure and function of the central nervous system (Zilles, 1992). Structural plasticity takes place during both development and adulthood. During development, brain structural plasticity is a fundamental element that generates the specificity of connections present in the mature nervous system, allowing morphogenetic processes such as cell proliferation, cell migration, axonal or dendritic growth and remodeling. This plastic ability diminishes with age being limited during adulthood to some specific regions (Bonfanti, 2006). During adulthood, the neurogenic aspect of structural plasticity is limited to the subventricular zone (SVZ), and the subgranular zone (SGZ) of the dentate gyrus. Plastic processes are crucial for learning and adaptability (Cotman et al., 1998; Gage, 2000).

One of the cerebral regions where brain structural plasticity remains specially active during adulthood is the hippocampus (Leuner and Gould, 2010). In adult animals, the pyramidal neurons of the CA1 and CA3 regions, and the granule neurons of the dentate gyrus undergo dynamic modifications of their dendritic profiles and synaptic contacts. The generation of neurons persists in the dentate gyrus until old age (Altman, 1962; Altman and Das, 1965; Eriksson et al., 1998; Hastings and Gould, 1999; van Praag et al., 1999) and the formation of these neurons implies the growth of axons and dendrites and the generation of new synapses. During adulthood, neurons are generated from a population of stem cells that display astroglial characteristics (Seri et al., 2001; Garcia et al., 2004). In the hippocampus, after their generation, newly born cells migrate and differentiate into granule neurons. They will generate dendritic processes with spines (van Praag et al., 2002; Laplagne et al., 2006; Ribak and Shapiro, 2007; Toni et al., 2007), receiving synaptic inputs (Kaplan and Hinds, 1977; Markakis and Gage, 1999) and will extend their axons to specific targets (Hastings and Gould, 1999; Markakis and Gage, 1999; Toni et al., 2008), releasing glutamate as a main neurotransmitter (Toni et al., 2008). However, it is important to note that many of these newly born neurons in the hippocampus die during the process of maturation and integration (Gould et al., 1999; Dayer et al., 2003). Survival of newly born neurons during adulthood is highly sensitive to environmental stimulus and learning, suggesting that adult neurogenesis allows the individuals to adapt to new environments (Doetsch and Hen, 2005).

The other region displaying neurogenesis in the adulthood is the SVZ (for a review see Alvarez-Buylla and Lim, 2004), that gives rise to neurons that migrate through the rostral migratory stream (RMS) and integrate in the olfactory bulb. In the SVZ, slow cycling stem cells (also called B cells) express the astrocytic marker glial-fibrillary acidic protein (GFAP) and give rise to rapidly dividing intermediate progenitor cells (also called C cells) which stop expressing GFAP and begin expressing distal-less homeobox (Dlx)-2 (Alvarez-Buylla and Garcia-Verdugo, 2002). These progenitors produce neuroblasts (called type A cells) that express the polysialylated neural cell adhesion molecule (PSA-NCAM) and neuronal markers such as doublecortin (DCX) (Alvarez-Buylla and Garcia-Verdugo, 2002). Chains of neuroblasts leave the SVZ, moving along the RMS before terminating in the olfactory bulb where they differentiate into GABAergic interneurons (Alvarez-Buylla and Garcia-Verdugo, 2002; Doetsch, 2003; Mignone et al., 2004; Brazel et al., 2005; Merkle et al., 2007; Kriegstein and Alvarez-Buylla, 2009).

Several animal models that mimic the alterations in DS are available. One of the most studied is the Ts65Dn mouse. This model is segmentally trisomic for a portion of the mouse chromosome 16 that is orthologous to the long arm of the human chromosome 21. This segment contains approximately 140 genes, many of which are highly conserved between mice and humans (Gardiner et al., 2003; Sturgeon and Gardiner, 2011; Rueda et al., 2012). These mice display a delay in the acquisition of a number of sensory and motor tasks (Holtzman et al., 1996; Costa et al., 1999), as well as defects in learning and in the execution of memory tasks mediated by the hippocampus (Reeves et al., 1995; Holtzman et al., 1996; Demas et al., 1998, 1999; Escorihuela et al., 1998; Sago et al., 2000; Hyde et al., 2001), and deficits in long-term potentiation (LTP) (Siarey et al., 1997, 1999; Kleschevnikov et al., 2004). Many of these deficiencies may be consequence of impairments in neuronal structural brain plasticity and related to adult neurogenesis. In fact, abnormalities in the dendritic arborization of pyramidal neurons have been observed in the neocortex of DS individuals and mice models for this syndrome (Takashima et al., 1981, 1989; Kaufmann and Moser, 2000; Dierssen et al., 2003). Our group has demonstrated a similar atrophy of dendritic arborization in the granule neurons of the hippocampus although CA1 pyramidal neurons remained unaltered (Villarroya et al., unpublished results).

Ts65Dn mice display reduction in the rate of cell proliferation from early postnatal stages in the SGZ: by day 2 (Contestabile et al., 2007) or by day 6 (Lorenzi and Reeves, 2006). This impairment continues into adulthood, but its magnitude is a matter of controversy (Rueda et al., 2005; Clark et al., 2006; Contestabile et al., 2007). Several hypotheses have been proposed to explain the impairment in neurogenesis. In fact, the cell cycle progresses more slowly due to an arrest in G2 phase, and consequently it is produced a lower number of cells (Contestabile et al., 2007). DS individuals display a reduction in cell proliferation (Mittwoch, 1972) and a reduction in the number of differentiated neurons although the number of astrocytes remains unaltered (Guidi et al., 2008). *In vitro* studies have shown a reduction in neuronal production from neurospheres obtained from neuronal precursors extracted from human fetuses with DS (Bahn et al., 2002; Esposito et al., 2008). Finally, it has been observed an increment of apoptotic cells in the hippocampus of DS fetuses (Guidi et al., 2008). Altogether, reduced cell proliferation and increased apoptosis may generate the hypocellularity observed in the brain of DS individuals (Guidi et al., 2008), or the lower number of dentate gyrus granule cells in Ts65Dn mice (Insausti et al., 1998; Lorenzi and Reeves, 2006). Studies in the SVZ, the RMS and the olfactory bulb have revealed a reduction in cell proliferation in the Ts65Dn mice model (Chakrabarti et al., 2011; Bianchi et al., 2014). Moreover olfactory learning is impaired in Ts65Dn mice (de Souza et al., 2011), similarly to the observed impairment in olfactory performance in adult with DS (Nijjar and Murphy, 2002). Activation of the olfactory system by odor exposition doesn't affect the number of proliferating cells; however the number of survival cells in the olfactory bulb is increased (Rochefort et al., 2002). This effect is different to the one observed in the hippocampus where the learning process, as it happens in an enriched environment, increases cell proliferation (reviewed in Kempermann et al., 2004).

In this study, we aim to characterize the processes of cell proliferation and neuronal maturation in the two main neurogenic regions of adult Ts65Dn mice: the SGZ and the SVZ (and also the RMS). We also want to characterize the survival rate and phenotype of the surviving cells in the hippocampus and the olfactory bulb of the adult Ts65Dn mice, in order to analyze whether these processes could be responsible for the hypocellularity and hypofunction observed in these two regions of this DS model.

MATERIALS AND METHODS

Experimental mice were generated by repeated backcrossing of Ts65Dn females to C57/6Ei 9 C3H/HeSnJ (B6EiC3) F1 hybrid males. The parental generation was obtained from the research colony of Jackson Laboratory. Euploid littermates of Ts65Dn mice served as controls. We have used a total of 17 trisomic mice and 24 euploid mice. For the characterization of proliferation and maturation we have used 4- to 5-month-old male mice (10 trisomic mice and 16 euploid mice). For the study of survival and characterization of newly born cells we have used 4-month old male mice (7 trisomic mice and 8 euploid mice). Mice were injected with 5′BrdU (50 mg/kg i.p.) twice per day (one injection every 12 h) during 2 days and were sacrificed 21 days after the last injection.

The genotypic characterization was established by qRT-PCR using SYBR Green PCR master mix (Applied Biosystems) from genomic DNA extracted from mice tails by mean of the phenol-chloroform method. The relative amount of each gene was quantified by the ABI PRISM 7700 (Applied Biosystems). The genes analyzed where APP (3 copies) and Apo-B (2 copies) as previously described (Liu et al., 2003; Hernández et al., 2012). All animal experimentation was conducted in accordance with the Directive 2010/63/EU of the European Parliament and of the Council of 22 September 2010 on the protection of animals used for scientific purposes and was approved by the Committee on Bioethics of the Universitat de València. Every effort was made to minimize the number of animals used and their suffering.

Animals were transcardially perfused under deep anesthesia (choral hydrate 4%, 1 ml/100 gw) using a solution containing 4% paraformaldehyde in phosphate buffer 0.1 M, pH 7.4. Brains were removed and cryoprotected using 30% sucrose. Fifty microns thick sections (6 subseries were collected for each brain) were obtained using a sliding freezing microtome.

Immunohistochemical Procedure

Tissue was processed "free-floating" for immunohistochemistry as follows. Briefly, sections were incubated with 10% methanol and 3% H2O2 in phosphate-buffered saline (PBS) for 10 min to block endogenous peroxidase activity.

After this, sections were treated for 1 h with 5% normal donkey serum (NDS) (Jackson ImmunoResearch Laboratories, West Grove, PA, USA) in PBS with 0.2% Triton- X100 (Sigma-Aldrich, St Louis, MO, USA) and were incubated overnight at room temperature either in polyclonal rabbit IgG anti-Ki67 (1:1000, Novocastra, NCL-Ki67p), polyclonal goat IgG anti-DCX (1:200, Santa Cruz, sc-8066), monoclonal mouse IgM anti-PSA-NCAM (1:700, Chemicon, MAB5324) or polyclonal goat IgG anti-NeuroD (1:1000; Santa Cruz, sc-1084) antibodies. After washing, sections were incubated for 2 h with donkey anti-rabbit IgG, donkey anti-mouse IgM or donkey anti-goat IgG biotinylated antibodies (1:250; Jackson ImmunoResearch Laboratories, West Grove, PA, USA), followed by avidin–biotin–peroxidase complex (ABC; Vector Laboratories, Peterborough, UK) diluted in PBS, for 30 min. Color development was achieved by incubating with 0.05% 3,3-diaminobenzidine tetrahydrochloride (Sigma-Aldrich) and 0.033% hydrogen peroxide in PB for 4 min. Finally, sections were mounted on slides, dried for 1 day at room temperature, dehydrated with ascending alcohols and rinsed in xylene. After this, sections were coverslipped using Eukitt mounting medium (PANREAC). All studied sections passed through all procedures simultaneously in order to minimize any difference from the immunohistochemical staining itself. To avoid any bias in the analysis, all slides were coded prior to analysis and remained so until the experiment was completed.

Detection of Apoptotic Cells (Cleaved Caspase-3 Positive)

Tissue was processed "free-floating" for immunofluorescence as follows. Briefly, sections were incubated with citrate buffer (0.01M, pH 6.0) for 1 min at 100°C. After this, sections were treated for 1 h with 5% normal donkey serum (NDS) (Jackson ImmunoResearch Laboratories, West Grove, PA, USA) in PBS with 0.2% Triton- X100 (Sigma-Aldrich, St Louis, MO, USA) and were incubated overnight at room temperature in polyclonal rabbit IgG anti-cleaved caspase-3 (1:500, Cell Signaling, 9661) antibody. After washing, sections were incubated for 2 h with donkey anti-rabbit IgG conjugated with DL549 (1:200, Jackson Immunoresearch) for 2 h. After washing, sections were mounted on slides using Dako fluorescent medium (Dako North America, California). The sections were counterstained with 4′, 6-Diamidino-2-phenylindole (DAPI) (dilution 1/500)

(Sigma-Aldrich, St Louis, MO, USA) to identify cellular nuclei. The analysis of sections was performed using a confocal microscope (Leica TSC-SPE) using 40X objective. Serial stacks of the different regions (granule layer of dentate gyrus, RMS and olfactory bulb) were analyzed using ImageJ software. Interval between z planes was 1.15 μm.

Cell Quantification of Proliferating, Immature Neurons, and Apoptotic Cells

We have analyzed the number of cells proliferating (Ki67 positive), the number of neurons in process of maturation (DCX positive) and the number of caspase 3 positive cells in two regions: the SGZ of the dentate gyrus in the hippocampus and the SVZ and RMS. Moreover we have analyzed the number of neurons in process of maturation using other markers, NeuroD and PSA-NCAM in the SGZ.

For the SGZ of dentate gyrus we have estimated the total number of cells expressing these markers. The number of cells expressing these markers in each region was estimated using a modified version of the fractionator method (West, 1993) as described before (Nacher et al., 2002). We counted cells covering 100% of the sample area, that is, within each section, all labeled cells were counted. The fractionator sampling scheme refers to the methodology of examining one out of every 6 brain sections. Thus, our modification of the optical dissector combined with a 1:6 fractionator sampling is truly a modification of the optical fractionator method. 1:6 systematic series of sections covering the whole rostral to caudal extension of this structure were viewed under an Olympus CX41 microscope. Cell somata were identified and counted with a 40X objective (NA 0.65). Cells appearing in the upper focal plane were omitted to prevent overcounting. The volume of the different areas analyzed was determined for each animal using the Cavalieri's principle (Gundersen and Jensen, 1987).

For the SVZ, RMS and olfactory bulb we have analyzed the cell density. We have analyzed 3–4 sections per animal covering the whole rostral to caudal extension (Bregma 1.3, 0.98, 0.5, and 0.14 mm, for SVZ and RMS and Bregma 4.28, 3.92, and 3.56 mm for the olfactory bulb). Cells were observed under an Olympus CX41 microscope. Cell somata were identified and counted with a 40X objective. The volume of the different areas analyzed, as pointed out before, was determined for each animal using the Cavalieris's principle (Gundersen and Jensen, 1987). The areas of the analyzed regions were measured using ImageJ software (NIH). Results were expressed as cells per square millimeter. Ratio values (DCX/Ki67 and RMS/SVZ) were obtained for each animal. For the case of caspase 3 positive cells, due to the low number of cells presents, we have counted all the cells presents in the regions analyzed in one to six sections. Data were reported as mean ± sem. Means were determined for each experimental group and the data were statistically analyzed using the SPSS software package (version 15). Differences between groups were analyzed with one way ANOVA followed by Student–Newman–Keuls *post-hoc* test. Nissl-stained sections adjacent to the measured ones were used to determine the location and borders of the analyzed regions.

Phenotipic Characterization of Newly Born Cells

In order to characterize the phenotype of the newly born cells in the dentate gyrus and the olfactory bulb, we have performed a triple immunolabeling using antibodies against 5′BrdU, NeuN (neurons) and GFAP (astrocytes). The triple labeling was performed following the "free-floating" procedure described previously with some changes.

Sections were incubated in PBS during 60 min to 60°C. After cooling down, sections were incubated with HCl 2N for 30 min. After washing, sections were incubated with a blocking solution containing 10% NDS for 1 h and overnight with a mix of monoclonal rat IgG anti-5′BrdU (1:1000, Inmunological Direct, OBT0030), polyclonal rabbit IgG anti-GFAP (1:500 Sigma Aldrich, G9269) and monoclonal mouse IgG anti-NeuN (1:100, Millipore, MAB377) antibodies. After washing, sections were incubated with a mix of secondary antibodies containing: Donkey anti-rat IgG conjugated with Alexa 488 (1:200, Molecular Probes), donkey anti-rabbit IgG conjugated with DL649 (1:200, Jackson Immunoresearch) and donkey anti-mouse IgG conjugated with DL549 (1:200, Jackson Immunoresearch) for 2 h. After washing, sections were mounted on slides using Dako fluorescent medium (Dako North America, California). The analysis of sections was performed using a confocal microscope (Leica TSC-SPE) using 40X objective. Stacks (z-step 1.15 μm) of the different regions (granule layer of dentate gyrus and olfactory bulb) and were analyzed using ImageJ software. A minimum of 50 cells were analyzed for each animal. Percentages for every marker were obtained and mean for each group and region was determined and analyzed using SPSS software.

RESULTS

We analyzed the cell proliferation, neuronal maturation and phenotype of the surviving cells in the two major neurogenic areas during adulthood, the SGZ of the dentate gyrus (including the granule layer for the analysis of cell survival) and the SVZ (including here also the RMS and the olfactory bulb for the analysis of cell survival).

Subgranular Zone and Dentate Gyrus

We studied the number of proliferating cells using the marker Ki67 (**Figures 1A,C,D**). In the SGZ we observed that Ki67 labeled nuclei often appeared in clusters (**Figures 1C,D**). Trisomic mice displayed a reduction in the number of proliferating cells in the SGZ (878 ± 179 cells in the SGZ of Ts65Dn mice vs. 1479 ± 101 cells in the euploid littermates, $p < 0.01$) (**Figure 1A**).

We quantified the number of immature neurons using the marker doublecortin (DCX) (**Figures 1B,E,F**). This marker is present in the cytoplasm, both in the cell body and the proximal dendrites of newly generated neurons. DCX positive cells are located in the inner part of granule layer adjacent to the SGZ, where neurons are produced (**Figures 1E,F**). We have observed a reduction in the number of immature neurons in the dentate gyrus of the Ts65Dn model (5687 ± 1408 in Ts65Dn mice

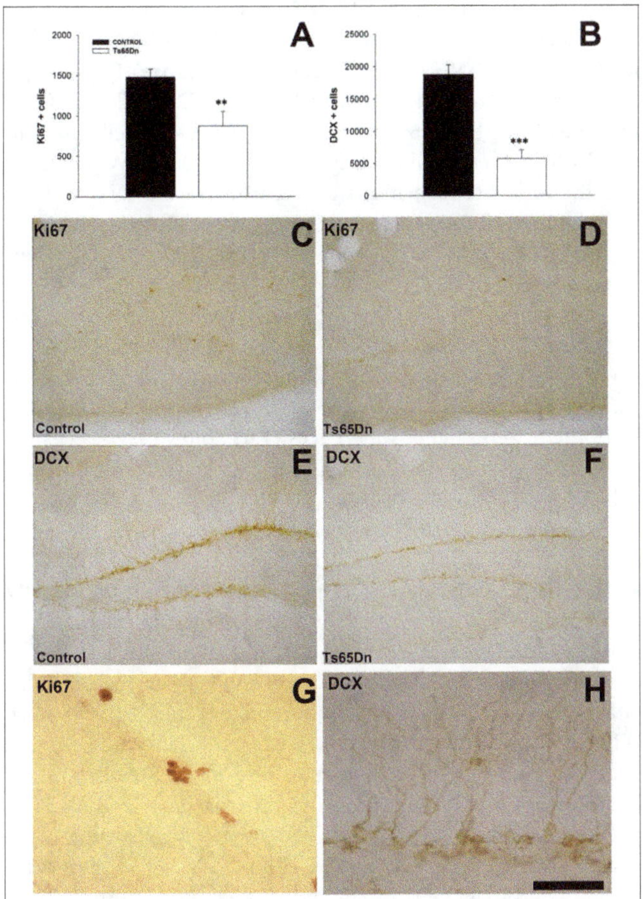

FIGURE 1 | Proliferating cells and immature neurons in the dentate gyrus of adult Ts65Dn mice. (A) Graph showing the changes in the number of proliferating cells (Ki67) between control (black bar) and Ts65Dn mice (white bar). **(B)** Graph showing the change in the number of immature neurons (DCX) in the dentate gyrus between control (black bar) and Ts65Dn mice (white bar). Representative images of the expression of Ki67 in the SGZ of control **(C)** and Ts65Dn mice **(D)** and DCX in the dentate gyrus of euploid **(E)** and Ts65Dn mice **(F)** Details of the expression of Ki67 **(G)** and DCX **(H)** in control mice. Scale bar: 250 microns **(B–F)** and 50 microns **(G,H)**. $^{**}p < 0.01$; $^{***}p < 0.001$).

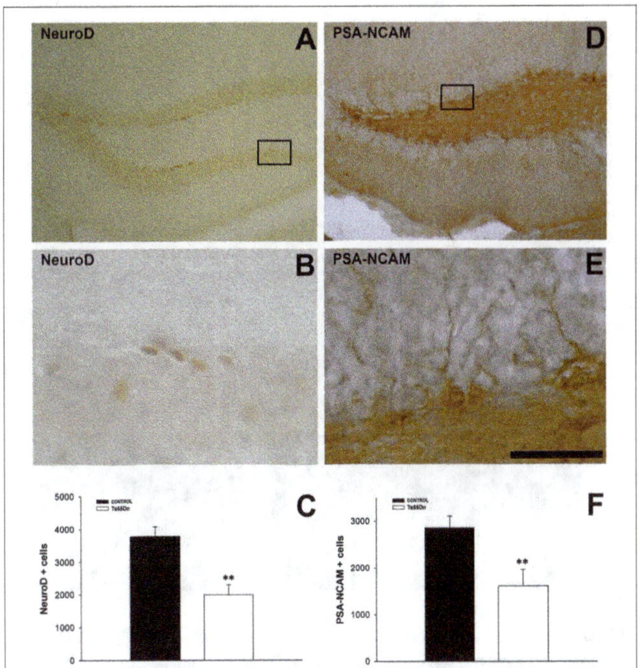

FIGURE 2 | Immature neurons in the dentate gyrus of adult Ts65Dn mice. (A) Representative image of the expression of NeuroD in the SGZ. **(B)** High magnification image of the region boxed in **(A)**. **(C)** Graph showing the changes in the number of immature neurons in the SGZ (NeuroD) between control (black bar) and Ts65Dn mice (white bar). **(D)** Representative image of the expression of PSA-NCAM in the SGZ. **(E)** High magnification image of the region boxed in **(D)**. **(F)** Graph showing the changes in the number of immature neurons in the SGZ (PSA-NCAM) between control (black bar) and Ts65Dn mice (white bar). Scale bar: 350 microns for **(A,D)** and 75 microns for **(B,E)**. $^{**}p < 0.01$.

vs. 18713 ± 1518 in their euploid littermates, $p < 0.001$) (**Figure 1B**). Similar results were obtained with other markers for immature neurons such as the transcription factor NeuroD (**Figures 2A–C**), a protein involved in the differentiation of hippocampal granule neurons (Schwab et al., 2000), which is also expressed in some progenitor cells in the rodent SGZ (Seri et al., 2004), or the polysialylated form of the Neural Cell Adhesion Molecule (PSA-NCAM (**Figures 2D–F**). For NeuroD, we have observed a moderate but significant reduction in the number of immature neurons (1998 ± 303 in the Ts65Dn mice vs. 3788 ± 291 in their euploid littermates, $p < 0.01$) (**Figure 2C**) or the polysialylated form of the Neural Cell Adhesion Molecule (PSA-NCAM) (1616 ± 350 immature neurons in the granule layer of Ts65Dn mice vs. 2857 ± 254 immature neurons in their euploid littermates, $p < 0.01$) (**Figure 2F**).

We analyzed the number of surviving cells from this population of newly generated cells using 5′BrdU injection and allowing mice to survive for 21 days (**Figure 3**). After this period, we analyzed the number of cells that had incorporated 5′BrdU. We observed that, in the hippocampus, labeled nuclei were mainly restricted to the granule layer. The quantification of the total number of surviving cells in the granule layer of the dentate gyrus reflected no changes between euploid and Ts65Dn mice (**Figure 3A**). Therefore, despite the difference in cell proliferation, the percentage of cells surviving is higher in Ts65Dn mice. We observed 643 ± 75 cells in the Ts65Dn granule layer and 704 ± 67 in the granule layer of the euploid littermates ($p = 0.57$). Using triple immunohistochemistry, we have characterized the phenotype of the surviving cells (**Figures 3B–H**). Surviving cells were characterized mainly as neurons (NeuN+) (60.4% in euploid mice and 68.6% in Ts65Dn mice), whereas those idenfied as astrocytes (GFAP+) represented less than one third of them (28.2% in euploid mice and 20.2% in Ts65Dn mice). The rest of cells were negative for GFAP or NeuN and their percentages were similar in both groups (11.4% in euploid mice and 11.2% in Ts65Dn mice). There were no statistical differences between groups.

Subventricular Zone, Rostral Migratory Stream, and Olfactory Bulb

We studied the density of cells proliferating in the SVZ and proximal region of RMS using the marker Ki67. The volume analysis revealed no changes between control and trisomic mice

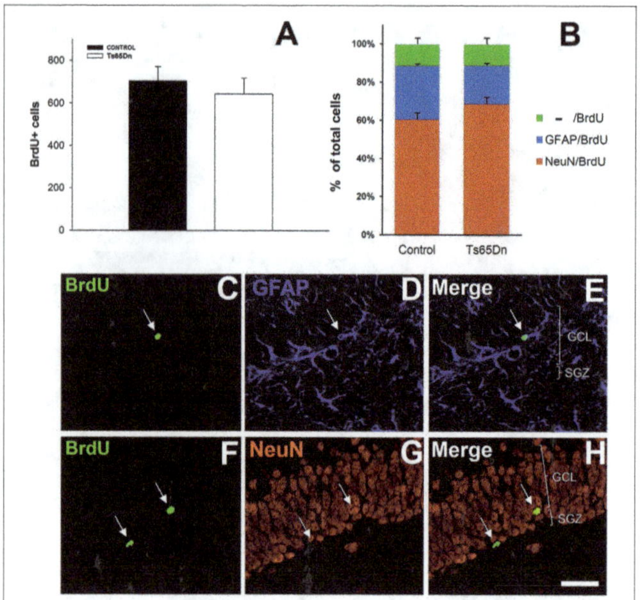

FIGURE 3 | Number and phenotype of surviving cells in the granule layer of the dentate gyrus of the adult Ts65Dn mice. (A). Graph showing the total number of 5′BrdU positive cells in the granule layers of control (black bar) and Ts65Dn mice (white bar). **(B)** Graph showing the phenotype of the surviving cells in the granule layer of dentate gyrus: NeuN/BrdU positive cells (red bar), GFAP/BrdU positive cells (blue bar) and BrdU-only positive cells (green bar). **(C–H)** Representative confocal images showing colocalization between BrdU and GFAP **(C–E)** and BrdU and NeuN **(F–H)**. Scale bar: 50 microns.

in the SVZ (0.34 ± 0.01 mm^3 for euploid mice vs. 0.32 ± 0.02 mm^3 for trisomic mice) neither in the RMS (0.61 ± 0.03 mm^3 in euploid mice vs. 0.58 ± 0.06 mm^3 for Ts65Dn mice). We observed clusters of stained nuclei in the SVZ and in the RMS (**Figures 4D,E**). Trisomic mice displayed a reduction in the density of proliferating cells in the SVZ (**Figure 4A**) (162 ± 48 cells/mm^2 in Ts65Dn mice vs. 296 ± 55 cells/mm^2 in their euploid littermates, $p < 0.05$). However, when we quantified the density of proliferating cells in the proximal RMS (**Figure 4A**), we failed to observe differences between groups (413 ± 49 cells/mm^2 in Ts65Dn mice vs. 477 ± 57 cells/mm^2 in their euploid littermates, $p = 0.4714$). We also analyzed the ratio between the density of proliferating cells in the SVZ and the RMS (**Figure 4C**). We observed that trisomic mice displayed a higher proportion of proliferating cells in the RMS vs. the SVZ than their euploid littermates (3.54 ± 0.75 times for Ts65Dn mice vs. 1.81 ± 0.22 times for their euploid littermates, $p < 0.01$). This result suggests that cells proliferate slowly in the trisomic mice and that the proliferative process continues into the RMS during the migrating process in a higher proportion than in the control mice.

We quantified the density of immature neurons in the SVZ and the RMS using the marker DCX. This molecule is present in the cytoplasm in both the cell body and the proximal dendrites of newly generated neurons (**Figures 4F,G**). We observed a reduction (**Figure 4B**) in the number of immature neurons in the SVZ of the Ts65Dn model (891 ± 221 cells/mm^2 in the SVZ of the Ts65Dn mice vs. 1483 ± 253 cells/mm^2 in their euploid littermates, $p < 0.01$). When we analyzed the density of immature neurons in the RMS of the Ts65Dn mice (**Figure 4B**), we have also observed a reduction in their density (2472 ± 315 cells/mm^2 in the RMS of the Ts65Dn mice vs. 3564 ± 332 cells/mm^2 in the RMS of their euploid littermates, $p < 0.01$). We checked also the ratio between immature neurons in the SVZ and the RMS (**Figure 4C**), in this case there were not differences between groups (2.72 ± 0.74 for the Ts65Dn mice vs. 2.23 ± 0.24 for their euploid littermates).

The analysis of the ratio between proliferating (ki67) and immature (DCX) cells in SVZ reflected no differences (5.02 ± 0.34 DCX cells for each Ki67 cell in controls vs. 5.55 ± 1.23 in Ts65Dn mice), however when we analyzed the same ratio in the RMS there were higher differences (7.69 ± 0.95 DCX cells for each Ki67 cell in controls vs. 6.25 ± 1.42 in Ts65Dn mice) but still not statistically significant.

As described before, we analyzed the survival of the adult generated cells using 5′BrdU injection and allowing mice to survive for 21 days. After this period we analyzed the density of 5′BrdU cells (**Figure 5A**). We observed that, in the olfactory bulb they were present in the granule and glomerular layers. The quantification of the density of surviving cells in the olfactory bulb reflected no changes between euploid and Ts65Dn mice (**Figure 5A**). We have observed 101 ± 18 cells/mm^2 in the olfactory bulb of the Ts65Dn mice and 95 ± 8 cells/mm^2 in the olfactory bulb of their euploid littermates ($p = 0.73$). The phenotypical characterization of the surviving cells using triple immunofluorescence (**Figures 5C–F**) revealed that they were mainly neurons (91.8% in euploid mice and 91.5% in Ts65Dn mice) (**Figure 5B**), whereas astrocytes represented less than one tenth of surviving cells (7.4% in euploid mice and 7.2% in Ts65Dn mice). The rest of the cells were negative for GFAP or NeuN and their percentage was similar in both groups (0.8% in euploid mice and 1.3% in Ts65Dn mice). As it happened in the hippocampus, there were no statistical differences between groups.

Apoptotic Cells in the Hippocampus, RMS and Olfactory Bulb

Cell proliferation is impaired in SGZ and SVZ in the Ts65Dn mice model, however there are no differences in the final number of surviving cells (BrdU+). To understand this paradox, we analyzed the number of apoptotic cells (positive for cleaved caspase 3) in the dentate gyrus of the hippocampus, the RMS and the olfactory bulb (**Figure 6**). In the dentate gyrus, we have observed cells with different morphologies (**Figures 6B,C**). Cleaved caspase 3 cells have been also observed in the RMS (**Figure 6D**) and in the granular layer of the olfactory bulb (**Figure 6E**). We quantified the number of cells positive for cleaved caspase 3 in the different regions (**Figure 6A**). There was a lower number of apoptotic cells in the dentate gyrus of the Ts65Dn mice model (542 ± 63 cells in the dentate gyrus of Ts65Dn mice vs. 794 ± 56 in their euploid litteramates, $p < 0.05$). In the olfactory system, we quantified the number of apoptotic cells in the RMS and the olfactory bulb. For the

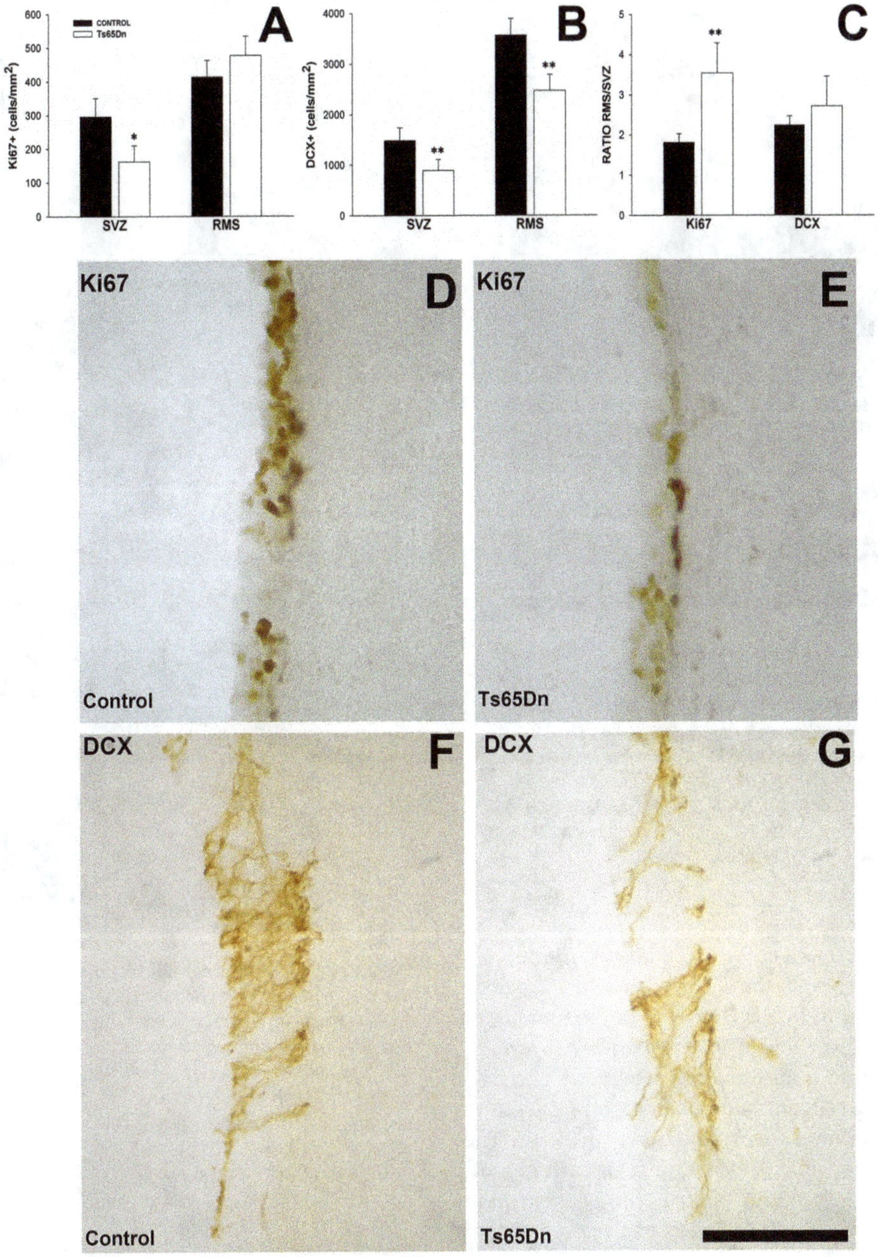

FIGURE 4 | Proliferating cells and immature neurons in the SVZ and the RMS of adult Ts65Dn mice. (A) Graph showing the changes in the density of proliferating cells (Ki67) in the SVZ and RMS between control (black bar) and Ts65Dn mice (white bar). **(B)** Graph showing the change in the density of immature neurons (DCX) in the SVZ abd RMS between control (black bar) and Ts65Dn mice (white bar). **(C)** Graph showing the ratio of proliferative and immature neurons between the SVZ and RMS. Representative images of the expression of Ki67 in the SVZ of control **(D)**, and Ts65Dn mice **(E)** and DCX in the SVZ of euploid **(F)** and Ts65Dn mice **(G)**. Scale bar: 100 microns. $^{*}p < 0.05$; $^{**}p < 0.01$).

RMS we observed a lower number but not statistically significant (302 ± 50 cells in the RMS of the Ts65Dn mice vs. 537 ± 101 for their euploid littermates, $p = 0.067$). In the olfactory bulb, we observed a lower number of apoptotic cells in the Ts65Dn mice model (823 ± 82 cells in the olfactory bulb of the Ts65Dn mice model vs. 1538 ± 241 for their euploid littermates, $p < 0.05$).

DISCUSSION

In this study, we analyzed the proliferation and maturation rate in the SGZ, SVZ, and RMS of the DS mice model Ts65Dn and the integration of the newly born cells in the dentate gyrus and olfactory bulb. We have observed a reduction in the number of (Ki67 positive) proliferative cells in the SGZ and

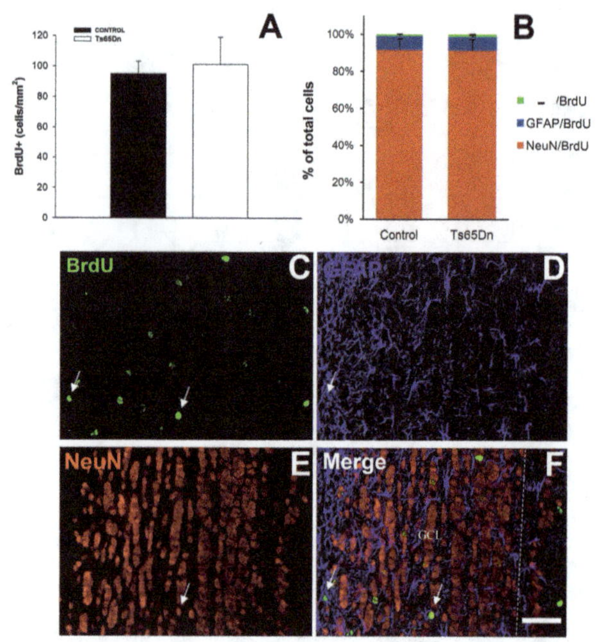

FIGURE 5 | Number and phenotype of surviving cells in the olfactory bulb of the adult Ts65Dn mice. (A) Graph showing the density of BrdU positive cells in the olfactory bulb of control (black bar) and Ts65Dn mice (white bar). **(B)** Graph showing the phenotype of surviving cells in the olfactory bulb: NeuN/BrdU positive cells (red bar), GFAP/BrdU positive cells (blue bar) and BrdU only positive cells (green bar). **(C–F)** Representative confocal images showing colocalization between BrdU **(C)**, NeuN **(D)** and GFAP **(E)** and the merged image **(F)** arrow in **(D)** show a neuron and in E an astrocyte. Dashed line marks the limit of granule layer. Scale bar: 50 microns.

SVZ. The analysis of the number of (DCX positive) immature neurons indicated a decrease in the Ts65Dn mice in all regions analyzed (SGZ, SVZ, and RMS). The analysis of the number of apoptotic cells, reflects that Ts65Dn mice have a lower level of cells death in all the regions analyzed. Moreover, we analyzed the number of surviving cells and their phenotype 21 days after their generation using intraperitoneal injections of 5′BrdU. The absolute number of surviving cells was similar in both groups; their characterization reflected that the majority of them were neurons in both trisomic and euploid mice, and the proportion of them did not change between groups. So, we can conclude that Ts65Dn mice display impairment in cell proliferation during adulthood, but due to the reduced apoptotic rate, the number of cells surviving after 21 days is similar in both groups and their phenotype is similar in Ts65Dn mice and their euploid littermates.

First of all, we analyzed the density (SVZ and RMS) and the total number of proliferating cells (DG) in the adulthood using the marker Ki67; this protein is present during G1, S, G2 and mitosis phases but it is absent during G0 phase (Gerdes et al., 1984). We have observed a 41% reduction in cell proliferation in the adult SGZ. Our results are in accordance with previous studies showing a reduction in cell proliferation in this region (Clark et al., 2006). However, other studies have found that the number of proliferating cells is maintained in the SGZ of adult

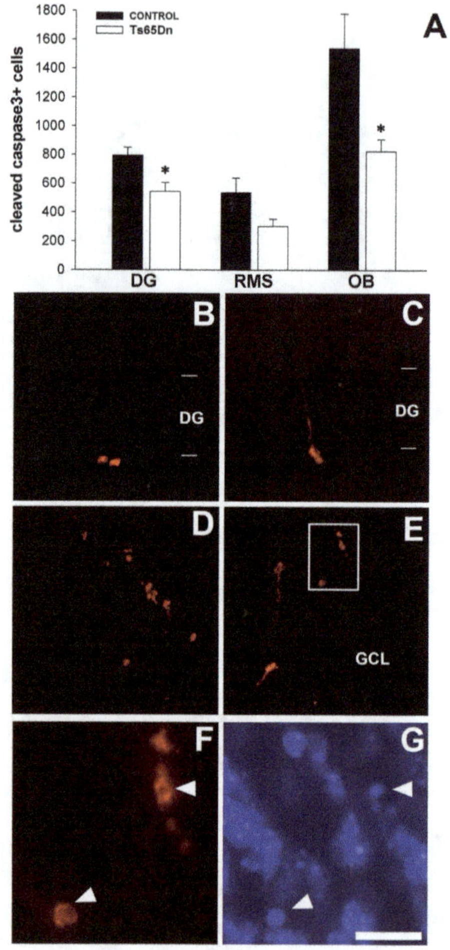

FIGURE 6 | Apoptotic cells (cleaved-caspase 3 positive cells) in the dentate gyrus of the hippocampus and the olfactory bulb of the adult Ts65Dn mice. (A) Graph showing the changes in the number of cleaved-caspase 3 cells in the dentate gyrus (DG), RMS and olfactory bulb (OB) between control (black bar) and Ts65Dn mice (white bar). Representative images of the expression of cleaved-caspase 3 positive cells in the dentate gyrus **(B,C)**. **(D)** Cleaved-caspase 3 positive cells along the RMS, observe their morphological aspect. **(E)** Apoptotic cells in the granule layer of the olfactory bulb (GCL). **(F)** High magnification image of the region boxed in **(E)**. **(G)** DAPI counterstaining of the area showed in **(F)**. Observe the presence of condensed nuclei in the cells displaying cleaved caspase 3 expression (arrowheads). Images are taken from a Ts65Dn animal, presenting similar morphologies in controls. Scale bar: 75 microns **(B–E)** and 20 microns **(F–G)**. $^{*}p < 0.05$.

Ts65Dn mice (Rueda et al., 2005). This discrepancy could be explained because of the fine regulation of adult neurogenesis and the high sensitivity to external and internal factors that could induce drastic changes in cell proliferation (for a detailed review see Balu and Lucki, 2009). In Rueda's study (Rueda et al., 2005), mice are subjected to BrdU injection during 12 days and surviving neurons are quantified at 30 days. They observe changes in old but no young animals. Our study has been performed in mouse of a similar age but our procedure is different (2 days BrdU injection, 21 days survival). We have observed an impairment in cell proliferation and this study observe no change. Perhaps the manipulation during 12 days has induced stress of mice and trisomic mice are less sensitive to this manipulation. Supporting this possibility our group has observed a lower sensitivity (analyzed as a reduction in cell proliferation) to manipulation in trisomic mice than control (Ballestín et al., unpublished results).

Rodents living in an enriched environment show increased the number of surviving cells in the SGZ (van Praag et al., 1999). However, stress conditions reduce drastically neurogenesis in the SGZ (for a review see Mirescu and Gould, 2006). Human DS fetuses also displayed a reduction in the cell proliferation in the SGZ (Contestabile et al., 2007).

The analysis of cell proliferation in the SVZ and RMS of the Ts65Dn mice reflects a reduction in the SVZ (46%) but no change in the RMS. Previous studies have shown similar results in 15 days-old mice (Bianchi et al., 2014). However, when the animals analyzed were old (13 months old) both regions displayed a similar reduction in cell proliferation (Bianchi et al., 2014). The animals used in our study are adults (4–5 months old) and consequently our results suggest that, at this age, the alterations in cell proliferation are similar to those observed in younger animals. Moreover, we have analyzed the ratio of this parameter in the RMS/SVZ in Ts65Dn and control mice and we have observed that it is higher in the trisomic mice. Our results support previous studies that claim that the proliferation process is slower in Ts65Dn mice (Contestabile et al., 2007). When we compared the ratio between proliferating (Ki67) and maturating (DCX) in SVZ we observed that there were no differences (5.02 ± 0.34 DCX cells for each Ki67 cell in controls vs. 5.55 ± 1.23 in Ts65Dn mice), however when we analyzed the same ratio in the RMS there is a trend toward a higher ratio in the control mice (7.69 ± 0.95 DCX cells for each Ki67 cell in controls vs. 6.25 ± 1.42 in Ts65Dn mice). It has been previously characterized that the cell cycle last longer (at least its G2 phase) in trisomic mice (Contestabile et al., 2007). Therefore, more cells could reach the RMS while they are still proliferating. The reason for this enlarged cell cycle can be connected with the fact that microtubules are altered in this model and this alteration may compromise the formation of the mitotic spindle (Liu et al., 2008).

In the second part of our study, we have analyzed the alteration in the number of immature neurons in the SGZ, SVZ, and RMS. We have used the marker doublecortin (DCX). This protein acts as a microtubule associated protein (Moores et al., 2003). DCX is transiently expressed by immature neurons and is absent from glial cells (Rao and Shetty, 2004); it participates in neuronal migration (Feng and Walsh, 2001; Brown et al., 2003; Couillard-Despres et al., 2005). The analysis of the DCX cells in the different regions showed a reduction in number and density of positive cells in the Ts65Dn mice in all the regions analyzed (70% in the SGZ, 40% in the SVZ and 31% in the RMS).

There is a discrepancy between the reduction in cell proliferation (41%) and that of immature neurons (70%) in the SGZ. There are, at least, four possible explanations for this difference: an increase in apoptosis only in the SGZ, an accelerated maturation process, an effect over an specific type of DCX cells or an affectation specifically in the marker analyzed, DCX, in this model.

The analysis of the number of apoptotic cells, using the marker cleaved-caspase 3, revealed a reduction in the number of apoptotic cells in both the olfactory bulb and the dentate gyrus of the hippocampus. Previous studies have shown controversial results. The analysis of P6 animals revealed no changes in the number of apoptotic cells (Lorenzi and Reeves, 2006). However, 12 month old Ts65Dn display lower number of apoptotic cells in the SVZ (Bianchi et al., 2010b). Our results are in accordance with the data observed in old animals, however the reduction is similar in the SGZ and the OB. An alternative explanation could be an accelerated maturation process or affectation of an specific subtype of DCX positive cells (Plümpe et al., 2006). This explanation must be discarded because of the results observed with other markers for immature neurons, such as PSA-NCAM or NeuroD. Using these markers, there is only a reduction of around 45% in the number of immature neurons, similar to the 41% observed in proliferating cells. Differences in the total number of cells between these markers are due to methodology (different sensibility of antibodies). Therefore, the loss of DCX expressing cells could be due to an alteration in the expression of this protein in the hippocampus of trisomic mice. Supporting this possibility, Ts65Dn mice (and individuals with DS) have an extra copy of the gene Dyrk1A (Gardiner et al., 2003). Dyrk1A phosphorylates tau (Liu et al., 2008) and this phosphorylation induces destabilization of the microtubules. DCX binds microtubules and their alteration can also affect its expression. This can explain the lower intensity of staining observed in the Ts65Dn DCX positive dendrites.

A surprising result from our study is that the number of surviving mature neurons after 21 days is similar in both Ts65Dn and control mice. However, our study agrees with the literature in that the number of proliferating and immature neurons are lower in trisomic mice. Therefore, the proportion of cells surviving is higher in trisomic mice than in euploid mice. Moreover, the analysis of the phenotype of the surviving cells reflects that the vast majority are neurons in the two analyzed regions (dentate gyrus and olfactory bulb) and in a similar proportion in control and trisomic. It has been pointed that NeuN is not a reliable marker for mature neurons in the glomerular layer of the olfactory bulb (Bagley et al., 2007). In our study we can overcome this inconvenient due to the fact that only around one per cent of BrdU positive cells in the olfactory bulb were negative for both NeuN and GFAP. Perhaps these cells could be neurons unmarked by NeuN but the results are similar.

There are two critical periods in adult neurogenesis when the number of dying cells is high, the first point is during the transient amplifier progenitor and neuroblast stages (1–4 days after mitosis) (Platel et al., 2010; Sierra et al., 2010), whereas the second is during the immature neuron stage (around the second week postmitosis) (Tashiro et al., 2006; Mouret et al., 2008). Thus, 21 days after mitosis the number of surviving cells must approximate the number of cells that will finally survive and integrate into the circuitry. Similar results have been observed analyzing the integration of newly born neurons in the olfactory bulb (Winner et al., 2002) Our results suggest that the total number of surviving cell remains unaltered independently of the number of proliferative cells. One possibility could be that the availability of trophic factors may be similar in both groups and as a consequence of that the number of cells able to survive would be similar in both cases. This possibility could be supported by the fact that the number of apoptotic cells is reduced in Ts65Dn mice as we mentioned above. Another possible scenario is that the lower cell density in the trisomic animals may offer higher opportunities for the newly generated cells of establish the proper connectivity and integrate.

Regarding the dentate gyrus, previous studies (Contestabile et al., 2007) have analyzed the survival rate of the cells generated in the SGZ, but in younger animals. 5′BrdU was injected at P2 and sacrifice was done at P30. In this case, there was a reduction in the number of cells surviving in the dentate gyrus and the phenotypical characterization of them reflects a higher amount of astrocytes than neurons. It must be taken into account that the vast majority of granule neurons of the dentate gyrus are produced during the first two postnatal weeks (for a review see Seress, 2007). Thus, the results observed in that study cannot be compared with our study at 4–5 months.

In the case of the olfactory bulb, previous studies (Bianchi et al., 2014) have observed a reduction in the survival rate, but only in old animals (13 months old). Therefore, the reduction in cell survival in the olfactory bulb observed in that study correlates with impairment in the olfactory function in these mice (de Souza et al., 2011), but can be the effect of premature aging. Similar impairment in odor discrimination has been observed in elderly individuals with DS (Nijjar and Murphy, 2002). On the contrary, in our animals (4–5 month old) cell survival is similar to controls.

Possible Consequences of the Impairment in Adult Neurogenesis

The cognitive impairment observed in Ts65Dn mice suggest that the hippocampal function is impaired. A possible explanation for this alteration can be impairment in neuronal structural plasticity (neurogenesis, synaptogenesis and neuritogenesis). Thus, the reduction in neurogenesis observed in this study shows that these processes are affected in adult trisomic mice. However, during adulthood the number of new neurons incorporated is similar to controls. Therefore, is probable that other aspects of structural plasticity are involved more directly in the impairment observed in cognitive performance. Some studies have treated to increase cell proliferation in Ts65Dn during the early period of life. The use of fluoxetine (Clark et al., 2006; Bianchi et al., 2010a; Stagni et al., 2013) is an example of this approach. These studies were able to increase the density of proliferating cells in the SGZ and, in many cases, to improve the cognitive capabilities of Ts65Dn mice. However, it should be considered that fluoxetine increases not only cell proliferation but also the other aspects of structural plasticity such as synaptogenesis and neuritogenesis (Varea et al., 2007a,b; Guirado et al., 2012) and also increases the activity of many neurons in the brain (Guirado et al., 2009). Therefore, we cannot exclude that the improvement in cognitive performance observed as a consequence of fluoxetine treatment could be due to changes in cellular activity and synaptic and dendritic remodeling rather than to the increase in cell proliferation.

Cell proliferation in the hippocampus has been shown to be dependent of extracellular glutamate (Nácher et al., 2007). Since in DS models there is an excess of inhibition, the lower cell proliferation may be due to lower levels of extracellular glutamate in the neurogenic niches. If this hypothesis is correct, adult neurogenesis would be a consequence of the level of activity of the system (Piatti et al., 2011). DS individuals and the Ts65Dn mice model showed overinhibition in several regions of the brain such the somatosensory cortex (Pérez-Cremades et al., 2010) and the hippocampus (Belichenko et al., 2004; Hernández-González et al., 2015), Thus, overinhibition would lead to a decrease in the level of activity of the system and consequently to a reduction in cell proliferation (as we have observed in this study).

Although there is a reduction in the number of proliferating cells in trisomic mice, the final number of neurons integrated in the system is the same. Therefore, the reduction of adult proliferation cannot be held responsible for neuronal hypocellularity in the hippocampus or for the olfactory learning deficit.

AUTHOR CONTRIBUTIONS

RL performed the experiments, discussed results and participated in the writing of the manuscript. RB performed the experiments, discussed results and participated in the writing of the manuscript. JV performed the experiments, discussed results and participated in the writing of the manuscript. JB discussed results and participated in the writing of the manuscript. CC discussed results and participated in the writing of the manuscript. JG performed the genotyping of mice, discussed results and participated in the writing of the manuscript. JN discussed results and participated in the writing of the manuscript. EV designed the experiments, discussed results and participated in the writing of the manuscript.

ACKNOWLEDGMENTS

This study has been funded by the Jerome Lejeune Foundation, the Spanish Ministry of Science and Innovation BFU2012-32512, and Generalitat Valenciana PROMETEO 2013/069.

REFERENCES

Altman, J. (1962). Are new neurons formed in the brains of adult mammals? *Science* 135, 1127–1128.

Altman, J., and Das, G. D. (1965). Autoradiographic and histological evidence of postnatal hippocampal neurogenesis in rats. *J. Comp. Neurol.* 124, 319–335. doi: 10.1002/cne.901240303

Alvarez-Buylla, A., and Garcia-Verdugo, J. M. (2002). Neurogenesis in adult subventricular zone. *J. Neurosci.* 22, 629–634.

Alvarez-Buylla, A., and Lim, D. A. (2004). For the long run:maintaining germinal niches in the adult brain. *Neuron* 41, 683–686. doi: 10.1016/S0896-6273(04)00111-4

Bagley, J., LaRocca, G., Jimenez, D. A., and Urban, N. N. (2007). Adult neurogenesi and specific replacement of interneuron subtypes in the mouse main olfactory bulb. *BMC Neurosci.* 8:92. doi: 10.1186/1471-2202-8-92

Bahn, S., Mimmack, M., Ryan, M., Caldwell, M. A., Jauniaux, E., Starkey, M., et al. (2002). Neuronal target genes of the neuron-restrictive silencer factor in neurospheres derived from fetuses with Down's syndrome: a gene expression study. *Lancet* 359, 310–315. doi: 10.1016/S0140-6736(02)07497-4

Ball, M. J., and Nuttall, K. (1980). Neurofibrillary tangles, granulovacuolar degeneration, and neuron loss in Down Syndrome: quantitative comparison with Alzheimer dementia. *Ann. Neurol.* 7, 462–465. doi: 10.1002/ana.410070512

Balu, D. T., and Lucki, I. (2009). Adult hippocampal neurogenesis: regulation, functional implications, and contribution to disease pathology. *Neurosci. Biobehav. Rev.* 33, 232–252. doi: 10.1016/j.neubiorev.2008.08.007

Belichenko, P. V., Masliah, E., Kleschevnikov, A. M., Villar, A. J., Epstein, C. J., Salehi, A., et al. (2004). Synaptic structural abnormalities in the Ts65Dn mouse model of Down syndrome. *J. Comp. Neurol.* 480, 281–298. doi: 10.1002/cne.20337

Bianchi, P., Bettini, S., Guidi, S., Ciani, E., Trazzi, S., Stagni, F., et al. (2014). Age-related impairment of olfactory bulb neurogenesis in the Ts65Dn mouse model of Down syndrome. *Exp. Neurol.* 251, 1–11. doi: 10.1016/j.expneurol.2013.10.018

Bianchi, P., Ciani, E., Contestabile, A., Guidi, S., and Bartesaghi, R. (2010b). Lithium restores neurogenesis in the subventricular zone of the Ts65Dn mouse, a model for Down syndrome. *Brain Pathol.* 20, 106–118. doi: 10.1111/j.1750-3639.2008.00246.x

Bianchi, P., Ciani, E., Guidi, S., Trazzi, S., Felice, D., Grossi, G., et al. (2010a). Early pharmacotherapy restores neurogenesis and cognitive performance in the Ts65Dn mouse model for Down syndrome. *J. Neurosci.* 30, 8769–8779. doi: 10.1523/JNEUROSCI.0534-10.2010

Bonfanti, L. (2006). PSA-NCAM in mammalian structural plasticity and neurogenesis. *Prog. Neurobiol.* 80, 129–164. doi: 10.1016/j.pneurobio.2006.08.003

Brazel, C. Y., Limke, T. L., Osborne, J. K., Miura, T., Cai, J., Pevny, L., et al. (2005). Sox2 expression defines a heterogeneous population of neurosphere-forming cells in the adult murine brain. *Aging Cell* 4, 197–207. doi: 10.1111/j.1474-9726.2005.00158.x

Brown, J. P., Couillard-Després, S., Cooper-Kuhn, C. M., Winkler, J., Aigner, L., and Kuhn, H. G. (2003). Transient expression of doublecortin during adult neurogenesis. *J. Comp. Neurol.* 467, 1–10. doi: 10.1002/cne.10874

Chakrabarti, L., Scafidi, J., Gallo, V., and Haydar, T. F. (2011). Environmental enrichment rescues postnatal neurogenesis defect in the male and female Ts65Dn mouse model of Down syndrome. *Dev. Neurosci.* 33, 428–441. doi: 10.1159/000329423

Clark, S., Schwalbe, J., Stasko, M. R., Yarowsky, P. J., and Costa, A. C. S. (2006). Fluoxetine rescues deficient neurogenesis in hippocampus of the Ts65Dn mouse model for Down syndrome. *Exp. Neurol.* 200, 256–261. doi: 10.1016/j.expneurol.2006.02.005

Contestabile, A., Fila, T., Ceccarelli, C., Bonasoni, P., Bonapace, L., Santini, D., et al. (2007). Cell cycle alteration and decreased cell proliferation in the hippocampal dentate gyrus and in the neocortical germinal matrix of fetuses with Down syndrome and in Ts65Dn mice. *Hippocampus* 17, 665–678. doi: 10.1002/hipo.20308

Costa, A. C., Walsh, K., and Davisson, M. T. (1999). Motor dysfunction in a mouse model for Down syndrome. *Physiol. Behav.* 68, 211–220. doi: 10.1016/S0031-9384(99)00178-X

Cotman, C. W., Hailer, N. P., Pfister, K. K., Soltesz, I., and Schachner, M. (1998). Cell adhesion molecules in neural plasticity and pathology: similar mechanisms, distinct organizations? *Prog. Neurobiol.* 55, 659–669. doi: 10.1016/s0301-0082(98)00025-2

Couillard-Despres, S., Winner, B., Schaubeck, S., Aigner, R., Vroemen, M., Weidner, N., et al. (2005). Doublecortin expression levels in adult brain reflect neurogenesis. *Eur. J. Neurosci.* 21, 1–14. doi: 10.1111/j.1460-9568.2004.03813.x

Dayer, A. G., Ford, A. A., Cleaver, K. M., Yassaee, M., and Cameron, H. A. (2003). Short-term and long-term survival of new neurons in the rat dentate gyrus. *J. Comp. Neurol.* 460, 563–572. doi: 10.1002/cne.10675

Demas, G. E., Nelson, R. J., Krueger, B. K., and Yarowsky, P. J. (1998). Impaired spatial working and reference memory in segmental trisomy (Ts65Dn) mice. *Behav. Brain Res.* 90, 199–201. doi: 10.1016/S0166-4328(97)00116-2

Demas, G. E., Nelson, R. J., Krueger, B. K., and Yarowsky, P. J. (1999). Spatial memory deficits in segmental trisomic Ts65Dn mice. *Behav. Brain Res.* 82, 85–92. doi: 10.1016/S0166-4328(97)81111-4

de Souza, F. M., Busquet, N., Blatner, M., Maclean, K. N., and Restrepo, D. (2011). Galatamine improves olfactory learning in the Ts65Dn mouse model of Down syndrome. *Sci. Rep.* 1:137. doi: 10.1038/srep00137

Dierssen, M., Benavides-Piccione, R., Martínez-Cué, C., Estivill, X., Flórez, J., Elston, G. N., et al. (2003). Alterations of neocortical pyramidal cell phenotype in the Ts65Dn mouse model of Down syndrome: effects of environmental enrichment. *Cereb. Cortex* 13, 758–764. doi: 10.1093/cercor/13.7.758

Doetsch, F. (2003). A niche for adul tneural stem cells. *Curr. Opin. Genet. Dev.* 13, 543–550. doi: 10.1016/j.gde.2003.08.012

Doetsch, F., and Hen, R. (2005). Young and excitable: the function of new neurons in the adult mammalian brain. *Curr. Opin. Neurobiol.* 15, 121–128. doi: 10.1016/j.conb.2005.01.018

Eriksson, P. S., Perfilieva, E., Björk-Eriksson, T., Alborn, A. M., Nordborg, C., Peterson, D. A., et al. (1998). Neurogenesis in the adult human hippocampus. *Nat. Med.* 4, 1313–1317. doi: 10.1038/3305

Escorihuela, R. M., Vallina, I. F., Martínez-Cué, C., Baamonde, C., Dierssen, M., Tobeña, A., et al. (1998). Impaired short- and long-term memory in Ts65Dn mice, a model for Down syndrome. *Neurosci. Lett.* 247, 171–174.

Esposito, G., Imitola, J., Lu, J., De Filippis, D., Scuderi, C., Ganesh, V. S., et al. (2008). Genomic and functional profiling of human Down syndrome neural progenitors implicates S100B and aquaporin 4 in cell injury. *Hum. Mol. Genet.* 17, 440–457. doi: 10.1093/hmg/ddm322

Feng, Y., and Walsh, C. A. (2001). Protein–Protein interactions, cytoskeletal regulation and neuronal migration. *Nat. Rev. Neurosci.* 2, 408–416. doi: 10.1038/35077559

Folin, M., Baiguera, S., Conconi, M. T., Pati, T., Grandi, C., Parnigotto, P. P., et al. (2003). The impact of risk factors of Alzheimer's disease in the Down syndrome. *Int. J. Mol. Med.* 11, 267–270. doi: 10.3892/ijmm.11.2.267

Gage, F. H. (2000). Structural plasticity: cause, result, or correlate of depression. *Biol. Psychiatry* 48, 713–714. doi: 10.1016/S0006-3223(00)01019-2

Garcia, A. D. R., Doan, N. B., Imura, T., Bush, T. G., and Sofroniew, M. V. (2004). GFAP-expressing progenitors are the principal source of constitutive neurogenesis in adult mouse forebrain. *Nat. Neurosci.* 7, 1233–1241. doi: 10.1038/nn1340

Gardiner, K., Fortna, A., Bechtel, L., and Davisson, M. T. (2003). Mouse models of Down syndrome: how useful can they be? Comparison of the gene content of human chromosome 21 with orthologous mouse genomic regions. *Gene* 318, 137–147. doi: 10.1016/S0378-1119(03)00769-8

Gerdes, J., Lemke, H., Baisch, H., Wacker, H. H., Schwab, U., and Stein, H. (1984). Cell cycle analysis of a cell proliferation-associated human nuclear antigen defined by the monoclonal antibody Ki-67. *J. Immunol.* 133, 1710–1715.

Gould, E., Beylin, A., Tanapat, P., Reeves, A., and Shors, T. J. (1999). Learning enhances adult neurogenesis in the hippocampal formation. *Nat. Neurosci.* 2, 260–265. doi: 10.1038/6365

Guidi, S., Bonasoni, P., Ceccarelli, C., Santini, D., Gualtieri, F., Ciani, E., et al. (2008). Neurogenesis impairment and increased cell death reduce total neuron number in the hippocampal region of fetuses with Down syndrome. *Brain Pathol.* 18, 180–197. doi: 10.1111/j.1750-3639.2007.00113.x

Guirado, R., Sanchez-Matarredona, D., Varea, E., Crespo, C., Blasco-Ibáñez, J. M., and Nacher, J. (2012). Chronic fluoxetine treatment in middle-aged rats induces changes in the expression of plasticity-related molecules and in neurogenesis. *BMC Neurosci.* 13:5. doi: 10.1186/1471-2202-13-5

Guirado, R., Varea, E., Castillo-Gómez, E., Gómez-Climent, M. A., Rovira-Esteban, L., Blasco-Ibáñez, J. M., et al. (2009). Effects of chronic fluoxetine treatment on the rat somatosensory cortex: activation and induction of neuronal structural plasticity. *Neurosci. Lett.* 457, 12–15. doi: 10.1016/j.neulet.2009.03.104

Gundersen, H. J., and Jensen, E. B. (1987). The efficiency of systematic sampling in stereology and its prediction. *J. Microsc.* 147, 229–263. doi: 10.1111/j.1365-2818.1987.tb02837.x

Hastings, N. B., and Gould, E. (1999). Rapid extension of axons into the CA3 region by adult-generated granule cells. *J. Comp. Neurol.* 413, 146–154.

Hernández, S., Gilabert-Juan, J., Blasco-Ibáñez, J. M., Crespo, C., Nácher, J., and Varea, E. (2012). Altered expression of neuropeptides in the primary somatosensory cortex of the Down syndrome model Ts65Dn. *Neuropeptides* 46, 29–37. doi: 10.1016/j.npep.2011.10.002

Hernández-González, S., Ballestín, R., López-Hidalgo, R., Gilabert-Juan, J., Blasco-Ibáñez, J. M., Crespo, C., et al. (2015). Altered distribution of hippocampal interneurons in the murine down syndrome model Ts65Dn. *Neurochem. Res.* 40, 151–164. doi: 10.1007/s11064-014-1479-8

Hof, P. R., Bouras, C., Perl, D. P., Sparks, D. L., Mehta, N., and Morrison, J. H. (1995). Age-related distribution of neuropathologic changes in the cerebral cortex of patients with Down's syndrome. Quantitative regional analysis and comparison with Alzheimer's disease. *Arch. Neurol.* 52, 379–391. doi: 10.1001/archneur.1995.00540280065020

Holland, A. J., Hon, J., Huppert, F. A., and Stevens, F. (2000). Incidence and course of dementia in people with Down's syndrome: findings from a population-based study. *J. Intellect. Disabil. Res.* 44(Pt 2), 138–146. doi: 10.1046/j.1365-2788.2000.00263.x

Holtzman, D. M., Santucci, D., Kilbridge, J., Chua-Couzens, J., Fontana, D. J., Daniels, S. E., et al. (1996). Developmental abnormalities and age-related neurodegeneration in a mouse model of Down syndrome. *Proc. Natl. Acad. Sci. U.S.A.* 93, 13333–13338. doi: 10.1073/pnas.93.23.13333

Hyde, L. A., Frisone, D. F., and Crnic, L. S. (2001). Ts65Dn mice, a model for Down syndrome, have deficits in context discrimination learning suggesting impaired hippocampal function. *Behav. Brain Res.* 118, 53–60. doi: 10.1016/S0166-4328(00)00313-2

Insausti, A. M., Megías, M., Crespo, D., Cruz-Orive, L. M., Dierssen, M., Vallina, I. F., et al. (1998). Hippocampal volume and neuronal number in Ts65Dn mice: a murine model of Down syndrome. *Neurosci. Lett.* 253, 175–178. doi: 10.1016/S0304-3940(98)00641-7

Kaplan, M. S., and Hinds, J. W. (1977). Neurogenesis in the adult rat: electron microscopic analysis of light radioautographs. *Science* 197, 1092–1094. doi: 10.1126/science.887941

Kaufmann, W. E., and Moser, H. W. (2000). Dendritic anomalies in disorders associated with mental retardation. *Cereb. Cortex.* 10, 981–991. doi: 10.1093/cercor/10.10.981

Kempermann, G., Wiskott, L., and Gage, F. H. (2004). Functional significance of adult neurogenesis. *Curr. Opin. Neurobiol.* 14, 186–191. doi: 10.1016/j.conb.2004.03.001

Kleschevnikov, A. M., Belichenko, P. V., Villar, A. J., Epstein, C. J., Malenka, R. C., and Mobley, W. C. (2004). Hippocampal long-term potentiation suppressed by increased inhibition in the Ts65Dn mouse, a genetic model of Down syndrome. *J. Neurosci.* 24, 8153–8160. doi: 10.1523/JNEUROSCI.1766-04.2004

Kriegstein, A., and Alvarez-Buylla, A. (2009). The glial nature of embryonic and adult neural stem cells. *Annu. Rev. Neurosci.* 32, 149–184. doi: 10.1146/annurev.neuro.051508.135600

Laplagne, D. A., Espósito, M. S., Piatti, V. C., Morgenstern, N. A., Zhao, C., van Praag, H., et al. (2006). Functional convergence of neurons generated in the developing and adult hippocampus. *PLoS Biol.* 4:e409. doi: 10.1371/journal.pbio.0040409

Leuner, B., and Gould, E. (2010). Structural plasticity and hippocampal function. *Annu. Rev. Psychol.* 61, 111–140, C1-C3. doi: 10.1146/annurev.psych.093008.100359

Liu, D. P., Schmidt, C., Billings, T., and Davisson, M. T. (2003). Quantitative PCR genotyping assay for the Ts65Dn mouse model of Down syndrome. *Biotechniques* 35, 1170–1174, 1176, 1178 passim.

Liu, F., Liang, Z., Wegiel, J., Hwang, Y.-W., Iqbal, K., Grundke-Iqbal, I., et al. (2008). Overexpression of Dyrk1A contributes to neurofibrillary degeneration in Down syndrome. *FASEB J.* 22, 3224–3233. doi: 10.1096/fj.07-104539

Lorenzi, H. A., and Reeves, R. H. (2006). Hippocampal hypocellularity in the Ts65Dn mouse originates early in development. *Brain Res.* 1104, 153–159. doi: 10.1016/j.brainres.2006.05.022

Lott, I. T., and Head, E. (2005). Alzheimer disease and Down syndrome: factors in pathogenesis. *Neurobiol. Aging* 26, 383–389. doi: 10.1016/j.neurobiolaging.2004.08.005

Markakis, E. A., and Gage, F. H. (1999). Adult-generated neurons in the dentate gyrus send axonal projections to field CA3 and are surrounded by synaptic vesicles. *J. Comp. Neurol.* 406, 449–460.

Merkle, F. T., Mirzadeh, Z., and Alvarez-Buylla, A. (2007). Mosaic organization of neural stem cells in the adult brain. *Science* 317, 381–384. doi: 10.1126/science.1144914

Mignone, J. L., Kukekov, V., Chiang, A.-S., Steindler, D., and Enikolopov, G. (2004). Neural stem and progenitor cells in nestin-GFP transgenic mice. *J.Comp. Neurol.* 469, 311–324. doi: 10.1002/cne.10964

Mirescu, C., and Gould, E. (2006). Stress and adult neurogenesis. *Hippocampus* 16, 233–238. doi: 10.1002/hipo.20155

Mittwoch, U. (1972). Mongolism and sex: a common problem of cell proliferation? *J. Med. Genet.* 9, 92–95. doi: 10.1136/jmg.9.1.92

Moores, C. A., Francis, F., Perderiset, M., and Houdusse, A. (2003). A double-take on MAPs. *Nat. Struct. Biol.* 10, 314–316. doi: 10.1038/nsb0503-314

Mouret, A., Gheusi, G., Gabellec, M.-M., de Chaumont, F., Olivo-Marin, J.-C., and Lledo, P.-M. (2008). Learning and survival of newly generated neurons: when time matters. *J. Neurosci.* 28, 11511–11516. doi: 10.1523/JNEUROSCI.2954-08.2008

Nacher, J., Alonso-Llosa, G., Rosell, D., and McEwen, B. (2002). PSA-NCAM expression in the piriform cortex of the adult rat. Modulation by NMDA receptor antagonist administration. *Brain Res.* 927, 111–121. doi: 10.1016/S0006-8993(01)03241-3

Nácher, J., Varea, E., Miguel Blasco-Ibáñez, J., Gómez-Climent, M. A., Castillo-Gómez, E., Crespo, C., et al. (2007). N-methyl-d-aspartate receptor expression during adult neurogenesis in the rat dentate gyrus. *Neuroscience* 144, 855–864. doi: 10.1016/j.neuroscience.2006.10.021

Nadel, L. (2003). Down's syndrome: a genetic disorder in biobehavioral perspective. *Genes. Brain. Behav.* 2, 156–166. doi: 10.1034/j.1601-183X.2003.00026.x

Nijjar, R. K., and Murphy, C. (2002). Olfactory impairment increases as a function of age in persons with Down syndrome. *Neurobiol. Aging* 23, 65–73. doi: 10.1016/S0197-4580(01)00263-9

Pérez-Cremades, D., Hernández, S., Blasco-Ibáñez, J. M., Crespo, C., Nacher, J., and Varea, E. (2010). Alteration of inhibitory circuits in the somatosensory cortex of Ts65Dn mice, a model for Down's syndrome. *J. Neural Transm.* 117, 445–455. doi: 10.1007/s00702-010-0376-9

Piatti, V. C., Davies-Sala, M. G., Espósito, M. S., Mongiat, L. A., Trinchero, M. F., and Schinder, A. F. (2011). The timing for neuronal maturation in the adult hippocampus is modulated by local network activity. *J. Neurosci.* 31, 7715–7728. doi: 10.1523/JNEUROSCI.1380-11.2011

Platel, J.-C., Dave, K. A., Gordon, V., Lacar, B., Rubio, M. E., and Bordey, A. (2010). NMDA receptors activated by subventricular zone astrocytic glutamate are critical for neuroblast survival prior to entering a synaptic network. *Neuron* 65, 859–872. doi: 10.1016/j.neuron.2010.03.009

Plümpe, T., Ehninger, D., Steiner, B., Klempin, F., Jessberger, S., Brandt, M., et al. (2006). Variability of doublecortin-associated dendrite maturation in adult hippocampal neurogenesis is independent of the regulation of precursor cell proliferation. *BMC Neurosci.* 7:77. doi: 10.1186/1471-2202-7-77

Rao, M. S., and Shetty, A. K. (2004). Efficacy of doublecortin as a marker to analyse the absolute number and dendritic growth of newly generated neurons in the adult dentate gyrus. *Eur. J. Neurosci.* 19, 234–246. doi: 10.1111/j.0953-816X.2003.03123.x

Reeves, R. H., Irving, N. G., Moran, T. H., Wohn, A., Kitt, C., Sisodia, S. S., et al. (1995). A mouse model for Down syndrome exhibits learning and behaviour deficits. *Nat. Genet.* 11, 177–184. doi: 10.1038/ng1095-177

Ribak, C. E., and Shapiro, L. A. (2007). Dendritic development of newly generated neurons in the adult brain. *Brain Res. Rev.* 55, 390–394. doi: 10.1016/j.brainresrev.2006.12.005

Rochefort, C., Gheusi, G., Vincent, J. D., and Lledo, P. M. (2002). Enriched odor exposure increases the number of newborn neurons in the adult olfactory bulb and improves odor memory. *J. Neurosci.* 22, 2679–2689.

Roizen, N. J., and Patterson, D. (2003). Down's syndrome. *Lancet* 361, 1281–1289. doi: 10.1016/S0140-6736(03)12987-X

Rueda, N., Flórez, J., and Martínez-Cué, C. (2012). Mouse models of Down syndrome as a tool to unravel the causes of mental disabilities. *Neural Plast.* 2012:584071. doi: 10.1155/2012/584071

Rueda, N., Mostany, R., Pazos, A., Flórez, J., and Martínez-Cué, C. (2005). Cell proliferation is reduced in the dentate gyrus of aged but not young Ts65Dn mice, a model of Down syndrome. *Neurosci. Lett.* 380, 197–201. doi: 10.1016/j.neulet.2005.01.039

Sago, H., Carlson, E. J., Smith, D. J., Rubin, E. M., Crnic, L. S., Huang, T. T., et al. (2000). Genetic dissection of region associated with behavioral abnormalities in mouse models for Down syndrome. *Pediatr. Res.* 48, 606–613. doi: 10.1203/00006450-200011000-00009

Schwab, M. H., Bartholomae, A., Heimrich, B., Feldmeyer, D., Druffel-Augustin, S., Goebbels, S., et al. (2000). Neuronal basic helix-loop-helix proteins (NEX and BETA2/Neuro D) regulate terminal granule cell differentiation in the hippocampus. *J. Neurosci.* 20, 3714–3724.

Seress, L. (2007). Comparative anatomy of the hippocampal dentate gyrus in adult and developing rodents, non-human primates and humans. *Prog. Brain Res.* 163, 23–41. doi: 10.1016/S0079-6123(07)63002-7

Seri, B., García-Verdugo, J. M., Collado-Morente, L., McEwen, B. S., and Alvarez-Buylla, A. (2004). Cell types, lineage, and architecture of the germinal zone in the adult dentate gyrus. *J. Comp. Neurol.* 478, 359–378. doi: 10.1002/cne.20288

Seri, B., García-Verdugo, J. M., McEwen, B. S., and Alvarez-Buylla, A. (2001). Astrocytes give rise to new neurons in the adult mammalian hippocampus. *J. Neurosci.* 21, 7153–7160.

Siarey, R. J., Carlson, E. J., Epstein, C. J., Balbo, A., Rapoport, S. I., and Galdzicki, Z. (1999). Increased synaptic depression in the Ts65Dn mouse, a model for mental retardation in Down syndrome. *Neuropharmacology* 38, 1917–1920. doi: 10.1016/S0028-3908(99)00083-0

Siarey, R. J., Stoll, J., Rapoport, S. I., and Galdzicki, Z. (1997). Altered long-term potentiation in the young and old Ts65Dn mouse, a model for Down Syndrome. *Neuropharmacology* 36, 1549–1554. doi: 10.1016/S0028-3908(97)00157-3

Sierra, A., Encinas, J. M., Deudero, J. J. P., Chancey, J. H., Enikolopov, G., Overstreet-Wadiche, L. S., et al. (2010). Microglia shape adult hippocampal neurogenesis through apoptosis-coupled phagocytosis. *Cell Stem Cell* 7, 483–495. doi: 10.1016/j.stem.2010.08.014

Stagni, F., Magistretti, J., Guidi, S., Ciani, E., Mangano, C., Calzà, L., et al. (2013). Pharmacotherapy with fluoxetine restores functional connectivity from the dentate gyrus to field CA3 in the Ts65Dn mouse model of down syndrome. *PLoS ONE* 8:e61689. doi: 10.1371/journal.pone.0061689

Sturgeon, X., and Gardiner, K. J. (2011). Transcript catalogs of human chromosome 21 and orthologous chimpanzee and mouse regions. *Mamm. Genome* 22, 261–271. doi: 10.1007/s00335-011-9321-y

Takashima, S., Becker, L. E., Armstrong, D. L., and Chan, F. (1981). Abnormal neuronal development in the visual cortex of the human fetus and infant with down's syndrome. A quantitative and qualitative Golgi study. *Brain Res.* 225, 1–21. doi: 10.1016/0006-8993(81)90314-0

Takashima, S., Ieshima, A., Nakamura, H., and Becker, L. E. (1989). Dendrites, dementia and the Down syndrome. *Brain Dev.* 11, 131–133. doi: 10.1016/S0387-7604(89)80082-8

Tashiro, A., Sandler, V. M., Toni, N., Zhao, C., and Gage, F. H. (2006). NMDA-receptor-mediated, cell-specific integration of new neurons in adult dentate gyrus. *Nature* 442, 929–933. doi: 10.1038/nature05028

Toni, N., Laplagne, D. A., Zhao, C., Lombardi, G., Ribak, C. E., Gage, F. H., et al. (2008). Neurons born in the adult dentate gyrus form functional synapses with target cells. *Nat. Neurosci.* 11, 901–907. doi: 10.1038/nn.2156

Toni, N., Teng, E. M., Bushong, E. A., Aimone, J. B., Zhao, C., Consiglio, A., et al. (2007). Synapse formation on neurons born in the adult hippocampus. *Nat. Neurosci.* 10, 727–734. doi: 10.1038/nn1908

van Praag, H., Kempermann, G., and Gage, F. H. (1999). Running increases cell proliferation and neurogenesis in the adult mouse dentate gyrus. *Nat. Neurosci.* 2, 266–270. doi: 10.1038/6368

van Praag, H., Schinder, A. F., Christie, B. R., Toni, N., Palmer, T. D., and Gage, F. H. (2002). Functional neurogenesis in the adult hippocampus. *Nature* 415, 1030–1034. doi: 10.1038/4151030a

Varea, E., Blasco-Ibáñez, J. M., Gómez-Climent, M. A., Castillo-Gómez, E., Crespo, C., Martínez-Guijarro, F. J., et al. (2007a). Chronic fluoxetine treatment increases the expression of PSA-NCAM in the medial prefrontal cortex. *Neuropsychopharmacology* 32, 803–812. doi: 10.1038/sj.npp.1301183

Varea, E., Castillo-Gómez, E., Gómez-Climent, M. A., Blasco-Ibáñez, J. M., Crespo, C., Martínez-Guijarro, F. J., et al. (2007b). Chronic antidepressant treatment induces contrasting patterns of synaptophysin and PSA-NCAM expression in different regions of the adult rat telencephalon. *Eur. Neuropsychopharmacol.* 17, 546–557. doi: 10.1016/j.euroneuro.2007.01.001

West, M. J. (1993). New stereological methods for counting neurons. *Neurobiol. Aging* 14, 275–285. doi: 10.1016/0197-4580(93)90112-O

Winner, B., Cooper-Kuhn, C. M., Aigner, R., Winkler, J., and Kuhn, H. G. (2002). Long-term survival and cell death of newly generated neurons in the adult rat olfactory bulb. *Eur J Neurosci.* 16, 1681–1689. doi: 10.1046/j.1460-9568.2002.02238.x

Zilles, K. (1992). Neuronal plasticity as an adaptive property of the central nervous system. *Ann. Anat.* 174, 383–391. doi: 10.1016/S0940-9602(11)80255-4

21

Conditional Disabled-1 Deletion in Mice Alters Hippocampal Neurogenesis and Reduces Seizure Threshold

Matthew J. Korn [1], *Quinton J. Mandle* [1] *and Jack M. Parent* [1,2*]

[1] *Department of Neurology, University of Michigan Medical Center, Ann Arbor, MI, USA,* [2] *VA Ann Arbor Healthcare System, Ann Arbor, MI, USA*

Edited by:
Laura López-Mascaraque, Instituto Cajal-Consejo Superior de Investigaciones Científicas, Spain

Reviewed by:
Helen E. Scharfman, New York State Department of Health, USA
Ashok K. Shetty, Texas A&M Health Science Center College of Medicine at Scott & White, USA

***Correspondence:**
Jack M. Parent
parent@umich.edu

Many animal models of temporal lobe epilepsy (TLE) exhibit altered neurogenesis arising from progenitors within the dentate gyrus subgranular zone (SGZ). Aberrant integration of new neurons into the existing circuit is thought to contribute to epileptogenesis. In particular, adult-born neurons that exhibit ectopic migration and hilar basal dendrites (HBDs) are suggested to be pro-epileptogenic. Loss of reelin signaling may contribute to these morphological changes in patients with epilepsy. We previously demonstrated that conditional deletion of the reelin adaptor protein, disabled-1 (Dab1), from postnatal mouse SGZ progenitors generated dentate granule cells (DGCs) with abnormal dendritic development and ectopic placement. To determine whether the early postnatal loss of reelin signaling is epileptogenic, we conditionally deleted Dab1 in neural progenitors and their progeny on postnatal days 7–8 and performed chronic video-EEG recordings 8–10 weeks later. Dab1-deficient mice did not have spontaneous seizures but exhibited interictal epileptiform abnormalities and a significantly reduced latency to pilocarpine-induced status epilepticus. After chemoconvulsant treatment, over 90% of mice deficient for Dab1 developed generalized motor convulsions with tonic-clonic movements, rearing, and falling compared to <20% of wild-type mice. Recombination efficiency, measured by Cre reporter expression, inversely correlated with time to the first sustained seizure. These pro-epileptogenic changes were associated with decreased neurogenesis and increased numbers of hilar ectopic DGCs. Interestingly, neurons co-expressing the Cre reporter comprised a fraction of these hilar ectopic DGCs cells, suggesting a non-cell autonomous effect for the loss of reelin signaling. We also noted a dispersion of the CA1 pyramidal layer, likely due to hypomorphic effects of the conditional Dab1 allele, but this abnormality did not correlate with seizure susceptibility. These findings suggest that the misplacement or reduction of postnatally-generated DGCs contributes to aberrant circuit development and hyperexcitability, but aberrant neurogenesis after conditional Dab1 deletion alone is not sufficient to produce spontaneous seizures.

Keywords: neural stem cells, adult neurogenesis, temporal lobe epilepsy, pilocarpine

INTRODUCTION

Mesial temporal lobe epilepsy (mTLE) is a common and often intractable focal epilepsy (Bender et al., 2004; Dube et al., 2012). Structural changes in the hippocampal dentate gyrus (DG) are implicated in mTLE pathogenesis, though the mechanisms underlying these changes are poorly understood. Neurogenesis is markedly disrupted in rodent models of mTLE (Parent et al., 1997, 2006; Jessberger et al., 2005, 2007; Shapiro et al., 2005; Murphy et al., 2011, 2012), leading to the idea that aberrantly integrated adult-born neurons (namely dentate granule cells, DGCs) produce seizures (Parent and Kron, 2012; Pun et al., 2012; Bielefeld et al., 2014; Cho et al., 2015) and contribute to associated comorbidities such as cognitive dysfunction and depression (Groticke et al., 2007; Muller et al., 2009; Zhang et al., 2010; Lesting et al., 2011; Levin et al., 2012; Klein et al., 2015).

The role of adult DGC neurogenesis is complex and there are several competing hypotheses as to how continuous integration of new neurons might be implicated in seizure development. Intact adult neurogenesis may mitigate acute seizure susceptibility (Iyengar et al., 2015) and suppressing adult neurogenesis with brain irradiation can exacerbate kindling progression (Raedt et al., 2007; Pekcec et al., 2011). However, the development of epilepsy after an acute insult, such as status epilepticus (SE), is attenuated if the seizure-induced increase in adult neurogenesis is inhibited by antimitotic agents (Jung et al., 2006; Sugaya et al., 2010) or pharmacogenetic methods (Cho et al., 2015). Perhaps most compelling is the finding that disrupting the integration of a subset of postnatal-born DGCs by suppressing phosphatase and tensin homolog (PTEN) signaling is sufficient to produce spontaneous seizures in mice, and the affected DGCs exhibit many of the aberrant changes seen in animal models of mTLE (Pun et al., 2012). Thus, there is an interest in identifying signaling pathways that regulate DGC neurogenesis and whose disruption might produce mTLE.

Reelin-expressing interneurons persist throughout the adult DG (Alcantara et al., 1998; Pesold et al., 1998; Gong et al., 2007) and reelin expression is decreased in human and experimental mTLE (Gong et al., 2007; Haas and Frotscher, 2010). It is proposed that altered neurogenesis in mTLE may arise in part due to disrupted reelin signaling (Haas et al., 2002; Gong et al., 2007; Kobow et al., 2009; Haas and Frotscher, 2010; Freiman et al., 2011). Loss of the reelin adaptor protein, disabled-1 (Dab1), imparts a similar developmental phenotype to loss of reelin function (Howell et al., 1997a; Sheldon et al., 1997; Olson et al., 2006). In prior work, we conditionally deleted Dab1 from nestin-expressing neural stem cells (NSCs) in the postnatal mouse subgranular zone (SGZ) and found that NSCs deficient in Dab1 generate adult-born neurons that migrate ectopically and have abnormal dendritic development (Teixeira et al., 2012). Here we explore whether the disrupted integration of Dab1-deficient early postnatal- through adult-born neurons leads to altered seizure susceptibility or epilepsy.

MATERIALS AND METHODS

Animals and Tamoxifen Administration

All procedures and experiments were approved by the University of Michigan Institutional Committee on the Use and Care of Animals and were performed in accordance with guidelines developed by the National Institutes of Health. NestinCreER^{T2}/R26RYFP/Dab1$^{Flox/Flox}$ triple transgenic mice were derived and maintained as previously described (Teixeira et al., 2012). Briefly, mice harboring the Dab1-conditional allele (Pramatarova et al., 2008) were crossed with *Nestin-Cre-ER*^{T2} mice (Lagace et al., 2007; "Line K" in Sun et al., 2014) and a recombination reporter line, R26R-YFP, containing a floxed-stop followed by yellow fluorescent protein (YFP) in the *ROSA26* gene locus (Zambrowicz et al., 1997). Thus, tamoxifen (TMX)-inducible, cre-mediated recombination results in the deletion of Dab1 along with expression of YFP in nestin-expressing progenitors and their subsequent progeny. Bigenic mice with wild-type Dab1 treated with TMX and mice with mutant Dab1 but not treated with TMX were used as controls. Heterozygous mice (NestinCreER^{T2}/R26RYFP/Dab1$^{Flox/+}$) served as a gene dose comparison to the homozygous null mutants. We refer to homozygous mutants as Dab1$^{Flox/Flox}$, heterozygous as Dab1$^{Flox/+}$, and controls as Dab1$^{+/+}$. Experimenters were blind to genotype and pups were treated i.p. once daily with TMX at 100 mg/kg (dissolved in 10% EtOH/90% sunflower oil, 12.5 mg/ml) or vehicle on P7 and P8. Animals survived to P55 before any additional manipulations were performed (**Supplemental Figure 1**). Unless otherwise noted, mice were housed under a 12 h light/dark cycle and were given food and water *ad libitum*.

Epidural Electrode Placement and Video-EEG

To determine if Dab1-deficient mice exhibit spontaneous seizures or epileptiform activity, we monitored animals with continuous video-EEG. Mice were implanted with four epidural screw electrodes at 2 months after the last administration of TMX. Procedures for affixing electrodes were performed as previously described (Lee et al., 2012; Kehrl et al., 2014; Wagnon et al., 2015). Mice were anesthetized with ketamine and xylazine and placed in a stereotaxic mouse adaptor (Stoelting). Six burr holes were made in the skull using a 3.2 mm steel bit (Meisinger USA, Centennial, Colorado). Electrodes were positioned and fastened (left and right frontal, left and right parietal, one cerebellar, and one reference over the sinus cavity) using mounting screws (E363/20; PlasticsOne, Roanoke, VA). The sockets were fitted into a 6-pin electrode pedestal and the entire apparatus was secured with dental cement (Stoelting). Animals received buprenorphine (0.05 mg/kg) every 12 h for 3 days after surgery. Following recovery, animals were monitored continuously for 10 days by video/EEG recording (Ceegraph Vision; Natus, Middleton, WI). Recordings were sampled at 256 Hz and concurrent video was analyzed offline and synced with EEG data in Persyst 12 (Persyst, Prescott, AZ). Seizures and epileptiform activity were assessed manually in their entirety by an observer blind to the genotypes. Interictal epileptiform discharges (IEDs) were defined as paroxysmal waveforms lasting 20–200 ms having spike or sharp-wave and after-going slow wave morphology, identified visually to be independent of preceding behavioral activity. Spontaneous seizures were defined as the abrupt appearance of rhythmic waveforms or runs of spikes/sharp waves that persisted for a minimum of 10 s and displayed an unequivocal evolution in frequency and morphology, followed by postictal suppression and return to baseline. Detailed evaluation of EEG waveforms was performed by randomly selecting a 4-h epoch from each day during the 10 day recording period.

Pilocarpine Administration and Seizure Threshold

Mice were injected intraperitoneally with scopolamine methyl nitrate (5 mg/kg) to block peripheral cholinergic effects, followed 20 min later with pilocarpine hydrochloride (289 mg/kg), a muscarinic cholinergic agonist, to produce SE. Animals were monitored for 45 min and were given additional half-doses (not exceeding twice the original dose) of pilocarpine if no seizure activity was detected.

The clinical manifestation of SE was scored using a modified Racine scale (Racine, 1972). The scoring was: 0 for mice displaying no abnormal behavior; 1 for periods of freezing, chewing or nodding; 2–3 if tremors and shaking developed, along with straub tail; 4 for mice with seizures that included rearing or clonus, followed by a clear recovery; 5 was used for mice with rearing and clonus, along with running and falling; 6 for severe and repeated stage 5 seizures where animals either did not recover between events or expired.

Seizure threshold was defined as the latency (in minutes) from the administration of pilocarpine until the animal experienced the electrographic onset of SE, consisting of either a prolonged seizure lasting at least 3 min or 3 contiguous seizure events less than 2-min apart from one another without intervening complete behavioral recovery. Electrographic onset was defined by a distinctive shift in background activity whereby low-amplitude high frequency waves evolved into large, rhythmic epileptiform discharges, at least one standard deviation greater in amplitude compared to background activity.

Tissue Processing and Immunohistochemistry

Immediately after a 90-min SE episode, mice were injected with an overdose of sodium pentobarbital and perfused intracardially with 0.9% saline followed by 4% paraformaldehyde (PFA) in phosphate buffered saline (PBS), pH 7.4. Brains were fixed overnight, cryoprotected in 30% sucrose at 4°C, and cyrosectioned at 40 μm in the coronal plane using a Leica CM1850 cyrostat (Leica Microsystems, St. Louis, MO). Sections were collected into cyropreservative (sucrose and ethylene glycol in 50 mM phosphate buffer) as series of every 12th section through the entire extent of the septotemporal axis and stored at −20°C until processed for immunohistoschemistry (IHC). Tissues were rinsed thoroughly in Tris buffered saline (TBS, pH 7.6) and incubated for 90 min at room temperature in a blocking solution containing 10% normal goat serum, triton x-100, glycine, and bovine serum albumin in TBS. Floating sections were incubated overnight at 4°C with a cell type-specific antibody along with a chicken anti-GFP (1:2000, Aves Labs - GFP-1020; Cho et al., 2015) to enhance the endogenous YFP fluorescence and confirm colocalization. Cell-type specific antibodies included rabbit anti-doublecortin (DCX, 1:1000, AbCam - ab18723; Lee and Umemori, 2013), mouse anti-NeuN (1:2000, Chemicon - MAB377; Miltiadous et al., 2013), and rabbit anti-Prox1 (1:2000, Millipore - AB5475; Farrar et al., 2005; Parent et al., 2006). We verified deletion of Dab1 by using a rabbit anti-Dab1 antibody (1:1000, Sigma – ab-232; Howell et al., 1997b; Teixeira et al., 2012 and **Figures 3A,B'**). Rabbit anti-MAP2 (2a+2b) antibody (1:1000, Sigma-M2320; Quadrato et al., 2014) was used to visualize hippocampal dendritic organization. Rabbit Ki67 antibody was used to label actively dividing cells (1:1000, Vector Labs–VP-K451; Singer et al., 2009). Alexa secondary antibodies (1:600; ThermoFisher) were used for single or double immunofluorescence. In some instances tissue was briefly rinsed with Hoescht 33342 (1:5000) for a bisbenzimide nuclear counterstain. Low-magnification images were acquired on a Leica DMI 6000 inverted scope and higher magnification images for co-localization were collected as thin optical section (1–2 μm) z-stacks on a Nikon A-1 laser scanning confocal microscope.

Data Quantification

For colocalization with each cell type-specific antigen, we quantified the left or right hemisphere of 4–5 sections per animal. Three-dimensional stacks were viewed as a maximum intensity projection and a grid comprised of 100 × 100 μm squares was placed over the image in ImageJ 1.48 (NIH, Bethesda, MD). Squares containing the GCL and SGZ were numbered and at least three were selected at random for quantification. Cells expressing the reporter were identified in the z-stack and colocalization of the Alexa secondary was confirmed in x and y dimension using Nikon Element Viewer (Melville, NY). No fewer than 5 cells were counted per section and a minimum of 30 cells were counted per animal. Values are reported as cells that express YFP and cell type–specific antigen over total number of YFP-positive cells. For recombination efficiency, we estimated the number of YFP-labeled cells per 100 μm^2 by averaging the number of cells over three tissue sections for each animal. We verified localization of each cell type-specific antigen with bisbenzimide. Density of DCX+ cells was estimated with the aid of MicroBrightField Neurolucida (MBF, Williston, VT). For each animal, we selected a 500 μm linear region along the GCL and included cells within the SGZ and GCL. Only whole round or spherical cell bodies were counted and fragments of DCX labeling less than 5 μm were excluded. Cells were tagged with a digital marker through each optical section to prevent double-counting. Clusters of cells where one cell body merged into another were counted as one, thus our quantification underestimates the total number of DCX-positive cells. This number is reported as average number of DCX-expressing neurons per 500 μm. The density of hilar ectopic granule cells (HEGCs) was determined by counting all Prox1+ cells within a defined region of interest restricted to the hilar region of the DG, delineated as 20 μm from the bottom of the GCL. Representative images of labeling were exported as TIFF files and edited using

Corel PaintShop Pro X7 (Corel, Ottawa, Ontario, Canada). Images were cropped to fit the dimensions of each figure.

Statistical Analyses

All statistical analyses were made using JMP Pro 11 software (SAS, Cary, NC). Data sets were checked for normal distributions. ANOVA with *post-hoc* test was performed to assess differences across multiple comparisons. Individual comparisons were made using Tukey's HSD test to correct for sample number. We performed a non-parametric comparison using Wilcoxon's *t*-test for comparison between groups for latency and Spearman's ρ or Fisher's Exact Test (small sample sizes) for multivariate correlations. Values are reported as mean ± SEM, for all statistical comparisons: $^{*}p < 0.05$, $^{**}p < 0.02$.

RESULTS

Dab1–Deficient Adult Mice Exhibit Infrequent Interictal EEG Abnormalities and Rare Seizure-Like Events

We reviewed 10 day video-EEG records and found that no vehicle treated $Dab1^{Flox/Flox}$ ($n = 10$), vehicle or TMX treated $Dab1^{Flox/+}$ ($n = 5$) or TMX treated $Dab1^{+/+}$ ($n = 9$), exhibited seizures or IEDs (**Figure 1A**). A total of 3 of the 17 $Dab1^{Flox/Flox}$ mice that received TMX exhibited IEDs. One mouse exhibited brief myoclonic spasms, with preceding spike-wave discharges (black arrowheads, **Figure 1B**). We identified a second animal (**Figure 1C**) with recurrent epileptiform discharges at regular intervals with background suppression and slowing, coinciding with prolonged periods of immobility, tremors, and labored movement. A third mouse (**Figure 1D**) displayed intermittent 2–4 s discharges of large amplitude theta waves that were occasionally followed by brief spasms, not associated with an obvious epileptiform EEG discharge. Lastly, a single mouse exhibited intermittent spike-wave discharges (black arrowheads, **Figure 1E**) throughout the 10-day recording period but experienced no behavioral events. These observations indicate that deletion of Dab1 in postnatal NSCs does not cause overt spontaneous convulsive seizures, but leads to hyperexcitable network changes that can generate spike discharges and sporadic EEG patterns with behavioral events on an interictal-to-ictal continuum.

Adult Mice Deficient in Dab1 Exhibit More Severe Seizures and a Reduced Latency to the Onset of Pilocarpine-Induced SE

To probe whether postnatal Dab1 deletion in DGCs alters susceptibility to developing SE after pilocarpine administration, we injected drug while animals were still being monitored by

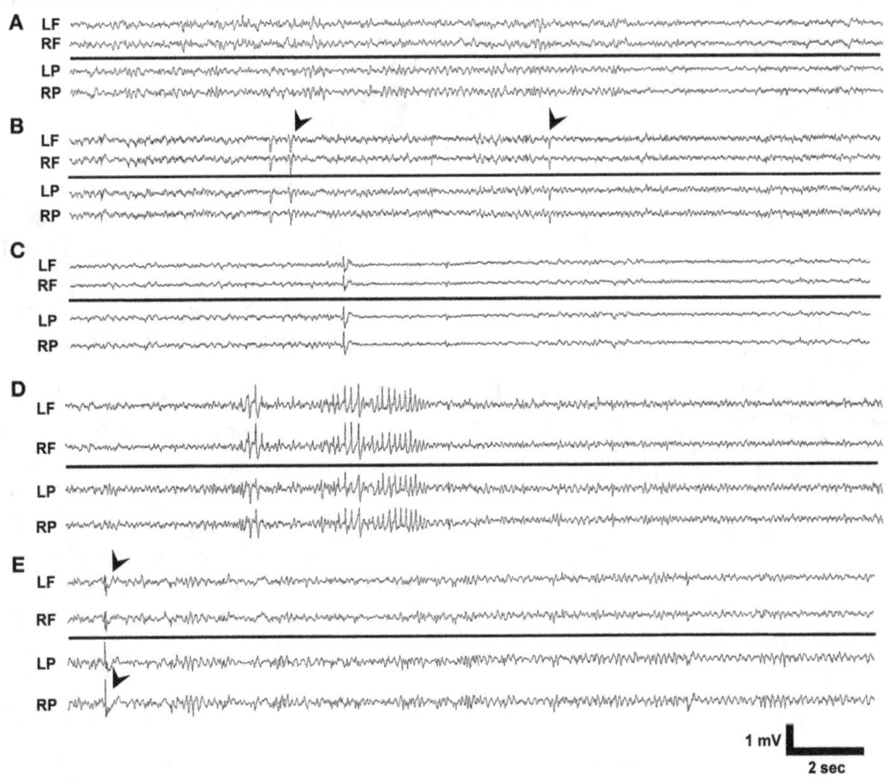

FIGURE 1 | EEG phenotypes of $Dab1^{Flox/Flox}$ mutants. (A) Typical interictal EEG which exhibits no abnormalities, interictal spikes, or epileptiform discharges. **(B)** Intermittent sharp waves and background slowing which occasionally was associated with a myoclonic spasm (black arrowheads). This patterned activity persisted for 3 min. **(C)** Prolonged periods of low amplitude beta with intermittent spikes coinciding with behavioral inactivity. **(D)** High amplitude, sharply contoured theta waveforms that preceded myoclonus. **(E)** Interictal spike discharges (black arrowheads) appeared throughout the 10 day recording period as the sole abnormality in this mouse. LF, left frontal; RF, right frontal; LP, left parietal; RP, right parietal.

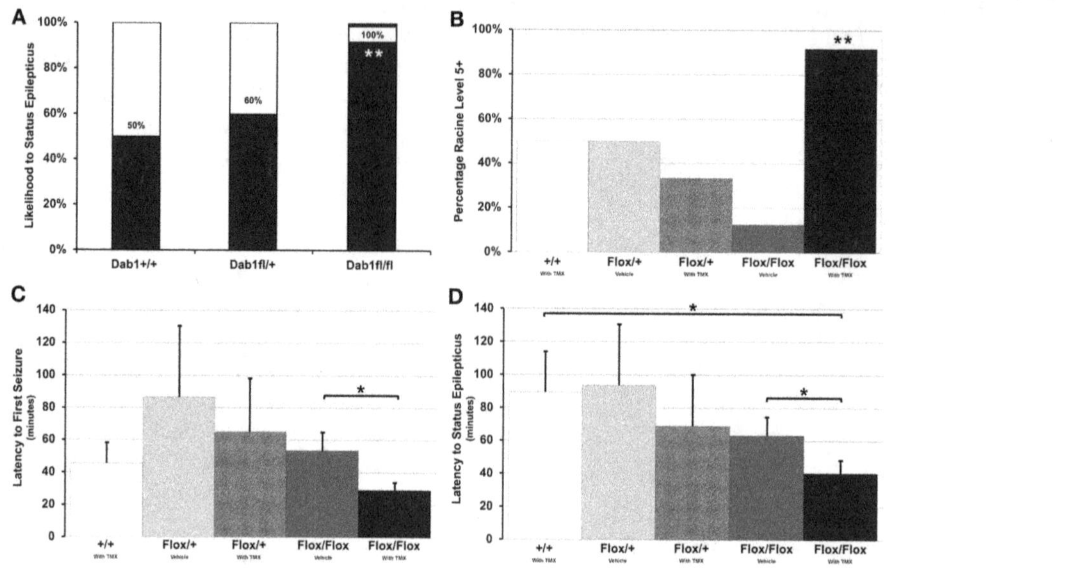

FIGURE 2 | Conditional deletion of Dab1 reduces SE latency and increases seizure severity. (A) Dab1$^{Flox/Flox}$ mice were significantly more likely to develop SE compared to Dab1$^{Flox/+}$ or Dab1$^{+/+}$ mice. **(B)** Compared to all other treatment groups, TMX treated Dab1$^{Flox/Flox}$ mice were significantly more likely to develop severe, Racine stage 5 or 6 seizures following the administration of pilocarpine. **(C)** TMX-treated Dab1$^{Flox/Flox}$ mice exhibited the shortest latency to the first seizure and **(D)** a significantly shorter latency to SE compared to vehicle treated Dab1$^{Flox/Flox}$ or Dab1$^{+/+}$mice. For all statistical comparisons: $^*p < 0.05$, $^{**}p < 0.02$.

video-EEG. In addition to scoring the severity of the seizures, we measured the latency to onset of the first seizure and to the beginning of SE.

All Dab1$^{Flox/Flox}$ mice, regardless of whether or not they were treated with TMX, developed SE (**Figure 2A**, $n = 20$). This was in contrast to only 50% of Dab1$^{+/+}$ ($n = 4$) and 67% of Dab1$^{Flox/+}$ ($n = 5$) mice, indicating that mutant mice are significantly more likely to develop SE (Fisher's Exact Test; $p < 0.02$). Mutants typically required less pilocarpine to develop SE, but we determined that this variability was not significant (Fisher's Exact Test; $p = 0.27$). In some cases, mice that failed to develop SE exhibited brief seizures. Of the animals that did develop behavioral and electrographic SE, only mutants that received TMX ($n = 12$) were likely to develop severe, stage 5 seizures (**Figure 2B**, Fisher's Exact Test; $p < 0.02$). Only three mice expired during the course of the experiments (1 each in Dab1$^{+/+}$ + TMX, Dab1$^{Flox/Flox}$ + vehicle, and Dab1$^{Flox/Flox}$ + TMX groups), and mortality did not differ between groups (Fisher's Exact Test; $p = 0.86$).

Dab1$^{Flox/Flox}$ mice treated with TMX consistently had the earliest onset to the first seizure (**Figure 2C**), which was significantly shorter compared to Dab1$^{Flox/Flox}$ given vehicle (Dab1$^{Flox/Flox}$ + TMX: $n = 12$, 29.4 ± 4.1; Dab1$^{Flox/Flox}$ + vehicle: $n = 8$, 53.6 ± 10.7; $p < 0.05$). Dab1$^{Flox/Flox}$ mice had a significantly reduced latency to SE (**Figure 2D**, 40.5 ± 7.4) compared to Dab1$^{Flox/Flox}$ animals treated with vehicle (63.3 ± 10.7; $p < 0.05$) and mice with WT Dab1 (89.3 ± 24.2; $p < 0.05$), but were not different than Dab1$^{Flox/+}$ mice given TMX (69.0 ± 30.6; $p = 0.17$) or vehicle (93.5 ± 36.5; $p = 0.08$). From these data we conclude that mice with conditional Dab1 deletion in postnatal DGCs develop seizures that evolve into SE more quickly than controls, and exhibit a greater seizure severity after pilocarpine treatment.

Recombination Efficiency and Deletion of Dab1 is Negatively Correlated with Latency to SE

Dab1 protein is predominately expressed throughout the SGZ of adult mice (white arrowheads, **Figure 3A**), and at lower levels in the GCL (white arrow, **Figure 3A**). Sporadic Dab1-positive neurons were also seen in the hilus and inner molecular layer. Treatment with TMX resulted in the expression of YFP (**Figure 3B**) and loss in the expression of virtually all Dab1 protein (**Figure 3B′**). YFP expression was limited to regions that exhibit postnatal neurogenesis.

Using reporter activity as a proxy for recombination efficiency, we sought to determine if latency to SE varied as a function of the loss of Dab1 protein (**Figure 3C**). We found a significant inverse correlation between recombination efficiency after TMX treatment and SE onset latency for Dab1$^{Flox/Flox}$ ($n = 12$; $\rho = -0.74$, $p < 0.02$), an inverse correlation for Dab1$^{Flox/+}$ ($n = 3$; $\rho = -1$), but not Dab1$^{+/+}$ ($n = 4$; $\rho = 0.41$) mice. This finding suggests that progressively greater loss of Dab1 results in a more pronounced susceptibility to pilocarpine-induced SE. Thus, despite the absence of definite spontaneous seizures, altered circuitry associated with the conditional deletion of Dab1 appears to be pro-epileptic.

Dab1$^{Flox/Flox}$ Mice Exhibit a Dispersed CA1 Pyramidal Cell Layer which does not Correlate with Seizure Phenotype

We next sought to examine structural alternations potentially underlying the increased seizure susceptibility caused by conditional Dab1 deletion in postnatal NSCs and their progeny. Mice homozygous for floxed *Dab1* have reduced Dab1 protein levels from P1-7, even without cre driven recombination

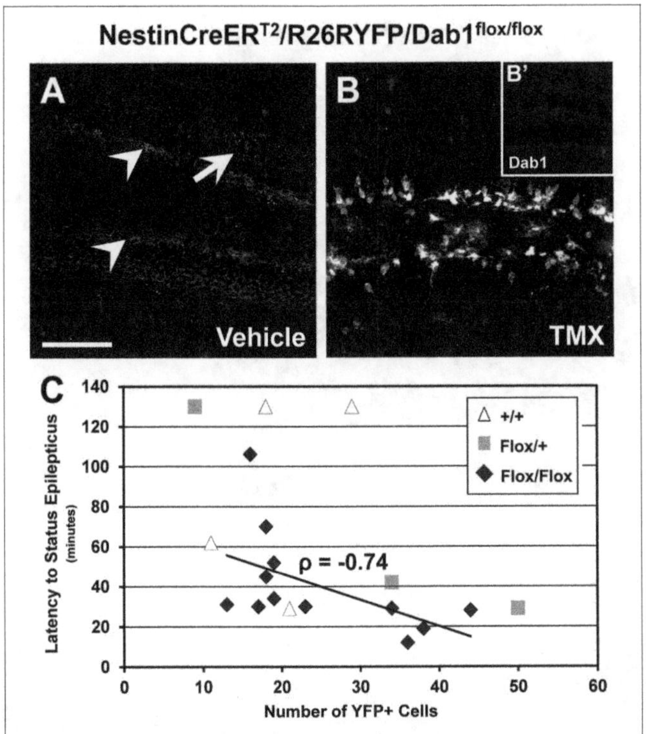

FIGURE 3 | Recombination efficiency and latency to status epilepticus in NestinCreER^{T2}/R26RYFP/Dab1$^{Flox/Flox}$ mice. (A–B′) Confocal images of sections through the DG immunostained for Dab1 **(A,B′)** or YFP **(B)**. **(A)** Dab1 expression is distributed through the SGZ (arrowheads) of the DG in untreated Dab1$^{Flox/Flox}$ mice. Scattered labeling is present in the GCL (arrow) and to a lesser extent within the molecular layer and hilus. **(B)** Two days of TMX treatment induces Cre activation and recombination in Dab1$^{Flox/Flox}$ mice, resulting in substantial YFP reporter expression 2 months later. **(B′)** Note that virtually no Dab1 expression remains in the DG after TMX treatment. **(C)** There is a significant inverse correlation between recombination efficiency and latency to SE in TMX treated Dab1$^{Flox/Flox}$ mice, indicating that the latency to SE is influenced by reelin signaling in postnatal- or adult-born DGCs. No correlation exists for Dab1$^{+/+}$ mice. Scale bar = 100 μm **(A,B)**, 250 μm in **(B′)**.

(Pramatarova et al., 2008; Teixeira et al., 2014). This coincides with the period of development when pyramidal neurons migrate away from the ventricular zone and the hippocampal primordium to stratify in the outer lamina of CA1 (Stanfield and Cowan, 1979; Nakahira and Yuasa, 2005). It is not surprising then that the CA1 pyramidal layer is disrupted in mutants whether treated with vehicle or TMX (**Figures 4A–C**). MAP2ab labeling, which allows for visualization of CA1 apical dendrites, revealed that the ectopic layer of pyramidal neurons maintain their apical arbors (**Figures 4D–F**). In contrast to the highly organized dendritic fields of the inner layer, dendrites emanating from ectopic pyramidal neurons were notably tortuous (white arrow in **Figure 4F′**). This phenotype did not appear to contribute to the reduced seizure latency as we found no correlation between the mean width of the CA1 layer and latency to SE (**Figure 4G**) in vehicle ($\rho = -0.36$, $p = 0.43$) or TMX treated ($\rho = -0.14$, $p = 0.66$) mice, regardless of genotype (data not shown).

Dab1-Deficient NSCs Produce Fewer Immature Neurons but More HEGCs, the Degree of which Correlates with Reduced Seizure Latency

Previous work suggests that loss of Dab1 in postnatal NSCs and their progeny alters DGC development and maturation (Teixeira et al., 2012). To assess the degree of neurogenesis and location of DGCs after conditional Dab1 deletion, we performed IHC to identify proliferating cells (Ki67), immature neurons (DCX), and post-mitotic granule cells (Prox1).

We found significantly fewer actively proliferating cells in Dab1$^{Flox/Flox}$ mice (**Figure 5A**, $n = 6$; 10.3 ± 1.0) compared to controls (**Figures 5B,C**; $n = 5$; 25.5 ± 5.5; $p < 0.02$). Consistent with the decreased cell proliferation, there were also less DCX-labeled immature neurons observed in TMX treated Dab1$^{Flox/Flox}$ mice compared to wild-type vehicle treated controls (**Figures 5D,E**), suggesting decreased neurogenesis. As with our previous findings (Teixeira et al., 2012), immature neurons exhibited stunted dendrites with atrophic apical branches (white arrowheads, **Figure 5E**). We found fewer DCX-positive immature neurons in TMX treated Dab1$^{Flox/Flox}$ mice (**Figure 5F**; $n = 14$; 19.6 ± 2.2 per 500 linear μm) compared to TMX treated Dab1$^{+/+}$ mice ($n = 8$; 32.6 ± 3.4; $p < 0.02$), but not Dab1$^{Flox/+}$ mice ($n = 3$; 22.2 ± 6.7; $p = 0.10$).

We then quantified the percentage of DCX-positive cells that co-expressed YFP to determine how loss of Dab1 directly affects neuronal differentiation (**Figures 5G,H**). We observed significantly fewer DCX+/YFP+ immature neurons in TMX-treated Dab1$^{Flox/Flox}$ (**Figure 5I**; $n = 17$; 22.3% $\pm$ 0.03) and Dab1$^{Flox/+}$ mice ($n = 3$; 18.6% $\pm$ 0.04) compared to TMX-treated controls ($n = 9$; 56.8% $\pm$ 0.05, $p < 0.02$). From these data we conclude that the loss of Dab1 reduces the proliferation of DG neural progenitors, which contributes to the decrease in the number of immature neurons.

We previously demonstrated that adult-born neurons generated from Dab1-deficient, nestin-expressing NSCs and their progeny migrate ectopically (Teixeira et al., 2012). Here we confirm the observation that mice deficient for Dab1 exhibit significantly more Prox1+ HEGCs (**Figures 6A–C**; $n = 12$, 6.48 ± 0.75 per 100 μm^2) than TMX-treated controls ($n = 6$, 1.20 ± 0.36 per 100 μm^2, $p < 0.02$) or Dab1$^{Flox/+}$ mice ($n = 2$, 1.83 ± 0.12 per 100 μm^2, $p < 0.05$). Notably, the number of HEGCs inversely correlated with the latency to onset of SE (**Figure 6D**; $n = 13$, $\rho = -0.56$, $p < 0.05$). Initially, we reasoned that it was the cell autonomous deletion of Dab1 from nestin-expressing NSCs that was responsible for causing Dab1-deficient neurons to migrate ectopically away from the GCL. In examining YFP+/Prox1+ granule cells (data not shown), we noted that the majority of HEGCs were negative for YFP reporter expression (**Figure 6E**, 83.95% $\pm$ 0.03). Taken together, the conditional deletion of Dab1 from postnatal nestin-expressing NSCs results in a non-cell autonomous ectopic migration of granule cells into the hilus, and their presence correlates with a reduced latency to SE onset.

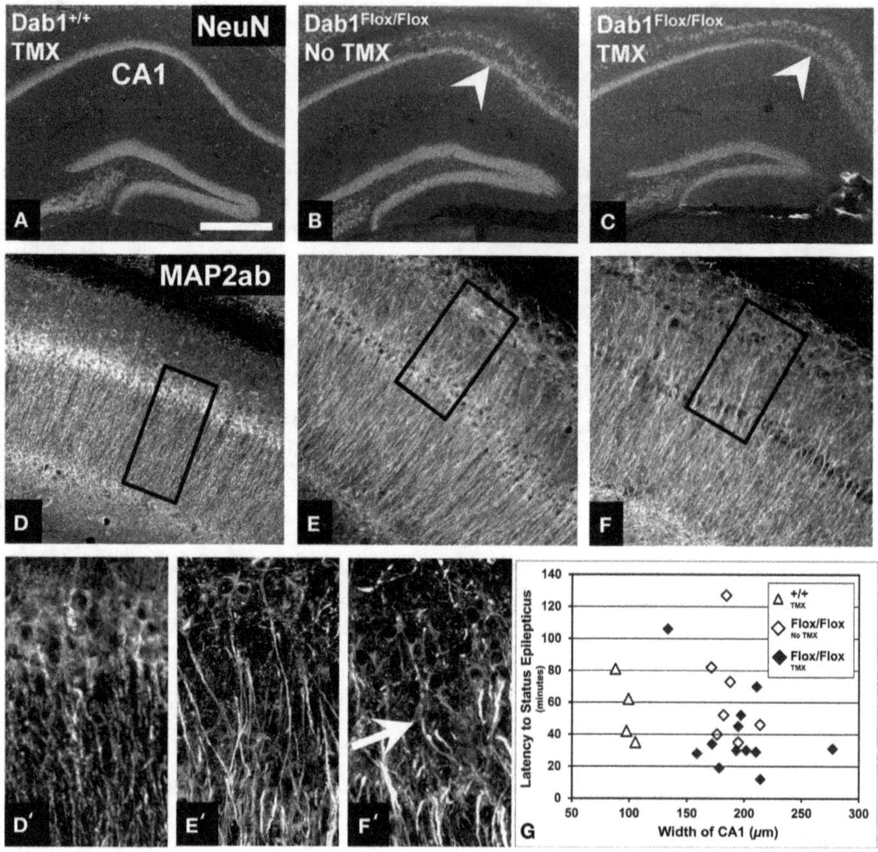

FIGURE 4 | Abnormalities of the CA1 pyramidal layer do not correlate with latency to SE. (A) Labeling for NeuN demonstrates that the CA1 pyramidal cell layer of mice with WT Dab1 is single layered compared to the ectopic layer (above the white arrowheads, which point to the "normal" layer) found in hypomorphic mice harboring floxed-Dab1, regardless if they are treated with vehicle **(B)** or TMX **(C)**. Similar to mice with WT Dab1 **(D)**, the primary pyramidal layer of Dab1$^{Flox/Flox}$ mice treated with vehicle **(E)** or TMX **(F)**, exhibit intact apical dendrites. **(D′)** Dendrites from pyramidal neurons of WT mice extend perpendicular to the long access of the cell layer. In contrast, dendrites of the ectopic pyramidal layer in mice with Floxed-Dab1, treated with vehicle **(E′)** or TMX **(F′)** have curved apical arbors (white arrow) with overlapping domains. **(D′–F′)** are the boxed regions in **(D–F)**, respectively. **(G)** Despite this pronounced phenotype, there was no correlation between overall width of the CA1 pyramidal layer and latency to SE. Scale bar = 500 μm **(A–C)**, 300 μm **(D–F)**, and 50 μm **(D′–F′)**.

DISCUSSION

We sought to determine if changes that arise following conditional deletion of Dab1 from postnatal NSCs and their progeny cause spontaneous seizures. We observed no definite behavioral or electrographic seizures, but some mice experienced single myoclonic spasms associated with EEG discharges, and others showed three different patterns of epileptiform or paroxysmal discharges among 4 of 17 TMX-treated mutant mice. These findings suggest that the conditional loss of reelin signaling in postnatally-generated DGCs does not result in a robust epilepsy phenotype. However, we did find that TMX-treated Dab1$^{Flox/Flox}$ mice are more likely to develop severe SE after administration of the chemoconvulstant pilocarpine, with a shorter latency than TMX-treated heterozygous or wild-type mice, as well as vehicle-treated homozygous littermates. Histological analyses confirmed that the postnatal loss of Dab1 in NSCs induces the ectopic migration of DGCs (Teixeira et al., 2012) and reduces ongoing adult neurogenesis. Possible mechanisms for this latter finding may involve promoting NSC quiescence, changing the phenotype of NSC progeny from neuronal to glial (Teixeira et al., 2012), or decreasing the proliferation or survival of transit amplifying progenitors or immature neurons.

The Development of HEGCs in Dab1$^{Flox/Flox}$ Mice is not Sufficient to Generate Spontaneous Seizures

Among the more notable changes in Dab1$^{Flox/Flox}$ mice is the ectopic placement of adult-born granule cells into the hilus and along the border between the GCL and the inner molecular layer of the dentate gyrus (**Figure 6**; Teixeira et al., 2012). Dispersion of the GCL and HEGCs are hallmark features in humans with mTLE (Lurton et al., 1998; Parent et al., 2006; Blumcke et al., 2009; Bae et al., 2010) and can be reproduced in models that induce SE with kainic acid, pilocarpine, or limbic kindling (Bouilleret et al., 1999; McCloskey et al., 2006; Botterill et al., 2015). Several studies have confirmed that the loss of reelin correlates with aberrant migration (Haas et al., 2002; Heinrich et al., 2006; Gong et al.,

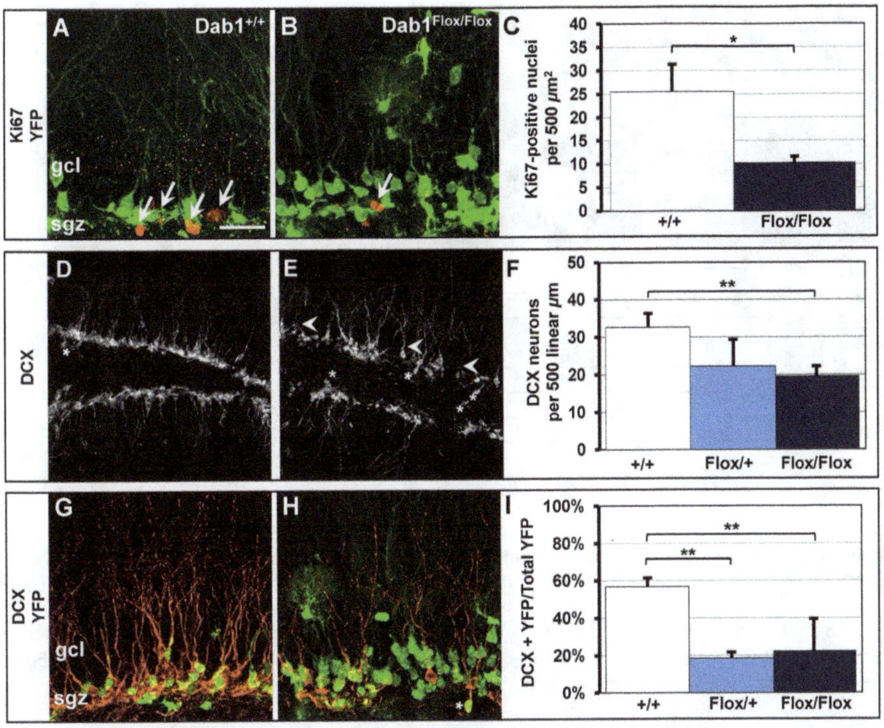

FIGURE 5 | Cell proliferation and DCX-positive immature neurons are reduced in Dab1-deficient mice. (A) Ki67-labeled nuclei are distributed throughout the SGZ of Dab1$^{+/+}$ mice treated with TMX and are often seen in clusters (white arrows). **(B)** In contrast, sparsely distributed Ki67-labeled nuclei (white arrow) are observed in Dab1$^{Flox/Flox}$ mice treated with TMX. **(C)** There are significantly fewer Ki67-labeled nuclei in Dab1$^{Flox/Flox}$ mice treated with TMX compared to controls treated with TMX. **(D)** DCX-expressing immature neurons are distributed throughout the SGZ and inner GCL of WT mice. Most have distinct apical dendrites (white arrowheads) and very few are found in the hilus (asterisk). **(E)** In contrast, we observe a sparse distribution of DCX-positive immature neurons in Dab1-deificient mice. Immature neurons exhibit fewer, atrophic, apical dendrites (white arrowheads) and several are located ectopically (asterisks). **(F)** There are significantly fewer DCX-expressing immature neurons throughout the SGZ and GCL of Dab1$^{Flox/Flox}$ mice treated with TMX compared to controls, but not Dab1$^{Flox/+}$ mice, treated with TMX. **(G)** DCX/YFP co-expressing immature neurons are distributed throughout the SGZ and inner third of the granule cell layer. **(H)** Despite the appearance of more YFP labeling, fewer YFP+ cells co-localized with DCX throughout the SGZ, and some appeared ectopic (asterisks). **(I)** Significantly fewer DCX/YFP double-labeled cells appeared in Dab1$^{Flox/+}$ and Dab1$^{Flox/Flox}$ mice compared to controls. Scale bar (in **A**) = 20 μm for **(A,B,G,H)** and 100 μm for **(D,E)**.

2007; Haas and Frotscher, 2010), but our study is unique in several ways. In contrast to the overt developmental phenotype of the *reeler* mutant mouse, conditional deletion of Dab1 from postnatal nestin-expressing NSCs allows us to explore whether the aberrant development of neonatal- and adult-born neurons disrupt an already established circuit. Secondly, our approach evaluates the contribution of displaced neonatal- or adult-born DGCs to a potential seizure phenotype, separate from the ectopic dispersion of mature DGCs in the DG (Heinrich et al., 2006). Another striking observation is the large percentage of ectopic Prox1+/YFP- DGCs, presumably those expressing normal levels of Dab1. Based upon this finding, we postulate that although the loss of Dab1 in the progeny of NSCs may contribute to a migration deficit, the majority of HEGCs migrate into the hilus due to a non-cell autonomous effect of postnatal Dab1 deletion.

A prevailing hypothesis is that HEGCs contribute to the development of spontaneous seizures and epilepsy (Scharfman and Pierce, 2012), but our observation that mice with ectopically located granule cells are largely seizure-free suggests that there are unaccounted for factors that promote seizure development. Our findings are similar to the study by Koyama et al. (2012) where they demonstrated that generating aberrantly located neurons without inducing seizures was not sufficient to produce rats with epilepsy. Deletion of the pro-apoptotic gene *BAX* generates mice with HEGCs, and though the mice are deficient in a pattern separation task, they also remain seizure-free (Myers et al., 2013). These observations, along with the current study, challenge the hypothesis that HEGCs are sufficient for driving spontaneous seizures.

This does not eliminate the possibility that HEGCs can act as "hub" cells within a seizure network (Morgan and Soltesz, 2008; Cameron et al., 2011). There is clear electrophysiological evidence that they are hyperexcitable and make aberrant connections (Scharfman et al., 2000; Zhan and Nadler, 2009; Althaus et al., 2015). There is also strong correlative evidence between the presence of HEGCs and seizure severity (McCloskey et al., 2006; Hester and Danzer, 2013). It is possible that our deletion is not sufficient enough to generate enough aberrantly placed GCs. In support of this idea, the mouse with the highest recombination efficiency and that also had the greatest density of HEGCs did not show abnormalities on video/EEG monitoring. However, this mouse did exhibit the shortest latency to SE. We

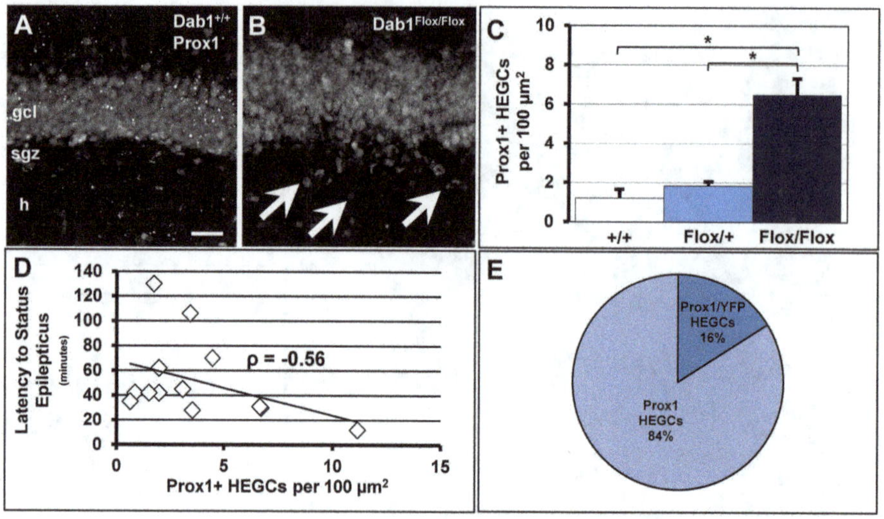

FIGURE 6 | Conditional deletion of Dab1 results in non-cell autonomous ectopic migration of Prox1+ granule cells that inversely correlates with latency to SE. (A) The GCL of Dab1$^{+/+}$ mice given TMX is compact with very few Prox1+ cells found outside the SGZ or GCL. **(B)** The overall structure of the GCL is disrupted in TMX-treated Dab1$^{Flox/Flox}$ mice, with many Prox1+ HEGCs evident (arrowheads). **(C)** The density of HEGCs in Dab1$^{Flox/Flox}$ mice was significantly greater compared to controls and Dab1$^{Flox/+}$ mice after TMX treatment. $^{*}p < 0.05$. **(D)** The density of Prox1 + HEGCs inversely correlated with latency to SE. **(E)** The majority of Prox1 + HEGCs were negative for YFP, supporting a non-cell autonomous effect of the loss of reelin signaling. Scale bar = 50 μm in **(A,B)**.

also considered the possibility that we did not allow enough time for the aberrant neurons to integrate. We addressed this by extending the period after TMX to 4 months, but these mice were also seizure-free. Though we cannot definitively exclude the possibility that there are subcortical seizures with a limited focal onset, HEGCs are not sufficient to cause epilepsy with clinical manifestations via cortical EEG, including generalized tonic-clonic seizures.

Notably, the study showing spontaneous seizure development after postnatal deletion of PTEN in murine DGCs also demonstrated substantial structural abnormalities in PTEN-deficient HEGCs and those in the GCL. These changes included increased soma size and an excess of dendritic spines, features that are likely important for the development of spontaneous seizures (Pun et al., 2012). We did not observe such structural abnormalities after postnatal Dab1 deletion. In summary, our findings suggest that HEGCs produce network instability, but additional aberrant structural or functional features are necessary to cause epilepsy.

CA1 Pyramidal Cell Layer Disruption in Dab1 Hypomorphs does not Contribute to Hyperexcitability in the Hippocampus

Mice expressing floxed *dab1* alleles, whether they are treated with vehicle or TMX, have been shown to express less protein during early postnatal development than the wild-type, and this hypomorphic effect causes abnormalities in the cerebellum and CA1, but not the dentate gyrus (Herrick and Cooper, 2002; Matsuki et al., 2008; Pramatarova et al., 2008). More recently, this structural phenotype was implicated in causing deficits in maternal behavior and spatial learning (Teixeira et al., 2014). Other genetic models that exhibit a similar heterotopia of CA1 exhibit deficits in long-term potentiation (Petrone et al., 2003). Occasionally, a bilayered CA1 pyramidal cell layer is even present in human mTLE hippocampal specimens (Sloviter et al., 2004). All of these observations are consistent with a role of this morphological abnormality in mTLE or its associated comorbidities. We noted that the CA1 phenotype was particularly severe in our Dab1$^{Flox/Flox}$ mice (**Figures 4A–C**), raising concerns that the ectopic CA1 may contribute to overall hyperexcitability. The strongest evidence to the contrary is the fact that Dab1$^{Flox/Flox}$ mice that exhibit a severe CA1 dispersion in the absence of TMX have a seizure latency which is significantly longer compared to Dab1$^{Flox/Flox}$ mice treated with TMX. This is particularly remarkable considering the dendritic disorganization found among the ectopically located CA1 pyramidal neurons (**Figures 4D–F**).

Recent work examining the onset of spontaneous seizure in the pilocarpine model of mTLE in the rat indicates that the firing rate of CA1 increases preictally and may indicate a focal ictal onset zone (Fujita et al., 2014). Despite the dramatic dispersion of CA1, the lack of hyperexcitability leads us to conclude that aberrant migration of CA1 pyramidal cells is not sufficient to drive spontaneous seizures. This further supports the role of the DG in seizure susceptibility and underscores the implications for aberrantly integrated adult-born neurons (Krook-Magnuson et al., 2015).

Reelin Signaling Modulates Adult Neurogenesis

Previous reports have demonstrated a role for reelin signaling in regulating embryonic (Won et al., 2006; Lakoma et al., 2011) and postnatal neurogenesis (Pujadas et al., 2010). We observed a significant decrease in DCX-expressing immature neurons in the adult DG of Dab1-deficient mice, which is novel in this context because the deletion of Dab1 targets NSCs that primarily contribute to ongoing adult neurogenesis. Interestingly, we found no difference in the number of NeuN+/YFP+ cells (data not shown), suggesting that Dab1-deficient NSCs differentiate into neurons at the same rate or higher than intact NSCs. One possible interpretation of these findings is that the percentage of neurons surviving after differentiation increases to compensate for the overall decrease in levels of cell proliferation (Tanapat et al., 2001). Another explanation, not necessary mutually exclusive, is that deletion of Dab1 causes newly-generated neurons to mature faster, resulting in a greater proportion of NeuN+/YFP+ neurons. Prolonged seizures have been shown to have this effect in a mouse model of mTLE (Overstreet-Wadiche et al., 2006), and together with our findings these data further implicate a role for the loss of reelin in structural DG abnormalities associated with mTLE. Future work should be directed at determining how Dab1 deletion influences the survival of newly generated neurons.

Recent work suggests that mice with reduced adult neurogenesis (by x-irradiation or pharmacogenetic deletion) exhibit a potentiated response to chemoconvulsants (Iyengar et al., 2015). Moreover, the pharmacogenetic suppression of adult neurogenesis leads to a potentially compensatory plasticity within the DG involving disinhibition of pre-existing DGCs (Singer et al., 2011). These observations are consistent with our findings that Dab1-deficent mice have dramatically fewer immature neurons and a reduced latency to pilocarpine-induced SE. Our results therefore highlight the importance of adult neurogenesis in maintaining network stability and suggest that this circuit is a potential target for anti-epileptogenic interventions.

AUTHOR CONTRIBUTIONS

MK and JP all contributed to the design and interpretation of the results. MK and QM collected, processed and quantified data included in this manuscript. MK and JP drafted and revised the contents of this manuscript; MK, QM, and JP approved the final version and its conclusions. MK, QM, and JP agreed to be accountable for the contents of this report.

ACKNOWLEDGMENTS

The authors would like thank Corey Powell and the Consulting for Statistics, Computing, and Analytics Research office at the University of Michigan for their assistance. These studies were supported by a NIH Grant to JP (NS058585) and Epilepsy Foundation Postdoctoral Fellowship to MK.

SUPPLEMENTARY MATERIAL

Supplemental Figure 1 | Flowchart of procedures and experimental time points. Animals were treated with TMX, 2 months later they were fitted for EEG and monitored for 10 days. At the end of the recording period, we challenged the seizure sensitivity with pilocarpine. Once in SE, mice were monitored for 90 min, at which time they were euthanized.

REFERENCES

Alcantara, S., Ruiz, M., D'arcangelo, G., Ezan, F., De Lecea, L., Curran, T., et al. (1998). Regional and cellular patterns of reelin mRNA expression in the forebrain of the developing and adult mouse. *J. Neurosci.* 18, 7779–7799.

Althaus, A. L., Sagher, O., Parent, J. M., and Murphy, G. G. (2015). Intrinsic neurophysiological properties of hilar ectopic and normotopic dentate granule cells in human temporal lobe epilepsy and a rat model. *J. Neurophysiol.* 113, 1184–1194. doi: 10.1152/jn.00835.2014

Bae, E. K., Jung, K. H., Chu, K., Lee, S. T., Kim, J. H., Park, K. I., et al. (2010). Neuropathologic and clinical features of human medial temporal lobe epilepsy. *J. Clin. Neurol.* 6, 73–80. doi: 10.3988/jcn.2010.6.2.73

Bender, R. A., Dube, C., and Baram, T. Z. (2004). Febrile seizures and mechanisms of epileptogenesis: insights from an animal model. *Adv. Exp. Med. Biol.* 548, 213–225. doi: 10.1007/978-1-4757-6376-8_15

Bielefeld, P., Van Vliet, E. A., Gorter, J. A., Lucassen, P. J., and Fitzsimons, C. P. (2014). Different subsets of newborn granule cells: a possible role in epileptogenesis? *Eur. J. Neurosci.* 39, 1–11. doi: 10.1111/ejn.12387

Blumcke, I., Kistner, I., Clusmann, H., Schramm, J., Becker, A. J., Elger, C. E., et al. (2009). Towards a clinico-pathological classification of granule cell dispersion in human mesial temporal lobe epilepsies. *Acta Neuropathol.* 117, 535–544. doi: 10.1007/s00401-009-0512-5

Botterill, J. J., Guskjolen, A. J., Marks, W. N., Caruncho, H. J., and Kalynchuk, L. E. (2015). Limbic but not non-limbic kindling impairs conditioned fear and promotes plasticity of NPY and its Y2 receptor. *Brain Struct. Funct.* 220, 3641–3655. doi: 10.1007/s00429-014-0880-z

Bouilleret, V., Ridoux, V., Depaulis, A., Marescaux, C., Nehlig, A., and Le Gal La Salle, G. (1999). Recurrent seizures and hippocampal sclerosis following intrahippocampal kainate injection in adult mice: electroencephalography, histopathology and synaptic reorganization similar to mesial temporal lobe epilepsy. *Neuroscience* 89, 717–729. doi: 10.1016/S0306-4522(98)00401-1

Cameron, M. C., Zhan, R. Z., and Nadler, J. V. (2011). Morphologic integration of hilar ectopic granule cells into dentate gyrus circuitry in the pilocarpine model of temporal lobe epilepsy. *J. Comp. Neurol.* 519, 2175–2192. doi: 10.1002/cne.22623

Cho, K. O., Lybrand, Z. R., Ito, N., Brulet, R., Tafacory, F., Zhang, L., et al. (2015). Aberrant hippocampal neurogenesis contributes to epilepsy and associated cognitive decline. *Nat. Commun.* 6:6606. doi: 10.1038/ncomms7606

Dube, C. M., Mcclelland, S., Choy, M. K., Brewster, A. L., Noam, Y., and Baram, T. Z. (2012). "Fever, febrile seizures and epileptogenesis," in *Jasper's Basic Mechanisms of the Epilepsies, 4th Edn.*, eds. J. L. Noebels, M. Avoli, M. A. Rogawski, R. W. Olsen, and A. V. Delgado-Escueta (Bethesda, MD: National Center for Biotechnology Information).

Farrar, C. E., Huang, C. S., Clarke, S. G., and Houser, C. R. (2005). Increased cell proliferation and granule cell number in the dentate gyrus of protein repair-deficient mice. *J. Comp. Neurol.* 493, 524–537. doi: 10.1002/cne.20780

Freiman, T. M., Eismann-Schweimler, J., and Frotscher, M. (2011). Granule cell dispersion in temporal lobe epilepsy is associated with changes in dendritic orientation and spine distribution. *Exp. Neurol.* 229, 332–338. doi: 10.1016/j.expneurol.2011.02.017

Fujita, S., Toyoda, I., Thamattoor, A. K., and Buckmaster, P. S. (2014). Preictal activity of subicular, CA1, and dentate gyrus principal neurons in the dorsal hippocampus before spontaneous seizures in a rat model of temporal lobe epilepsy. *J. Neurosci.* 34, 16671–16687. doi: 10.1523/JNEUROSCI.0584-14.2014

Gong, C., Wang, T. W., Huang, H. S., and Parent, J. M. (2007). Reelin regulates neuronal progenitor migration in intact and epileptic hippocampus. *J. Neurosci.* 27, 1803–1811. doi: 10.1523/JNEUROSCI.3111-06.2007

Groticke, I., Hoffmann, K., and Loscher, W. (2007). Behavioral alterations in the pilocarpine model of temporal lobe epilepsy in mice. *Exp. Neurol.* 207, 329–349. doi: 10.1016/j.expneurol.2007.06.021

Haas, C. A., Dudeck, O., Kirsch, M., Huszka, C., Kann, G., Pollak, S., et al. (2002). Role for reelin in the development of granule cell dispersion in temporal lobe epilepsy. *J. Neurosci.* 22, 5797–5802.

Haas, C. A., and Frotscher, M. (2010). Reelin deficiency causes granule cell dispersion in epilepsy. *Exp. Brain Res.* 200, 141–149. doi: 10.1007/s00221-009-1948-5

Heinrich, C., Nitta, N., Flubacher, A., Muller, M., Fahrner, A., Kirsch, M., et al. (2006). Reelin deficiency and displacement of mature neurons, but not neurogenesis, underlie the formation of granule cell dispersion in the epileptic hippocampus. *J. Neurosci.* 26, 4701–4713. doi: 10.1523/JNEUROSCI.5516-05.2006

Herrick, T. M., and Cooper, J. A. (2002). A hypomorphic allele of dab1 reveals regional differences in reelin-Dab1 signaling during brain development. *Development* 129, 787–796.

Hester, M. S., and Danzer, S. C. (2013). Accumulation of abnormal adult-generated hippocampal granule cells predicts seizure frequency and severity. *J. Neurosci.* 33, 8926–8936. doi: 10.1523/JNEUROSCI.5161-12.2013

Howell, B. W., Gertler, F. B., and Cooper, J. A. (1997a). Mouse disabled (mDab1): a Src binding protein implicated in neuronal development. *EMBO J.* 16, 121–132. doi: 10.1093/emboj/16.1.121

Howell, B. W., Hawkes, R., Soriano, P., and Cooper, J. A. (1997b). Neuronal position in the developing brain is regulated by mouse disabled-1. *Nature* 389, 733–737. doi: 10.1038/39607

Iyengar, S. S., Lafrancois, J. J., Friedman, D., Drew, L. J., Denny, C. A., Burghardt, N. S., et al. (2015). Suppression of adult neurogenesis increases the acute effects of kainic acid. *Exp. Neurol.* 264, 135–149. doi: 10.1016/j.expneurol.2014.11.009

Jessberger, S., Romer, B., Babu, H., and Kempermann, G. (2005). Seizures induce proliferation and dispersion of doublecortin-positive hippocampal progenitor cells. *Exp. Neurol.* 196, 342–351. doi: 10.1016/j.expneurol.2005.08.010

Jessberger, S., Zhao, C., Toni, N., Clemenson, G. D. Jr., Li, Y., and Gage, F. H. (2007). Seizure-associated, aberrant neurogenesis in adult rats characterized with retrovirus-mediated cell labeling. *J. Neurosci.* 27, 9400–9407. doi: 10.1523/JNEUROSCI.2002-07.2007

Jung, K. H., Chu, K., Lee, S. T., Kim, J., Sinn, D. I., Kim, J. M., et al. (2006). Cyclooxygenase-2 inhibitor, celecoxib, inhibits the altered hippocampal neurogenesis with attenuation of spontaneous recurrent seizures following pilocarpine-induced status epilepticus. *Neurobiol. Dis.* 23, 237–246. doi: 10.1016/j.nbd.2006.02.016

Kehrl, J. M., Sahaya, K., Dalton, H. M., Charbeneau, R. A., Kohut, K. T., Gilbert, K., et al. (2014). Gain-of-function mutation in Gnao1: a murine model of epileptiform encephalopathy (EIEE17)? *Mamm. Genome* 25, 202–210. doi: 10.1007/s00335-014-9509-z

Klein, S., Bankstahl, J. P., Loscher, W., and Bankstahl, M. (2015). Sucrose consumption test reveals pharmacoresistant depression-associated behavior in two mouse models of temporal lobe epilepsy. *Exp. Neurol.* 263, 263–271. doi: 10.1016/j.expneurol.2014.09.004

Kobow, K., Jeske, I., Hildebrandt, M., Hauke, J., Hahnen, E., Buslei, R., et al. (2009). Increased reelin promoter methylation is associated with granule cell dispersion in human temporal lobe epilepsy. *J. Neuropathol. Exp. Neurol.* 68, 356–364. doi: 10.1097/NEN.0b013e31819ba737

Koyama, R., Tao, K., Sasaki, T., Ichikawa, J., Miyamoto, D., Muramatsu, R., et al. (2012). GABAergic excitation after febrile seizures induces ectopic granule cells and adult epilepsy. *Nat. Med.* 18, 1271–1278. doi: 10.1038/nm.2850

Krook-Magnuson, E., Armstrong, C., Bui, A., Lew, S., Oijala, M., and Soltesz, I. (2015). *In vivo* evaluation of the dentate gate theory in epilepsy. *J. Physiol.* 593, 2379–2388. doi: 10.1113/JP270056

Lagace, D. C., Whitman, M. C., Noonan, M. A., Ables, J. L., Decarolis, N. A., Arguello, A. A., et al. (2007). Dynamic contribution of nestin-expressing stem cells to adult neurogenesis. *J. Neurosci.* 27, 12623–12629. doi: 10.1523/JNEUROSCI.3812-07.2007

Lakoma, J., Garcia-Alonso, L., and Luque, J. M. (2011). Reelin sets the pace of neocortical neurogenesiss. *Development* 138, 5223–5234. doi: 10.1242/dev.063776

Lee, C. H., Javed, D., Althaus, A. L., Parent, J. M., and Umemori, H. (2012). Neurogenesis is enhanced and mossy fiber sprouting arises in FGF7-deficient mice during development. *Mol. Cell. Neurosci.* 51, 61–67. doi: 10.1016/j.mcn.2012.07.010

Lee, C. H., and Umemori, H. (2013). Suppression of epileptogenesis-associated changes in response to seizures in FGF22-deficient mice. *Front. Cell. Neurosci.* 7:43. doi: 10.3389/fncel.2013.00043

Lesting, J., Geiger, M., Narayanan, R. T., Pape, H. C., and Seidenbecher, T. (2011). Impaired extinction of fear and maintained amygdala-hippocampal theta synchrony in a mouse model of temporal lobe epilepsy. *Epilepsia* 52, 337–346. doi: 10.1111/j.1528-1167.2010.02758.x

Levin, J. R., Serrano, G., and Dingledine, R. (2012). Reduction in delayed mortality and subtle improvement in retrograde memory performance in pilocarpine-treated mice with conditional neuronal deletion of cyclooxygenase-2 gene. *Epilepsia* 53, 1411–1420. doi: 10.1111/j.1528-1167.2012.03584.x

Lurton, D., El Bahh, B., Sundstrom, L., and Rougier, A. (1998). Granule cell dispersion is correlated with early epileptic events in human temporal lobe epilepsy. *J. Neurol. Sci.* 154, 133–136. doi: 10.1016/S0022-510X(97)00220-7

Matsuki, T., Pramatarova, A., and Howell, B. W. (2008). Reduction of Crk and CrkL expression blocks reelin-induced dendritogenesis. *J. Cell Sci.* 121, 1869–1875. doi: 10.1242/jcs.027334

McCloskey, D. P., Hintz, T. M., Pierce, J. P., and Scharfman, H. E. (2006). Stereological methods reveal the robust size and stability of ectopic hilar granule cells after pilocarpine-induced status epilepticus in the adult rat. *Eur. J. Neurosci.* 24, 2203–2210. doi: 10.1111/j.1460-9568.2006.05101.x

Miltiadous, P., Kouroupi, G., Stamatakis, A., Koutsoudaki, P. N., Matsas, R., and Stylianopoulou, F. (2013). Subventricular zone-derived neural stem cell grafts protect against hippocampal degeneration and restore cognitive function in the mouse following intrahippocampal kainic acid administration. *Stem Cells Transl. Med.* 2, 185–198. doi: 10.5966/sctm.2012-0074

Morgan, R. J., and Soltesz, I. (2008). Nonrandom connectivity of the epileptic dentate gyrus predicts a major role for neuronal hubs in seizures. *Proc. Natl. Acad. Sci. U.S.A.* 105, 6179–6184. doi: 10.1073/pnas.0801372105

Muller, C. J., Groticke, I., Bankstahl, M., and Loscher, W. (2009). Behavioral and cognitive alterations, spontaneous seizures, and neuropathology developing after a pilocarpine-induced status epilepticus in C57BL/6 mice. *Exp. Neurol.* 219, 284–297. doi: 10.1016/j.expneurol.2009.05.035

Murphy, B. L., Hofacer, R. D., Faulkner, C. N., Loepke, A. W., and Danzer, S. C. (2012). Abnormalities of granule cell dendritic structure are a prominent feature of the intrahippocampal kainic acid model of epilepsy despite reduced postinjury neurogenesis. *Epilepsia* 53, 908–921. doi: 10.1111/j.1528-1167.2012.03463.x

Murphy, B. L., Pun, R. Y., Yin, H., Faulkner, C. R., Loepke, A. W., and Danzer, S. C. (2011). Heterogeneous integration of adult-generated granule cells into the epileptic brain. *J. Neurosci.* 31, 105–117. doi: 10.1523/JNEUROSCI.2728-10.2011

Myers, C. E., Bermudez-Hernandez, K., and Scharfman, H. E. (2013). The influence of ectopic migration of granule cells into the hilus on dentate gyrus-CA3 function. *PLoS ONE* 8:e68208. doi: 10.1371/journal.pone.0068208

Nakahira, E., and Yuasa, S. (2005). Neuronal generation, migration, and differentiation in the mouse hippocampal primoridium as revealed by enhanced green fluorescent protein gene transfer by means of in utero electroporation. *J. Comp. Neurol.* 483, 329–340. doi: 10.1002/cne.20441

Olson, E. C., Kim, S., and Walsh, C. A. (2006). Impaired neuronal positioning and dendritogenesis in the neocortex after cell-autonomous Dab1 suppression. *J. Neurosci.* 26, 1767–1775. doi: 10.1523/JNEUROSCI.3000-05.2006

Overstreet-Wadiche, L. S., Bromberg, D. A., Bensen, A. L., and Westbrook, G. L. (2006). Seizures accelerate functional integration of adult-generated granule cells. *J. Neurosci.* 26, 4095–4103. doi: 10.1523/JNEUROSCI.5508-05.2006

Parent, J. M., Elliott, R. C., Pleasure, S. J., Barbaro, N. M., and Lowenstein, D. H. (2006). Aberrant seizure-induced neurogenesis in experimental temporal lobe epilepsy. *Ann. Neurol.* 59, 81–91. doi: 10.1002/ana.20699

Parent, J. M., and Kron, M. M. (2012). "Neurogenesis and Epilepsy," in *Jasper's Basic Mechanisms of the Epilepsies, 4th Edn.*, eds. J. L. Noebels, M. Avoli, M. A. Rogawski, R. W. Olsen, and A. V. Delgado-Escueta (Bethesda, MD: National Center for Biotechnology Information).

Parent, J. M., Yu, T. W., Leibowitz, R. T., Geschwind, D. H., Sloviter, R. S., and Lowenstein, D. H. (1997). Dentate granule cell neurogenesis is increased by seizures and contributes to aberrant network reorganization in the adult rat hippocampus. *J. Neurosci.* 17, 3727–3738.

Pekcec, A., Lupke, M., Baumann, R., Seifert, H., and Potschka, H. (2011). Modulation of neurogenesis by targeted hippocampal irradiation fails to affect kindling progression. *Hippocampus* 21, 866–876. doi: 10.1002/hipo.20802

Pesold, C., Impagnatiello, F., Pisu, M. G., Uzunov, D. P., Costa, E., Guidotti, A., et al. (1998). Reelin is preferentially expressed in neurons synthesizing gamma-aminobutyric acid in cortex and hippocampus of adult rats. *Proc. Natl. Acad. Sci. U.S.A.* 95, 3221–3226. doi: 10.1073/pnas.95.6.3221

Petrone, A., Battaglia, F., Wang, C., Dusa, A., Su, J., Zagzag, D., et al. (2003). Receptor protein tyrosine phosphatase alpha is essential for hippocampal neuronal migration and long-term potentiation. *EMBO J.* 22, 4121–4131. doi: 10.1093/emboj/cdg399

Pramatarova, A., Chen, K., and Howell, B. W. (2008). A genetic interaction between the APP and Dabl genes influences brain development. *Mol. Cell. Neurosci.* 37, 178–186. doi: 10.1016/j.mcn.2007.09.008

Pujadas, L., Gruart, A., Bosch, C., Delgado, L., Teixeira, C. M., Rossi, D., et al. (2010). Reelin regulates postnatal neurogenesis and enhances spine hypertrophy and long-term potentiation. *J. Neurosci.* 30, 4636–4649. doi: 10.1523/JNEUROSCI.5284-09.2010

Pun, R. Y., Rolle, I. J., Lasarge, C. L., Hosford, B. E., Rosen, J. M., Uhl, J. D., et al. (2012). Excessive activation of mTOR in postnatally generated granule cells is sufficient to cause epilepsy. *Neuron* 75, 1022–1034. doi: 10.1016/j.neuron.2012.08.002

Quadrato, G., Elnaggar, M. Y., Duman, C., Sabino, A., Forsberg, K., and Di Giovanni, S. (2014). Modulation of GABAA receptor signaling increases neurogenesis and suppresses anxiety through NFATc4. *J. Neurosci.* 34, 8630–8645. doi: 10.1523/JNEUROSCI.0047-14.2014

Racine, R. J. (1972). Modification of seizure activity by electrical stimulation. II. Motor seizure. *Electroencephalogr. Clin. Neurophysiol.* 32, 281–294. doi: 10.1016/0013-4694(72)90177-0

Raedt, R., Boon, P., Persson, A., Alborn, A. M., Boterberg, T., Van Dycke, A., et al. (2007). Radiation of the rat brain suppresses seizure-induced neurogenesis and transiently enhances excitability during kindling acquisition. *Epilepsia* 48, 1952–1963. doi: 10.1111/j.1528-1167.2007.01146.x

Scharfman, H. E., Goodman, J. H., and Sollas, A. L. (2000). Granule-like neurons at the hilar/CA3 border after status epilepticus and their synchrony with area CA3 pyramidal cells: functional implications of seizure-induced neurogenesis. *J. Neurosci.* 20, 6144–6158.

Scharfman, H. E., and Pierce, J. P. (2012). New insights into the role of hilar ectopic granule cells in the dentate gyrus based on quantitative anatomic analysis and three-dimensional reconstruction. *Epilepsia* 53(Suppl. 1), 109–115. doi: 10.1111/j.1528-1167.2012.03480.x

Shapiro, L. A., Korn, M. J., and Ribak, C. E. (2005). Newly generated dentate granule cells from epileptic rats exhibit elongated hilar basal dendrites that align along GFAP-immunolabeled processes. *Neuroscience* 136, 823–831. doi: 10.1016/j.neuroscience.2005.03.059

Sheldon, M., Rice, D. S., D'arcangelo, G., Yoneshima, H., Nakajima, K., Mikoshiba, K., et al. (1997). Scrambler and yotari disrupt the disabled gene and produce a reeler-like phenotype in mice. *Nature* 389, 730–733. doi: 10.1038/39601

Singer, B. H., Gamelli, A. E., Fuller, C. L., Temme, S. J., Parent, J. M., and Murphy, G. G. (2011). Compensatory network changes in the dentate gyrus restore long-term potentiation following ablation of neurogenesis in young-adult mice. *Proc. Natl. Acad. Sci. U.S.A.* 108, 5437–5442. doi: 10.1073/pnas.1015425108

Singer, B. H., Jutkiewicz, E. M., Fuller, C. L., Lichtenwalner, R. J., Zhang, H., Velander, A. J., et al. (2009). Conditional ablation and recovery of forebrain neurogenesis in the mouse. *J. Comp. Neurol.* 514, 567–582. doi: 10.1002/cne.22052

Sloviter, R. S., Kudrimoti, H. S., Laxer, K. D., Barbaro, N. M., Chan, S., Hirsch, L. J., et al. (2004). "Tectonic" hippocampal malformations in patients with temporal lobe epilepsy. *Epilepsy Res.* 59, 123–153. doi: 10.1016/j.eplepsyres.2004.04.001

Stanfield, B. B., and Cowan, W. M. (1979). The development of the hippocampus and dentate gyrus in normal and reeler mice. *J. Comp. Neurol.* 185, 423–459. doi: 10.1002/cne.901850303

Sugaya, Y., Maru, E., Kudo, K., Shibasaki, T., and Kato, N. (2010). Levetiracetam suppresses development of spontaneous EEG seizures and aberrant neurogenesis following kainate-induced status epilepticus. *Brain Res.* 1352, 187–199. doi: 10.1016/j.brainres.2010.06.061

Sun, M. Y., Yetman, M. J., Lee, T. C., Chen, Y., and Jankowsky, J. L. (2014). Specificity and efficiency of reporter expression in adult neural progenitors vary substantially among nestin-CreER(T2) lines. *J. Comp. Neurol.* 522, 1191–1208. doi: 10.1002/cne.23497

Tanapat, P., Hastings, N. B., Rydel, T. A., Galea, L. A., and Gould, E. (2001). Exposure to fox odor inhibits cell proliferation in the hippocampus of adult rats via an adrenal hormone-dependent mechanism. *J. Comp. Neurol.* 437, 496–504. doi: 10.1002/cne.1297

Teixeira, C. M., Kron, M. M., Masachs, N., Zhang, H., Lagace, D. C., Martinez, A., et al. (2012). Cell-Autonomous Inactivation of the Reelin Pathway Impairs Adult Neurogenesis in the Hippocampus. *J. Neurosci.* 32, 12051–12065. doi: 10.1523/JNEUROSCI.1857-12.2012

Teixeira, C. M., Masachs, N., Muhaisen, A., Bosch, C., Perez-Martinez, J., Howell, B., et al. (2014). Transient downregulation of Dabl protein levels during development leads to behavioral and structural deficits: relevance for psychiatric disorders. *Neuropsychopharmacology* 39, 556–568. doi: 10.1038/npp.2013.226

Wagnon, J. L., Korn, M. J., Parent, R., Tarpey, T. A., Jones, J. M., Hammer, M. F., et al. (2015). Convulsive seizures and SUDEP in a mouse model of SCN8A epileptic encephalopathy. *Hum. Mol. Genet.* 24, 506–515. doi: 10.1093/hmg/ddu470

Won, S. J., Kim, S. H., Xie, L., Wang, Y., Mao, X. O., Jin, K., et al. (2006). Reelin-deficient mice show impaired neurogenesis and increased stroke size. *Exp. Neurol.* 198, 250–259. doi: 10.1016/j.expneurol.2005.12.008

Zambrowicz, B. P., Imamoto, A., Fiering, S., Herzenberg, L. A., Kerr, W. G., and Soriano, P. (1997). Disruption of overlapping transcripts in the ROSA beta geo 26 gene trap strain leads to widespread expression of beta-galactosidase in mouse embryos and hematopoietic cells. *Proc. Natl. Acad. Sci. U.S.A.* 94, 3789–3794. doi: 10.1073/pnas.94.8.3789

Zhan, R. Z., and Nadler, J. V. (2009). Enhanced tonic GABA current in normotopic and hilar ectopic dentate granule cells after pilocarpine-induced status epilepticus. *J. Neurophysiol.* 102, 670–681. doi: 10.1152/jn.00147.2009

Zhang, Y., Cai, G. E., Yang, Q., Lu, Q. C., Li, S. T., and Ju, G. (2010). Time-dependent changes in learning ability and induction of long-term potentiation in the lithium-pilocarpine-induced epileptic mouse model. *Epilepsy Behav.* 17, 448–454. doi: 10.1016/j.yebeh.2010.02.008

22

Adult Olfactory Bulb Interneuron Phenotypes Identified by Targeting Embryonic and Postnatal Neural Progenitors

Maria Figueres-Oñate and Laura López-Mascaraque *

Molecular, Cellular, and Developmental Neurobiology, Instituto Cajal, Consejo Superior de Investigaciones Científicas, Madrid, Spain

Edited by:
Jack M. Parent,
University of Michigan, USA

Reviewed by:
Benedikt Berninger,
University Medical Center of the Johannes Gutenberg University Mainz, Germany
Harold Cremer,
Centre National de la Recherche Scientifique, France

****Correspondence:***
Laura López-Mascaraque
mascaraque@cajal.csic.es

Neurons are generated during embryonic development and in adulthood, although adult neurogenesis is restricted to two main brain regions, the hippocampus and olfactory bulb. The subventricular zone (SVZ) of the lateral ventricles generates neural stem/progenitor cells that continually provide the olfactory bulb (OB) with new granule or periglomerular neurons, cells that arrive from the SVZ via the rostral migratory stream. The continued neurogenesis and the adequate integration of these newly generated interneurons is essential to maintain homeostasis in the olfactory bulb, where the differentiation of these cells into specific neural cell types is strongly influenced by temporal cues. Therefore, identifying the critical features that control the generation of adult OB interneurons at either pre- or post-natal stages is important to understand the dynamic contribution of neural stem cells. Here, we used *in utero* and neonatal SVZ electroporation along with a transposase-mediated stable integration plasmid, in order to track interneurons and glial lineages in the OB. These plasmids are valuable tools to study the development of OB interneurons from embryonic and post-natal SVZ progenitors. Accordingly, we examined the location and identity of the adult progeny of embryonic and post-natally transfected progenitors by examining neurochemical markers in the adult OB. These data reveal the different cell types in the olfactory bulb that are generated in function of age and different electroporation conditions.

Keywords: *in utero* electroporation, postnatal neurogenesis, postnatal electroporation, periglomerular, lineage tracing

INTRODUCTION

In 1962, Joseph Altman revealed that tritiated thymidine could be incorporated into some neurons (based on their appearance under light microscopy) in the rat hippocampus (Altman, 1962; Altman and Das, 1965) and in the olfactory bulb (Altman, 1969). Electron microscopy confirmed the generation of neurons postnatally (Kaplan and Hinds, 1977; Bayer, 1983), a process that involves cell proliferation, neuronal differentiation, and integration into existing neural circuits. Newly generated cells originate in the SVZ of the lateral ventricle, which develops from the residual progenitors of the lateral ganglionic eminence (LGE) at embryonic stages (Bayer et al., 1994; Wichterle et al., 2001; Young et al., 2007). These develop into quite diverse interneurons (Price and Powell, 1970; Pinching and Powell, 1971), characterized morphologically and by their location, firing pattern and immunomarkers. Most of these newly generated interneurons are GABAergic granule cells (GCs: >90%), with a minority differentiating into periglomerular cells (PGCs: Altman, 1969; Luskin, 1993; Lois and Alvarez-Buylla, 1994). To date, PGCs have been characterized either as GABAergic, dopaminergic (Kosaka et al., 1998; Bagley et al., 2007; Batista-Brito et al., 2008), or as a subset of glutamatergic excitatory juxtaglomerular interneurons (Brill et al., 2009; Winpenny et al., 2011). All these PGCs can be incorporated into neural circuits during adulthood, albeit at a lower proportion than granular cells (De Marchis et al., 2007; Whitman and Greer, 2007). The identity of both granule and PGCs is regulated both spatially and temporally (Merkle et al., 2007; Sequerra, 2014; Fuentealba et al., 2015). Moreover, the heterogeneity among newly generated cells is determined in function of their location within the SVZ, defining whether they become granule cells or periglomerular interneurons. Neural progenitor cells (NPCs) in the dorsal adult SVZ give rise to superficial GCs, CR^+ cells, and periglomerular TH^+ cells, whereas the lateral and ventral regions generate mostly deep GCs and periglomerular $Calbindin^+$ cells (for a review, see Fiorelli et al., 2015). In addition, the diversity of olfactory bulb (OB) interneurons is also determined by their temporal origin (De Marchis et al., 2007). TH+ and Calbindin+ (PGCs) production are generated principally during embryogenesis and their production declines postnatally, when $Calretinin^+$ GCs and PGC generation increases (Batista-Brito et al., 2008). Specific subpopulations of adult newborn OB cells have also been characterized based on progenitor domains (Merkle et al., 2007, 2014). Adult born GCs have been classified into five different groups based on their maturational states (Petreanu and Alvarez-Buylla, 2002) and new subtypes are still being described (Merkle et al., 2014).

In order to fully capture the heterogeneity among the OB interneurons generated in the adult, embryonic, or postnatal cells were targeted by electroporation with a ubiquitous transposable vector expressing the enhanced green fluorescent protein (eGFP). Our data reveals this tool to be a powerful means to visualize the specific cell fate of different embryonic and postnatal progenitors in function of their age and on the placement of the electrodes for electroporation. Thus, in this analysis we are able to correlate, lineages, and cell dispersion within the different OB layers as a function of those parameters.

MATERIALS AND METHODS

Animals

Wild type C57BL/6 mice were obtained from the Cajal Institute animal facility, and the day the vaginal plug was detected was considered as the first embryonic day (E0) and day of birth as postnatal day 0 (P0). All procedures were carried out in compliance with the ethical regulations on the use and welfare of experimental animals of the European Union (2010/63/EU) and the Spanish Ministry of Agriculture (RD 1201/2005 and L 32/2007), and the CSIC's bioethical committee approved all the animal protocols. At least $N = 3$ animals were used per experimental condition.

Transposable Vectors

The pPB-UbC-eGFP integrable plasmid containing eGFP under the control of the human ubiquitous Ubiquitin C (UbC) promoter was used here (Yusa et al., 2009; Figueres-Oñate et al., 2015). The genomic integration of this construct was mediated by co-electroporation with a vector containing a hyperactive transposase of the PiggyBac system (hyPBase), kindly provided by Prof. Bradley (Yusa et al., 2011).

In utero Electroporation (IUE)

Briefly, E13 or E15 pregnant mice were anesthetized with 2% isofluorane (Isova vet, Centauro), which was maintained with 1.5% isofluorane/O_2 inhalation, and the mice were placed on a thermal plate at 37°C during the surgery. Before making the peritoneal excision, the mice were administered an antibiotic, enrofloxacin (5 mg/kg: Baytril Bayer), and an anti-inflammatory agent, meloxicam (300 μg/kg: VITA Laboratories). The uterine horns were exposed by midline laparotomy and the embryos maintained humid with physiological saline. Embryos were visualized by trans-illumination and up to 1 μl of the plasmid mixture was injected through a pulled glass capillary into the lateral ventricle of each embryo. The DNA mixture was comprised of the pPB-UbC-eGFP construct and hyPBase in a 3:1 ratio (1–2 μg/ml final concentration), with 0.1% Fast Green (SIGMA). Five consecutive electric square wave pulses (33 or 37 V, 50 ms duration, 950 ms interval) were then applied with 3 mm tweezer-type electrodes (Sonidel). Subsequently, the uterine horns were returned to the abdomen, and the abdominal muscle and skin were sutured. The mice were allowed to recover at 37°C with oxygen administration.

Postnatal Electroporation

Pups (P0/P1) were anesthetized by hypothermia and placed under a cold light to facilitate visualization of the lateral ventricles by trans-illumination. The DNA mixture (see above) was injected into the ventricular cavity and electroconductive LEM Gel (DRV1800, MORETTI S.P.A.) was placed on both electrode paddles to avoid damaging the pups and to achieve successful current flow. Five 100 V electric pulses were applied (50 ms duration, 950 ms intervals), with the positive electrode positioned in the dorso-lateral region to direct the negatively charged DNA to the subventricular zone. After the pulses, the pups were placed on a thermal plate and when they had recovered, they were returned to their mother.

Tissue Processing

Brains were analyzed at adult stages (from P25 onwards). Mice were deeply anesthetized by intraperitoneal injection of sodium pentobarbital (Dolethal, 40–50 mg/kg) and they were transcardially perfused with 4% paraformaldehyde (PFA). The brains were post-fixed in PFA overnight at 4°C and 50 μm thick free-floating coronal or sagittal vibratome sections were obtained.

Immunohistochemistry

To identify the phenotypes of the olfactory bulb cell population, we studied the immunohistochemical labeling of neuronal and glial antibodies. Sections were permeabilized with 0.1% Triton-X in PBS (PBS-T), blocked with 5% normal goat serum (NGS) and then they were incubated with the primary antibodies (see **Table 1**). The following day, the sections were washed and subsequently incubated with the appropriate conjugated secondary antibodies: red fluorophore (1:1000, Alexa Fluor 568 nm, Molecular Probes) or an infrared fluorochrome (1:1000, Alexa Fluor 633 or 647 Molecular Probes).

Imaging Processing

Green fluorescent labeling was examined under an epifluorescence microscope (Nikon, Eclipse E600) with the fluorescein filter cube (450–490 nm, Semrock). Immunohistochemical labeling was observed with the red and far-red filter cubes: rhodamine (569–610 nm) and Cy5 (628–640 nm). The final images were acquired on a Leica TCS-SP5 confocal microscope adjusting the settings so that there was no spectral overlap: eGFP (Ex: 488; Em: 498–550), Alexa 568 (Ex: 561; Em: 575–620), and Alexa 633/647 (Ex: 633; Em: 645–740). Confocal laser lines were used in-between 25 and 40% in all cases.

The maximum projection images were created using the confocal software (LASAF Leica) and other software, such as NIH-ImageJ software. Captured images were processed to adjust the contrast and brightness equally using Adobe Photoshop CS5 software.

Quantitative Analysis

After image acquisition the distribution of the OB cells after either postnatal or *in utero* electroporation was analyzed with ImageJ software. First, images were converted to 8-bits and to facilitate the analyses of both the cell's morphology and layer localization, ICA Lut was applied. Cells were counted using the Cell Counter plug-in analysis tool of the Image J software, analyzing four P25-30 mice animals per group (IUE or postnatal electroporation). Up to 1875 OB cells were counted following postnatal electroporation and 926 cells from the *in utero* electroporated animals. The somata area of DCX positive cells was analyzed with the ImageJ software (60 cells within the granular cell layer and 40 within the subependymal zone). Statistical analyses were performed with SigmaPlot 13 (Systat Software) and the values were represented as the mean ± SEM. *T*-tests were performed to determine the significance between different groups, or with the Mann-Whitney Rank Sum Test when the normality test failed. A confidence interval of 95% ($p < 0.05$) was required to considered values statistically significant.

RESULTS

Histochemical Phenotypes of Neural Olfactory Bulb Cells

To establish the profile of neurochemical markers expressed by OB interneurons, first we performed an immunohistochemical study for a battery of markers (**Table 1** and Supplementary Figures S1, S2). Both neuronal and glial markers were used to determine the heterogeneity of cell phenotypes from the glomerular layer (GL), external plexiform layer (EPL), mitral layer (ML), internal plexiform layer (IPL), granular cell layer (GCL) to the subependymal zone (SEZ; Supplementary

TABLE 1 | Primary antibodies used for the immunohistochemical analysis of newly generated cells in the adult olfactory bulb.

Antibody	Abbreviations	USE	SP.	Source
Adenomatous Polyposis Coli	APC/CC-1	1:200	MS	Calbiochem (OP80)
Calbindin	CB	1:500	Rb	Abcam (Ab11426)
Calretinin	CR	1:500	Rb	Abcam (Ab702)
2′,3′-Cyclic-nucleotide 3′phosphodiesterase	CNPase	1:200	Ms	Covance (SMI-91R)
Doublecortin	DCX	1:500	Rb	Cell signaling (4604)
DOPA decarboxylase	DDC	1:500	Rb	Abcam (Ab3905)
Gamma-Aminobutyric acid	GABA	1:500	Rb	Sigma (A2052)
Glutamate decarboxylase 67	GAD67	1:500	Ms	Millipore (MAB5406)
Glial fibrillary acidic protein	GFAP	1:1000	Ms	Millipore (MAB3402)
Myelin Basic Protein	MBP	1:500	Rat	Serotec (MCA409S)
Neuronal Nuclei	NeuN	1:500	Ms	Millipore (MAB377)
Neuron-glial antigen 2	NG2	1:500	Ms	Millipore (AB5320)
Oligodentrocyte transcription factor 2	Olig2	1:2000	Rb	Millipore (AB9610)
Alpha-type platelet-derived growth factor receptor	PDGFRα	1:300	Rb	Santa Cruz (C-20) (sc-338)
Parvalbumin	PV	1:500	Rb	Swant (PV-25)
Reelin	Reel	1:500	Ms	Millipore (MAB5364)
S100 calcium binding protein beta	S100β	1:300	Ms	Abcam (Ab66028)
Somatostatin	SOM/SST	1:500	Rb	Millipore (AB5494)
T-box, brain, 1	Tbr1	1:500	Rb	Abcam (AB31940)
T-box, brain, 2	Tbr2	1:500	Rb	Abcam (Ab23345)
Tyrosine hydroxylase	TH	1:500	Rb	Millipore (AB152)

Figure S1A). Calbindin (CB, Supplementary Figure S1B) immunoreactive cells appeared predominantly in both the GL and the external plexiform layer (EPL). However, tyrosine hydroxylase (TH) was exclusively expressed by a subset of PGCs (Supplementary Figure S1C). Calretinin (CR, Supplementary Figure S1D) immunolabeling was restricted to periglomerular and granular cells, while Parvalbumin$^+$ cells (PV, Supplementary Figure S1E) were located throughout the EPL and occasionally in the external granular cell layer (eGCL). Few somatostatin (SOM) interneurons were found in the EPL (Supplementary Figure S1F), while dopa decarboxylase (DDC) was expressed by a large number of periglomerular and granular cells (Supplementary Figure S1G). All the interneurons were generally labeled for either GABA (Supplementary Figure S1H) or GAD67 (Supplementary Figure S1I). The microtubule-associated protein doublecortin (DCX), that plays an important role in neuronal migration, labeled neuroblasts within the SEZ and throughout the GCL (Supplementary Figure S1J). The extracellular protein reelin was mainly detected around mitral cells but also, around some tufted and periglomerular cells (Supplementary Figure S1K). Interestingly, the regulatory T-box brain 1 and 2 genes (Tbr1 and Tbr2) were expressed by a few glutamatergic periglomerular OB cells. Indeed, while both were expressed at the same OB location, Tbr2 labeled a few more cells (Supplementary Figure S1L) than Tbr1 (Supplementary Figure S1M) as described previously (Winpenny et al., 2011). To tag all the neurons in the OB we used the marker of neuronal nuclei, NeuN, which was mostly expressed in the GCL and the mitral cell layer in the OB (Supplementary Figure S1N). As a large number of neurons, mostly in the GL, did not express NeuN, we assessed the neurochemical identity of NeuN by double staining with CB (Supplementary Figure S1O) and CR (Supplementary Figure S1P). Although most CB$^+$ cells in the GL did not express NeuN, both antibodies co-stained a population of GL neurons, (arrowheads in Supplementary Figure S1O magnification). Only a few cells were dual stained for CR and NeuN in the GCL (arrowheads in Supplementary Figure S1P magnification). To further address the phenotype of the cells expressing NeuN, dual NeuN, and DCX labeling was assessed, the later an early neural marker (Supplementary Figure S1Q). While most DCX cells concentrated in the SEZ, both markers co-localized in a subset of GCL cells close to the SEZ (arrowheads in Supplementary Figure S1Q magnification), indicating an overlap of those immunomarkers. Finally, to better understand the distribution of the mature interneurons and the neuroblasts migrating along the SVZ-RMS-OB pathway, double immunostaining with CR-DCX was performed. DCX positive cells were confined to the RMS and the SEZ, while CR$^+$ cells were located in the eGCL and GL, regions with weaker DCX labeling (Supplementary Figure S1R).

The distribution of glial cells in the OB was studied with markers for astrocytes (GFAP and S100β proteins), NG2 cells (antibodies against NG2 and PDGFRα), and oligodendrocytes (Olig2, MBP, APC, and CNPase). GFAP-positive cells were located throughout the OB layers except for the EPL, mostly concentrating in the SEZ (Supplementary Figure S2A). NG2 stained cells were homogeneously distributed throughout all the OB layers (Supplementary Figure S2B) and Olig2 immunoreactivity was equally widespread along the SVZ-RMS-OB pathway (Supplementary Figure S2C). Finally, CNPase expression was restricted to myelinating oligodendrocytes (Supplementary Figure S2D). Dual immunofluorescence for Olig2 and APC (Supplementary Figure S2E) indicated that the vast majority of APC$^+$ cells co-expressed Olig2 (arrowheads in Supplementary Figure S2E magnifications), although since Olig2 is a marker for the complete oligodendroglial lineage and APC only labels myelinating oligodendrocytes, not all cells with Olig2 expressed the APC marker (asterisks in Supplementary Figure S2E magnifications). Olig2 and MBP did not co-localize (Supplementary Figure S2F) as their expression in oligodendrocytes differs considerably: Olig2 labels the nucleus while MBP is found in myelin sheaths. Finally, we also analyzed the co-expression of oligodendroglial and astroglial lineages with the combinations of the S100β-Olig2 (Supplementary Figure S2G) and GFAP-PDGFRα (Supplementary Figure S2H) markers. S100β and Olig2 were expressed in different cell populations (asterisks in Supplementary Figure S2G magnifications), although the S100β astrocytic marker co-localized with some Olig2$^+$ oligodendrocytes (arrowheads in Supplementary Figure S2E magnifications). By contrast, the GFAP and PDGFRα immunomarkers (Supplementary Figure S2H) did not co-localize along the SVZ-RMS-OB pathway (Supplementary Figure S2Ha magnification). In fact, GFAP was expressed strongly within the RMS (Supplementary Figure S2Hb magnification) while PDGFRα maintained a uniform cell density through this migratory channel.

Tracking Different Olfactory Bulb Cell Lineages with Different Electroporation Conditions

We followed the cell progeny in the OB by targeting neural progenitors using *in utero* or postnatal electroporation of the following vectors: a plasmid ubiquitously expressing eGFP flanked by two terminal repeat sequences (TRs); the PiggyBac transposase (mPBase). The mPBase transposase integrates the vector including the reporter gene directly into the genome of the transfected cell (**Figure 1A**), allowing the entire progeny of a single cell to be analyzed, regardless of its mitotic activity. To label the different OB populations, IUE was performed (E13–E15) varying electrode positions and with distinct orientations along rostro-caudal axis. Interestingly, neural populations labeled were located at different positions in the OB depending on the embryonic area electroporated. First, IUE was performed at E15 to target progenitors from the dorso-lateral area of the ventricular surface (**Figure 1B**). Analyzing brains 30 days post-electroporation (dpe), labeled cells corresponding to glial and neuronal lineages were located within the dorsal cortex (**Figure 1Ba**). After electroporation on E15, neurons were located within cortical layers II-III, whilst glial cells were widespread throughout cerebral cortex (**Figure 1Ba′**). Moreover, neuronal precursors and labeled oligodendrocytes were located within the corpus callosum, near to the ventricular surface (**Figure 1Ba″**). Furthermore, a large population of labeled neurons was also

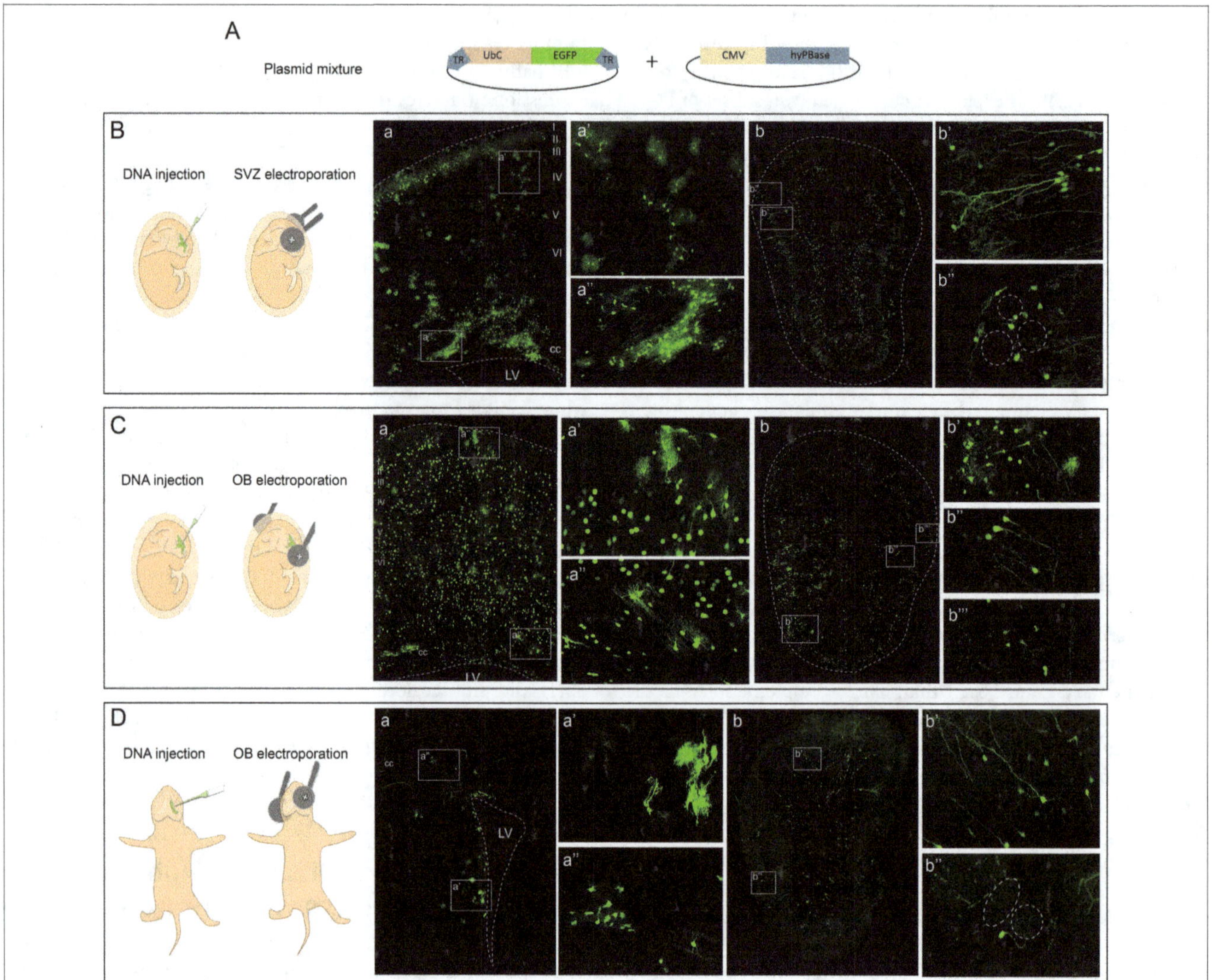

FIGURE 1 | Targeting cells in the olfactory bulb by electroporation. (A) *In vivo* electroporation after ventricular injection of a plasmid mixture containing an integrable vector expressing the eGFP reporter and the transposase of the PiggyBac system. **(B)** Dorso-lateral *in utero* electroporation (IUE) after injection of the plasmid mixture into the lateral ventricles. **(a)** Transfected cells occupying several layers of the cerebral cortex and the corpus callosum (cc) in adult mice. In particular, glial cells with different morphologies are shown, astrocytes in **(a′)** and oligodendrocytes in **(a″)**. After IUE of the subventricular zone (SVZ) OB cells were found in the OB **(b)** corresponding to granular **(b′)** and periglomerular **(b″)** phenotypes. **(C)** Rostral IUE after injection of the plasmid mixture into the lateral ventricles labeled cells in the cerebral cortex **(a)**. Neurons were widespread throughout the cerebral cortex, as were astrocytes **(a′)**. Cells corresponding to oligodendrocytes were positioned in the cc **(a″)**. Cells in the OB **(b)** with a glial **(b′)** and neuronal morphology corresponding to granular **(b″)** and periglomerular cells **(b‴)**. **(D)** Postnatal (P1) electroporation of dorso-lateral SVZ-progenitors. Labeled cells were surrounding the ventricular surface **(a)** with astroglial **(a′)** and oligodendroglial **(a″)** morphologies. In the OB **(b)** cells with a neuronal phenotype were situated in the granular **(b′)** and glomerular **(b″)** layers.

evident in the OB (**Figure 1Bb**). Transfected neurons were widespread along the rostro-caudal and ventro-lateral OB axis at 30 dpe, mostly located within the GCL (**Figure 1Bb′**) and GL (**Figure 1Bb″**). Remarkably, no glial cells were detected in the OB when performing dorso-lateral electroporations.

To assess the potentiality of progenitors at the OB ventricular surface, E13 IUE was performed directing the electrodes to the most rostral part of the LV (**Figure 1C**). At adult stages (30 dpe), labeled cells were distributed within the cerebral cortex of E13 electroporated brains (**Figure 1Ca**), with neurons distributed within layers II-VI of the cerebral cortex and glial cells also occupying several cortical areas (**Figure 1Ca′**). Progenitors remained labeled in the SVZ, as well as recognizable oligodendroglial cells (**Figure 1Ca″**). In contrast to dorso-lateral electroporation, labeled glia, and neurons were evident in the OB (**Figure 1Cb**). Thus, OB glial cells were produced by progenitors from the rostral part of the ventricular surface (**Figure 1Cb′**) but not by dorso-lateral progenitors after *in utero* electroporation (**Figure 1Bb**). The identity of the OB glia was addressed by studying different markers, corroborating the presence of astrocytes through the co-localization of eGFP with GFAP (Supplementary Figure S3A) and S100β (Supplementary

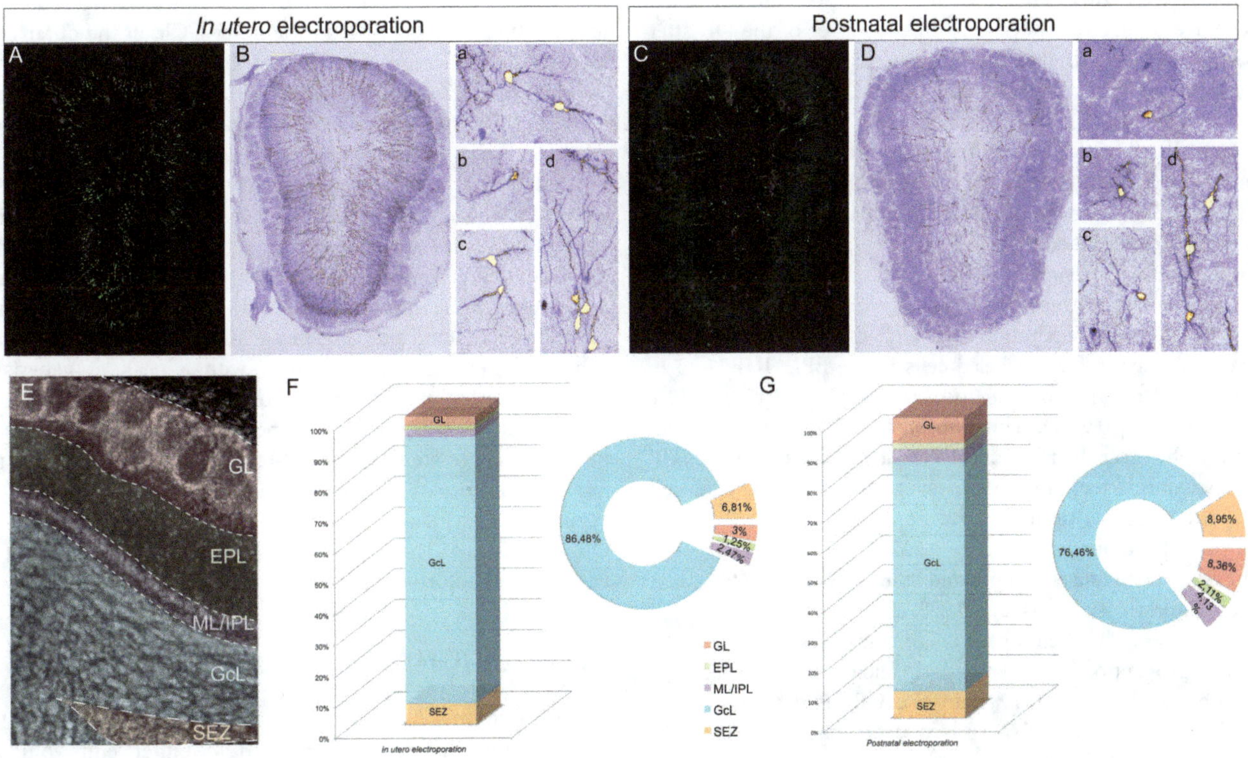

FIGURE 2 | Distribution of electroporated cells within the OB. The percentage of electroporated cells occupying different layers of the OB was studied after electroporation at E15 IUE or P1. **(A)** Representative coronal section of a P30 animal electroporated at E15. **(B)** To quantify the distribution the images were analyzed with ICA Lut (ImageJ software). Representative morphologies of periglomerular **(Ba)** and granular **(Bb–d)** electroporated cells. **(C)** Representative slice of a P30 OB after P1 electroporation. **(D)** Different cell morphologies and dispersion analysis was performed by applying the ICA Lut. Particular morphologies of periglomerular **(Da,b)** and granular **(Db–d)** electroporated cells are showed. **(E)** Different layers of analyzed OB: GL, glomerular layer; EPL, external plexiform layer; ML/IPL, mitral and internal plexiform layer; GCL, granular cell layer; SEZ, subependymal zone. **(F,G)** The percentage of P30 labeled cells after E15 IUE (1875 cells in 4 animals) and P1 electroporation (926 cells in 4 different animals) are shown in **(F,G)**, respectively.

Figure S3B). The oligodendroglial lineage was identified by either Olig2 (Supplementary Figure S3C) or PDGFRα (Supplementary Figure S3D), and electroporated cells that co-expressed both were present in the adult OB after such electroporations. Moreover, granular (**Figure 1Cb″**) and periglomerular cells (**Figure 1Cb‴**) were also labeled in the GCL and GL of the adult OB. Regarding their distribution, it is important to note that glial cells were located only within a lateral region of the OB, while neurons were broadly dispersed across the whole OB. Thus, neurons and glia generated from embryonic progenitors appear to have a different distribution pattern. Labeled SVZ progenitors remained at the adult ventricular surface (**Figure 1Ca″**), suggesting that some interneurons may still originate from these SVZ-transfected progenitors in the adult brain.

Finally, to specifically analyze the postnatal contribution of SVZ progenitors to the OB, we performed postnatal (P1) electroporations positioning the electrodes in the dorso-lateral region (**Figure 1D**). Transfected progenitors were evident in the dorso-lateral area of the ventricular surface of adult brains (30 dpe: **Figure 1Da**). Moreover, glial cells surrounded the electroporated area near the ventricular surface, with astrocytes (**Figure 1Da′**) and oligodendrocytes (**Figure 1Da″**) readily recognized. Targeting postnatal progenitors in the dorso-lateral region labeled interneurons in the OB (**Figure 1Db**). These postnatally labeled interneurons were mostly GCs located in the GCL (**Figure 1Db′**) and PGCs surrounding the glomeruli (**Figure 1Db″**).

Cell Phenotypes after Embryonic and Postnatal Electroporation

To assess the distribution and heterogeneity among the eGFP-transfected cells after *in utero* or postnatal electroporation, the cell dispersion within the OB layers was quantified at P30 (**Figure 2**). To focus exclusively on the extrabulbar origin of OB interneurons, only dorso-lateral electroporations of the SVZ were studied, examining a total of four animals with similar electroporations for both analyses (**Figures 2A,C**). A gross morphological analysis with ICA Lut (ImageJ) distinguished different arbor morphologies (**Figures 2B,D**) mainly associated with the glomerular (**Figures 2Ba,b,2Da,b**) and granule cell (**Figures 2Bc,d,2Dc,d**) layers. Glomerular cells have oval or round-shaped cell bodies, giving rise to a spiny apical dendritic tree that arborizes within the glomerulus (**Figures 2Ba,b,2Da,b**). However, most cells were overwhelmingly restricted to the GCL and they had dendritic arbors with a characteristic GC morphology (**Figures 2Bc,d,2Dc,d**). We also quantified the percentage of electroporated cells in each layer of the OB after *in utero* or neonatal electroporation. Cells were arranged into five groups regarding their position within the GL, EPL, ML/IPL, GCL, or SEZ (**Figure 2E**). In general, eGFP-positive cells were similarly distributed after *in utero* or postnatal electroporation (**Figures 2F,G**). The proportion of the adult labeled cells in the different OB layers was quantified following *in utero* ($n = 4$ animals, 1875 eGFP-adult cells) and P1 ($n = 4$ animals, 926 eGFP-adult cells) electroporation. The vast majority of cells were located within the GCL (IUE 86.48 ± 0.59 and 76.46 ± 3.2% postnatal electroporation), with E15 and P1 electroporated animals displaying fewer labeled cells in the EPL (IUE: 1.25 ± 0.18% and P1: 2.11 ± 0.31%) and ML/IPL (IUE: 2.47 ± 0.32% and P1: 4.13 ± 0.96%). Thus, no significant differences were found in the layer distribution of the labeled cells between IUE and postnatal electroporation. However, the percentage of labeled cells in the GL was significantly different between E15 and P1 electroporated animals (*t*-test, $P = 0.022$), with more labeled cells in the GL of postnatal electroporated animals (8.36 ± 1.65%) than in electroporated embryos (3 ± 0.22%).

To address the heterogeneity of the cells generated by targeted progenitors we analyzed the neurochemical markers expressed by labeled cells within the OB (**Figure 3**). As our specific aim was to analyze interneurons that contribute to the olfactory bulb from an extra bulbar origin throughout life, electroporation was performed to target the dorso-lateral SVZ in either embryos (**Figure 1B**) or postnatal (**Figure 1D**) mice. The eGFP expressing cells analyzed in P30 mice represented a heterogeneous population of interneurons that expressed CR (**Figures 3A,B**), CB (**Figures 3C,D**), TH (**Figures 3E,F**), DDC (**Figures 3G,H**) and DCX (**Figures 3I,J**), yet not reelin (**Figures 4A,B**) or glial markers (**Figures 4C–J**).

According to the literature, the dorso-lateral area targeted is the origin of TH positive PGCs and thus, after electroporation, labeled cells were distributed in the glomerular area of the OB (**Figures 2F,G**). The number of $EGFP^+$ periglomerular cells was significantly higher in postnatal electroporated animals. However, the vast majority of eGFP-labeled cells were located within the GCL and SEZ as electroporation was directed toward the most dorso-lateral ventricular zones. In the OB, the labeled cells corresponded to a highly heterogeneous population, as reflected by the co-expression of the selected neuronal markers (arrowheads in **Figures 2A–H** magnifications), although interestingly in low numbers. The distribution of the labeled cells did not significantly vary after embryonic or postnatal electroporation, excluding PGCs. Regarding to the maturation of targeted cells, eGFP-DCX cells were found within the SEZ layer after either embryonic or postnatal electroporation (**Figures 3I,J** arrowheads). There were significant differences in the soma size of DCX positive cells in the SEZ (white region in Figure S4A) and GCL (pink area in Figure S4A), the former representing significantly smaller cells within the SEZ (mean 23.02 ± 0.89 μm^2, Supplementary Figure S4B) than those in the GCL (mean 51.97 ± 1.12 μm^2, Supplementary Figure S4C: Mann–Whitney test, $P < 0.001$, Supplementary Figure S4D). This suggests some maturation of the SEZ output when it reaches its final destination.

In addition, after E15 IUE eGFP-DCX positive cells at P30 were found either near the SEZ, in the inner GCL, in the outer GCL or in the GL, reflecting the wide distribution of immature cells at the stages analyzed (Supplementary Figures S4E–G).

After IUE and postnatal electroporation transfected cells were rarely located in the EPL (IUE 1.25 ± 0.18 and 2.11 ± 0.31% postnatal electroporation) where PV and SOM are expressed widely. Moreover, the few eGFP-labeled cells in this layer did not express either PV (arrowheads in **Figures 3K,L** magnification) or SOM (arrowheads in **Figures 3M,N** magnification). We also performed reelin immunostaining to verify that no projection neurons were targeted (**Figures 4A,B**). Since mitral cells are generated between E10 and E13, with a peak of genesis at E11 (Blanchart et al., 2006), no eGFP-positive mitral cells were detected when IUE was performed at E15, as shown by reelin expression (**Figures 4A,B**). As expected, eGFP did not co-localize with any of the glial markers analyzed (S100β, **Figures 4C,D**; PDGFRα, **Figures 4E,F**; GFAP, **Figures 4G,H**; Olig2, **Figures 4I,J**) as electroporation did not target progenitors within the olfactory ventricle (**Figure 1C**).

DISCUSSION

This study addressed the distribution and neurochemical identity of adult OB interneurons targeted at either embryonic or postnatal ages with a ubiquitously expressed transposable reporter vector encoding eGFP. Through this approach, a stable tag is introduced into the genome of targeted progenitor cells that is inherited by all their progeny (Figueres-Oñate et al., 2015). Our results showed that the age of the mice and the electrode placement was critical for the targeting of different cell lineages in the OB, particularly for glial lineages and projection neurons. Moreover, the targeted cells represented a heterogeneous population of interneurons, both in animals electroporated as embryos or postnatally. The distribution of the progeny of either embryonic or postnatal dorso-lateral progenitors was similar in all the OB layers, except in the glomerular area where more PGCs were labeled by postnatal electroporation.

A Comparison of Embryonic and Postnatal OB Interneuron Generation

We previously reported that after *in vivo* embryonic electroporation of SVZ progenitors, several labeled OB interneurons undergo rounds of cell divisions before they differentiate (Figueres-Oñate et al., 2015). The progenitors of these interneurons were present in the SVZ at embryonic stages and the embryonic time at which the different OB populations of projection neurons and interneurons are generated has been addressed through *in utero* electroporation (Chen and LoTurco, 2012; Imamura and Greer, 2013, 2014; Siddiqi et al., 2014). OB interneurons originate from E13 progenitors located in the sub-pallium, specifically in the LGE (Wichterle et al., 2001; Kohwi et al., 2007). These LGE progenitors later distribute along the ventricular surface and some of them become adult neural stem cells, this destiny being specified before E15 (Fuentealba

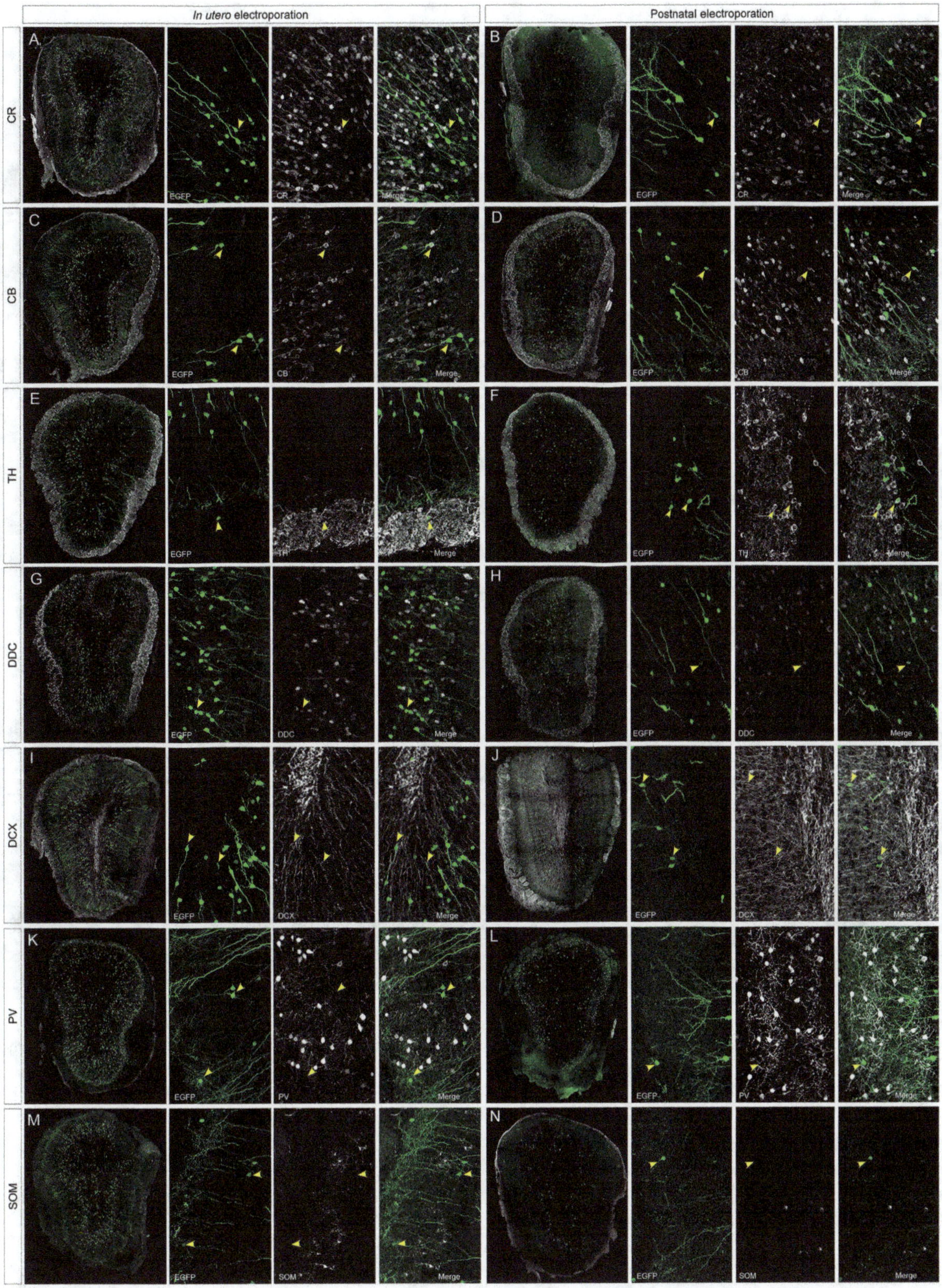

FIGURE 3 | Neuronal immunolabeling after IUE (E15) or postnatal (P1) electroporation. At P30, EGFP labeled cells immunostained for: CR, calretinin **(A,B)**; CB, calbindin **(C,D)**; TH, tyrosine hydroxylase **(E,F)**; DDC, dopa decarboxylase **(G,H)**; DCX, doublecortin **(I,J)**. Arrowheads in magnifications show targeted cells that co-express the respective markers. **(K–N)** After IUE or postnatal electroporation, analyzed cells targeted in the OB (arrowheads in **K,L**) did not contain parvalbumin (PV, arrowheads in **K,L** magnifications) or somatostatin (SOM, arrowheads in **M,N** magnifications).

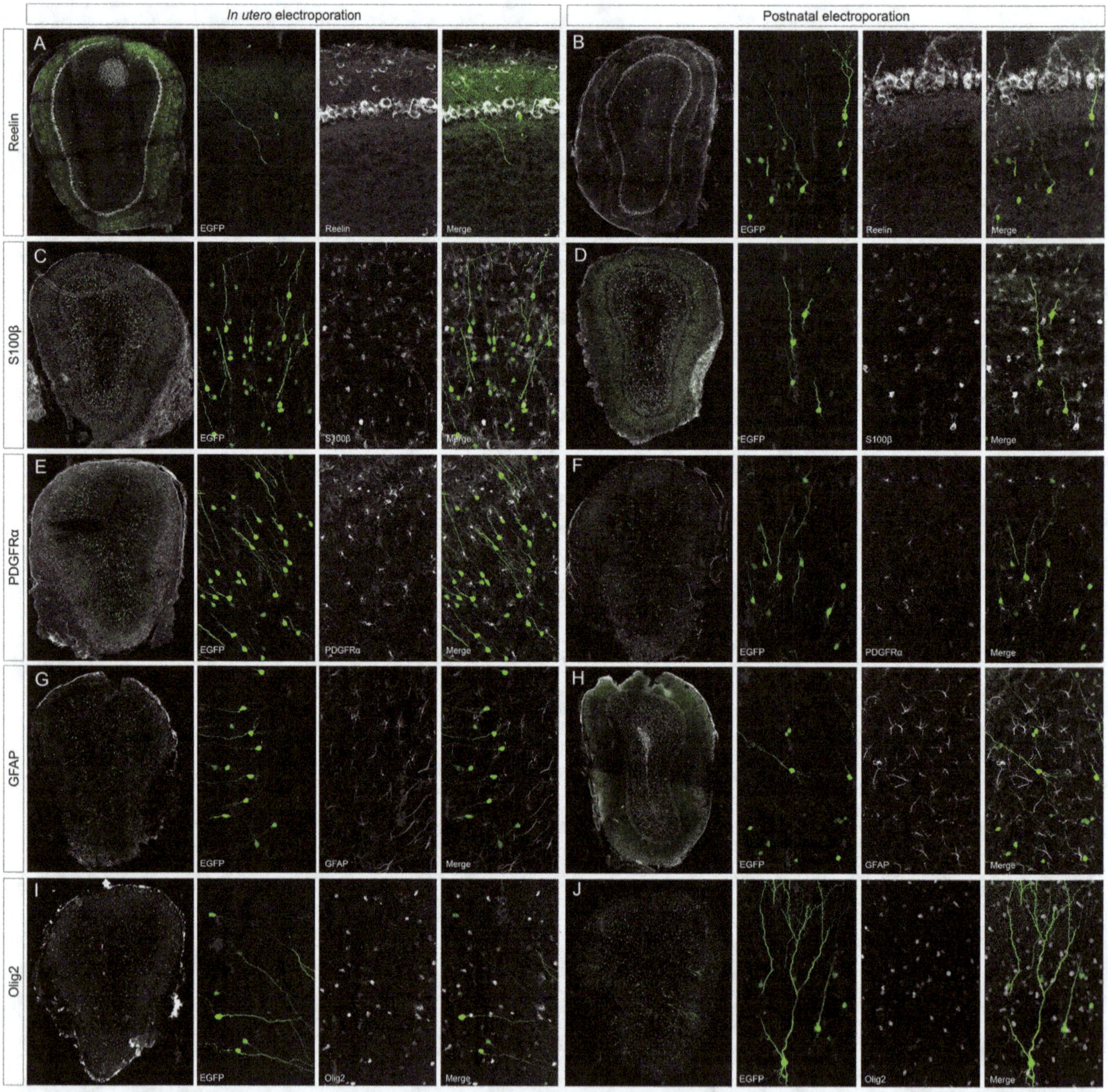

FIGURE 4 | Negative immunomarkers after IUE or postnatal electroporations. (A,B) After E15 or P1 electroporation, adult targeted cells (P30) did not express reelin (reel). **(C–J)** The analyzed glial markers, S100β **(C,D)**, PDGFRα **(E,F)**, GFAP **(G,H)**, or Olig2 **(I,J)**, did not co-localized with P30 $EGFP^+$ cells. Thus, neither projection nor glial cells were targeted after electroporation of the dorso-lateral progenitors from the ventricular zone at embryonic or postnatal stages.

et al., 2015). Accordingly, our dorso-lateral electroporation at E15 labeled SVZ progenitors that were already compromised to establish certain OB interneuron subtypes. The temporal pattern of interneuron generation from embryonic to postnatal stages has been studied by tracing the lineages derived from specific progenitors in transgenic mice (Calzolari et al., 2015). In this way it became clear that different OB interneuron populations are generated from DLX1/2 progenitors at different times (Batista-Brito et al., 2008). Different adult new-born subpopulations are generated at different ages, the most heterogeneous being generated around the time of the animal's birth, when olfactory sensation begins (Brann and Firestein, 2014). For example, CB-positive PGCs are preferentially generated during the early postnatal period, whereas CR and TH neurons are mainly produced later in life (De Marchis et al., 2007). To measure the potential differences between OB interneurons generated at postnatal or embryonic ages, we used *in utero* and postnatal electroporation. However, at P30 there were no significant differences between the populations of transfected cells after dorso-lateral embryonic or postnatal electroporation. The postnatal generation of specific granular or periglomerular interneuron subpopulations that originate from specific Pax6, Tbr2, 5HT3, or Neurog2 progenitors has previously been studied in the OB (Kohwi et al., 2005; Inta et al., 2008; Brill et al., 2009; Winpenny et al., 2011). Two weeks after postnatal electroporation at the ventricular surface, OB cells that were labeled expressed markers of interneurons and they were electrically excitable (Chesler et al., 2008). Moreover, the heterogeneity and specific regionalization of these interneurons in the OB can be addressed changing the orientation of the electrodes (Fernández et al., 2011). Thus, the SVZ represents a heterogeneous pool of neural progenitors at both embryonic or postnatal stages, highlighting that a correlation exists between OB neuron-type and SVZ regionalization (Hack et al., 2005; Merkle et al., 2007).

With regards location, our data showed that there were few transfected cells within the EPL and ML/IPL, the vast majority occupying either the most external or internal part of the granular cell layer. The increase in the proportion of transfected PGCs after postnatal electroporation may be related to the precise location of the SVZ progenitors that differentially contribute to distinct types of periglomerular interneurons (Lledo et al., 2008).

Targeted Cells Do Not Co-Localize with a Large Number of Markers

Our data show that newborn cells represent a heterogeneous population, since the transfected eGFP-cells expressed most of the markers analyzed. Actually, the large variety of markers for newly generated cells contrasts with the lower number of newborn cells expressing each when compared with the total number of eGFP transfected cells. In fact, after virus infection (Merkle et al., 2007), *in utero* electroporation (Fernández et al., 2011), or tamoxifen administration in transgenic mice (Batista-Brito et al., 2008), the percentages of labeled GCs that express immunohistochemical markers is also really low. Those different approaches to label adult newborn cells in the OB established that the percentage of CR and CB expressing neurons in the GCL is no more than 20% (Bagley et al., 2007). However, the percentage of positive CR cells in relation to the total population of cells in the GCL of the adult OB is around 10% (Parrish-Aungst et al., 2007). Therefore, despite the large diversity of markers used there are relatively few newly generated cells with regards the total proportion of those cells types in the OB. In this respect, and due to the lack of markers, new cells occupying the internal part of the granular layer were described by their morphology, layering, and origin (Merkle et al., 2014). This highlights the need for new markers to define these populations of newborn interneurons that are generated in the OB throughout adulthood.

Another possibility is that those cells remained immature at the time of analysis (P30), although newly generated cells display electrical properties 2 weeks after postnatal electroporation (Chesler et al., 2008). Similarly, Tbr1-Tbr2 expression is evident in dopaminergic cells 21 days after labeling (Winpenny et al., 2011). In other studies the immunochemical nature of OB interneurons arising from ventricular-targeted progenitors can be defined 15–30 days post progenitor targeting (Fernández et al., 2011; de Chevigny et al., 2012; Merkle et al., 2014). Otherwise, we found labeled cells that expressed immature markers like DCX at 20 dpe, widely spread across the OB, although there were too few to assume that analyzed cells did not express mature markers because they were undifferentiated. Moreover, our dual immunohistochemistry studies using markers of mature (NeuN, CB, CR) and immature (DCX) cells showed some overlap within these populations, indicating a gradual maturation of these cells.

Ontogeny of Glial Cells in the Olfactory Bulb

We recently analyzed the clonal dispersion and migratory routes of NG2 cells in the OB (García-Marqués et al., 2014) using the StarTrack method (García-Marqués and López-Mascaraque, 2013). We also described the large heterogeneity within the glial lineages in the OB (Figueres-Oñate et al., 2014; García-Marqués and López-Mascaraque, 2016) and cerebral cortex (Bribián et al., 2016). However, the origin of glial cells in the OB is not as well understood as that of neurons. Most studies describe the glial populations in the OB through their morphology (De Castro, 1920; Valverde and Lopez-Mascaraque, 1991) or using immunohistochemical markers (Bailey and Shipley, 1993; Chiu and Greer, 1996; Emsley and MacKlis, 2006), while the origin and heterogeneity this lineage within the OB is still unclear. A general analysis of the GFAP and S100β expression throughout the brain showed a high density of astrocytes in the OB (Emsley and MacKlis, 2006) and thus, considering OB astrocytes in functional studies is important to understand the specific role of glial cells in the SVZ-RMS-OB pathway (García-Marqués et al., 2010). Moreover, our data show that after postnatal or embryonic electroporation of the dorso-lateral part of the lateral ventricles there was no labeled glial cells within the OB. However, we could trace glial lineages in the OB, such as astrocytes, oligodendrocytes, and Ng2 cells after performing electroporations at E13 directed to the most rostral part of the lateral ventricles. Thus, these glial cells would appear to come from progenitors located within the OB. In addition, the distribution of glial cells within the OB in just one lateral region suggests that they may be generated following the radial glial processes, as in the cortex (García-Marqués and López-Mascaraque, 2013).

In summary, a better understanding of the neural cells generated in adulthood and the factors that control their proliferation, migration, and integration into neural circuits is crucial. Moreover, it is also essential to use clonal analysis so that single progenitor cells can be labeled and their progeny tracked in order to match progenitor cells to specific neural populations in the adult OB, including glial lineages.

AUTHOR CONTRIBUTIONS

LM, Conceived and designed the experiments, writing the paper and obtained funding. MF, help in the design of the study, performed the experiments and writing the paper.

ACKNOWLEDGMENTS

This work was supported by research Grant BFU2013-48807-R from the Spanish Ministry of Economy and Competitiveness. We thank Dr. Mark Sefton for helpful editorial assistance.

REFERENCES

Altman, J. (1962). Are new neurons formed in the brains of adult mammals? *Science* 135, 1127–1128. doi: 10.1126/science.135.3509.1127

Altman, J. (1969). Autoradiographic and histological studies of postnatal neurogenesis. IV. Cell proliferation and migration in the anterior forebrain, with special reference to persisting neurogenesis in the olfactory bulb. *J. Comp. Neurol.* 137, 433–457. doi: 10.1002/cne.901370404

Altman, J., and Das, G. D. (1965). Post-natal origin of microneurones in the rat brain. *Nature* 207, 953–956. doi: 10.1038/207953a0

Bagley, J., LaRocca, G., Jimenez, D. A., and Urban, N. N. (2007). Adult neurogenesis and specific replacement of interneuron subtypes in the mouse main olfactory bulb. *BMC Neurosci.* 8:92. doi: 10.1186/1471-2202-8-92

Bailey, M. S., and Shipley, M. T. (1993). Astrocyte subtypes in the rat olfactory bulb: morphological heterogeneity and differential laminar distribution. *J. Comp. Neurol.* 328, 501–526. doi: 10.1002/cne.903280405

Batista-Brito, R., Close, J., Machold, R., and Fishell, G. (2008). The distinct temporal origins of olfactory bulb interneuron subtypes. *J. Neurosci.* 28, 3966–3975. doi: 10.1523/JNEUROSCI.5625-07.2008

Bayer, S. (1983). 3H-thymidine-radiographic studies of neurogenesis in the rat olfactory bulb. *Exp. Brain Res.* 50, 329–340. doi: 10.1007/bf00239197

Bayer, S. A., Zhang, X., Russo, R. J., and Altman, J. (1994). Three-dimensional reconstructions of the developing forebrain in rat embryos. *Neuroimage* 1, 296–307. doi: 10.1006/nimg.1994.1014

Blanchart, A., De Carlos, J. A., and López-Mascaraque, L. (2006). Time frame of mitral cell development. *J. Comp. Neurol.* 543, 529–543. doi: 10.1002/cne.20941

Brann, J. H., and Firestein, S. J. (2014). A lifetime of neurogenesis in the olfactory system. *Front. Neurosci.* 8:182. doi: 10.3389/fnins.2014.00182

Bribián, A., Figueres-Oñate, M., Martín-López, E., and López-Mascaraque, L. (2016). Decoding astrocyte heterogeneity: new tools for clonal analysis. *Neuroscience* 323, 10–19. doi: 10.1016/j.neuroscience.2015.04.036

Brill, M. S., Ninkovic, J., Winpenny, E., Hodge, R. D., Ozen, I., Yang, R., et al. (2009). Adult generation of glutamatergic olfactory bulb interneurons. *Nat. Neurosci.* 12, 1524–1533. doi: 10.1038/nn.2416

Calzolari, F., Michel, J., Baumgart, E. V., Theis, F., Götz, M., and Ninkovic, J. (2015). Fast clonal expansion and limited neural stem cell self-renewal in the adult subependymal zone. *Nat. Neurosci.* 18, 490–492. doi: 10.1038/nn.3963

Chen, F., and LoTurco, J. (2012). A method for stable transgenesis of radial glia lineage in rat neocortex by piggyBac mediated transposition. *J. Neurosci. Methods* 207, 172–180. doi: 10.1016/j.jneumeth.2012.03.016

Chesler, A. T., Le Pichon, C. E., Brann, J. H., Araneda, R. C., Zou, D.-J., and Firestein, S. (2008). Selective gene expression by postnatal electroporation during olfactory interneuron neurogenesis. *PLoS ONE* 3:e1517. doi: 10.1371/journal.pone.0001517

Chiu, K., and Greer, C. A. (1996). Immunocytochemical analyses of astrocyte development in the olfactory bulb. *Dev. Brain Res.* 95, 28–37. doi: 10.1016/0165-3806(96)00055-7

De Castro, F. (1920). Estudios sobre la neuroglia de la corteza cerebral del hombre y de los animales. *Trab. Lab. Invest. Biol.* 18, 1–35.

de Chevigny, A., Core, N., Follert, P., Wild, S., Bosio, A., Yoshikawa, K., et al. (2012). Dynamic expression of the pro-dopaminergic transcription factors Pax6 and Dlx2 during postnatal olfactory bulb neurogenesis. *Front. Cell Neurosci.* 6:6. doi: 10.3389/fncel.2012.00006

De Marchis, S., Bovetti, S., Carletti, B., Hsieh, Y. C., Garzotto, D., Peretto, P., et al. (2007). Generation of distinct types of periglomerular olfactory bulb interneurons during development and in adult mice: implication for intrinsic properties of the subventricular zone progenitor population. *J. Neurosci.* 27, 657–664. doi: 10.1523/JNEUROSCI.2870-06.2007

Emsley, J. G., and MacKlis, J. D. (2006). Astroglial heterogeneity closely reflects the neuronal-defined anatomy of the adult murine CNS. *Neuron Glia Biol.* 2, 175–186. doi: 10.1017/S1740925X06000202

Fernández, M. E., Croce, S., Boutin, C., Cremer, H., and Raineteau, O. (2011). Targeted electroporation of defined lateral ventricular walls: a novel and rapid method to study fate specification during postnatal forebrain neurogenesis. *Neural Dev.* 6:13. doi: 10.1186/1749-8104-6-13

Figueres-Oñate, M., García-Marqués, J., Pedraza, M., De Carlos, J. A., and López-Mascaraque, L. (2015). Spatiotemporal analyses of neural lineages after embryonic and postnatal progenitor targeting combining different reporters. *Front. Neurosci.* 9:87. doi: 10.3389/fnins.2015.00087

Figueres-Oñate, M., Gutiérrez, Y., and López-Mascaraque, L. (2014). Unraveling Cajal's view of the olfactory system. *Front. Neuroanat.* 8:55. doi: 10.3389/fnana.2014.00055

Fiorelli, R., Azim, K., Fischer, B., and Raineteau, O. (2015). Adding a spatial dimension to postnatal ventricular-subventricular zone neurogenesis. *Development* 142, 2109–2120. doi: 10.1242/dev.119966

Fuentealba, L. C., Rompani, S. B., Parraguez, J. I., Obernier, K., Romero, R., Cepko, C. L., et al. (2015). Embryonic origin of postnatal neural stem cells. *Cell* 161, 1644–1655. doi: 10.1016/j.cell.2015.05.041

García-Marqués, J., De Carlos, J. A., Greer, C. A, and López-Mascaraque, L. (2010). Different astroglia permissivity controls the migration of olfactory bulb interneuron precursors. *Glia* 58, 218–230. doi: 10.1002/glia.20918

García-Marqués, J., and López-Mascaraque, L. (2013). Clonal identity determines astrocyte cortical heterogeneity. *Cereb. Cortex* 23, 1463–1472. doi: 10.1093/cercor/bhs134

García-Marqués, J., and López-Mascaraque, L. (2016). Clonal mapping of astrocytes in the olfactory bulb and rostral migratory stream. *Cereb. Cortex.* [Epub ahead of print].

García-Marqués, J., Núñez-Llaves, R., and López-Mascaraque, L. (2014). NG2-glia from pallial progenitors produce the largest clonal clusters of the brain: time frame of clonal generation in cortex and olfactory bulb. *J. Neurosci.* 34, 2305–2313. doi: 10.1523/JNEUROSCI.3060-13.2014

Hack, M. A., Saghatelyan, A., de Chevigny, A., Pfeifer, A., Ashery-Padan, R., Lledo, P.-M., et al. (2005). Neuronal fate determinants of adult olfactory bulb neurogenesis. *Nat. Neurosci.* 8, 865–872. doi: 10.1038/nn1479

Imamura, F., and Greer, C. A. (2013). Pax6 regulates Tbr1 and Tbr2 expressions in olfactory bulb mitral cells. *Mol. Cell. Neurosci.* 54, 58–70. doi: 10.1016/j.mcn.2013.01.002

Imamura, F., and Greer, C. A. (2014). Segregated labeling of olfactory bulb projection neurons based on their birthdates. *Eur. J. Neurosci.* 41, 1–10. doi: 10.1111/ejn.12784

Inta, D., Alfonso, J., von Engelhardt, J., Kreuzberg, M. M., Meyer, A. H., van Hooft, J., et al. (2008). Neurogenesis and widespread forebrain migration of distinct GABAergic neurons from the postnatal subventricular zone. *Proc. Natl. Acad. Sci. U.S.A.* 105, 20994–20999. doi: 10.1073/pnas.0807059105

Kaplan, M. S., and Hinds, J. W. (1977). Neurogenesis in the adult rat: electron microscopic analysis of light radioautographs. *Science* 197, 1092–1094 doi: 10.1126/science.887941

Kohwi, M., Osumi, N., Rubenstein, J. L. R., and Alvarez-Buylla, A. (2005). Pax6 is required for making specific subpopulations of granule and periglomerular neurons in the olfactory bulb. *J. Neurosci.* 25, 6997–7003. doi: 10.1523/JNEUROSCI.1435-05.2005

Kohwi, M., Petryniak, M. A., Long, J. E., Ekker, M., Obata, K., Yanagawa, Y., et al. (2007). A subpopulation of olfactory bulb GABAergic interneurons is derived from Emx1- and Dlx5/6-expressing progenitors. *J. Neurosci.* 27, 6878–6891. doi: 10.1523/JNEUROSCI.0254-07.2007

Kosaka, K., Toida, K., Aika, Y., and Kosaka, T. (1998). How simple is the organization of the olfactory glomerulus?: the heterogeneity of so-called periglomerular cells. *Neurosci. Res.* 30, 101–110. doi: 10.1016/S0168-0102(98)00002-9

Lledo, P.-M., Merkle, F. T., and Alvarez-Buylla, A. (2008). Origin and function of olfactory bulb interneuron diversity. *Trends Neurosci.* 31, 392–400. doi: 10.1016/j.tins.2008.05.006

Lois, C., and Alvarez-Buylla, A. (1994). Long-distance neuronal migration in the adult mammalian brain. *Science* 264, 1145–1148. doi: 10.1126/science.8178174

Luskin, M. B. (1993). Restricted proliferation and migration of postnatally generated neurons derived from the forebrain subventricular zone. *Neuron* 11, 173–189. doi: 10.1016/0896-6273(93)90281-U

Merkle, F. T., Fuentealba, L. C., Sanders, T. A., Magno, L., Kessaris, N., and Alvarez-Buylla, A. (2014). Adult neural stem cells in distinct microdomains generate previously unknown interneuron types. *Nat. Neurosci.* 17, 207–214. doi: 10.1038/nn.3610

Merkle, F. T., Mirzadeh, Z., and Alvarez-Buylla, A. (2007). Mosaic organization of neural stem cells in the adult brain. *Science* 317, 381–384. doi: 10.1126/science.1144914

Parrish-Aungst, S., Shipley, M. T., Erdelyi, F., Szabo, G., and Puche, A. C. (2007). Quantitative analysis of neuronal diversity in the mouse olfactory bulb. *J. Comp. Neurol.* 501, 825–836. doi: 10.1002/cne.21205

Petreanu, L., and Alvarez-Buylla, A. (2002). Maturation and death of adult-born olfactory bulb granule neurons: role of olfaction. *J. Neurosci.* 22, 6106–6113.

Pinching, A. J., and Powell, T. P. S. (1971). The neuropil of the glomeruli of the olfactory bulb. *J. Cell Sci.* 9, 347–377.

Price, J. L., and Powell, T. P. (1970). The synaptology of the granule cells of the olfactory bulb. *J. Cell Sci.* 7, 125–155.

Sequerra, E. B. (2014). Subventricular zone progenitors in time and space: generating neuronal diversity. *Front. Cell. Neurosci.* 8:434. doi: 10.3389/fncel.2014.00434

Siddiqi, F., Chen, F., Aron, A. W., Fiondella, C. G., Patel, K., and LoTurco, J. (2014). Fate mapping by piggybac transposase reveals that neocortical GLAST+ progenitors generate more astrocytes than Nestin+ progenitors in rat neocortex. *Cereb. Cortex* 24, 508–520. doi: 10.1093/cercor/bhs332

Valverde, F., and Lopez-Mascaraque, L. (1991). Neuroglial arrangements in the olfactory glomeruli of the hedgehog. *J. Comp. Neurol.* 307, 658–674.

Whitman, M. C., and Greer, C. A. (2007). Adult-generated neurons exhibit diverse developmental fates. *Dev. Neurobiol.* 67, 1079–1093. doi: 10.1002/dneu.20389

Wichterle, H., Turnbull, D. H., Nery, S., Fishell, G., and Alvarez-Buylla, A. (2001). *In utero* fate mapping reveals distinct migratory pathways and fates of neurons born in the mammalian basal forebrain. *Development* 128, 3759–3771.

Winpenny, E., Lebel-Potter, M., Fernandez, M. E., Brill, M. S., Götz, M., Guillemot, F., et al. (2011). Sequential generation of olfactory bulb glutamatergic neurons by Neurog2-expressing precursor cells. *Neural Dev.* 6:12. doi: 10.1186/1749-8104-6-12

Young, K. M., Fogarty, M., Kessaris, N., and Richardson, W. D. (2007). Subventricular zone stem cells are heterogeneous with respect to their embryonic origins and neurogenic fates in the adult olfactory bulb. *J. Neurosci.* 27, 8286–8296. doi: 10.1523/JNEUROSCI.0476-07.2007

Yusa, K., Rad, R., Takeda, J., and Bradley, A. (2009). Generation of transgene-free induced pluripotent mouse stem cells by the piggyBac transposon. *Nat. Methods* 6, 363–369. doi: 10.1038/nmeth.1323

Yusa, K., Zhou, L., Li, M. A., Bradley, A., and Craig, N. L. (2011). A hyperactive piggyBac transposase for mammalian applications. *Proc. Natl. Acad. Sci. U.S.A.* 108, 1531–1536. doi: 10.1073/pnas.1008322108

Permissions

All chapters in this book were first published in 50AANOHB, by Frontiers; hereby published with permission under the Creative Commons Attribution License or equivalent. Every chapter published in this book has been scrutinized by our experts. Their significance has been extensively debated. The topics covered herein carry significant findings which will fuel the growth of the discipline. They may even be implemented as practical applications or may be referred to as a beginning point for another development.

The contributors of this book come from diverse backgrounds, making this book a truly international effort. This book will bring forth new frontiers with its revolutionizing research information and detailed analysis of the nascent developments around the world.

We would like to thank all the contributing authors for lending their expertise to make the book truly unique. They have played a crucial role in the development of this book. Without their invaluable contributions this book wouldn't have been possible. They have made vital efforts to compile up to date information on the varied aspects of this subject to make this book a valuable addition to the collection of many professionals and students.

This book was conceptualized with the vision of imparting up-to-date information and advanced data in this field. To ensure the same, a matchless editorial board was set up. Every individual on the board went through rigorous rounds of assessment to prove their worth. After which they invested a large part of their time researching and compiling the most relevant data for our readers.

The editorial board has been involved in producing this book since its inception. They have spent rigorous hours researching and exploring the diverse topics which have resulted in the successful publishing of this book. They have passed on their knowledge of decades through this book. To expedite this challenging task, the publisher supported the team at every step. A small team of assistant editors was also appointed to further simplify the editing procedure and attain best results for the readers.

Apart from the editorial board, the designing team has also invested a significant amount of their time in understanding the subject and creating the most relevant covers. They scrutinized every image to scout for the most suitable representation of the subject and create an appropriate cover for the book.

The publishing team has been an ardent support to the editorial, designing and production team. Their endless efforts to recruit the best for this project, has resulted in the accomplishment of this book. They are a veteran in the field of academics and their pool of knowledge is as vast as their experience in printing. Their expertise and guidance has proved useful at every step. Their uncompromising quality standards have made this book an exceptional effort. Their encouragement from time to time has been an inspiration for everyone.

The publisher and the editorial board hope that this book will prove to be a valuable piece of knowledge for researchers, students, practitioners and scholars across the globe.

List of Contributors

José R. Pineda
Laboratory of Neural Stem Cells and Neurogenesis, Achucarro Basque Center for Neuroscience, Zamudio, Spain

Juan M. Encinas
Laboratory of Neural Stem Cells and Neurogenesis, Achucarro Basque Center for Neuroscience, Zamudio, Spain
IKERBASQUE, The Basque Foundation for Science, Bilbao, Spain

Simona Gradari, Anna Pallé, Kerry R. McGreevy, Ángela Fontán-Lozano and José L. Trejo
Laboratory of Adult Neurogenesis, Department of Molecular, Cellular and Developmental Neurobiology, Cajal Institute, Consejo Superior de Investigaciones Científicas, Madrid, Spain

Vanesa Nieto-Estévez, Çağla Defterali and Carlos Vicario-Abejón
Consejo Superior de Investigaciones Científicas (CSIC), Instituto Cajal, Madrid, Spain
Centro de Investigación Biomédica en Red sobre Enfermedades Neurodegenerativas (CIBERNED), Madrid, Spain

Carolyn Hollands, Nancy Bartolotti and Orly Lazarov
Department of Anatomy and Cell Biology, College of Medicine, The University of Illinois at Chicago, Chicago, IL, USA

Felipe Ortega
Biochemistry and Molecular Biology Department, Faculty of Veterinary Medicine, Complutense University, Madrid, Spain

Marcos R. Costa
Brain Institute, Federal University of Rio Grande do Norte, Natal, Brazil

Elena W. Adlaf
Department of Cell Biology, Duke University School of Medicine, Durham, NC, USA

Aaron Mitchell-Dick
Department of Cell Biology, Duke University School of Medicine, Durham, NC, USA
Cellular and Molecular Biology Graduate Training Program, Duke University School of Medicine, Durham, NC, USA

Chay T. Kuo
Department of Cell Biology, Duke University School of Medicine, Durham, NC, USA
Cellular and Molecular Biology Graduate Training Program, Duke University School of Medicine, Durham, NC, USA
Brumley Neonatal Perinatal Research Institute, Duke University School of Medicine, Durham, NC, USA
Department of Neurobiology, Duke University School of Medicine, Durham, NC, USA
Preston Robert Tisch Brain Tumor Center, Duke University School of Medicine, Durham, NC, USA
Duke Institute for Brain Sciences, Duke University, Durham, NC, USA

Marçal Vilar
Neurodegeneration Unit, Unidad Funcional de Investigación de Enfermedades Crónicas-Instituto de Salud Carlos III, Madrid, Spain

Helena Mira
Molecular Neurobiology Unit, Unidad Funcional de Investigación de Enfermedades Crónicas-Instituto de Salud Carlos III, Madrid, Spain

Nancy M. Unda, Wendy Portillo, Rebeca Corona and Raúl G. Paredes
Neurobiología Conductual y Cognitiva, Instituto de Neurobiología, Universidad Nacional Autónoma de México, Juriquilla, Mexico

Archana Gengatharan and Rodrigo R. Bammann
Cellular Neurobiology Unit, Centre de Recherche de l'Institut Universitaire en Santé Mentale de Québec, Quebec, QC, Canada

Armen Saghatelyan
Cellular Neurobiology Unit, Centre de Recherche de l'Institut Universitaire en Santé Mentale de Québec, Quebec, QC, Canada

Department of Psychiatry and Neuroscience, Université Laval, Quebec, QC, Canada

Sei-ichi Yoshihara, Hiroo Takahashi and Akio Tsuboi
Laboratory for the Molecular Biology of Neural Systems, Advanced Medical Research Center, Nara Medical University, Kashihara, Japan

Serena Bovetti
Department of Neuroscience and Brain Technologies, Istituto Italiano di Tecnologia, Genova, Italy

Carlos De la Rosa-Prieto, Daniel Saiz-Sanchez, Isabel Ubeda-Banon, Alicia Flores-Cuadrado and Alino Martinez-Marcos
Neuroplasticity and Neurodegeneration Laboratory, CRIB, Ciudad Real Medical School, Universidad de Castilla-La Mancha, Ciudad Real, Spain

Margarita Pérez-Martín
Departamento de Biología Celular, Genética y Fisiología, Instituto de Investigación Biomédica de Málaga, Universidad de Málaga, Málaga, Spain

Patricia Rivera, Juan Decara, Francisco J. Pavón, Antonia Serrano, Fernando Rodríguez de Fonseca and Juan Suárez
UGC Salud Mental, Instituto de Investigación Biomédica de Málaga, Universidad de Málaga-Hospital Universitario Regional de Málaga, Málaga, Spain

Eduardo Blanco
UGC Salud Mental, Instituto de Investigación Biomédica de Málaga, Universidad de Málaga-Hospital Universitario Regional de Málaga, Málaga, Spain
Departament de Pedagogia i Psicologia, Facultat d'Educació, Psicologia i Treball Social, Universitat de Lleida, Lleida, Spain

Clara Lorefice
Departamento de Biología Celular, Genética y Fisiología, Instituto de Investigación Biomédica de Málaga, Universidad de Málaga, Málaga, Spain
UGC Salud Mental, Instituto de Investigación Biomédica de Málaga, Universidad de Málaga-Hospital Universitario Regional de Málaga, Málaga, Spain

Quentin Marlier, Sebastien Verteneuil, Renaud Vandenbosch and Brigitte Malgrange
GIGA-Neurosciences, University of Liege, C.H.U. Sart Tilman, Liege, Belgium

Sara Bonzano, Paolo Peretto and Silvia De Marchis
Department of Life Sciences and Systems Biology, University of Turin, Torino, Italy
Neuroscience Institute Cavalieri Ottolenghi, University of Turin, Orbassano, Italy

Claudio Gendusa
Department of Life Sciences and Systems Biology, University of Turin, Torino, Italy

Kasum Azim and Benedikt Berninger
Focus Translational Neuroscience, Institute of Physiological Chemistry, University of Mainz, Mainz, Germany

Olivier Raineteau
Inserm U1208, Stem Cell and Brain Research Institute, Université Lyon 1, Bron, France

Luca Bonfanti
Neuroscience Institute Cavalieri Ottolenghi, Orbassano, Italy
Department of Veterinary Sciences, University of Turin, Torino, Italy

Rachele Salvi, Jürgen Winkler and Zacharias Kohl
Department of Molecular Neurology, Friedrich-Alexander University Erlangen-Nürnberg, Erlangen, Germany

Tobias Steigleder
Department of Neurology, Friedrich-Alexander University Erlangen-Nürnberg, Erlangen, Germany
Department of Palliative Medicine, Friedrich-Alexander University Erlangen-Nürnberg, Erlangen, Germany

Johannes C. M. Schlachetzki
Department of Molecular Neurology, Friedrich-Alexander University Erlangen-Nürnberg, Erlangen, Germany
Department of Cellular and Molecular Medicine, University of California, San Diego, CA, USA

Elisabeth Waldmann
Department of Medical Informatics, Biometry and Epidemiology, Friedrich-Alexander University Erlangen-Nürnberg, Erlangen, Germany

Stefan Schwab
Department of Neurology, Friedrich-Alexander University Erlangen-Nürnberg, Erlangen, Germany

Beate Winner
IZKF Junior Research Group III and BMBF Research Group Neuroscience, Friedrich-Alexander University Erlangen-Nürnberg, Erlangen, Germany

Rebeca Corona, Wendy Portillo and Raúl G. Paredes
Instituto de Neurobiología, Universidad Nacional Autónoma de México, Mexico, Mexico

Socorro Retana-Márquez
Departamento de Biología de la Reproducción, Universidad Autónoma Metropolitana-Iztapalapa, Mexico, Mexico

María Llorens-Martín and Jesús Ávila
Molecular Neurobiology, Function of Microtubular Proteins, Centro de Biología Molecular Severo Ochoa (Consejo Superior de Investigaciones Científicas-Universidad Autónoma de Madrid), Madrid, Spain
Centro de Investigación Biomédica en Red sobre Enfermedades Neurodegenerativas (Instituto de Salud Carlos III), Madrid, Spain

Matthew J. Korn and Quinton J. Mandle
Department of Neurology, University of Michigan Medical Center, Ann Arbor, MI, USA

Alberto Rábano
Centro de Investigación Biomédica en Red sobre Enfermedades Neurodegenerativas (Instituto de Salud Carlos III), Madrid, Spain
Neuropathology Department, CIEN Foundation, Madrid, Spain

Rosa López-Hidalgo, Raul Ballestín, Jessica Vega, José M. Blasco-Ibáñez, Carlos Crespo and Emilio Varea
Neurobiology Unit and Program in Basic and Applied Neurosciences, Cell Biology Department, Universitat de València, València, Spain
Estructura de Recerca Interdisciplinar en Biotecnologia i Biomedicina (BIOTECMED), Universitat de València, València, Spain

Jack M. Parent
Department of Neurology, University of Michigan Medical Center, Ann Arbor, MI, USA
VA Ann Arbor Healthcare System, Ann Arbor, MI, USA

Javier Gilabert-Juan and Juan Nácher
Neurobiology Unit and Program in Basic and Applied Neurosciences, Cell Biology Department, Universitat de València, València, Spain
Estructura de Recerca Interdisciplinar en Biotecnologia i Biomedicina (BIOTECMED), Universitat de València, València, Spain
Fundación Investigación Hospital Clínico de Valencia, INCLIVA, València, Spain
CIBERSAM, Spanish National Network for Research in Mental Health, València, Spain
Genetics Department, CIBERSAM, Universitat de València, València, Spain

Maria Figueres-Oñate and Laura López-Mascaraque
Molecular, Cellular, and Developmental Neurobiology, Instituto Cajal, Consejo Superior de Investigaciones Científicas, Madrid, Spain

Index

www.ingramcontent.com/pod-product-compliance
Lightning Source LLC
LaVergne TN
LVHW081018210926
848485LV00004B/899